Joint Loading

JOINT LOADING

BIOLOGY AND HEALTH OF ARTICULAR STRUCTURES

Edited by

H J Helminen	I Kiviranta	A-M Säämänen
M Tammi	K Paukkonen	J Jurvelin

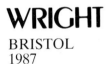

WRIGHT

BRISTOL
1987

John Wright
is an imprint of Butterworth Scientific

First published 1987

© **Butterworth & Co. (Publishers) Ltd, 1987**
Borough Green, Sevenoaks, Kent TN15 8PH, England

British Library Cataloguing in Publication Data
Joint loading: biology and health of articular structures.
  1. Joints
  I. Helminen, H.J.
  612'.75   QP301

ISBN 0 7236 07249

Typeset by
KEYTEC, Bridport, Dorset

Printed in Great Britain by
Butler & Tanner Ltd., Frome and London

Preface

This book is devoted to the clarification of joint loading effects on the properties and behaviour of articular cartilage and other joint structures. Sequelae of weight-bearing, physical exercise, unloading, immobilization, and amputation of the distal part of a limb on the physiology, biological properties and health of the joints are described in light of the present state of knowledge. We believe this to be the first book ever published aiming at fulfilling this specific goal.

From June 25th to 27th, 1986, a symposium under the title 'Articular Cartilage and Other Joint Structures in relation to Loading and Movement' was held in Kuopio, Finland. The papers printed in this book have been written by the authors who gave the main lectures at the symposium. We have also invited a few additional authors to contribute in order to cover the area of interest as well as possible. Most of the contributing authors are well known and highly appreciated by scientists and experts of joint research all over the world. We thank our authors heartily for their contributions.

Joints are the weakest points in the musculoskeletal system. Muscles and bones are not as vulnerable and not as prone to be affected by permanently disabling diseases as joints are. Exposed to considerable forces during motion, the joints require sufficient support and stability. Congruent joint surfaces with adequate lubrication, integrity of ligaments, active muscles, correct biomechanical alignment of movements and joint loading are needed to maintain the health of the joint. Lack of any of these components, due to injury, disease or disuse of the joint, will ultimately lead to the degradation of articular cartilage and the clinical signs of osteoarthrosis, the most common of the rheumatic diseases.

The goal of scientists is to find means for the prevention of joint diseases and for the improvement of routine clinical therapy. This ambitious aim is particularly important today when the world's population is not only growing but also getting relatively older, urbanized, and more sedentary than ever before during the history of man. This is probably a threat to the health of joints. However, before effective action for prevention can be taken, we must know much more about the biological properties of the joint structures and their responses to mechanical stress. This book is dedicated to the review of these aspects of joint biology.

The chapters treat, in detail, the biological, biomechanical, and clinical aspects of joint loading. The **biological part** opens with a historical survey of the research area, followed by chapters examining the effects of joint instability, physical training, load bearing, and immobilization on the articular cartilage. The interrelationship between physical exercise and ageing on the articular cartilage is also reviewed. The influences of articular cartilage loading *in vitro* and effects on the chondrocytes, at the cellular and molecular level, have been treated in separate chapters. Reviews on the synovial fluid and its flow in normal and in moving joints, effects of physical exercise on the intervertebral disc, and genetic and mechanical factors in the growth and development of epiphyseal cartilage close the biological section of the book.

The **biomechanical part** contains chapters dealing with the adaptation of the articular cartilage and bone to mechanical stress and fluid transport properties of articular cartilage exposed to loading. A treatise on the response of tendons and ligaments to joint loading and movements is included in this section of the book.

An essay on the significance of occupational and ergonomic aspects in the epidemiology of degenerative joint diseases begins the **clinical part** of the book. The role of endogenous and exogenous mechanisms in the pathogenesis of osteoarthritis is reviewed. Separate chapters are devoted to the physiology and therapeutic value of passive motion, drugs and physical therapy in the treatment of rheumatoid arthritis patients.

The book concludes with the review of Professor Leon Sokoloff, giving an account of the implications of current knowledge for prevention and treatment of osteoarthritis with special reference to the roles of joint loading and motion.

We wish you rewarding moments of study!

ACKNOWLEDGEMENTS

The editorial group expresses its gratitude to John Wright and Sons, Ltd., Publishers, for their never-failing interest and support during the editorial work of this book. Especially, the helpful comments of Mr. Roy Baker, Senior Acquisitions Editor, are gratefully acknowledged.

Kuopio, July 1987

Heikki J. Helminen
Ilkka Kiviranta
Anna-Marja Säämänen
Markku Tammi
Kari Paukkonen
Jukka Jurvelin

Contributors

W. H. Akeson Division of Orthopaedics and Rehabilitation, University of California, 225 Dickinson Street, San Diego, CA 92103-9981, USA

D. Amiel Division of Orthopaedics and Rehabilitation, University of California, 225 Dickinson Street, San Diego, CA 92103-9981, USA

S. Bernick Department of Cell Biology and Anatomy, School of Medicine, University of Southern California, 1333 San Paulo St., Los Angeles, CA 90033, USA

S. L. Carney Division of Biochemistry, The Kennedy Institute of Rheumatology, 6 Bute Gardens, Hammersmith, London W6 7DW, UK

H. G. Fassbender Zentrum für Rheuma-Pathologie, WHO Centre, Kleine Windmühlenstrasse 2A, D-6500 Mainz, FRG

H. J. Helminen Department of Anatomy, University of Kuopio, P.O. Box 6, SF-70211 Kuopio, Finland

S. H. Holm Department of Orthopaedic Surgery I, University of Gothenburg, Sahlgren Hospital, S-413 45 Gothenburg, Sweden

M. H. Holmes Department of Mathematical Sciences, Rensselaer Polytechnic Institute, Troy, NY 12180, USA

D. R. Johnson Department of Anatomy, School of Medicine, Medical and Dental Building, University of Leeds, Leeds LS2 9JT, UK

J. Jurvelin Department of Anatomy, University of Kuopio, P.O. Box 6, SF-70211 Kuopio, Finland

G. P. J. van Kampen Jan van Breemen Instituut, Center for Rheumatology and Rehabilitation, Dr. Jan van Breemenstraat, 1056 AB Amsterdam, Netherlands

I. Kiviranta Department of Anatomy, University of Kuopio, P.O. Box 6, SF-70211 Kuopio, Finland

I. V. Knets Institute of Polymer Mechanics, 23 Aizkraukles St., Riga 226006, Latvian SSR, USSR

W. M. Lai Orthopaedic Research Laboratory, College of Physicians and Surgeons, Columbia University, Black Medical Research Building, 168th St., New York, NY 10032, USA

J. S. Lawrence 386 Worsley Road, Swinton, Manchester M27 3FH, UK

J. R. Levick Department of Physiology, St. George's Hospital Medical School, Cranmer Terrace, Tooting, London SW17 0RE, UK

V. C. Mow Orthopaedic Research Laboratory, College of Physicians and Surgeons, Columbia University, Black Medical Research Building, 168th St., and New York Orthopaedic Hospital Research Laboratory of Columbia-Presbyterian Medical Center, New York, NY 10032, USA

H. Muir Division of Biochemistry, The Kennedy Institute of Rheumatology, 6 Bute Gardens, Hammersmith, London W6 7DW, UK

K. Paukkonen Department of Anatomy, University of Kuopio, P.O. Box 6, SF-70211 Kuopio, Finland

H. E. Paulus Department of Medicine, Division of Rheumatology, UCLA School of Medicine, 1000 Veteran Avenue, Los Angeles, CA 90024, USA

S. L. Silverman Department of Medicine, Division of Rheumatology, UCLA School of Medicine, 1000 Veteran Avenue, Los Angeles, CA 90024, USA

L. Sokoloff Department of Pathology, Health Sciences Center, State University of New York at Stony Brook, Stony Brook, New York, NY 11794–8691, USA

J. S. Spiegel Department of Medicine, Division of Rheumatology, UCLA School of Medicine, 1000 Veteran Avenue, Los Angeles, CA 90024, USA

T. M. Spiegel Department of Medicine, Division of Rheumatology, UCLA School of Medicine, 1000 Veteran Avenue, Los Angeles, CA 90024, USA

R. J. van de Stadt Jan van Breemen Instituut, Center for Rheumatology and Rehabilitation, Dr. Jan van Breemenstraat, 1056 AB Amsterdam, Netherlands

R. A. Stockwell Department of Anatomy, University Medical School, Teviot Place, Edinburgh EH8 9AG, UK

A.-M. Säämänen Department of Anatomy, University of Kuopio, P.O. Box 6, SF-70211 Kuopio, Finland

M. Tammi Department of Anatomy, University of Kuopio, P.O. Box 6, SF-70211 Kuopio, Finland

J. P. G. Urban University Laboratory of Physiology, Oxford University, Park Road, Oxford, UK

J. M. Walker School of Physiotherapy, Dalhousie University, Forrest Bldg., 5869 University Ave., Halifax, Nova Scotia, Canada B3H 3J5

S. L-Y. Woo School of Medicine, Department of Surgery, Division of Orthopaedics and Rehabilitation, University of California, M-030, La Jolla, CA 92093, USA

Contents

Chapter 1

Joint Loading Effects on Articular Cartilage: A Historical Review

H.J. Helminen, J. Jurvelin, I. Kiviranta, K. Paukkonen, A. -M. Säämänen and M. Tammi

CONTENTS

INTRODUCTION

The prerequisite for planning new research experiments and coping with future trends in science is a thorough analysis of the present state of knowledge, and finding the ways of thinking which have led to the situation of today. On this basis new research hypotheses and strategies can be built. This chapter aims at presenting a short historical review of the accumulation of scientific knowledge on the structure and properties of articular cartilage; special attention is paid to the reactions of the cartilage tissue towards altered joint loading. The current interest in loading effects is quite understandable since we know little of the aetiology of osteoarthrosis (osteoarthritis, OA, or degenerative joint disease, DJD) (1, 2, 3), the most common of the crippling rheumatic diseases.

1

The goal of research in this area is to find effective measures to prevent and cure rheumatic diseases such as OA. This objective of medical research is highly ambitious, but both basic research and therapeutic work need high ideals; setting goals low gives meagre results and, conversely, goals set high give new relevant results. Therefore, far off as it may be, the prevention of the disease must be our ultimate objective. Additional basic and clinical knowledge is needed to improve the routine therapy of our sick fellow citizens.

Under these conditions research activities are necessary for increasing our understanding about the biology of joint structures, pathology of the disease, and factors supporting and maintaining joint health. Genetic and hereditary aspects must be studied too. The overwhelming character of the problem compels us to seek the causes and the means of prevention of the disease beyond the specific synovial joint and even the human body. It is in society and its culture that the causes for the onset of OA must also be sought. Therefore, our whole lifestyle deserves scrutiny.

This idea emphasizes the importance of elimination of those factors in our everyday life that threaten our health, in this particular case the health of our joints. We should ask ourselves whether or not our lifestyle is conducive to the health of our joints. Do our daily working conditions degrade or maintain the health of our joints and musculoskeletal system in general? Does increased leisure time mean increased participation in sports and related activities? Are modern sports and physical culture beneficial or harmful to joint health?

Proper answers to the above questions must be received before practical steps, possibly altering our current lifestyles substantially, can be taken to prevent the disease. The necessary steps may be so far-reaching that their justification must be shown by the results of scientific investigation. This kind of thinking may strike against our basic values of life because we come to the question: is joint health – or health in general – so important that other aspects of life should be sacrificed at its altar? Probably not, but would it be possible to find a compromise which corrects our lifestyle in such a way that it would still satisfy most of us? This might be a realistic strategy.

AREAS OF SPECIAL IMPORTANCE IN PREVIOUS RESEARCH ON ARTICULAR CARTILAGE

From Exudate to Organized Tissue

Before the advent of modern biology very little was known about the structure, composition and properties of articular cartilage. Ancient physicians considered articular cartilage as cold exudate of the blood which covered the bone ends. According to Hunter (1743, *Fig.* 1.1), the bone ends were 'covered with a smooth elastic Crust, to prevent mutual Abrasion; connected with strong Ligaments, to prevent Dislocation; and inclosed in a Bag that contains a proper Fluid deposited there, for lubricating the Two contiguous Surfaces' (5). Lieutaud (1742) was of the opinion that cartilage was made of a special kind of bone, which was softer and more fragile than true bone (6). According to Bichat (1801, *Fig.* 1.2), cartilage tissue consisted of a mucinous substance infiltrated by

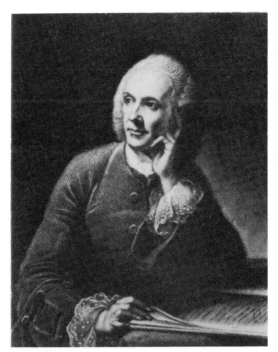

Fig. 1.1. William Hunter (1718–1783), surgeon, communicated to the Royal Society in 1743 an important work entitled: 'Of the Structure and Diseases of Articulating Cartilages'. In this communication he described the perpendicular striation of the tissue and its lack of blood vessels. He wrote on diseased articular cartilage: '. . . ulcerated cartilage is universally allowed to be a very troublesome Disease; that it admits of a Cure with more Difficulties than a carious Bone; and that, when destroyed, it is never recovered'. [Portrait from Talbott, 1970 (4), with permission.]

gelatin (7, 8). Cartilage yielded jelly or glue after boiling (8, 9). Velpeau (1837) considered articular cartilage to consist of varnish secreted by the bone ends (10). Cruveilhier (1824) and Velpeau did not believe that cartilage was an organized tissue (10, 11). Cruveilhier stated cogently that articular cartilage is not a living unit (11).

Articular cartilage first appeared to be an amorphous substance. However, Hunter (1743), Florman (1820), Weber (1830) and Lauth (1835) described fibres lying side by side in the tissue (5, 9, 12, 13). Bruns (1841) and Leidy (1849) observed zones or cell layers in the articular cartilage on the basis of cell shape (14, 15), the superficial zone containing flattened cells and the deep zone cells having their long axes perpendicular to the articular surface. According to Bock (1851), Purkinje was the first to describe cartilage cells or *corpuscula cartilaginum* (16). The fibrous structure of the cartilage was explained as being due to cell rows (13, 14). According to Kölliker (1850) there was a layer of calcified cartilage at the junction between cartilage and bone (17); the matrix of this layer appeared fibrous and calcified although it contained cartilage cells (*Fig.* 1.3). Already in 1743, Hunter had shown that articular cartilage was free of blood vessels (5). This view was substantiated by Toynbee (1841) (18).

At the beginning of the 19th century it was first thought that the synovial

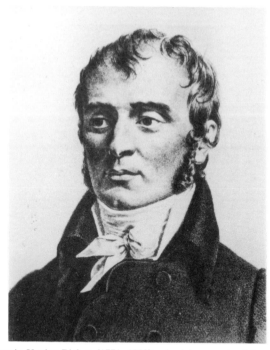

Fig. 1.2. Marie Francois Xavier Bichat (1771–1802), physician, anatomist and physiologist who wrote 4 major publications; one was 'Anatomie générale', also translated into German and English. Bichat has been considered the founder of histology – although without benefit of the microscope. He used deduction, dissection, putrefaction, desiccation, maceration, boiling, and chemical action in the study of tissue components. Treatment with boiling water of the cartilage from moving bones yielded a kind of glue; remnants of articular cartilage were scanty after prolonged boiling. [Portrait from Talbott, 1970 (4), with permission.]

membrane was also present on the surface of the articular cartilage (5, 9, 19). However, Bruns (1841), Todd and Bowman (1845), Kölliker (1848), Leidy (1849) and later Hueter (1866) reported that neither the synovial 'epithelium' nor the areolar connective tissue could be found on the load-bearing articular cartilage (14, 15, 20, 21, 22, 23)(*Fig.* 1.4).

Characteristic of the second part of the 19th century was the rapid development of histology and histochemistry. Compound microscopes with improved lens systems and light sources were available (24). At the same time new varieties of stains, such as haematoxylin (25, 26) and carmine (27, 28) as well as synthetic ones were developed. Two or more stains were usually used either together or in succession (29).

Hansen (1905) postulated that the histochemical basophilia of cartilage was due to chondroitin–sulphuric acid which could be demonstrated with methylene blue (30). He also observed that the surface zone of articular cartilage contained smaller amounts of chondroitin–sulphuric acid than the rest of the cartilage. In 1922, Benninghoff suggested the term 'chondrone' for structures consisting of groups of isogenous chondrocytes and territorial matrix (31).

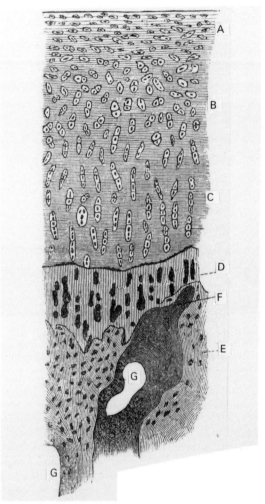

Fig. 1.3. A diagram showing microscopic details of human metacarpal articular cartilage (× 90). A, superficial flat chondrocytes; B, middle roundish chondrocytes; C, innermost cells in rows and cell axis at right angles to the articular surface; D, outermost layer of the bone with ossified, fibrous ground substance with dark chondrocytes; E, true bone substance; F, blind end of marrow space; G, marrow space. [From Kölliker, 1850 (17).]

In 1950 a specific stain for mucins utilizing alcian blue 8GS was introduced by Steedman (32). However, it was particularly the modification of Scott and Dorling (1965) which made use of the critical electrolyte concentration in the ensuing differential staining of the glycosaminoglycans (33). By this method Stockwell and Scott (34) studied the distribution of chondroitin and keratan sulphates in the human articular cartilage. It appeared that in mature articular cartilage chondroitin sulphate was predominantly territorial, while keratan sulphate was characteristically interterritorial. Earlier Lison (1935) had sug-

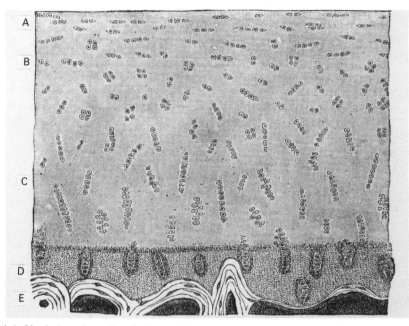

Fig. 1.4. Vertical section of articular cartilage covering the lower end of the tibia (human). Magnified about 30 diameters. A, cells and cell-groups flattened conformably with the surface; B, cell-groups irregularly arranged; C, cell-groups disposed perpendicularly to the surface; D, layer of calcified cartilage; E, bone. [From Thomson *et al.*, 1882 (23).]

gested that the basic metachromatic stains (35), e.g. toluidine blue, reacted with sulphuric acid esters of high molecular weight, making possible the study of the intercellular substance of tissue. The PAS (Periodic acid–Schiff) technique was taken into use in histology by McManus in 1946 (36) and Lillie *et al.* (37). While this method demonstrates the most likely oligosaccharides of glycoproteins and other structural proteins, the modified PAS method of Scott and Dorling (38) shows uronic acid containing carbohydrate components (chondroitin sulphate) after prolonged periodic acid treatment. The use of safranin O as a histochemical stain for proteoglycans was proposed by Rosenberg in 1971 (39).

Chondrin, Chondrosin and Proteoglycans

The long march towards the era of molecular biology of proteoglycans was initiated by Wharton who, in 1656, isolated hyaluronic acid in crude form ('Wharton's jelly') (41).

The next important observation was made by Müller (1836; *Fig.* 1.5), who steamed cartilage obtaining a solution called 'chondrin'. The properties of chondrin (Knorpelleim) were distinctly different from those of 'colla' (gewöhnlichen Leim, Tischlerleim, etc.) (42). Krukenberg (1884) isolated the chief component of chondrin, calling it 'Chondroitsäure' (chondroitin–sulphuric acid) (43). Morochowetz (44) and Krukenberg observed that extraction of the

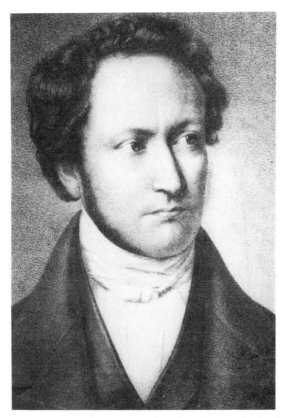

Fig. 1.5. Johannes Peter Müller (1801–1858), physiologist and anatomist, has been regarded as the founder of modern physiology. He coined the name 'Bindegewebe' about 1830 and published an important paper: 'Ueber die Structur and die chemischen Eigenschaften der thierischen Bestand- theile der Knorpel und Knochen', in which he separated 'Knorpelleim, Chondrin' from 'gewöhnlichen Leim, Tischlerleim, Colla' on basis of their chemical properties. We now know that the former substance contained proteoglycans and the latter collagen. [Portrait from Schadewaldt, 1986 (40).]

cartilage with a mild base solubilized most of the tissue chondrin or chondroitin sulphate. Chondroitin sulphate was purified by Mörner (45) and subsequently hydrolysed to 'chrondrosin', 'Glykuronsäure', and 'Glykosamin' by Schmiedeberg (46). In 1913 Levene and La Forge isolated the glucuronic acid component of chondroitin–sulphuric acid and also found evidence that the second component would be glucosamine (47).

The idea of the coexistence of carbohydrate and protein in one molecular species is probably derived from the studies of Eichwald in 1865 (48). Some years earlier, Fischer and Boedeker found sugar in the yield after the steaming of hyaline cartilage with strong hydrochloric acid (49). The differences between 'chondrosin' and the saccharide units of glycoproteins became gradually apparent in the 1920s (50).

The components of hyaluronic acid were discovered by Meyer and Palmer in 1934 (51). Also the viscoelastic properties of the molecule became apparent.

Meyer and Chaffee described the dermatan sulphate molecule in 1941 (52). The method for uronic acid determination was published by Dische in 1947 (53). In 1956 Meyer *et al.* described chondroitin sulphates A, B and C (54). Davidson and Meyer showed that chondroitin is a repeating disaccharide with *N*-acetyl galactosamine (chondrosamine) and glucuronic acid as repeating units (55). Meyer *et al.* (1953) showed that galactose and *N*-acetyl glucosamine formed the repeating disaccharide units in keratan sulphate (keratosulphate) (56). Shatton and Schubert (1954) showed that in cartilage the chondroitin sulphate was associated with a particular type of protein molecule (57). It was concluded that the material was a mucoprotein.

A few years later, Muir demonstrated that chondroitin sulphate was attached to serine residues of protein (58). Gregory *et al.* (1964) showed that the linkage region of the polysaccharide chain contained xylose and galactose molecules linked to serine (59). The term 'proteoglycans' was introduced in the 1960s (60). Caesium chloride density gradient centrifugation for fractionation of the protein–polysaccharide preparations was introduced by Franek and Dunstone in 1967 (61). A new era in the molecular biology of articular cartilage began when Sajdera and Hascall (1969) were able to extract intact proteoglycan molecules (62). In 1972 Hardingham and Muir discovered the specific interaction of proteoglycans with hyaluronic acid on which proteoglycan aggregation depends (63).

Gelatin and Collagen

In the 19th century collagen, the molecule that in many contexts has been considered to be the main agent controlling the distribution of both externally and internally applied forces, was defined as 'that constituent of connective tissue which yields gelatin on boiling' (Oxford Dictionary, 1893). The term 'collagen' was introduced in the English language around 1865 and was probably influenced by the French denotation 'collagéne' deriving from the Greek word for glue (=κολλα) (64). At the beginning of the 19th century, Bichat, Beclard, Florman and others knew that cartilage tissue yielded gelatin (jelly or glue) when treated with boiling water (8, 9, 42). By 1900, 13 amino acids had been discovered by biochemists (64); hydroxyproline was separated by Fischer in 1902 (65).

Collagen of the cartilage has been studied by the aid of the polarizing microscope for more than 100 years (66, 67). The optical phenomenon generated in a cartilage specimen by the polarizing microscope was, according to von Ebner (1882), most probably due to the 'cartilaginous fibres' (Fibrillen des Knorpels) (68). In the 1880s Mörner acknowledged in his histochemical papers on cartilage that collagen was known at least to Morochowetz, Landtwehr, and Krukenberg (45, 69). Hultkrantz (1898) demonstrated the so-called 'split lines' (Spaltrichtungen) of the articular cartilage (70). His view that the orientation of collagen might be dependent on frictional forces in the joint received little support from Benninghoff (1925), who made extensive observations on the system and orientation of collagen fibres in the articular cartilage, especially in relation to joint loading (71). Our basic idea of the arrangement of collagen in cartilage rests mainly on the work of Benninghoff (*Figs.* 1.6, 1.7).

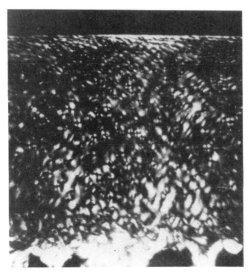

Fig. 1.6. Cartilage of the human femoral condyle under polarized light. The planes of the Nicol's prisms were parallel to the edges of the micrograph. [From Benninghoff, 1925 (71).]

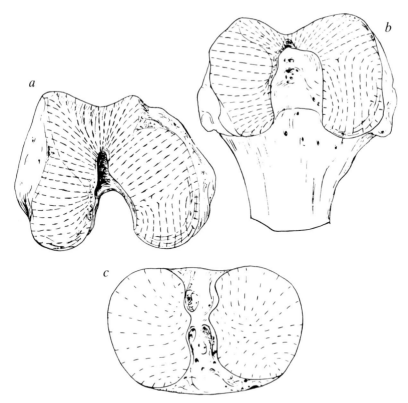

Fig. 1.7. Articular surfaces of the lower end of femur. *a*, Frontal view. *b*, View from below. Atypical path of the split lines in the lower part of the medial condyle. *c*, Proximal end of tibia. [From Benninghoff, 1925 (71).]

Still, up to the 1940s, the term collagen implied a gluelike, viscous protein solution. An accurate analysis of the 13 amino acids of gelatin was carried out by Dakin (72). Nageotte (1927) demonstrated that collagen could be dissolved in dilute acetic acid, forming a solution from which collagen could be reconstituted by the addition of salt (73). Somewhat earlier, both Van Slyke and Hiller (74) and Schryver et al. (75) reported the presence of a hitherto undiscovered amino acid in the hydrolysates of gelatin. This proved to be hydroxylysine. In the 1940s thorough chemical analysis of ox hide collagen was performed by Bowes and Kenten (76).

In 1942, Hall et al. (77) and in 1943 Wolpers (78) showed the bands of collagen by transmission electron microscopy. Bucher came to the conclusion that collagenous fibres of hyaline cartilage were S-shaped and that they were adapted to withstand not only pressure but also stretching (79, 80). Later, ultrastructural studies showed that the superficial zone of articular cartilage contained tangentially oriented collagen bundles of closely spaced unit collagen fibres separated by amorphous ground substance (81, 82). This arrangement appeared to affect significantly the permeability of articular cartilage (83). Pauwels (1959) was of the opinion that the collagen orientation was not that proposed by Benninghoff (1925). In Pauwels' opinion the fibres were oriented along the tension trajectories of the joint surface (84). This view corroborates the observations of Hultkrantz (70). Also, Zarek and Edwards (1963) supported the idea that the surface collagen fibres were predominantly oriented in the direction of principal tensile stress trajectories (85). This orientation of collagen is possibly settled during embryonic life (86).

In the 1950s a new era in collagen research began when the 'tropocollagen' molecule (87) and its components (88, 89) were detected. At the same time the helical structure of the molecule was resolved by X-ray diffraction studies (90, 91). We now know of several types of collagen molecules. Type II collagen is the principal collagen type found in the cartilaginous tissues; it was discovered by Miller and Matukas in 1969 (92).

Mechanical Testing of Articular Cartilage

Rauber (1876) and Triepel (1902) investigated the elasticity of rib cartilage (93, 94). Fürbringer (1888) reported that the articular head of the humerus had firmer cartilage than the socket (95). Lubosch (1910) came to the same conclusion (96). Braune and Fischer (1891) studied movements of the knee joint, pointing out the property of deformation of the articular cartilage under load and discussing the significance of this observation to cartilage and joint physiology (97).

Hirsch (98) constructed an elastometer on the principles developed earlier by Schade (99), Bär (100), and Göcke (101) (Figs. 1.8, 1.9, 1.10). He utilized Hooke's Law and Herz's theory in the calculation of the relative elasticity modulus. He also investigated the histology and metachromatic staining of the tissue from points tested for elasticity. The cartilage showing chondromalacia was smoother and exhibited reduced metachromasia, particularly in the superficial zone of the cartilage (98). Benninghoff (1925) had already stated that 'reduction of hyaline makes cartilage softer' (71).

Elmore et al. (1963) and Sokoloff (1966) further improved the methodology of

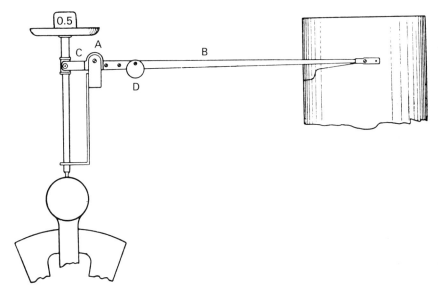

Fig. 1.8. Elastometer for the estimation of elasticity of the articular cartilage. A, rotational axis; B, drawing arm; C, weight arm; D, movable weight. [From Bär, 1926 (100).]

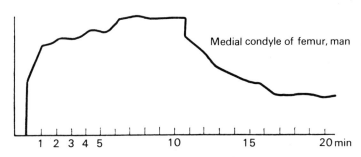

Medial condyle of femur, man

Fig. 1.9. Typical response of articular cartilage to loading followed by unloading (from 10 min on). [From Bär, 1926 (100).]

elasticity determination (102, 103). Elmore *et al.* pointed out that the previous measurements were performed in air, which gave erroneous results (102). Linn and Sokoloff (1965) reported that, immediately after loading, cartilage shows a springlike deformation which is independent of water expulsion (104). Sokoloff observed that few or no differences were found as a function of age, either in the deformability or recovery of adult articular cartilage (103).

A creep modulus at 2 s after load application was designed by Kempson (105). A highly significant relationship existed between the creep modulus and the total mucopolysaccharide content (for review *see* 106). Kempson *et al.* showed that the area with the lowest indentation coincided with the contact area, whilst the non-contact areas presented the largest indentation (106). Indentation increased with degeneration of the cartilage. A recent comprehensive history on the mechanical testing of articular cartilage has been published by Mow *et al.* (107).

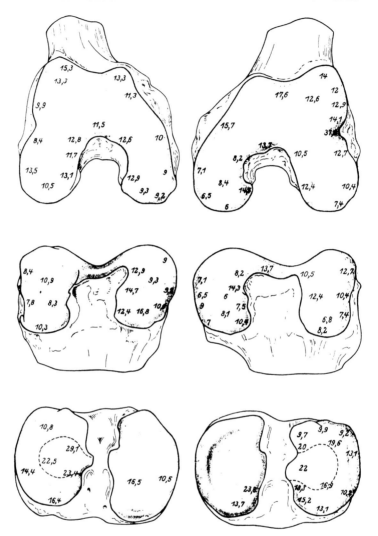

Fig. 1.10. Right and left knee joint of the same individual. The numbers refer to the elasticity of the cartilage; the higher the value, the softer is the cartilage. *Note*: the meniscus-free area of the tibia appears softer than the cartilage covered by menisci. [From Bär, 1926 (100).]

The Problem of Nutrition: from Synovial Fluid or Underlying Bone?

Nutrition and metabolism of articular cartilage has posed problems to research workers ever since the work of Hunter (1743), who observed that articular cartilage was devoid of blood vessels (5). This observation was later confirmed by many authors, e.g. Beclard 1823 (8), Toynbee 1841 (18) and Leidy 1849 (16). According to Hunter, nutrition of the articular cartilage came from the *circulus articuli vasculosus*, located close to the margins of cartilage tissue. Toynbee (1841) stated that the nutrients come from the plasma transuded from the underlying cancellous bone (18). In 1939 Fisher wrote that the deeper strata are nourished by subarticular vessels, the superficial and central areas by synovial fluid, and the cartilage near the edges receive nutrition from the *circulus articuli vasculosus* which is the principal source of nutrition (108). Gradually, however, support was given to the idea that synovial fluid was the main, if not the only, route of nutrition of articular cartilage (109–111). Ito (1924) demonstrated that a loose body in the joint cavity could be supported solely by synovial fluid (112). Earlier, Schmieden (1900) had held this view (113). Ekholm (1951) utilized radioactive gold in his studies on articular cartilage nutrition (114). He concluded that the nutrition of rabbit joint cartilage 'most probably takes place partly from synovial fluid and partly via the direct contacts between the epiphyseal marrow spaces and the basal layers of the cartilage' (114). He also suggested that nutrition was improved by increased joint function. Brodin (1955), using a fluorescent probe, obtained the same results as Ekholm (115). Although Collins denied the subchondral route of nutrition in adult articular cartilage on account of its calcified basal zone (116), Brower *et al.* (117) and Mankin (118) showed that intravital dyes and isotope-labelled amino acids rapidly reached all parts of the developing articular cartilage. The idea that immature articular cartilage receives nutrition via the subchondral route was substantiated by McKibbin and Holdsworth (119).

Clinical and Epidemiological Assessment of Osteoarthritis

It was at the beginning of the 20th century (1907–9) that the clinical pictures of osteoarthrosis (osteoarthritis) and rheumatoid arthritis were irrevocably separated from each other (120–122). Modern usage of the term 'osteo-arthritis', (OA), and differentiation of the disease process from rheumatoid arthritis, was advocated by Garrod (120). He also related Heberden's nodes to osteoarthritis. The term osteoarthritis had already been used in the 1880s by Spender (123). The term 'arthrose' was suggested by von Müller in 1913 (124). This term has dominated in continental Europe since then.

It must be remembered, however, that although the two disease entities were distinguished from each other this recently, observations on articular cartilage lesions were made very early indeed. Brodie (1822) described (originally in 1818) the non-inflammatory erosion of articular cartilage (125), Ecker (1843) observed wearing away of the joint surface (126), and Ziegler (1877; *Fig.* 1.11) made observations on subchondral bone changes and cysts present in arthritis deformans (127). The term 'arthritis deformans', given by Virchow, covered subchondral bone changes of both osteoarthrosis and rheumatoid arthritis, which to some extent caused a delay in the clearcut separation of the two disease entities (128–130).

The role of mechanical factors as one (or the only) reason for OA was actively discussed during the first decades of our century. Preiser (1911) emphasized the significance of abnormal statics (patterns of loading) in the development of the disease (131). Pommer (132–134) stressed that the joint could not resist the mechanical and functional demands it was exposed to, e.g. in work, and the joint was therefore diseased. The idea was earlier (1897) presented by Beneke (135). According to Heine (1926) the theories of Pommer ('Die funktionelle Theorie')

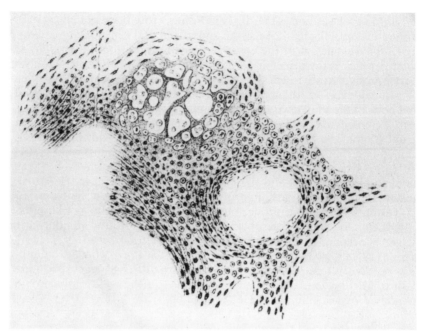

Fig. 1.11. Subchondral bone. The bone in the upper left corner is transformed into fibrous tissue and fibrocartilage. Hyaline cartilage is located in the central area where initial moulding of a cyst with enlarged lacunae can be observed. Some of the chondrocytes undergo proliferation, others show necrosis. In the right lower part of the illustration there is a cyst within fibrous bone. [From Ziegler, 1877 (127).]

was valid only as regards to the pathogenesis of osteoarthrosis, not in the aetiology of the disease (136). Burckhardt (137) proposed that the lack of correct proportion between the power of resistance of the tissue and the demands put upon it caused osteoarthrosis. Freund (138) treated the same problem. He was of the opinion that 'functional stimuli below or above the physiologic optimum, if active over a long period, are deleterious to joint cartilage' (138). Slightly earlier (1936), Baetzner published a large monograph on sports and work injuries advocating the practise of optimal sports activities within individually set limits to avoid injury of articular structures (139). Later, the Leeds hypothesis states that 'cartilage becomes conditioned to transmit, without sustaining damage, the stresses to which it is most regularly subjected' (140). Cartilage regularly subjected to high stresses is stiffer than cartilage which is regularly exposed to low stresses (141).

The adoption of epidemiological methods in rheumatological research has been extremely valuable for the determination of the prevalence of rheumatic diseases in populations (142, 143). Earlier studies on prevalence were more or less extensive autopsy studies (136, 144). The prevalence of rheumatic diseases in ageing populations (145, 146), different ethnic groups, and rural and urban populations (147–150) have been investigated.

At present, nationwide estimations of the prevalence of rheumatic diseases are continously compiled and published (151–153). The significance of biomechanical factors in the aetiology of osteoarthrosis has also been studied by epidemiological methods. The roles played by occupation and sports have been under especially close scrutiny (142, 154–157). Genetic factors in osteoarthrosis have also been investigated (158). Although the investigations have so far given conflicting results to some extent, epidemiological methods have already proved to be invaluable tools in the assessment of the total impact of rheumatic diseases in society and in populations.

THE ROLE OF MOVEMENTS IN THE EMBRYOLOGICAL DEVELOP-MENT OF JOINTS

Since the second half of the 19th century detailed knowledge has been available of the principles and timetable of human skeletal and joint development (22, 159–169). In 1878 Bernays drew attention to the adult appearance of the human embryo joint before any apparent joint activity existed (170). Animal embryos (chick and rabbit) were used in the experimental investigations of joint formation (160, 162). Kollmann stressed the importance of hereditary factors in the development of the contours of joint surfaces (167). On the other hand, Kölliker was of the opinion that the final form of the articulating surfaces was primarily influenced by the mechanical factors active during growth and development (163). He also emphasized the role of these factors in joint cavitation. According to him, mechanical factors were the primary stimuli for the development of a joint cavity. Kölliker did not support the idea of 'softening' of the interzonal tissue (the tissue between the two cartilaginous epiphyses) as the true cause for joint cavity formation. It is possible that the ideas of Roux (171) on the 'functionellen Anpassung' of tissues had influenced Kölliker's thinking.

Very early, joint development was divided into 2 stages; during the first stage the joint became distinguishable and displayed 3 tissue layers under the light microscope (161, 162, 170). Two peripheral articular surfaces were separated by an intervening zone of mesenchymal tissue. During the second stage, the joint cavity appeared. During the first half of this century, experimental work by Murray and Selby (172), Fell and Canti (173), and others (174–176) showed that the first stage (gross form of articular structures) also took place in vitro, which confirmed the genetic control of this stage, while mechanical factors, e.g. joint movements on account of muscle contractions, were necessary to elicit the development and maintenance of a joint cavity and the final form and size of the articular surfaces.

The importance of the intermittent compression and tension regimen to the formation of the avian secondary (adventitious) cartilage was clearly demonstrated by Murray and Smiles (177), and Hall (178). Continuous compression was not an appropriate stimulus for cartilage production (178). The thickness of the avian scleral cartilage, which surrounds the ocular bulb, proved to be inversely proportional to the amount of tension exposure (179). Strong tensile forces inhibited cartilage formation and reduced tension induced the development of thick sclerae.

Recent accounts on the development of cartilage and joints have been published by O'Rahilly and Gardner (180), Hall (181), and Thorogood (182).

OSTEOARTHROTIC LESIONS IN WILD AND DOMESTIC ANIMAL JOINTS

There is evidence that the Cretaceous dinosaur *Diplodocus* and the aquatic reptile *Platecarpus*, both living more than 100 million years ago (183, 184), and the cave bears, sabre-toothed tigers, and *Bos primigenius* of the Pleistocene Epoch (about 2 million years ago) suffered from chronic arthritis, reminiscent of human OA (185, 186). In 1893 Shufeldt pointed out that the pollex metacarpals showed osteophytes in several species of fossil, but in no contemporary species of anserine birds (187).

It is obvious that, to a certain extent, the arthritis of these specimens was due to trauma or other injury of the joint. This could be deduced from the conformation of the skeletal remains. In a study on arthritis of wild wolves (188), injuries of paws and bones could be shown concomitantly with arthritic lesions of limb joints.

In his extensive investigation on chronic arthritis in wild animals, Fox (189) concluded that 'the distribution of lesions in the different kinds of animals suggests that there may be a relationship of function and localization of disease, possibly related to locomotion and the jolt shock associated therewith' (189). Notably macrosomic animals showed many arthritic lesions; the anterior limbs were more often affected than the posterior ones. Animals with small bodies showed arthritis to a negligible degree. Anthropoid apes and baboons, Felidae (e.g. tiger), Hyaenidae (hyena), Ursidae (bears), Bovidae (antelopes), and Cervidae (deer, moose, elk) had conspicuous OA lesions. Few or no lesions were observed in some families of Carnivora, e.g. Canidae (wolves, foxes, etc.) and some orders of Rodentia (rats, mice, etc.) and Chiroptera (bats) (189). The first signs of arthritis were in the spinal column, but it was also observed extensively in the appendicular skeleton.

At this point, it is pertinent to repeat the words of Hildebrand, who stated: 'each animal adapts . . . to a coordinated life style. Manner of locomotion is nearly always related to feeding habits, and reproductive, defensive, and other behavior are usually correlated with manner of feeding and locomotion' (190). Locomotion thus forms the basis for the existence and behaviour of all animals. Therefore, the skeletal remains of any animal population may tell us how the animals have been able to adapt to the preponderant climatic and nutritive conditions and to competition within its own and between other species. In short, the success or failure of the species to cope with the external physical conditions can be read from the bones and joints with great reliability.

In a series of papers, Sokoloff and his co-workers have investigated the natural history of degenerative joint disease (DJD) in small laboratory animals and birds (191–194). In mice, he found DJD much like, although not identical with, human OA in several joints, particularly the knee joint, and there was a clear difference in the susceptibility of different murine strains to DJD (191). Severe lesions of the knee joint were observed e.g. in male STR/IN strain; strain differences were also shown regarding predilection of lesion localization. Sokoloff states that 'the involvement of the knee may be related mechanically to the fact that the animal frequently supports itself on the hind extremities' (191). He also comments on the very localized distribution of the changes on the articular surfaces: 'indeed, this very localized distribution of the changes constitutes one of the main pillars of the widely held view that osteoarthritis is a traumatic or destructive lesion, rather than a degenerative one' (191). That osteoarthritic lesions can occur in mice under certain conditions was reported earlier by Silberberg and Silberberg (195). Silberberg et al. also reported the occurrence of OA in the Syrian hamster (196).

The rat proved to be very resistant to spontaneous development of OA (192). However, a high fat (60%) diet increased the amount of DJD in the rat and in two strains of mice (197), but the lower fat content (37.4%) diet did not cause an increase of OA. Some years later, Sokoloff and Mickelsen reported the lack of deleterious effects on joints of strain DBA/2JN mice after a dietary supplement of saturated fats (198). Guinea-pigs were demonstrated to be susceptible to knee, shoulder, and vertebral column OA (193). Sokoloff states that, in the case of guinea-pigs, 'gross weight bearing independent of other mechanical or constitutional factors is not sufficient to account for development of the osteoarthrosis' (193). Avian primary OA, although milder than that of mammals, was found both in captive birds and those of zoological parks (194). The fibrous nature of the avian articular cartilage and the kinetics of volant movement might explain this observation.

Domestic animals also show OA lesions. In 1938 Callender and Kelser concluded after investigating specimens from man, horse, and mule that the lesions of degenerative arthritis were nearly identical (199). They suggested that the symptomatic disease occurred in Equidae from less advanced lesions than in man. This could be due to the greater physical activity of the animals. Fox (189) also pointed out that both draught and circus horses exhibit arthritis. In prehistoric wild horses the dorsal region of the spine was affected by OA, whereas riding and working horses showed lesions in the lumbar region (185). Ploughing increased the incidence of OA changes in the cannon (metapodial) bones of oxen (185). In contrast to the observation of Fox (189) that the forelimbs of wild macrosomic animals were most often affected, Young et al. (200) stressed that, in cattle, the highest incidence of OA involved the posterior limbs, even though the forelimbs support the majority of the body weight. Not only augmented, but also diminished, physical activity and locomotion has been considered to cause harm to the joints of domestic animals. The inactivity of turkeys seemed to cause continuous pressure at the distal end of the tibiotarsal bone, causing OA, severe pain, and an inability to stand and move (201).

Comprehensive accounts of the comparative pathology of arthritis have been written by Sokoloff (202), on comparative arthrology by Van Sickle and Kincaid (203), and on animal models in the study of OA by Young et al. (200).

ANTHROPOLOGICAL INVESTIGATIONS OF OSTEOARTHRITIS IN HUMAN JOINTS

Archaeologists and palaeopathologists have studied ancient disease to learn about the behaviour and environment of early men and animals. Infections, fractures of bones and dental erosions or deficit tell of the living conditions of the population with great fidelity (185, 204, 205). The commonest of the palaeopathological conditions is OA; it can affect almost every joint of the body (185). Most palaeopathologists have considered OA to be, essentially, a reaction to repeated trauma (185, 204, 206, 207) or functional stress (208), although the influences of systemic factors such as sex, ageing, endocrine and metabolic factors and heredity have also been taken into consideration in the aetiology of the disease (204, 208). 'As a sensitive indicator of occupational and behavioural stresses, arthritis is unrivalled and many inferences about ancient patterns of activity have been made from it', states Wells (185). It is probably not insignificant that the frequency of severe OA in Alaskan Eskimo skeletons was 13.5% in the right knee and 18.0% in the elbow, while the corresponding figures for American Whites were 3.0% and 5.8%, respectively (205).

OA is of great antiquity even in the history of man. Evidence of the disease has been recorded in the remains of Neanderthal man living about 70 000–125 000 years ago (204). Mandibular condyles, scapulae, patellae, and cervical vertebrae show lesions of OA. Mild to severe OA was also observed in more recent skeletons of *Homo neanderthalensis*, living about 46 000–60 000 years ago (209, 210). The vertebral OA changes of the La Chapelle-aux-Saints Neanderthal were so grave that the first description of Neanderthal posture was erroneously semi-erect and joint-bent instead of being about identical with the posture of the *Homo sapiens* of today (211, 212).

Trinkaus (212) gives a detailed description of the La Chapelle-aux-Saints remains including, among others, the following diagnoses: 'lower cervical, upper thoracic, and lower thoracic intervertebral DJD, a distal fracture of mid-thoracic rib, extensive DJD of the left hip, DJD of the right proximal interphalangeal articulation, bilateral humeral head eburnation, and minor exostosis formation on the right humerus, ulna, and radius'. The Neanderthals buried their dead and this may account for evidence of OA being first reported in this species (204).

Bronze and Iron Age skeletal remains of *Homo sapiens* have signs of OA of the temporomandibular joint (213), femoral head (eburnation and osteophytes) and acetabulum (osteophytic growth) (214). In general, however, the Bronze Age inhabitants of Britain appeared to have little arthritis (185). The explanation might be that the people were mostly pastoralists grazing their herds within reach of relatively short daily circuits (185).

Arthritis is also a well known disease in ancient Indian literature, with a description of the malady occurring in the Atharvaveda, which was written about 1000 BC (215). Another text, Caraka Samhita, written in the post-vedic period, deals more accurately with the then prevailing views of the aetiology, symptomatology, diagnosis, and treatment of arthritis (215). Caraka also prescribes local and systemic medicaments for the treatment of arthritis. Caraka explained that arthritis was born due to the disturbances of vata, the humor of air or wind: 'If the vata located in the bone and bone marrow gets provoked, there occurs cracking pain in bones and joints, arthralgia, loss of flesh and strength, loss of sleep and constant pain' (215). Instead of trauma or mechanical stress, philosophy and religion furnished an aetiology of the disease to the minds of people. This kind of tradition continues even today.

In the ancient Egyptians, extensive vertebral column OA was common, maybe due to the custom of carrying heavy loads on the head (206) but, curiously enough, their feet were almost completely free of the disease (185). Wells attributed this to walking barefoot or wearing light sandals only. On the other hand, bony remains of soldiers of Alexander the Great showed changes which might have been caused by repeated minor injuries due to long periods of marching in bad shoes (206). In a more recent Anglo-Saxon population, the wearing of somewhat clumsy boots might have accounted for the increased incidence of OA in joints of the feet (185). This population led a hard agricultural lifestyle with digging, plowing and timberjacking, which might explain the differences from the Egyptian remains (185).

In a recent study on the pattern of arthritis in Roman Britain, Thould and Thould (216) noticed a high prevalence of OA for a relatively young community with particularly severe changes in the vertebral column. The pattern of joint affection was different from that seen now. Severe spinal OA was seen in many young people. These people were farmers and artisans, and they were considered to lead physically hard lives, with a life expectancy of 40 years or less. A recent study of OA in the present British population shows knees being most often affected, then the hands, lumbar spine, hips, ankles, shoulders, elbows, and first metatarsophalangeal joints, in this decreasing order (217). The order was different among the Roman Britons. Most affected was the lumbar spine, and then the thoracic spine, cervical spine, patella, shoulder, hip, wrist together with knee and first metatarsophalangeal joint (216). The pattern is most probably related to the lifestyle of these people.

Griffin *et al.* (213) investigated the incidence of OA in the temporomandibular joint in the cranial remains of different cultures from the Bronze and Iron Ages to the 17th–20th centuries. They came to the conclusion that cultures which were exposed to more stringent living conditions and which had well worn teeth (i.e. Bronze Age and Early Iron Age British, East Coast Australian aborigines, and Christian Norse) had about twice the incidence of temporomandibular joint OA involvements as the more sophisticated cultures (Romano-British, medieval British,17th–20th century British and German).

Descriptions of the incidence of OA/DJD in the skeletal remains of the American continent have been published by Chapman (207), Jurmain (205, 208), and Minugh (204). In these papers, the appearance of OA was also interpreted to reflect the contemporary lifestyle of the population. On the other hand, it is of interest to note that Hudson *et al.* (218) have stressed the significance of *Erysipelothrix insidosa* infection as the cause for a rheumatoid arthritis-like disease in many animals, including deer and man.In their opinion this could be one reason for arthritis in the skeletal remains of ancient American populations (218). In general, however, the palaeopathologists appear to share the thoughts of Wells (185), who concludes: 'features of archaic osteoarthritis, in both man and animals, leave little doubt that its frequency and severity fluctuated at different times in response to many influences. These include: the general standard of hygiene, nutritional levels, the climatic and geographical background, the choice of dwelling sites, and the design of houses. If a main object of palaeopathology is to reconstruct vanished ways of living, it can be said that osteoarthritis is the most rewarding of all diseases to study.'

PRESENT HUMAN CULTURE AND HEALTH OF THE JOINTS

Joint Health and Mechanical Stress in Work

In 1901, Stempel drew attention to the fact that the prevalence of OA seemed to be exceptionally high in the hip joints of farmers (219). He suggested that the heavy work of these rural people, beginning in the fields at the age of 5 or 6 or so, was the primary reason for the disease. According to Pommer (220), excluding traumatic injuries and ageing, occupational conditions were the primary external cause for the degeneration of articular cartilage and OA. The first statistics on rheumatic diseases in some European countries were published in the early 1930s (221–223; see 142 for review).

During the last few decades, adoption of both epidemiological and clinical methods in the study of the prevalence of disease has made it possible to prove that OA of the spine, hips, and knees was indeed higher among workers engaged in heavy manual work than among those in lighter occupations (142). For example, miners (224), porters (225), dock workers (155), farmers (226, 227), forestry and foundry workers (228), were shown to have more OA of the spine and joints of the lower extremity than workers in the reference groups.

In the 1930s, some papers were published where OA of the elbow was regarded to be the consequence of pneumatic drilling (229, 230) or strenuous muscular work (231). Later studies have shown an increase of OA in the hands of cotton workers (232), farmers (233, 234), and professional musicians (235). OA appeared to be associated with the intensity of the physical stress of the work (234). In both the general population and cotton workers, there was more OA in the dominant hand (234, 236, 237).

It is held that trauma can result in OA of the joint. But, until now, we do not know whether strenuous joint usage can elicit cartilage degeneration and be a primary aetiological factor of OA or not. Non-injured articular cartilage has been reported to resist normal or even strenuous loading (238). Therefore, to overcome this problem, research workers have paid attention to the analysis of posture and specific joint movements and their role in the emanation of rheumatic complaints and OA (239–241). The high prevalence of OA among miners has been attributed to the forward inclination of the working men. It is anticipated that repetitive stress, even of a minor degree, to the articular cartilage when the joint is flexed, extended, or rotated to or near an extreme position, may cause trauma or give rise to fatigue of the articular cartilage (242).

Sports and Joint Health

In the 1920s Baetzner claimed that strenuous and repetitive sports activities caused overstrain injuries ('Sportschäden') in the locomotory system (243, 244). He started from the principle that use supports, exercise improves, but strenuous training worsens the qualities of the tissue. He considered joints and articular cartilage to be especially susceptible to overstrain injury and OA (139).

It has been commonly recognized that devotion to strenuous sports activities may increase risk of early OA. OA of the knee in runners (245), hip, knee, or ankle in football players (246– 251), femoropatellar joint of cyclists (252), spine, shoulder and elbow of gymnasts (253), elbow of baseball (254) and tennis (255) players, and hand of judo wrestlers (256) have been reported (for review see 257).

At first sight, therefore, the reasoning of Baetzner more than 50 years ago seems reasonable. In addition, in walking man the supporting limb bears slightly more than one body weight of the individual, while during running the heel strike generates forces about twice that amount and a moment later, when the weight has been transferred to the forefoot, forces 3–4 times the body weight are generated (258). Each heel strike gives rise to shock waves which travel along the limb and axial skeleton, the vibrations being gradually attenuated. In recreational athletes, running 20 miles a week sends approximately 1·7 million extra shock waves a year to the locomotory system (258). In middle and long distance runners the number of waves exceeds 3 million (257). This has been considered a risk factor for the health of joints (156, 258). It is the muscle stiffness together with bony deformation, joint movement, and cartilage compression that receive the shock waves. Radin *et al.* have suggested that resilience of the subchondral bone is the crucial factor in the aetiology of OA (259). In their opinion, microfractures and thickening, followed by stiffening of the subchondral plate after exposure of the bone to mechanical stress, is the reason for degeneration of the articular cartilage and OA. Recently, Radin *et al.* demonstrated changes of the bone and of the hexosamine content of articular cartilage in the weight-bearing joints of sheep who had been walking over a concrete floor for long periods (260). Sheep walking on wood chips showed no corresponding changes.

The possibility of the direct overstrain effect of repetitive loading on articular cartilage as the cause for OA has been discussed by several authors (238, 247, 248, 257). However, the majority of recent authors lay emphasis on the significance of earlier trauma or post-traumatic or inherent biomechanical misalignment between the joint surfaces, which cause excessive stress concentration upon the articular surface, as being the primary reason for OA (238, 247, 257). In addition, several research groups have pointed out that prior sports activities, even at the championship and international level, do not increase the incidence of OA in former athletes (261–263). Therefore, the prevailing view is that repetitive, even strenuous, loading of the normal healthy articular cartilage and joint does not bring forth OA (238).

X-ray pictures of athletes show signs of 'periarthropathie sportive' (264). Periarticular bone changes and calcification of ligament and tendon insertions can be found. The joint space is normal in weight-bearing X-ray studies. The marginal lips or 'osteophytes' in the X-rays have been considered as being signs of joint and bone remodelling (264). These alterations seem to represent an independent entity distinct from OA (257).

Epidemiological Data on the Prevalence of Osteoarthritis

There is no doubt that rheumatic diseases, and particularly OA, form a major social and health problem in modern societies. Estimates of the prevalence of OA in the USA range from 16–24 million to 40·5 million individuals (265). The overall prevalence is 37% for both males and females. OA incapacitates 2–6 subjects out of 1000 in the general population (157). British statistics show that, in 1974, 2·3% of men and 1·3% of women in the working population had to retire from work on account of OA or allied conditions (157). According to Swedish statistics from 1975, the prevalence of osteo- and spondyloarthritis was 2·4% in men and 3·0% in women (266). In Finland, the prevalence rate of OA was 3·2% in 1976 (153).

Although it is pertinent to state that only a fraction of the individuals having OA have clinically significant complaints or suffer from physical disability (267, 268), the total effect of this disease on the social welfare and health care systems is massive in all countries.

In 1973, OA was the second ranking cause of permanent incapacity of individuals over 50 years of age in the USA (157). It was estimated in 1975 that 1·7 million US citizens would have benefited from hip arthroplasties and 4·6 million by knee arthroplasties (157). In Finland, every fifth woman and every tenth man over 30 has peripheral OA, one half of these need therapy and one third of the treated require more active therapy (269). The problem of OA seems not to be as prominent in the developing countries (270). Whether this is due to genetic or environmental factors, working conditions, other selective forces like excessive mortality at early ages, or deficient statistics, is not known.

Future Prospects of Joint Health

Arthritis does not kill, but it cripples numerous people each year. No other group of diseases appears to cause as much suffering by so many for so long (184). OA is the disease of the aged, its prevalence increasing rapidly after 40 years of age. In one study, the OA of hands and feet increased from 4% at ages 18–24 to 85% at ages 75–79 (1, 265, 267).

The world population is expected to exceed 6000 million by the year 2000; then about 80% of the world's population will live in developing countries; today the figure is about 70% (271). The absolute number of the population at ages 65 or more will increase from 227 million to 395 million, a 75% increase within the 25-year period. In developed countries the increase is from 119 million to 168 million elderly persons. Thus by the year 2000, two-fifths of the world's elderly will live in the developed, and three-fifths (227 million) in the developing countries. By the year 2000, the population residing in urban areas will increase from the present 39% to 50%: in the developed countries the figures will be 69% and 81%, respectively (271). In short, the world's population will increase, grow older, and become urbanized. This also means a more sedentary lifestyle. Inevitably, the population suffering from rheumatic complaints will markedly increase.

Are there any measures that can be taken to prevent rheumatic diseases, OA in particular? The situation is problematical. According to WHO, 'the most fundamental difficulty with rheumatic diseases today is that the problem is insufficiently appreciated and understood' (271).

Prevention from traumas in traffic (accidents), work, sports activities, leisure time, home, etc. will support the joint health of the population. Proper physical education and moderate training of the young will probably aid in strengthening the locomotory apparatus (272, 273). Static and dynamic exercises, both in work and everday life, build up the health of the joints. Expert ergonomic planning will ward off joint lesions at the workplace, whether in factories, fields, or offices. Individual biomechanical conditions should be taken into account for both work and sports. Endocrine and metabolic diseases as well as the whole variety of rheumatic conditions should be treated most actively to prevent further articular cartilage lesions and OA. Bed rest and unloading of the skeletal system, or joint immobilization, increase the risk of OA. Many studies, but not all, point out that trauma to the weight-bearing joints, particularly knees, would be one sequel of obesity (147, 274, 275). However, the hands of obese persons are also involved by OA, giving the impression of an underlying metabolic disease (234, 276).

It has been stated that OA is an ancient paleozoic system of repair and represents altered physiology amenable to correction and control (277). The justification of this argument can be questioned in the light of present knowledge of articular cartilage repair. Its capacity of regeneration and repair is very limited indeed (278). On the other hand, all clinical measures available for treatment and cure of OA should be adopted, and the whole potential of the healing capacity of the articular cartilage should be brought into use (277, 279, 280). Seen from the global perspective, however, preventive measures are the only realistic possibility to alleviate the massive health problem. Our culture, our working and living conditions all deserve close scrutiny. In the first place it is outside the human body, in our everyday environment, where reasons for cartilage injury and OA should be sought and identified.

ARTICULAR CARTILAGE AFTER INCREASED LOAD BEARING AND MOTION

In the early years of this century, Retterer investigated the effects of increased load bearing on the development and microscopic structure of the articular cartilage in the guinea-pig shoulder joint (281). He amputated one forelimb of young (2-month-old) guinea-pigs at the distal humerus, causing increased weight-bearing on the non-operated side. After periods of 4, 6, 8, 12 months, 2 years and 3 years, the animals were killed and specimens of articular cartilage were taken for microscopic examination. Retterer observed that the elevated functional stress (suractivité fonctionelle) increased cartilage thickness (from 300 μm to 400 μm) and caused hypertrophy of the superficial cartilage cells. The superficial cells changed their shape, becoming reminiscent of cells of the intermediate zone. The 'bands' of intercellular matrix increased in thickness from 10–20 μm to 40–50 μm. The subchondral bone increased in thickness. Retterer stated that the results also supported Sappey's hypothesis of bone formation: augmented compression between joint surfaces inhibits bone formation (281).

Freund (1939) examined the joints of a youth with spastic quadriplegia and athetosis (138). He came to the conclusion that 'any marked function for a long period (infraphysiologic and ultraphysiologic demands) is certain to lead to degenerative changes of the joint cartilage and may be followed by the whole syndrome of fully developed arthritis deformans, the more probably the joint is exposed to unphysiologic use' (138).

In 1941, Sääf published results on the effects of physical training on the femoral head articular cartilage of guinea-pigs (282). Sääf used a motor-driven treadmill to make the animals run. The microscopic examination of the loaded areas revealed enlarged cells and chondrones containing more cells than in the controls. The basophilia of the intercellular matrix was increased. Just the opposite changes were observed in animals which were kept in narrow cages restricting free movements. The chondrocytes were small and only 1–2 cells were observed in each chondrone. The matrix basophilia was reduced. In a later communication, Sääf gave more details of his experimental system (283). The running distance was 1000 m/day for 20–100 days. Utilizing morphometric microscopical methods, Sääf was able to show that the sizes of cells in all zones of the cartilage grew larger during the course of the running exercise. Sääf concluded that the articular tissue of adult guinea-pigs reacted to the increased functioning of the joint. He also made a point of the continuous regeneration of articular cartilage at the joint surface, the intermediate zone playing a dominant role as a centre of reproduction of cartilage cells. This idea of Sääf, originally presented by Hammar (284), has not been confirmed later.

Lanier subjected mice to moderate, daily, forced exercise from the age of 6 weeks for a period of 12·5 months (285). After microscopic evaluation of the histological sections, he came to the conclusion that control mice had more minor lesions in the articular cartilage than exercised ones. Lanier also concluded that exercise was not an important factor in the occurrence of articular degeneration in mice.

In a series of papers Holmdahl, Ingelmark and Ekholm studied the effects of physical training on the properties of articular cartilage in rabbits (286–289). It turned out that the rabbit articular cartilage tissue showed pronounced functional adaptability, expressing itself in an increase in the thickness of articular cartilage after running exercise, relative increase of the intercellular substance, a tendency towards increase of cells in each chondrone, and possibly an enlargement of cartilage cells. Ingelmark and Ekholm claimed that the thickness of articular cartilage was increased by 10% immediately after running training (289). This increase declined to the control level within 1 h after running. This experiment has not been repeated and the results have not been substantiated. In general, the results of this group showed that physical training can have positive, anabolic effects on the articular cartilage.

The first observations that physical training can have negative, catabolic influences on the articular cartilage were those of Krause who, after exposing mice to a strenuous running programme, could show decreased staining of mucosubstances in the articular cartilage matrix (290). He made mice run on a treadmill approximately 6000–12 000 m/day with a total running distance of 450–800 km in 63 days. The stainability of the cartilage matrix for acid mucopolysaccharides, i.e. with alcian blue, Hale's dialysed iron, and methylene blue stains, was reduced in 11 of 13 runners but not in any of the controls. Krause concluded that excessive functional strain on normal articular cartilage can cause a pathological condition of the cartilage. Krause obtained histochemical but not morphological evidence in favour of the theory of Pommer, who claimed that the mechanical stress on the articular surface was the main reason for OA. Subsequently, degenerative alterations of the articular cartilage after physical exercise have been observed by Vasan in the femoral heads of dogs (291) and by Stofft and Graf and Ender and Lessel on the articular surfaces of exercised guinea-pigs and rabbits (292, 293).

In the 1970s Kostenszky and Oláh were able to show that the articular cartilage of canine load-bearing knee joints (the contralateral limb did not bear weight due to operation) showed a 19·4% increase of hexosamine and a 50% elevation of glucosamine content (294). It was suggested that the increased weight-bearing led to an accumulation of keratan sulphate and an acceleration of the ageing process in the articular cartilage tissue. These authors also demonstrated that increased load bearing brought about augmented levels of glycoproteins, but not collagen, in the articular cartilage tissue (295). Increased content of keratan sulphate after augmented weight bearing was later reported to take place in rabbit articular cartilage (296).

While Kostenszky and Oláh were unable to register any change, Caterson and Lowther observed an increase of chondroitin sulphate and total proteoglycans after a 4-week increased load bearing period of sheep (297). In the non-load-bearing joint there was a corresponding decrease of both chondroitin sulphate and total proteoglycans. The molecular weight of the proteoglycans was decreased. The alterations were interpreted to take place partly because of changes in the biosynthesis of the cartilage proteoglycans in response to altered functional demand.

After studying articular cartilage of exercised adult dogs, Kincaid and Van Sickle concluded, on the basis of histochemical results, that 'the exercise protocol did not produce significant variability in the metabolic pathways associated with respiration, anaerobic glycolysis, chemical energy transformation, or proteoglycan synthesis of the articular chondrocyte based on the indicator enzymatic reaction studied' (298). They suggested that lipid synthesis served to store excessive quantities of hydrogen ions in an innocuous form.

The consequences of repetitive impact loadings on the articular cartilage were studied by Radin et al. (299). The knee joints of adult rabbits were subjected to daily 1 h intervals of impulsive loading equivalent to their body weight at the rate of 60 impulses/min. The articular cartilage showed signs of degenerative joint disease. However, preceding microfractures with healing and stiffening of the subchondral bone were observed. When the experiment was repeated, the subchondral bone was first found to contain an increase of ^{99m}Tc labelling, followed by tetracycline labelling, bone formation, and relative stiffening of the bone (300). Horizontal splitting and deep fibrillation of the overlying articular cartilage followed the early bone changes. Radin et al. emphasized the primary role of the subchondral bone and its stiffening in the development of OA. Broom, on the other hand, demonstrated that repeated impact loading of articular cartilage brought about crimped radial texture in the cartilage matrix, which was very similar to that found in the softened cartilage of the central weight-bearing region of the tibial plateaux of large mammals (301). Human osteoarthrotic cartilage also showed a similar crimped radial pattern of texture.

ARTICULAR CARTILAGE AFTER RETAINED JOINT MOVEMENTS BUT WITH AN ABSENCE OF LOADING

This kind of situation is brought about by amputation of the distal part of the extremity. Retterer studied the shoulder joint of guinea-pigs after amputation of the forelimb above the elbow joint (302). The thickness of the humeral head cartilage was reduced to 120 μm instead of 300 μm in the control animals. The flat superficial cells and the true cartilaginous cells lying deeper in the tissue could be discerned. The amount of intercellular matrix was scanty. The normal orientation of cells in the deeper zones of the cartilage was disturbed. The subchondral plate was thinned. Retterer concluded that the chondrocytes survived the prolonged non-load-bearing, but the cells were incapable of forming solid 'bands' of intercellular matrix substance (302). This articular cartilage cannot resist heavy loading. If it is subjected to loading, the faint trabeculations of the matrix would be disrupted, walls of the lacunae broken and their contents liberated into the joint cavity. This kind of process would lead to OA with complete eburnation of the joint surface and development of other sequelae of the disease (302).

More than 60 years later, Oláh and Kostenszky relieved canine hind limbs from weight-bearing by osteotomy of the tibia and rejoining the bone ends with medullary nailing (303). As a consequence, the dogs (n = 8) avoided loading due to pain. After 40 days, tissue specimens were collected for analysis. Oláh and Kostenszky found that the hexosamine content was 58·4%, galactosamine 51·6%, and glucosamine 65·5% of the respective content in the contralateral load-bearing leg (303). The observed figures were still clearly below the values obtained from control dogs (n = 9) which were allowed to move freely. Oláh and Kostenszky concluded that loss of function caused marked reduction of the glycosaminoglycan content of the articular cartilage (303).

Palmoski et al. amputated the paws of 4 dogs below the knee joint. They showed that movement, but not weight bearing, took place in the amputated leg after the operation (304). On the operated side, the knee joint articular cartilage showed a decrease in thickness, safranin O staining, and uronic acid content (about 24%) and a slight increase in water content (about 6%). Incorporation of ^{35}S into proteoglycans was 34–67% less than on the contralateral side and there was an aggregation defect of proteoglycans (304). The results were almost identical with those occurring in the canine knee after immobilization of the leg in a cast. Palmoski et al. concluded that 'the loading of the joint which occurs from contraction of the muscles that span the knee and stabilize the limb in stance, and not merely joint movement, may be required to maintain the integrity of the articular cartilage.'

In 1975, Salter et al. reported that, by the aid of continuous passive movements, new hyaline cartilage developed in over half the full-thickness drill holes of the articular cartilage within 4 weeks (305). Further details were published a few years later (306). Healing of the defects (drill holes) by hyaline cartilage occurred in 8% of the defects in immobilized rabbits, 9% of the defects in rabbits permitted intermittent active motion, and 52% of defects in animals treated by passive continuous motion. The observation period ranged from 1 to 3 weeks. The above results were obtained with adolescent rabbits; with adult animals, healing was somewhat inferior. There is no certainty about the fate of the newly synthesized hyaline cartilage after the animals resumed normal load bearing. Salter et al. concluded that the metaplasia of the healing tissue from mesenchymal tissue to hyaline cartilage was not only more rapid but also more complete with continuous passive motion. Recently, O'Driscoll et al. published results showing that cartilage was the predominant tissue in only 9% of the free intra-articular periosteal autografts maintained in immobilized joints but in 59% of the grafts exposed to continuous passive motion (307). At present, principles of continuous passive motion are applied to clinical orthopaedic practice (308).

In human amputees, the amputated side characteristically shows osteoporosis, i.e. loss of bone substance (309). It is possible that the osteoporosis has a protective effect on joints on the amputated side. This is in line with the observations of Glyn *et al.* who observed a low prevalence of OA in hips and knees of poliomyelitis patients (310). Benichou and Wirotius reported reduced thickness of hip articular cartilage on the amputated side in 27 out of 53 patients (311). The reduced thickness appeared to correlate with the stump length, since it occurred in 11 of 13 upper-third amputees but in none of the lower-third amputees. It is of interest to note that in 42 lower limb amputees there was a significant increase of OA in the knee of the unamputated leg compared with the amputated side (309).

CHANGES IN ARTICULAR CARTILAGE DUE TO JOINT IMMOBILIZATION

The first experimental approach to clarify the consequences of joint immobilization on articular cartilage was made by Menzel in 1871 (312). Menzel used Plaster of Paris to immobilize one extremity of the experimental animals (2 adult dogs, 6 young rabbits) for 5–68 days, and observed the changes both macroscopically and microscopically. In dogs, the extremity was immobilized in flexion, in rabbits in extension. In Menzel's opinion, continuous immobilization of the normal joint caused decubitus ulcer at the contact site. The changes were first observed and were most severe at places where the heaviest compressive load occurred. He suggested that the pressure brought about deficient nutrition of the articular cartilage. Menzel mentioned that the first clinical observations on the influences of immobilization-induced compression on articular cartilage were published by Cloquet (1821), Teissier (1841), and Bonnet (1855) (312). Their specimens were from surgical patients whose limbs had been immobilized due mainly to fracture. The joints showed local signs of cartilage lesions with altered colour and softness, superficial ulcers, and deep defects.

In 1873 Reyher published the results of his experiments on the same problem, claiming that when immobilization was carried out by aid of Plaster of Paris the regions of contact between the articulating surfaces were not affected, whereas non-contact areas showed alterations including cartilage defects filled with connective tissue (313). Reyher used dogs in his experiments, both young and adult. The limbs were immobilized either in flexion or in extension. The first alterations were evident after 62 days and they were more pronounced after 127 days. Some years later, Moll splinted hind limbs of young and adult rabbits in extension and found articular cartilage lesions only in those regions which were devoid of continuous joint contact (314). Thus, Moll's results supported the observations of Reyher. The connective tissue covering the non-load-bearing cartilage seemed to be partly derived from local metaplasia of the cartilage tissue, the rest growing from the connective tissue at the cartilage–synovium junction.

In the 1920s Müller conducted further investigations on the influences of joint immobilization on articular cartilage (315, 316). He came to the conclusion that the degree of joint fixation was the most critical factor determining the response of the articular cartilage. With the prerequisite that the fixation was completely rigid, disintegration and lesions of the articular cartilage occurred at the site of contact. The non-contact areas were covered by connective tissue probably derived from the cartilage–synovium junction. This connective tissue was first loosely bound to the cartilage surface. For a long period the articular cartilage beneath this layer appeared intact; gradually, however, connective tissue was stacked closer to the cartilage surface, initiating erosion of the tissue. Müller considered that the mere disintegration or ulcer of the articular cartilage was not enough to evoke OA (317). Motion and load bearing was also needed to call forth the whole symptom complex of OA.

Koch showed that when two large articular surfaces in rabbits were in contact and compressed each other for 6 weeks, only superficial necroses of the cartilage occurred, or were completely absent (318). On the other hand, when a small and restricted bone end compressed the articular surface, severe necrosis of the cartilage took place within 3 weeks. After another 2 weeks, the destroyed cartilage was replaced by connective tissue. In joints where the articulating surfaces were separated from each other by forceful traction, the joint cavity was invaded by loose connective tissue within a few weeks and the cavity disappeared (318).

Ely and Mensor carried out further experiments with dogs (319). They could not entirely agree with the statement of Müller (315) that only extreme grades of immobilization gave distinct changes to cartilage structure. They could not achieve complete and constant immobilization of the joint during their experiment. In spite of this, they could observe thinning, irregularity, fibrillation, and at places vacuolization of the articular cartilage. This result was later confirmed by Evans *et al.* and others (320–323).

Evans *et al.* studied immobilization effects on the rat knee joint (320). The proliferation of intracapsular connective tissue and the formation of adhesions were the primary responses of the joint to limitation of motion; these changes were reversible to some degree. Major cartilage alterations such as matrix fibrillation, cleft formation and ulceration, as well as adjacent subchondral lesions, were the result of abnormal friction and pressure in the joint; these changes were no longer reversible. Notably, in the young rats immobilization periods between 27 and 123 days only increased cartilage thickness at the contact area and caused no degeneration (324). This was probably due to the fact that rigid fixation was not achieved. The knee was held mid-way between full flexion and full extension. When the adult rat knee was immobilized in extension for 23–186 days, the pressure-bearing articular cartilage portion degenerated, while in the non-pressure zone there was an increase in cell size, density, and deposition of basophilic material forming a territory around the cells (322). Similar results were achieved by Thaxter *et al.* (323).

Salter and Field investigated the effects of continuous compression on the rabbit and monkey articular cartilages (325). They found pressure necrosis of the articular cartilage after 6 days of continuous compression of the opposing joint surfaces and also after simple immobilization of the joints into forced positions (force was required to place the joint in a given position). Since then, several authors have investigated details of the degeneration of rabbit articular cartilage after experimental immobilization (326–333).

During the last few years, interesting new data have been obtained which elucidate the molecular mechanisms of cartilage atrophy. Palmoski *et al.* observed a 41% decrease in proteoglycan synthesis after a 6-day immobilization period of canine knee joint; after 3 weeks, proteoglycan aggregation was no longer demonstrable (334). Palmoski and Brandt showed that immobilization of the knee for 12 weeks after anterior cruciate ligament transection prevented OA of the knee joint developing, although articular cartilage atrophy ensued (335). In dogs ambulating freely in the pen after ligament transection, signs of OA developed with osteophytes, cartilage fibrillation, and a decrease of proteoglycan (uronic acid) content. The cartilage thickness remained unaltered and proteoglycan synthesis increased by 80% as compared to the non-operated knee (335). Williams and Brandt observed in guinea-pigs that temporary (3-week) immobilization led to a reduction in chondrocyte death and prevented both the formation of osteophytes and cartilage fibrillation following intra-articular injection of sodium iodoacetate (336). Thus, a brief period of immobilization after an injury seemed to protect the joint against further damage.

Interestingly, Bullough and co-workers observed in human hips and elbows that chondromalacia and fibrillation were early and universal in the unloaded areas of the joints (337, 338). In the dog, they found that the unloaded, inactive and effete tissue was very different from the overactive cartilage of the loaded area, which had increased cellularity and matrix synthesis, increased lysosomal enzyme activity and cell replication characteristic of the cartilage of established arthritis. Earlier, Harrison *et al.* had suggested that the early lesions of OA on the femoral head were in the unloaded and not in the loaded part of the joint (339). Most research workers, however, appear to have adopted as true the statement that the lesions leading to OA first appear in the areas representing greatest load bearing (for review *see* 130, 340).

REMOBILIZATION EFFECTS ON THE JOINT AND ARTICULAR CARTILAGE

In 1886, Moll published results of experiments in which he studied remobilization effects on the rabbit knee joint after an initial immobilization period of 29–98 days (314). The knee joint was immobilized in extension. The total number of animals was 4. In 2 cases he found complete healing after a remobilization period of 47–51 days, whereas the restoration was incomplete in 2 cases. In all cases, however, the normal lustre of the cartilage was altered in the regions devoid of cartilage-to-cartilage contact in an extended joint. The articular cartilage of non-contact regions was more or less injured, while the contact areas appeared preserved. In Moll's opinion, the majority of the changes appeared during the remobilization period, because they could not be found during or immediately after immobilization. In one case a deep ulcer appeared on the articular surface. Remobilization probably caused ruptures and irritation of the synovial tissue, with blood-stained synovial fluid calling up an inflammatory reaction (314).

More than 80 years later, Sood immobilized knee joints of adult rabbits in flexion for a period of 7–12 weeks before remobilization (327). The animals could move freely in their cages. The stainability of the intercellular matrix was only slightly, if at all, reduced after 12 weeks' remobilization. In 5 of the 6 femoral specimens, the articular surface appeared intact in histological sections. Sood's observations gave rise to the idea that after flexion-immobilization, regressive changes in the articular cartilage were completely reversible. On the other hand, Finsterbush and Friedman reported only partial restoration of knee motion in rabbits whose hind limbs were immobilized in semi-flexion for 6 weeks (329). Only 9 of the 14 rabbits regained normal or partial knee motion. Also, in joints where the motion was restored, the previous articular lesions were coated with a fibrous type of tissue and remnants of adhesions were observed.

Evans *et al.* studied remobilization effects in rats after an immobilization period of 45–110 days (320). The connective tissue which invaded the joint cavity persisted, although it adapted to joint movements by elongation and splitting into bundles. The joint cavity was restored to a limited degree and the synovial membrane was re-established through modification of the surface connective tissue of the new joint space. Only small areas of articular cartilage were free from adhesions after the remobilization period, but in all cases the underlying cartilage seemed viable and identifiable. There was no evidence after 35 days of remobilization that healing of the articular cartilage lesions was taking place (320).

Palmoski *et al.* observed in dogs that immobilization-induced aggregation defect of proteoglycans was reversible in 2 weeks after removal of a cast that had been worn for 6 weeks (334). After 3 weeks of free ambulation, the cartilage thickness, safranin O staining of the matrix, uronic acid content, and net proteoglycan synthesis of the articular cartilage were normalized. However, knee cartilage from dogs which had been exposed to vigorous running exercise (6 miles/day, 3 mph) for 3 weeks after removal of the casts showed a continuing decrease in thickness, safranin O staining, and uronic acid content, although the net proteoglycan synthesis was increased (341). On the other hand, in beagle dogs only partial restoration of the proteoglycans and physical properties of articular cartilage was observed after 15 weeks' remobilization following an initial immobilization period of 11 weeks (342–344). In guinea-pigs, temporary joint immobilization facilitated repair of chemically induced articular cartilage injury (336).

Rubak *et al.* investigated the influences of immobilization and remobilization on chondrogenesis in a periosteal graft transplanted into an artifical defect of the articular cartilage (345). They found that immobilization for 3–6 weeks had an inhibitory effect on chondrogenesis. However, chondrogenesis partially recovered after remobilization. Mooney and Ferguson found evidence that the primitive mesenchymal cells can furnish fibrocartilage to the repair granuloma, depending on the timing and duration of immobilization and subsequent motion (346).

IN VITRO LOADING OF ARTICULAR CARTILAGE

In 1975, Rodan *et al.* presented evidence for reduction of both cAMP and cGMP after exposing epiphyses of the tibiae from 16-day-old chick embryos to continuous compressive forces of physiological magnitude (60 g/cm^2, equal to 5.865 kPa) (347). The effect appeared to be mediated by translocation of calcium through enhanced cellular uptake (348). Using the same model, Veldhuizen *et al.* showed that, contrary to the effect of continuous pressure, intermittent compression above the threshold equivalent to weight bearing raised cAMP levels and reduced DNA synthesis (349). In nanomelic chickens, characterized by an almost complete absence of cartilage-specific proteoglycan but with the cartilage-specific collagen unaffected, the tissue responded to pressure like normal cartilage except that the overall cAMP content was lower and response to somatomedin was significantly different from that observed in normal animals (350).

When an intermittent compressive force regimen (0·3 Hz, pressure differential 130 mbar) was applied to chicken epiphyseal high density chondrocyte culture, incorporation of $^{35}SO_4$ into glycosaminoglycans increased 40% whereas DNA synthesis showed a 20% decrease (351, 352). The aggregation property of proteoglycans improved and the amount of proteoglycans not extractable with guanidinium–HCl increased. It was concluded that the regimen not only increased the synthesis of proteoglycans but also improved the aggregating property of the molecules and their coherence with other matrix components. When the same kind of culture was subjected to cyclical stretching (5·5% at a frequency of 0·2 Hz) a similar increase in glycosaminoglycan (proteoglycan) synthesis was observed (353). However, cyclical stretching also caused a 2·4-fold increase in ^3H-thymidine incorporation into DNA, which was a strikingly different result from that of the former experiment. The discrepant results can be explained by differences in the experimental set-ups.

In 1980 Kaye *et al.* reported increased (11–15%) uptake of labelled substrates ($^{35}SO_4$, ^3H-uridine, ^3H-glycine) in calf articular cartilage after exposure to continuous hydrostatic pressure 2587 kPa (354). A decrease in incorporation to values less than 50% of non-pressurized tissue resulted from exposure to lower pressures 517–2070 kPa (355). The recovery phase following exposure to pressure included initial release or rebound phenomenon, whereby a burst of metabolic rate to a normal level was observed following an initial treatment with low pressure (517–2070 kPa), and acceleration by 60% in tissue whose metabolism was stimulated with higher pressure 2587 kPa. Jones *et al.* investigated fragments of calf and human articular cartilage under continuous mechanical pressure (356). The authors found significant decreases in both proteoglycan breakdown and incorporation of $^{35}SO_4$ into glycosaminoglycans when a heavy pressure (30 kgf cm^{-2}) was applied to the cartilage fragments.

The influence of both static and intermittent stress on full-thickness plugs of canine articular cartilage was investigated by Palmoski and Brandt (357). When the plugs were exposed to static stress with a duty cycle of 60 s on/60 s off, the glycosaminoglycan synthesis was reduced to 30–60% of the controls. However, when the duty cycle of 4 s on/11 s off was used, the glycosaminoglycan synthesis increased 34% although protein synthesis and contents of DNA, uronic acid, and water remained unaltered. Judged from the uptake of ^{14}C-aminoisobutyric acid and ^{14}C-xylose, the change in glycosaminoglycan synthesis did not appear to be due to altered diffusion of nutrients through the articular cartilage tissue (357).

Copray *et al.* found that, after exposing mandibular condyles from 4-day-old rats to continuous and intermittent compression, light continuous force (0·5 g) stimulated proliferation of cartilage cells but reduced the synthesis of sulphated glycosaminoglycans and collagen (358). When an intermittent force (0·5–1·0 g, 0·7 Hz) was used, proliferative activity was reduced but synthesis of matrix components was stimulated. A continuous compressive force below 3 g did not affect cartilage growth, while a weight above 3 g ceased the growth (359). On the other hand, growth continued, although at a lower rate, under intermittent compressive forces with weights up to 8 g, the growth stopped when the weight exceeded 8 g. After removal of growth-restricting weight, reactivation of growth occurred until a new balance was achieved.

PRESENT STATE OF KNOWLEDGE AND FUTURE PROSPECTS

The pattern of locomotion is a characteristic of each species and related primarily to feeding habits. The species is adapted to cope with a certain range of environmental conditions such as climate, access to nutrients and water. The features of behaviour are carried into effect by the locomotory system. On the other hand, the body, particularly the locomotory system, needs the characteristic behaviour to maintain its normal level of adaptation and functional and structural integrity. Extreme variations in locomotory pattern will cause harm. The joints, especially the articular cartilage, form a *locus minoris resistentiae* (a weak point) in the musculoskeletal system. This is also true with man. Change from a rural to an urban lifestyle probably means a more sedentary way of living, threatening the normal dynamic loading pattern of the joints. Instead, the muscloskeletal system is exposed to a more static type of loading, which may risk its functional capacity and health. In short, the motion pattern of modern man draws ever farther away from the original one of our ancestors.

Joint movements and compressive forces exert influences of fundamental importance during embryonic and postnatal development of the locomotory system. Combined with the hereditary factors, state of health, and nutrition, the mechanical factors determine the properties of the musculoskeletal system. In developed countries, cultural aspects like working habits and conditions, sports and leisure-time activities, exert a most important impetus for the maintenance of health and functional capacity of the system of bones and joints. The same will also be true in the developing countries, provided that the problems of under-nutrition and infectious diseases can be overcome. The joints and articular cartilage need proper stress and use. This is probably threatened by the modern sedentary lifestyle and static working patterns.

In joints, the hyaline cartilage forms the bearing surface. The chondrocytes supply the tissue with its main macromolecular constituents, proteoglycans and collagen. The cells are largely dependent for their nutrition on the diffusion of molecules from the synovial fluid. Articular cartilage is devoid of nerves, blood and lymphatic vessels. The cartilage matrix is mainly composed of water held by the negative charge of the proteoglycans (glycosaminoglycans) linked to hyaluronic acid, forming large proteoglycan aggregates. The Type II collagen fibres serve as fine ropes having specific orientations in each zone of the articular cartilage, entrapping the proteoglycans and resisting the tension generated by these hydrated molecules. Articular cartilage obeys Wolff's Law (360). Both increased and decreased joint loading alter the biological properties of the cartilage tissue, although the changes are not as apparent as in bone. Immobilization of the joint severely deteriorates the joint, causing either atrophy or pressure-induced necrosis of the articular cartilage, depending on the mode of the experimental system.

OA is ancient disease, having affected dinosaurs 100 million years ago and ancient man 10000–100000 years ago. It is a ubiquitous condition in both wild and domestic animals. In man, OA is the most common of the rheumatic complaints. In future, its prevalence will show a further increase with an increase in the elderly population. The aetiology of OA is not known. Besides heredity, and some diseases, mechanical factors are most important in the aetiology and pathogenesis of the disease. It is also clear that a preceding trauma jeopardizes the joints to OA. At present, functional stress of the normal joint cannot be regarded as a traumatizing factor which would predispose the articular cartilage to OA. However, there is evidence that strenuous functional stress degrades the biological properties of articular cartilage, indicating its potential ability to cause trauma to it. Future research work will show whether functional stress alone can cause injury to the articular cartilage or not.

Alleviation of the health problem caused by OA has to be sought from prevention of the disease. Joints need appropriate motion and functional stress to maintain their health. Therefore, the access to non-static, ergonomically fit working conditions and leisure-time physical activities should be granted to everyone. Naturally, further actions should also be taken to improve the results of clinical therapy so that the present palliative care could be exchanged for therapeutic treatment. The same is true with rehabilitation. Seen from global perspective, preventive measures need to be far more effective and to reach all people. The accomplishment of this strategy does not need to depend on monetary resources but rather on proper education and legislation of the nations.

Continued research work is required to find new and powerful ways to prevent and cure OA. The history of science clearly shows that the acquisition of new discoveries largely depends on the development and adoption of new research methods. To a great extent, the progress of medical and biological research hitherto has been due to the contribution of mathematicians, physicists, and chemists to these branches of science. We believe that one day both research workers and clinicians can reach a unanimous opinion on the aetiology and pathogenesis of OA, which will make a solid basis for further work for the prevention and therapy of the disease.

CONCLUSIONS

Compared to the age of other aspects of human culture, science is still in its youth. Not more than 240 years has elapsed since Hunter (1743) published his famous observations on the structure of articular cartilage. One hundred and fifty years ago, Müller (in the 1830s) introduced the term 'Bindegewebe' (connective tissue) and made his first observations on chondrin, the substance derived from cartilage which we now know contained proteoglycans. At about the same time Cloquet (1821) and somewhat later Teissier (1841) and Bonnet (1855) investigated injuries of the articular cartilage of patients after long-term bed rest. Menzel (1871) and Reyher (1873) were the first to do experimental work on joint immobilization, and Moll (100 years ago) published his results on the effects of remobilization of joints after various periods of immobilization. At the beginning of this century, Retterer (1908) did experiments with guinea-pigs on the influences of increased weight bearing on articular cartilage. These research workers were the pioneers in the scientific field which has been surveyed in detail on the preceding pages. Great respect is due to their work and ideas.

Research work has shown that the articular cartilage also obeys Wolff's law; increased or decreased functional stress affects the biological properties of the cartilage tissue. Although this principle was initially established to apply to bone (360), it has become apparent that the rule also concerns other connective tissues of the locomotory system. During the last few decades, the progress of research on articular cartilage has been extremely rapid, largely due to innovations in research methods, resulting in a deeper understanding of the molecular, biophysical, structural, and biomechanical properties of the tissue.

PRACTICAL SIGNIFICANCE

Successful solution of future research problems rests on the life's work of past and present scientists. This chapter gives a historical account of the highlights of past research of connective tissue, especially articular cartilage. Emphasis has been laid on the clarification of influences and significance of joint motion and loading on the biological properties and health of the articular cartilage. The results of the most important investigations are reviewed. They are the cornerstone of our present knowledge of the biology of articular cartilage. This review clearly demonstrates the importance of the availability of new methods for the advancement of science. Alert and ingenious brains must be supplied with qualified research equipment. The methods of traditional light microscopy and organic chemistry of the 19th century have today been substituted for the latest methods of molecular biology, electron microscopy, biophysics, and biomechanics. After another 100 years, our present methods will probably still be appreciated but regarded as old-fashioned and insufficient. This is as it should be. The problem remains, but the knowledge and solutions will be fresh and new.

ACKNOWLEDGEMENTS

We are greatly indebted to Professor Hans Schadewaldt of Institut für Geschichte der Medizin, Düsseldorf, FRG, for the portrait of Johannes Müller; Mr Hindrik Strandberg of the Department of History of Medicine and Museum, University of Helsinki, for supplying important literary sources; personnel of the Library of the University of Kuopio for valuable assistance in acquisition of the old literature; Mr Daniel Williams, MSc, for linguistic assistance; and Ms Teija Koponen for typing the manuscript. This work has been supported by grants from the Academy of Finland, the Finnish Research Council for Physcial Education and Sports, Ministry of Education, the North Savo Fund of the Finnish Cultural Foundation, the Duodecim Foundation, the Yrjö Jahnsson Foundation, the Oskar Öflund Foundation, the Research Foundation of Orthopaedics and Traumatology, the Emil Aaltonen Foundation, the Paulo Foundation, the Heikki and Hilma Honkanen Foundation and the Sigrid Jusélius Foundation.

REFERENCES

1. Cooke T D V (1985) Pathogenetic mechanisms in polyarticular osteoarthritis. *Clin Rheum Dis* **11**: 203–38.
2. Gardner D L (1983) The nature and causes of osteoarthrosis. *Br Med J* **286**: 418–24.
3. Eyanson S and Brandt K D (1984) Osteoarthritis. *Primary Care* **11**: 259–69.
4. Talbott J H (1970) *A Biographical History of Medicine. Excerpts and Essays on the Men and their Work*. New York: Grune & Stratton.
5. Hunter W (1743) Of the structure and diseases of articulating cartilages. *Phil Trans R Soc Lond* **42**: 514–21.
6. Retterer E (1908) Structure du cartilage diarthrodial de l'adulte. *C R Soc Biol (Paris)* **64**: 45–8.
7. Bichat X (1801) *Anatomie Générale, appliquée à la Physiologie et à la Médecine*. Paris: Brosson, Gabon et Cie.
8. Beclard F A (1823) *Xavier Bichat Allgemeine Anatomie angewandt auf die Physiologie und Arzneywissenschaft und Uebersicht der neuern Entdeckungen in der Anatomie und Physiologie*. Leipzig: Hartmann.
9. Florman A H (1823) *Anatomisk Handbok för Läkare och Zoologer, Första Delen*. Lund: Berlingska.
10. Velpeau A A L M (1837) *Manuel d'anatomie chirurgicale, générale et topographique*. Paris: Méquignon-Marvis.
11. Cruveilhier J (1824) Observations sur les cartilages diarthrodiaux et les maladies des articulations diarthrodiales. *Arch Gen Med (Paris)*, 2ᵐᵉ *Année*, **IV**: 161–98.
12. Weber E H (1830) *Friedrich Hildebrandt's Handbuch der Anatomie des Menschen, Ausgabe 4, Band 2*. Braunschweig: Verlag der Schulbuchhandlung.
13. Lauth E A (1835) Neues Handbuch der Praktischen Anatomie, Band I. Stuttgart and Leipzig: Rieger.
14. Bruns V (1841) *Lehrbuch der allgemeinen Anatomie des Menschen*. Braunschweig: Vieweg.
15. Leidy J (1849) On the intimate structure and history of the articular cartilages. *Am J Med Sci* **34**: 277–94.
16. Bock C E (1851) *Anatomisches Taschenbuch, enhaltend die Anatomie des Menschen, systematisch, im ausführlichen und übersichtlichen Auszuge*, Auflage 4. Leipzig: Renger'sche Buchhandlung.
17. Kölliker A (1850) *Mikroskopische Anatomie*. Leipzig: Engelmann.
18. Toynbee J (1841) Researches, tending to prove the Non-vascularity and the peculiar uniform Mode of Organisation and Nutrition of certain Animal Tissues, etc. *Phil Trans R Soc Lond*. **131**: 159–92.
19. Henle J (1838) Ueber die Ausbreitung des Epithelium in menschlichen Körper. *Müllers Arch* 1838: 103–28.
20. Todd R B and Bowman W (1845) *The Physiological Anatomy and Physiology of Man, Vol I*. London: Parker.
21. Kölliker A (1848) Ueber den Bau der Synovialhäute. *Mitth Naturforsch Gesellsch Zuerich* **1**: 93–6.
22. Hueter C (1866) Zur Histologie der Gelenkflächen und Gelenkkapseln, mit einem kritischen Vorwort über die Versilberungsmethode. *Virchow's Arch* **36**: 25–80.
23. Thomson A, Schäfer E A and Thane G D (eds) (1882) *Quain's Elements of Anatomy, 9th Ed.* London: Longmans, Green and Co.
24. Gardner D L (1972) The influence of microscopic technology on knowledge of cartilage surface structure. *Ann Rheum Dis* **31**: 235–57.
25. Böhmer F (1865) Zur pathologischen Anatomie der Meningitis Cerebromedullaris epidemica. *Aerztl Intelligenzbl (Munich)* **12**: 539–50.
26. Frey H (1868) Die Hämatoxylinfärbung. *Arch Mikr Anat* **4**: 345–6.
27. Goeppert H R and Cohn F (1849) Ueber die Rotation des Zellinhaltes in *Nitella flexilis*. *Bot Zeitg* **7**: 665–73, 681–91, 697–705, 713–9.
28. Corti A (1851) Recherches sur l'organe de l'ouïe des mammifêres. *Z Wiss Zool* **3**: 109–69.
29. Schwartz E (1867) Ueber eine Methode doppelter Färbung mikroscopischer Objecte und ihre

Anwendung zur Untersuchung der Musculatur des Darmtraktes, der Milz, Lymphdrüsen und andere Organe. *Sitzber Acad Wiss Wien* **55**: 671–89.

30. Hansen F C C (1905) Untersuchungen über die Gruppe der Bindesubstanzen. I. Der Hyalinknorpel. *Anat Hefte* **83** (27, 3): 535–820.
31. Benninghoff A (1922) Ueber den funktionellen Bau des Knorpels. *Verh Anat Gesellsch* **55**: 250–67.
32. Steedman H F (1950) Alcian blue 8GS; a new stain for mucin. *Q J Microsc Sci* **91**: 477–9.
33. Scott J E and Dorling J (1965) Differential staining of acid glycosaminoglycans (mucopolysaccharides) by alcian blue in salt solution. *Histochemie* **5**: 22–33.
34. Stockwell R A and Scott J E (1967) Distribution of acid glycosaminoglycans in human articular cartilage. *Nature* **215**: 1376–8.
35. Lison L (1935) La signification histochimique de la métachromasie. *C R Séanc. Soc Biol (Paris)* **118**: 821–4.
36. McManus J F A (1946) Histological demonstration of mucin after periodic acid. *Nature* **158**: 202.
37. Lillie R D, Laskey A, Greco J and Jacquier H (1947) Reticulum staining with Schiff reagent after oxidation by acidified sodium periodate. *J Lab Clin Med* **32**: 910–2.
38. Scott J E and Dorling J (1969) Periodate oxidation of acid polysaccharides. III. A PAS method for chondroitin sulphates and other glycosamino-glycuronans. *Histochemie* **19**: 295–301.
39. Rosenberg L (1971) Chemical basis for the histological use of safranin O in the study of articular cartilage. *J Bone Joint Surg [Am]* **53**: 69–82.
40. Schadewaldt H (1986) Personal communication.
41. Wharton T (1656) Adenographia: Sive Glandularum Totius Corpores Descripto. London.
42. Müller J (1836) Ueber die Structur und die chemischen Eigenschaften der thierischen Bestandtheile der Knorpel und Knochen. *Poggendorf Annalen* **38**: 295–353.
43. Krukenberg C F W (1884) Die chemischen Bestandtheile des Knorpels. *Z Biol* **20**: 307–26.
44. Morochowetz L (1877) Zur Histochemie des Bindegewebes. *Verhandl Nat Hist Med Ver Heidelberg* **1**: 480–3.
45. Mörner C T (1889) Chemische Studien über den Trachealknorpel. *Skand Arch Physiol* **1**: 210–43.
46. Schmiedeberg O (1891) Ueber die chemische Zusammensetzung des Knorpels. *Arch Exp Pathol Pharmakol* **28**: 355–404.
47. Levene P A and Forge F B (1913) On chondroitin sulphuric acid. *J Biol Chem* **15**: 69–79, 155–60.
48. Eichwald E (1865) Beiträge zur Chemie der gewebbildenden Substanzen und ihrer Abkömmlinge. I. Ueber das Mucin, besonders der Weinbergschnecke. *Ann Chem Pharm* **134**: 177–211.
49. Fischer G and Boedeker C (1861) Künstliche Bildung von Zucker aus Knorpel (Chondrogen), und über die Umsetzung des genossenen Knorpels im menschlichen Körper. *Ann Chem Pharm* **117**: 111–8.
50. Rimington C (1929) The isolation of a carbohydrate derivative from serum-proteins. *Biochem J* **23**: 430–43.
51. Meyer K and Palmer J W (1934) The polysaccharide of the vitreous humor. *J Biol Chem* **107**: 629–34.
52. Meyer K and Chaffee E (1941) The mucopolysaccharides of skin. *J Biol Chem* **138**: 491–9.
53. Dische Z (1947) A new specific color reaction for hexuronic acids. *J Biol Chem* **167**: 189–98.
54. Meyer K, Davidson E, Linker A and Hoffman P (1956) The acid mucopolysaccharides of connective tissue. *Biochim Biophys Acta* **21**: 506–18.
55. Davidson E A and Meyer K (1954) Chondroitin, a new mucopolysaccharide. *J Biol Chem* **211**: 605–11.
56. Meyer K, Linker A, Davidson E A and Weissmann B (1953) The mucopolysaccharides of bovine cornea. *J Biol Chem* **205**: 611–6.
57. Shatton J and Schubert M (1954) Isolation of a mucoprotein from cartilage. *J Biol Chem* **211**: 565–73.
58. Muir H (1958) The nature of the link between protein and carbohydrate of a chondroitin sulphate complex from hyaline cartilage. *Biochem J* **69**: 195–204.
59. Gregory J D, Laurent T C and Rodén L (1964) Enzymatic degradation of chondromucoprotein. *J Biol Chem* **239**: 3312–20.
60. Kennedy J F (1979) *Proteoglycans – Biological and Chemical Aspects in Human Life.* Amsterdam: Elsevier.

61. Franek M D and Dunstone J R (1967) Connective tissue proteinpolysaccharides. Fractionation of the proteinpolysaccharides from bovine nasal cartilage. *J Biol Chem* **242**: 3460–7.
62. Sajdera S W and Hascall V C (1969) Proteinpolysaccharide complex from bovine nasal cartilage. A comparison of low and high shear extraction procedures. *J Biol Chem* **244**: 77–87.
63. Hardingham T E and Muir H (1972) The specific interaction of hyaluronic acid with cartilage proteoglycans. *Biochim Biophys Acta* **279**: 401–5.
64. Eastoe J E (1967) Composition of collagen and allied proteins. In: *Treatise on Collagen, Vol 1* (GN Ramachandran, ed), pp. 1–72. London: Academic Press.
65. Fischer E (1902) Ueber eine neue Aminosäure aus Leim. *Ber Dt Chem Ges* **35**: 2660–5.
66. Müller W (1861) Beiträge zur Kenntnis der Molekularstruktur thierischer Gewebe. *Z Rat Med* **3** (10): 173–94.
67. Ranvier L (1877) *Technisches Lehrbuch der Histologie.* Leipzig: Vogel.
68. v. Ebner V (1882) *Untersuchungen über die Ursachen der Anisotropie organisierter Substanzen.* Leipzig: Engelmann.
69. Mörner C T (1888) Histochemische Beobachtungen über die hyaline Grundsubstanz des Trachealknorpels. *Hoppe-Seyler's Z Physiol Chem* **12**: 396–404.
70. Hultkrantz W (1898) Ueber die Spaltrichtungen der Gelenkknorpel. *Verh Anat Ges* **12**: 248–56.
71. Benninghoff A (1925) Form und Bau der Gelenkknorpel in ihren Beziehungen zur Funktion. 2. Der Aufbau des Gelenkknorpels in seinen Beziehungen zur Funktion. *Z Zellforsch* **2**: 783–862.
72. Dakin H D (1920) Amino-acids of gelatin. *J Biol Chem* **44**: 499–529.
73. Nageotte J (1927) Sur la constitution du caillot de collagène formé dans l'eau distillée, faiblement acidifilée; fibrilles, sol et gel. *C R Soc Biol (Paris)* **96**: 464–8.
74. Van Slyke D D and Hiller A (1921) An unidentified base among the hydrolytic products of gelatin. *Proc Natl Acad Sci USA* **7**: 185–6.
75. Schryver S B, Buston H W and Mukherjee D H (1925) The isolation of a product of hydrolysis of the proteins hitherto undescribed. *Proc R Soc Lond [Biol]* **98**: 58–65.
76. Bowes J H and Kenten R H (1948) The amino-acid composition and titration curve of collagen. *Biochem J* **43**: 358–65.
77. Hall C E, Jakus M A and Schmitt F O (1942) Electron microscope observations of collagen. *J Am Chem Soc* **64**: 1234.
78. Wolpers C (1943) Kollagenquerstreifung und Grundsubstanz. *Klin Wochenschr* **22**: 624.
79. Bucher O (1942) Beitrag zum funktionellen Bau des hyalinen Knorpels (auf Grund von Untersuchungen im polarisierten Lichte). *Z Zellforsch* **32**: 281–300.
80. Bucher O (1942) Zur Architektur des hyalinen Knorpels. *Anat Anz* **93**: 306–13.
81. Bullough P and Goodfellow J (1968) The significance of the fine structure of articular cartilage. *J Bone Joint Surg [Br]* **50**: 852–7.
82. Weiss C, Rosenberg L and Helfet A J (1968) An ultrastructural study of normal young adult human articular cartilage. *J Bone Joint Surg [Am]* **50**: 663–74.
83. Maroudas A and Bullough P (1968) Permeability of articular cartilage. *Nature* **219**: 1260–1.
84. Pauwels F (1959) Die Struktur der Tangentialfaserschicht des Gelenkknorpels der Schulterpfanne als Beispiel für ein verkörpertes Spannungsfeld. *Z Anat Entwicklungsgesch* **121**: 188–240.
85. Zarek J M and Edwards J (1963) The stress–structure relationship in articular cartilage. *Med Electron Biol Eng* **1**: 497–507.
86. Little K, Pimm L H and Trueta J (1958) Osteoarthritis of the hip. An electron microscope study. *J Bone Joint Surg [Br]* **40**: 123–31.
87. Gross J, Highberger J H and Schmitt F O (1954) Collagen structures considered as states of aggregation of a kinetic unit. The tropocollagen particle. *Proc Natl Acad Sci USA* **40**: 679–88.
88. Orekhovitch V N and Shpikiter V O (1955) Study of some properties of denatured procollagen with the ultracentrifuge (in Russian). *Dokl Akad Nauk SSSR* **101**: 529–30.
89. Piez K A, Lewis M S, Martin G R and Gross J (1961) Subunits of the collagen molecule. *Biochim Biophys Acta* **53**: 596–8.
90. Ramachandran G N and Kartha G (1955) Structure of collagen. *Nature* **176**: 593–5.
91. Rich A and Crick F H C (1955) The structure of collagen. *Nature* **176**: 915–6.
92. Miller E J and Matukas V J (1969) Chick cartilage collagen: a new type of α1 chain not present in bone or skin of the species. *Proc Natl Acad Sci USA* **64**: 1264–8.
93. Rauber A A (1876) *Elasticität und Festigkeit der Knochen.* Leipzig: Engelmann.

94. Triepel H (1902) *Einführung in die physikalische Anatomie.* Wiesbaden: Bergmann.
95. Fürbringer M (1888) *Untersuchungen zur Morphologie und Systematik der Vögel, zugleich ein Beitrag zur Anatomie der Stütz- und Bewegungsorgane.* Amsterdam: van Holkema.
96. Lubosch W (1910) *Bau und Entstehung der Wirbeltiergelenke. Eine morphologische und histogenetische Untersuchung.* Jena: Fischer.
97. Braune W and Fischer O (1891) Die Bewegungen des Kniegelenks nach einer neuen Methode am lebenden Menschen. *Abhandl K S Ges Wiss* **29**: 75–150.
98. Hirsch C (1944) A contribution to the pathogenesis of chondromalacia of the patella. *Acta chir Scand* **90** (Suppl 83): 1–106.
99. Schade H (1912) Untersuchungen zur Organfunction des Bindegewebes. I. Mittheilung: Die Elasticitätsfunktion des Bindegewebes und die intravitale Messung ihrer Störungen. *Z Exp Path Therap* **11**: 369–99.
100. Bär E (1926) Elastizitätsprüfungen der Gelenkknorpel. *Wilhelm Roux' Arch Entwicklungsmech Org* **108**: 739–60.
101. Göcke C (1928) Elastizitätsstudien am jungen und alten Gelenkknorpel. *Z Orthop Chir* **49**: (Beilageheft): 130–47.
102. Elmore S M, Sokoloff L, Norris G and Carmeci P (1963) Nature of 'imperfect' elasticity of articular cartilage. *J Appl Physiol* **18**: 393–6.
103. Sokoloff L (1966) Elasticity of aging cartilage. *Fed Proc* **25**: 1089–95.
104. Linn F C and Sokoloff L (1965) Movement and composition of interstitial fluid of cartilage. *Arthritis Rheum* **8**: 481–94.
105. Kempson G E (1970) Mechanical properties of human articular cartilage. Thesis: University of London.
106. Kempson G E (1979) Mechanical properties of articular cartilage. *In: Adult Articular Cartilage, 2nd Ed* (MAR Freeman, ed), pp. 333–414. Tunbridge Wells: Pitman.
107. Mow V C, Holmes M H and Lai W M (1984) Fluid transport and mechanical properties of articular cartilage: a review. *J Biomech* **17**: 377–94.
108. Fisher A G T (1939) The structure and functions of synovial membrane and articular cartilage. *Br Med J* **2**: 390–3.
109. Bier A (1919) Beobachtungen über Regeneration beim Menschen. *Dtsch Med Wochenschr* **45**: 225–8.
110. Strangeways T S P (1920) The nutrition of articular cartilage. *Br Med J* **1**: 661–3.
111. Bauer W, Ropes M W and Waine H (1940) The physiology of articular structures. *Physiol Rev* **20**: 271–312.
112. Ito J K (1924) The nutrition of articular cartilage and its method of repair. *Br J Surg* **12**: 31–42.
113. Schmieden V (1900) Ein Beitrag zur Lehre von den Gelenkmäusen. *Arch Klin Chir* **62**: 542–72.
114. Ekholm R (1951) Articular cartilage nutrition. *Acta Anat (Basel)* **11**: (Suppl 15–2): 1–76.
115. Brodin H (1955) Paths of nutrition in articular cartilage and intervertebral discs. *Acta Orthop Scand* **24**: 177–83.
116. Collins D H (1949) *The Pathology of Articular and Spinal Diseases.* London: Arnold.
117. Brower T D, Akahoshi Y and Orlic P (1962) The diffusion of dyes through articular cartilage *in vivo. J Bone Joint Surg [Am]* **44**: 456–63.
118. Mankin H J (1963) The calcified zone (basal layer) of articular cartilage of rabbits. *Anat Rec* **145**: 73–87.
119. McKibbin B and Holdsworth F W (1966) The nutrition of immature joint cartilage in the lamb. *J Bone Joint Surg [Br]* **48**: 793–803.
120. Garrod A E (1907) Rheumatoid arthritis, osteo-arthritis, arthritis deformans. *In: A System of Medicine, Vol 3* (T C Allbutt and H D Rolleston, eds), pp. 3–43. London: Macmillan.
121. Hoffa A and Wollenberg G A (1908) *Arthritis deformans und sogenannter chronischer Gelenkrheumatismus.* Stuttgart: Enke.
122. Nichols E H and Richardson F L (1909) Arthritis deformans. *J Med Res* **21**: 149–221.
123. Spender J K (1889) *The Early Symptoms and the Early Treatment of Osteo-Arthritis (commonly called Rheumatoid Arthritis) with Special Reference to the Bath Thermal Waters.* London: Lewis.
124. v. Müller F (1913) Differentiation of the diseases included under chronic arthritis. *17th Int Congr Med*, London.
125. Brodie B C (1822) *Pathological and Surgical Observations on the Diseases of the Joints, 2nd Ed.* London: Longman, Hurst, Rees, Orme and Brown.

126. Ecker A (1843) Ueber Abnützung and Zerstörung der Gelenkknorpel. *Arch Physiol Heilkd* **2**: 235–48.
127. Ziegler E (1877) Ueber die subchondralen Veränderungen der Knochen bei Arthritis deformans und über Knochencysten. *Virchow's Arch* **70**: 502–20.
128. Virchow R (1869) Zur Geschichte der Arthritis deformans. *Virchow's Arch* **47**: 298–303.
129. Gardner D L (1965) *Pathology of the Connective Tissue Diseases*. London: Arnold.
130. Sokoloff L (1969) *The Biology of Degenerative Joint Disease*. Chicago: University of Chicago Press.
131. Preiser G (1911) *Statische Gelenkerkrankungen*. Stuttgart: Enke.
132. Pommer G (1913) Mikroskopische Befunde bei Arthritis deformans. *Sitzber Akad Wiss Wien* **89**: 65–315.
133. Pommer G (1920) Die funktionelle Theorie der Arthritis deformans vor dem Forum des Tierversuches und der pathologischen Anatomie. *Arch Orthop Unfall-Chir* **17**: 573–93.
134. Pommer G (1927) Ueber die mikroskopischen Kennzeichen un die Entstehungsbedingungen der Arthritis deformans (nebst neuen Beiträgen zur Kenntnis der Knorpelknötchen). *Virchow's Arch* **263**: 434–514.
135. Beneke R (1897) Zur Lehre von Spondylitis deformans. *In: Beiträge zur wissenschaftlichen Medizin*. Braunschweig: Bruhn.
136. Heine J (1926) Ueber die Arthritis deformans. *Virchow's Arch* **260**: 521–663.
137. Burckhardt H (1930) Ueber die Ursache und das Wesen der Arthritis deformans. *Arch Klin Chir* **162**: 192–4.
138. Freund E (1939) Joint cartilage under infraphysiologic, ultraphysiologic and euphysiologic demands. *Arch Surg* **39**: 596–623.
139. Baetzner W (1936) *Sport-und Arbeitsschäden*. Leipzig: Thieme.
140. Seedhom B B, Takeda T, Tsubuku M and Wright V (1979) Mechanical factors and patellofemoral osteoarthrosis. *Ann Rheum Dis* **38**: 307–16.
141. Swann A C and Seedhom B B (1986) The relationship between the stiffness of normal articular cartilage and the predominant acting stress levels. *Publ Univ Kuopio Med Orig Rep* **6**: Miniposter C3.
142. Lawrence J S (1977) *Rheumatism in Populations*. London: Heinemann.
143. Lawrence J S and Sebo M (1980) The geography of osteoarthrosis. *In: The Aetiopathogenesis of Osteoarthrosis* (G Nuki, ed), pp. 155–183. Tunbridge Wells: Pitman.
144. Bennett G A, Waine H and Bauer W (1942) *Changes in the Knee Joint at Various Ages*. New York: The Commonwealth Fund.
145. Wilcock G K (1979) The prevalence of osteoarthritis of the hip requiring total hip replacement in the elderly. *Int J Epidemiol* **8**: 247–50.
146. Wood P H N and Badley E M (1983) An epidemiological appraisal of bone and joint disease in the elderly. *In: Bone and Joint Disease in the Elderly* (V Wright, ed), pp. 1–22. Edinburgh: Churchill Livingstone.
147. Kellgren J H and Lawrence J S (1958) Osteo-arthrosis and disk degeneration in an urban population. *Ann Rheum Dis* **17**: 388–97.
148. Blumberg B S, Bloch K J, Black R L and Dotter C (1961) A study of the prevalence of arthritis in Alaskan Eskimos. *Arthritis Rheum* **4**: 325–41.
149. Bremner J M, Lawrence J S and Miall W E (1968) Degenerative joint disease in a Jamaican rural population. *Ann Rheum Dis* **27**: 326–32.
150. Solomon L, Beighton P and Lawrence J S (1976) Osteoarthrosis in a rural South African Negro population. *Ann Rheum Dis* **35**: 274–8.
151. Kelsey J L, Pastides H, Bisbee G E jr and White AA (1978) *Musculo-skeletal disorders. Their frequency of occurrence and their impact on the population of the United States*. New York: Prodist.
152. Bjelle A (1980) Epidemiological aspects of osteo-arthritis. *Scand J Rheumatol [Suppl]* **43**: 1–48.
153. Klaukka T, Sievers K and Takala J (1982) Epidemiology of rheumatic diseases in Finland in 1964–76. *Scand J Rheumatol [Suppl]* **47**: 5–15.
154. Wright V (1981) Biomechanical factors in the development of osteoarthrosis, epidemiological studies. *In: Epidemiology of Osteoarthritis* (J G Peyron, ed), pp. 140–6. Paris: Geigy.
155. Partridge R E H and Duthie J J R (1968) Rheumatism in dockers and civil servants. A comparison of heavy manual and sedentary workers. *Ann Rheum Dis* **27**: 559–68.
156. Murrary R O and Duncan C (1971) Athletic activity in adolescence as an aetiological factor in degenerative hip disease. *J Bone Joint Surg* [Br] **53**: 406–19.

157. Peyron J G (1984) The epidemiology of osteoarthritis. In: Osteoarthritis (R W Moskowitz, D S Howell, V M Goldberg and H J Mankin, eds), pp. 9–27. Philadelphia: Saunders.
158. Harper P and Nuki G (1980) Genetic Factors in Osteoarthrosis. In: The Aetiopathogenesis of Osteoarthrosis (G Nuki, ed), pp. 184–201. Tunbridge Wells: Pitman.
159. Luschka H (1855) Zur Entwickelungsgeschichte der Gelenke. Müllers Arch 1855: 481–88.
160. Bentzen G E (1875) Bidrag til ledhulernes udviklingshistorie. Nord Med Ark VII (25): 1–6.
161. Henke W and Reyher C (1874) Studien über die Entwickelung der Extremitäten des Menschen, insbesondere der Gelenkflächen. Sitzber Kais Akad Wiss Wien 3: 217–73.
162. Hagen-Torn O (1882) Entwickelung und Bau der Synovialmembranen. Arch Mikr Anat 21: 591–663.
163. Kölliker A (1884) Grundriss der Entwickelungsgeschichte des Menschen und der höheren Tiere, 2. Auflage. Leipzig: Engelmann.
164. Kazzander J (1894) Ueber die Entwickelung des Kniegelenkes. Arch Anat Physiol (Anat Abtlg) 1894: 161–76.
165. Retterer E (1894) Sur le mode de formation des articulations. C R Soc Biol (Paris) 1894: 862–5.
166. Minot C S (1894) Lehrbuch der Entwickelungsgeschichte des Menschen. Leipzig: Von Veit.
167. Kollman J (1898) Lehrbuch der Entwickelungsgeschichte des Menschen. Jena: Fischer.
168. v. Korff K (1914) Uber die Histogenese and Struktur der Knorpelgrundsubstanz. Arch Mikr Anat 84: 263–99.
169. Kajava Y (1919) Beitrag zur Kenntnis der Entwicklung des Gelenkknorpels. Acta Soc Sci Fenn 48 (3): 1–127.
170. Bernays A (1878) Die Entwicklungsgeschichte des Kniegelenkes des Menschen, mit Bemerkungen über die Gelenke im Allgemeinen. Gegenbaur's Morphol Jahrb 4: 403–46.
171. Roux W (1881) Der Kampf der Theile im Organismus. Leipzig: Engelmann.
172. Murray P D F and Selby D (1930) Intrinsic and extrinsic factors in the primary development of the skeleton. Wilhelm Roux' Arch Entwicklungsmech Org 122: 629–62.
173. Fell H B and Canti R G (1934) Experiments on the development in vitro of the avian knee joint. Proc R Soc Lond Ser B 116: 316–51.
174. Drachman D B and Sokoloff L (1966) The role of movement in embryonic joint development. Dev Biol 14: 401–20.
175. Murray P D F and Drachmann D B (1969) The role of movement in the development of joints and related structures: the head and neck in the chick embryo. J Embryol Exp Morphol 22.: 349–71.
176. Lelkes G (1958) Experiments in vitro on the role of movement in the development of joints. J Embryol Exp Morphol 6: 183–6.
177. Murray P D F and Smiles M (1965) Factors in the evocation of adventitious (secondary) cartilage in the chick embryo. Aust J Zool 13: 351–81.
178. Hall B K (1968) In vitro studies on the mechanical evocation of adventitious cartilage in the chick. J Exp Zool 168: 283–306.
179. Weiss P and Amprino R (1940) The effect of mechanical stress on the differentiation of scleral cartilage in vitro and in the embryo. Growth 4: 245–58.
180. O'Rahilly R and Gardner E (1978) The embryology of movable joints. In: The Joints and Synovial Fluid. Vol I (L Sokoloff, ed), pp. 49–103. New York: Academic Press.
181. Hall B K, (ed) (1983) Cartilage, Vol. 2, Development, Differentiation, and Growth. New York: Academic Press.
182. Thorogood P (1983) Morphogenesis of Cartilage. In: Cartilage, Vol. 2, Development, Differentiation, and Growth (B K Hall, ed), pp. 223–54. New York: Academic Press.
183. Blumberg B S and Sokoloff L (1961) Coalescence of caudal vertebrae in the giant dinosaur Diplodocus. Arthritis Rheum 4: 592–601.
184. Hollander J L (1979) Introduction to arthritis and the rheumatic diseases. In: Arthritis and Allied Conditions, 9th Ed (D J McCarty, ed), pp. 3–7. Philadelphia: Lea and Febiger.
185. Wells C (1972) Ancient arthritis. M & B Pharm Bull 21: 67–70.
186. Virchow R (1895) Knochen von Höhlenbären mit krankhaften Veränderungen. Z Ethnol 27: 706–8.
187. Shufeldt R W (1893) Notes on palaeopathology. Popul Sci Month 42: 679–84.
188. Cross E C (1939) Arthritis among wolves. Can Field-Naturalist 54: 2–4.
189. Fox H (1939) Chronic arthritis in wild mammals. Trans Am Philos Soc 31: 73–124.
190. Hildebrand M (1974) Analysis of Vertebrate Structure. New York: Wiley.
191. Sokoloff L (1956) Natural history of degenerative joint disease in small laboratory animals. I. Pathologic anatomy of degenerative joint disease in mice. Arch Pathol 62: 118–28.

192. Sokoloff L and Jay G E jr (1956) Natural history of degenerative joint disease in small laboratory animals. 4. Degenerative joint disease in the laboratory rat. *Arch Pathol* **62**: 140–2.
193. Silverstein E and Sokoloff L (1958) Natural history of degenerative joint disease in small laboratory animals. 5. Osteoarthritis in guinea pigs. *Arthritis Rheum* **1**: 82–6.
194. Sokoloff L (1963) Degenerative joint disease in birds. *Lab Invest* **12**: 531–7.
195. Silberberg M and Silberberg R (1941) Age changes of bones and joints in various strains of mice. *Am J Anat* **68**: 69–95.
196. Silberberg R, Saxton J, Sperling G and McCay C (1952) Degenerative joint disease in Syrian hamsters. *Fed Proc* **11**. 427.
197. Sokoloff L, Mickelsen O, Silverstein E, Jay G E jr and Yamamoto R S (1960) Experimental obesity and osteoarthritis. *Am J Physiol* **198**: 765–70.
198. Sokoloff L and Mickelsen O (1965) Dietary fat supplements, body weight and osteoarthritis in DBA/2JN mice. *J Nutr* **85**: 117–21.
199. Callender G R and Kelser R A (1938) A comparison of the pathological changes in man and equines. *Am J Pathol* **14**: 253–71.
200. Young D M, Fetter A W and Johnson L C (1979) Osteoarthritis (osteoarthrosis); degenerative joint disease. *In: Spontaneous Animal Models of Human Disease, Vol II* (E J Andrews, B C Ward and N H Altman, eds), pp. 257–61. New York: Academic Press.
201. Julian R J and Bhatnagar M K (1985) Cartilage lesions associated with shaky-leg lameness in turkeys. *Avian Dis* **29**: 218–32.
202. Sokoloff L (1960) Comparative pathology of arthritis. *Adv Vet Sci Comp Med* **6**: 193–250.
203. Van Sickle D C and Kincaid S A (1978) Comparative Arthrology. *In: The Joints and Synovial Fluid, Vol I* (L Sokoloff, ed), pp. 1–47. New York: Academic Press.
204. Minugh N S (1982) A brief survey of osteoarthritis outside modern human populations. *J Am Pediatr Med Ass* **72**: 217–21.
205. Jurmain R D (1980) The involvement of appendicular degenerative joint disease. *Am J Phys Anthropol* **53**: 143–50.
206. Zivanovic S (1982) Ancient diseases. The elements of palaeopathology. London: Methuen.
207. Chapman F H (1963) The incidence and age distribution of osteoarthritis in an archaic American indian population. *Proc Indiana Acad Sci* **73**: 64–6.
208. Jurmain R D (1977) Stress and the etiology of osteoarthritis. *Am J Phys Anthropol* **46**: 353–66.
209. Trinkaus E and Zimmerman M R (1979) Paleopathology of the Shanidar Neanderthals. *Am J Phys Anthropol* **50**: 487.
210. Stewart T D (1977) The Neanderthal skeletal remains from Shanidar Cave, Iraq: a summary of findings to date. *Proc Am Philos Soc* **121**: 121–65.
211. Straus W and Cave A J E (1957) Pathology and the posture of Neanderthal man. *Q Rev Biol* **32**: 348–63.
212. Trinkaus E (1985) Pathology and the posture of the La Chapelle-aux-Saints Neandertal. *Am J Phys Anthropol* **67**: 19–41.
213. Griffin C J, Powers R and Kruszynski R (1979) The incidence of osteoarthritis of the temporomandibular joint in various cultures. *Aust Dent J* **24**: 94–106.
214. Pitt-Rivers G H L F (1965) Osteoarthritis of a Bronze-Age pelvic skeleton. *J Coll Gen Practit* **9**: 266–9.
215. Sharma J N, Sharma J N and Arora R B (1972) Arthritis in ancient Indian literature. *Indian J Hist Sci* **8**: 37–42.
216. Thould A K and Thould B T (1983) Arthritis in Roman Britain. *Br Med J* **287**: 1909–11.
217. Huskisson E C, Dieppe P A, Tucker A K and Cornell I B (1979) Another look at osteoarthritis. *Ann Rheum Dis* **38**: 423–9.
218. Hudson C, Butler R and Sikes D (1975) Arthritis in the prehistoric Southeastern United States: biological and cultural variables. *Am J Phys Anthropol* **43**: 57–62.
219. Stempel W (1901) Das Malum coxae senile als Berufskrankheit und in seinen Beziehungen zur socialen Gesetzgebung. *Dtsch Z Chir* **60**: 265–345.
220. Pommer G (1915) *Ueber die Beziehungen der Arthritis Deformans zu den Gewerbekrankheiten. Das Österreichische Sanitätswesen*. Wien: Hölder.
221. Glover J A (1930) Incidence of rheumatic diseases. *Lancet* **1**: 499–505.
222. Danischewski G (1930) Akuter und chronischer Rheumatismus in der UdSSR. *Acta Rheumatol (Amst)* **2** (5): 16–8.
223. Kahlmeter G (1932) Du role joué en suède par le rhumatisme articulaire chronique comme cause d'incapacité permanente de travail dans les divers groupes professionnels. *Acta Rheumatol (Amst)* **4** (14): 34–5.
224. Kellgren J H and Lawrence J S (1952) Rheumatism in miners. Part II: X-ray study. *Brit J Ind*

Med **9**: 197–207.
225. Schlomka G and Schröter G (1953) Ueber die Bedeutung der beruflichen Belastung für die Entstehung der degenerativen Gelenkleiden. *Z Inn Med* **8**: 473–6.
226. Bjelle A (1981) Osteoarthrosis and back disorders in Sweden. *In: Epidemiology of Osteo-arthritis.* (J G Peyron, ed), pp. 17–29. Paris: Geigy.
227. Typpö T (1985) Osteoarthritis of the hip. Radiologic findings and etiology. *Ann Chir Gynaecol [Suppl]* **201**: 1–38.
228. Wickström G (1978) Effect of work on degenerative back disease. A review. *Scand J Work Environ Health* **Suppl 1**: 1–12.
229. Holtzmann F (1929) Erkrankungen durch Arbeit mit Pressluftwerkzeugen. *Umschau* **33**. 1002–3.
230. Meiss W C (1933) Gelenksveränderungen durch die Benutzung von durch Pressluft getriebenen Werkzeugen. *Monatschr Unfallheilkd* **40**: 453–62.
231. Eichelbaum K (1930) Doppelseitige Arthritis deformans des Ellenbogengelenks als Berufskrankheit. *Zentralbl Chir* **25**: 1534–7.
232. Lawrence J S (1961) Rheumatism in cotton operatives. *Br J Ind Med* **18**: 270–6.
233. Gordon T (1968) Osteoarthrosis in US adults. *In: Population Studies of the Rheumatic Diseases. Proceedings of the third international symposium in Amsterdam* (Bennet P H and Wood H N, eds), pp. 391–7. Amsterdam: Excerpta Medica.
234. Kärkkäinen A (1985) Osteoarthrosis of the hand in the Finnish population aged 30 years and over (in Finnish, English summary). *Kansaneläkel Julk ML*: **52**: 1–110.
235. Bard C C, Sylvestre J J and Dussault R G (1984) Hand osteoarthropathy in pianists. *J Can Assoc Radiol* **35**: 154–8.
236. Acheson R M, Chan Y-K and Clemett A R (1970) New Haven survey of joint diseases. XII: Distribution and symptoms of osteoarthrosis in the hands with reference to handedness. *Ann Rheum Dis* **29**: 275–86.
237. Hadler N M, Gillings D B, Imbus H R, Levitin P M, Makuc D, Utsinger P D, Yount W J, Slusser D and Moskovitz N (1978) Hand structure and function in an industrial setting. Influence of three patterns of stereotyped repetitive usage. *Arthritis Rheum* **21**: 210–20.
238. Stulberg S D and Keller C S (1984) Exercise and osteoarthritis. *In: Osteoarthritis. Diagnosis and Management* (R W Moskowitz, D S Howell, V M Goldberg and H J Mankin, eds), pp. 561–8. Philadelphia: Saunders.
239. Hadler N M (1977) Industrial rheumatology. Clinical investigations into the influence of the pattern of usage on the pattern of regional musculoskeletal disease. *Arthritis Rheum* **20** 1019–25.
240. Anderson J A D (1984) Arthrosis and its relation to work. *Scand J Work Environ Health* **10**: 429–33.
241. Wickström G, Niskanen T and Riihimäki H (1985) Strain on the back in concrete reinforcement work. *Br J Ind Med* **42**: 233–9.
242. Weightman B and Kempson G E (1979) Load carriage. *In: Adult Articular Cartilage, 2nd Ed* (MAR Freeman, ed), pp. 291–329. Tunbridge Wells: Pitman.
243. Baetzner W (1926) Sportschäden am Bewegungsapparat. *Klin Wochenschr* **5**: 653–4.
244. Baetzner W (1927) Ueber Sportschäden am Bewegungsapparat. *Med Klin* **5**: 173–6.
245. McDermott M and Freyne P (1983) Osteoarthrosis in runners with knee pain. *Br J Sports Med* **17**: 84–7.
246. Brodelius Å (1961) Osteoarthrosis of the talar joints in footballers and ballet dancers. *Acta Orthop Scand* **30**: 309–14.
247. Arens W (1959) Arthrosis bei Leistungssportlern. *Hefte Unfallheilkd* **48**: 101–5.
248. Schneider P G (1962) Die Früharthrose im Femoropatellargelenk des Leistungssportlers. *Arch Orthop Unfall-Chir* **54**: 401–16.
249. Solonen K A (1966) The joints of the lower extremeties of football players. *Ann Chir Gynaecol Fenn* **55**: 176–80.
250. Klünder K B, Rud B and Hansen J (1980) Osteoarthritis of the hip and knee joint in retired football players. *Acta Orthop Scand* **51**: 925–7.
251. Chantraine A (1985) Knee joint in soccer players: osteoarthritis and axis deviation. *Med Sci Sports Exerc* **17**: 434–9.
252. Bagneres M (1967) Lesions ostéo-articulaires chroniques des sportifs. *Rhumatologie* **19**: 41–50.
253. Szot Z, Boron Z and Galaj Z (1985) Overloading changes in the motor system occurring in elite gymnasts. *Int J Sports Med* **6**: 36–40.
254. Adams J E (1965) Injury to the throwing arm. *Calif Med* **102**: 127–32.
255. Priest J D, Jones H H, Tichenor C J C and Nagel D A (1977) Arm and elbow changes in expert

tennis players. *Minnesota Med* **60**: 399–404.

256. Frey A and Müller W (1984) Heberden-Arthrosen bei Judo-Sportlern. *Schweiz Med Wochenschr* **114**: 40–7.

257. Adams I D (1976) Osteoarthrosis and sport. *Clin Rheum Dis* **2**: 523–41.

258. Dickinson J A, Cook S D and Leinhardt T M (1985) The measurement of shock waves following heel strike while running. *J Biomech* **18**: 415–22.

259. Radin E L, Paul I L, and Rose R M (1972) Role of mechanical factors in pathogenesis of primary osteoarthritis. *Lancet* **i**: 519–22.

260. Radin E L, Orr R B, Kelman J L, Paul I L and Rose R M (1982) Effect of prolonged walking on concrete on the knees of sheep. *J Biomech* **15**: 487–92.

261. Puranen J, Alaketola L, Peltokallio P and Saarela J (1975) Running and primary osteoarthritis of the hip. *Br Med J* **276**: 424–5.

262. Nettles J L, Whelan E and Filson E (1981) Does long-term long-distance running cause osteoarthritis? *XV Congress Internat Rhum. Rev Rhum Mal Osteoartic*: Abstract **794**.

263. Sohn R S and Micheli L J (1985) The effects of running on the pathogenesis of osteoarthritis. *Clin Orthop* **198**: 106–9.

264. Cabot J R (1964) Lésions chroniques dans le sport (1) au niveau des extrémités inférieures. *Med Educ Phys Sport* **4**: 277–302.

265. Neuberger J S and Neuberger G B (1984) Epidemiology of the rheumatic diseases. *Nurs Clin North Am* **19**: 713–25.

266. Bjelle A and Allander E (1981) Regional distribution of rheumatic complaints in Sweden. *Scand J Rheumatol* **10**: 9–15.

267. Hadler N M (1985) Osteoarthritis as a public health problem. *Clin Rheum Dis* **11**: 175–185.

268. Isomäki H A (1983) Prevalence and social impact of rheumatic diseases in Finland. *J Rheumatol [Suppl]* **10**: 29–31.

269. Heliövaara M (1986) Mini-Suomi tutkimus. *Lääkintöhallitus tiedottaa* **1**: 5.

270. Valkenburg H A (1983) Osteoarthritis in some developing countries. *J Rheumatol [Suppl]* **10**: 20–22.

271. World Health Organization (1980) *Sixth Report on the World Health Situation. Part 1: Global Analysis*. Geneva: WHO.

272. Malina R M (1980) Physical activity, growth, and functional capacity. In: *Human Physical Growth and Maturation. Methodologies and Factors*. (F E Johnston, A F Roche and C Susanne, eds), pp. 303–27. New York: Plenum.

273. LeVeau B F and Bernhardt D B (1984) Developmental biomechanics. Effects of forces on the growth, development, and maintenance of the human body. *Phys Ther* **64**: 1874–82.

274. Leach R E, Baumgard S and Broom J (1973) Obesity: its relationship to osteoarthritis of the knee. *Clin Orthop* **93**: 271–3.

275. Bray G A (1985) Complications of obesity. *Ann Intern Med* **103**: 1052–62.

276. Acheson R M and Collart A B. New Haven survey of joint diseases. XVII. Relationship between some systemic characteristics and osteoarthrosis in a general population. *Ann Rheum Dis* **34**: 379–87.

277. Bland J H (1983) The reversibility of osteoarthritis: a review. *Am J Med* **74** (6A): 16–26.

278. Mankin H J (1982) The response of articular cartilage to mechanical injury. *J Bone Joint Surg [Am]* **64**: 460–6.

279. Perry G H, Smith M J G and Whiteside C G (1972) Spontaneous recovery of the joint space in degenerative hip disease. *Ann Rheum Dis* **31**: 440–8.

280. Radin E L and Burr D B (1984) Hypothesis: Joints can heal. *Semin Arthritis Rheum* **13**: 293–302.

281. Retterer E (1908) De l'influence de la suractivité fonctionelle sur la structure du cartilage diarthrodial. *C R Soc Biol (Paris)* **64**: 117–20.

282. Sääf J (1941) Präliminares Resultat eines Studiums über die funktionelle Anpassung des Gelenkknorpels. *Acta Soc Med Ups* **46**: 349–53.

283. Sääf J (1950) Effects of exercise on adult articular cartilage. *Acta Orthop Scand [Suppl]* **7**: 1–86.

284. Hammar J A (1892) *Bidrag till Ledgångarnes histologi*. Upsala: Akademiska.

285. Lanier R (1946) The effects of exercise on the knee-joints of inbred mice. *Anat Rec* **94**: 311–21.

286. Holmdahl D E and Ingelmark B E (1947) Hauptresultate einer experimentellen, morphophysiologischen Gelenkuntersuchung. *Zool Bidr Upsala* **25**: 91–101.

287. Holmdahl D E and Ingelmark B E (1948) Der Bau des Gelenkknorpels unter verschiedenen funktionellen Verhältnissen. *Acta Anat (Basel)* **6**: 309–75.

288. Ingelmark B E (1957) Morpho-physiological aspects of gymnatic exercises. *Bull Fed Int D'Educ*

Phys **27**: 37–44.
289. Ingelmark B E and Ekholm R (1948) A study on variations in the thickness of articular cartilage in association with rest and periodical load. *Acta Soc Med Ups* **53**: 61–74.
290. Krause W-D (1969) *Mikroskopische Untersuchungen am Gelenkknorpel extrem funktionell belasteter Mäuse*. Thesis, Köln: Gouder & Hansen.
291. Vasan N (1983) Effects of physical stress on the synthesis and degradation of cartilage matrix. *Connect Tissue Res* **12**: 49–58.
292. Stofft E and Graf J (1983) Rasterelektronmikroskopische Untersuchung des hyalinen Gelenkknorpels. *Acta Anat (Basel)* **116**: 114–25.
293. Ender A and Lessel W (1983) Stadien im Arthroseprozess–eine rasterelektronmikroskopische Studie am Kaninchenkniegelenk. *Beitr Orthop Traumatol* **30**: 662–7.
294. Kostenszky K S and Oláh E H (1972) Effect of increased functional demand on the glycosaminoglycan (mucopolysaccharide) content of the articular cartilage. *Acta Biol Hung* **23**: 75–82.
295. Kostenszky K S and Oláh E H (1975) Functional adaptation of the articular cartilage. *Acta Biol Hung* **26**: 157–64.
296. Tammi M, Säämänen A-M, Jauhiainen A, Malminen O, Kiviranta I and Helminen H (1983) Proteoglycan alterations in rabbit knee articular cartilage following physical exercise and immobilization. *Connect Tissue Res* **11**: 45–55.
297. Caterson B and Lowther D A (1978) Changes in the metabolism of the proteoglycans from sheep articular cartilage in response to mechanical stress. *Biochim Biophys Acta* **540**: 412–22.
298. Kincaid S A and Van Sickle D C (1982) Effects of exercise on the histochemical changes of articular chondrocytes in adult dogs. *Am J Vet Res* **43**: 1218–26.
299. Radin E L, Parker H G, Pugh J W, Steinberg R S, Paul I L and Rose R M (1973) Response of joints to impact loading, III. Relationship between trabecular microfractures and cartilage degeneration. *J Biomech* **6**: 51–7.
300. Radin E L, Martin R B, Burr D B, Caterson B, Boyd R D and Goodwin C (1984) Effects of mechanical loading on the tissues of the rabbit knee. *J Orthop Res* **2**: 221–34.
301. Broom N D (1986) Structural consequences of traumatising articular cartilage. *Ann Rheum Dis* **45**: 225–34.
302. Retterer E (1908) Influence de l'inactivité sur la structure du cartilage diarthrodial. *C R Soc Biol (Paris)* **64**: 155–8.
303. Oláh E H and Kostenszky K S (1972) Effect of altered functional demand on the glycosaminoglycan content of the articular cartilage of dogs. *Acta Biol Hung* **23**: 195–200.
304. Palmoski M J, Colyer R A and Brandt K D (1980) Joint motion in the absence of normal loading does not maintain normal articular cartilage. *Arthritis Rheum* **23**: 325–34.
305. Salter R B, Simmonds D F, Malcolm B W, Rumble E J and Macmichael D (1975) The effects of continuous passive motion on the healing of articular cartilage defects–an experimental investigation in rabbits. *J Bone Joint Surg [Am]* **57**: 570–1.
306. Salter R B, Simmonds D F, Malcolm B W, Rumble E J, Macmichael D and Clements N D (1980) The biological effect of continuous passive motion on the healing of full-thickness defects in articular cartilage. *J Bone Joint Surg [Am]* **62**: 1232–51.
307. O'Driscoll S W and Salter R B (1984) The induction of neochondrogenesis in free intra-articular periosteal autografts under the influence of continuous passive motion. *J Bone Joint Surg [Am]* **66**: 1248–57.
308. Frank C, Akeson W H, Woo SL-Y, Amiel D and Coutts R D (1984) Physiology and therapeutic value of passive joint motion. *Clin Orthop* **185**: 113–125.
309. Burke M J, Roman V and Wright V (1978) Bone and joint changes in lower limb amputees. *Ann Rheum Dis* **37**: 252–4.
310. Glyn J H, Sutherland I, Walker G F and Young A C (1966) Low incidence of osteoarthrosis in hip and knee after anterior poliomyelitis: a late review. *Br Med J* **2**: 739–42.
311. Benichou C and Wirotius J M (1982) Articular cartilage atrophy in lower limb amputies. *Arthritis Rheum* **25**: 80–2.
312. Menzel A (1871) Ueber die Erkrankung der Gelenke bei dauernder Ruhe derselben. Ein experimentelle Studie. *Arch Klin Chir* **12**: 990–1009.
313. Reyher C (1873) Ueber die Veränderungen der Gelenke bei dauernder Ruhe. *Dtsch Z Chir* **3**: 189–255.
314. Moll A (1886) Experimentelle Untersuchungen über den anatomischen Zustand der Gelenke bei andauernder Immobilisation derselben. *Virchow's Arch* **105**: 466–85.
315. Müller W (1924) Experimentelle Untersuchungen über die Wirkung langdauernder Immobilisierung auf die Gelenke. *Z Orthop Chir* **44**: 478–88.

316. Müller W (1929) *Biologie der Gelenke*. Leipzig: Ambrosius Barth.
317. Müller W (1924) Experimentelle Untersuchungen über Druckusuren am Gelenkknorpel und ihre Beziehungen zur Arthritis deformans. *Z Klin Chir* **131**: 642–55.
318. Koch H (1927) Uber Schädigungen des Gelenkknorpels durch übermässige Druckeinwirkungen. *Dtsch Z Chir* **201**: 367–87.
319. Ely L W and Mensor M C (1933) Studies on the immobilization of the normal joints. *Surg Gynecol Obstet* **37**: 212–5.
320. Evans E B, Eggers G W N, Butler J K and Blumel J (1960) Experimental immobilization and remobilization of rat knee joints. *J Bone Joint Surg [Am]* **42**: 737–58.
321. Roy S (1970) Ultrastructure of articular cartilage in experimental immobilization. *Ann Rheum Dis* **29**: 634–42.
322. Hall M C (1964) Articular changes in the knee of the adult rat after prolonged immobilization in extension. *Clin Orthop* **34**: 184–95.
323. Thaxter T H, Mann R A and Anderson C E (1965) Degeneration of immobilized knee joints in rats. *J Bone Joint Surg [Am]* **47**: 567–85.
324. Hall M C (1963) Cartilage changes after experimental immobilization of the knee joint of the young rat. *J Bone Joint Surg [Am]* **45**: 36–44.
325. Salter R B and Field P (1960) The effects of continuous compression on living articular cartilage. *J Bone Joint Surg [Am]* **42**: 31–49.
326. Crelin E S and Southwick W O (1964) Changes induced by sustained pressure in the knee joint articular cartilage of adult rabbits. *Anat Rec* **149**: 113–33.
327. Sood S C (1971) A study of the effects of experimental immobilisation on rabbit articular cartilage. *J Anat* **108**: 497–507.
328. Thompson R C jr and Bassett C A L (1970) Histological observations on experimentally induced degeneration of articular cartilage. *J Bone Joint Surg [Am]* **52**: 435–43.
329. Finsterbush A and Friedman B (1975) Reversibility of joint changes produced by immobilization in rabbits. *Clin Orthop* **111**: 290–8.
330. Refior H J and Hackenbroch M H jr (1976) Die Reaktion des hyalinen Gelenkknorpels unter Druck, Immobilisation und Distraktion. *Hefte Unfallheilkd* **127**: 23–36.
331. Videman T (1982) Experimental osteoarthritis in the rabbit. Comparison of different periods of repeated immobilization. *Acta Orthop Scand* **53**: 339–47.
332. Paukkonen K, Helminen H J, Tammi M, Jurvelin J, Kiviranta I and Säämänen A-M (1984) Quantitative morphological and biochemical investigations on the effects of physical exercise and immobilization on the articular cartilage of young rabbits. *Acta Biol Hung* **35**: 293–304.
333. Paukkonen K, Jurvelin J and Helminen H J (1986) Effects of immobilization on the articular cartilage in young rabbits. A quantitative light microscopic stereological study. *Clin Orthop* **206**: 270–280.
334. Palmoski M, Perricone E and Brandt K D (1979) Development and reversal of a proteoglycan aggregation defect in normal canine knee cartilage after immobilization. *Arthritis Rheum* **22**. 508–17.
335. Palmoski M J and Brandt K D (1982) Immobilization of the knee prevents osteoarthritis after anterior cruciate ligament transection. *Arthritis Rheum* **25**: 1201–8.
336. Williams J M and Brandt K D (1984) Temporary immobilisation facilitates repair of chemically induced articular cartilage injury. *J Anat* **138**: 435–46.
337. Bullough P, Goodfellow J and O'Connor J (1973) The relationship between degenerative changes and load-bearing in the human hip. *J Bone Joint Surg [Br]* **55**: 746–58.
338. Bullough P G (1984) Osteoarthritis: pathogenesis and etiology. *Br J Rheumatol* **23**: 166–9.
339. Harrison M H M, Schajowicz F and Trueta J (1953) Osteoarthritis of the hip: a study of the nature and evolution of the disease. *J Bone Joint Surg [Br]* **35**: 598–626.
340. Gardner D L (1980) General pathology of the peripheral joints. In: *The Joints and Synovial Fluid, Vol II* (L Sokoloff, ed), pp. 315–425. New York: Academic Press.
341. Palmoski M and Brandt K D (1981) Running inhibits the reversal of atrophic changes in canine knee cartilage after removal of a leg cast. *Arthritis Rheum* **24**: 1329–37.
342. Säämänen A-M, Tammi M, Kiviranta I, Jurvelin J and Helminen H J (1986) Remobilization of the canine knee after joint immobilization does not restore the proteoglycan matrix of articular cartilage. *Publ Univ Kuopio Med Orig Rep* **6**: Miniposter E 22.
343. Kiviranta I, Jurvelin J, Arokoski J, Säämänen A-M, Tammi M and Helminen H J (1986) Diminished content of articular cartilage proteoglycans in the immobilized knee joint of young beagle dogs is only partially recovered during remobilization of the limb. *Publ Univ Kuopio Med Orig Rep* **6**: Miniposter E 21.
344. Jurvelin J, Kiviranta I, Säämänen A-M and Helminen H J (1986) Remobilization period of 15

weeks only partially restores stiffness of the softened articular cartilage in the immobilized canine knee. *Publ Univ Kuopio Med Orig Rep* **6**: Miniposter E 19.

345. Rubak J M, Poussa M and Ritsilä V (1982) Effect of joint motion on the repair of articular cartilage with free periosteal grafts. *Acta Orthop Scand* **53**: 187–91.

346. Mooney V and Ferguson A B (1966) The influence of immobilization and motion on the formation of fibrocartilage in the repair granuloma after joint resection in the rabbit. *J Bone Joint Surg [Am]* **48**: 1145–55.

347. Rodan G A, Bourret L A, Harvey A and Mensi T (1975) Cyclic AMP and cyclic GMP: mediators of the mechanical effects of bone remodelling. *Science* **189**: 467–9.

348. Bourret L A and Rodan G A (1976) The role of calcium in the inhibition of cAMP accumulation in epiphyseal cartilage cells exposed to physiological pressure. *J Cell Physiol* **88**: 353–62.

349. Veldhuizen J P, Bourret L A and Rodan G A (1979) *In vitro* studies of the effect of intermittent compressive forces on cartilage cell proliferation. *J Cell Physiol* **98**: 299–306.

350. Bourret L A, Goetinck P F, Hintz R and Rodan G A (1979) Cyclic 3', 5'-AMP changes in chondrocytes of the proteoglycan-deficient chick embryonic mutant, *Nanomelia*. *FEBS Lett* **108**: 353–5.

351. van Kampen G P J (1983) *Modulation of Chondrocyte Metabolism in vitro*. Thesis, Amsterdam: Academische Pers.

352. van Kampen G P J, Veldhuizen J P, Kuijer R, van de Stadt R J and Schipper C A (1985) Cartilage response to mechanical force in high-density chondrocyte cultures. *Arthritis Rheum* **28**: 419–24.

353. De Witt M T, Handley C J, Oakes B W and Lowther D A (1984) *In vitro* response of chondrocytes to mechanical loading. The effect of short term mechanical tension. *Connect Tissue Res* **12**: 97–109.

354. Kaye C F, Lippiello L, Mankin H and Numata T (1980) Evidence for a pressure sensitive stimulus receptor system in articular cartilage. *Trans Orthop Res Soc* **5**: 1.

355. Lippiello L, Kaye C, Neumata T and Mankin H J (1985) *In vitro* metabolic response of articular cartilage segments to low levels of hydrostatic pressure. *Connect Tissue Res* **13**: 99–107.

356. Jones I L, Klämfeldt A and Sandström T (1982) The effect of continuous mechanical pressure upon the turnover of articular cartilage proteoglycans *in vitro*. *Clin Orthop* **165**: 283–9.

357. Palmoski M J and Brandt K D (1984) Effects of static and cyclic compressive loading on articular cartilage plugs *in vitro*. *Arthritis Rheum* **27**: 675–81.

358. Copray J C V M, Jansen H W B and Duterloo H S (1985) Effects of compressive forces on proliferation and matrix synthesis in mandibular condylar cartilage of the rat *in vitro*. *Arch Oral Biol* **30**: 299–304.

359. Copray J C V M, Jansen H W B and Duterloo H S (1985) An *in vitro* system for studying the effect of variable compressive forces on the mandibular condylar cartilage of the rat. *Arch Oral Biol* **30**: 305–11.

360. Wolff J (1892) *Das Gesetz der Transformation der Knochen*. Berlin: Hirschwald.

Chapter 2

Pathological and Biochemical Changes in Cartilage and Other Tissues of the Canine Knee Resulting from Induced Joint Instability

H. Muir and S. L. Carney

CONTENTS

INTRODUCTION

Diarthrodial joints are designed for a variety of movements under load, and tissues of the joint are subjected to compressive, tensile, and shearing forces. In the last few years there has been considerable progress in explaining how mechanical properties, especially of cartilage, are related to composition and structure.

Cartilage is a hydrated, fibre-reinforced composite where collagen fibres embedded in a gel of proteoglycans provide architectural framework and strength. Proteoglycans play a complementary role in modulating the properties of the collagenous framework. They are extremely large hydrophilic polyanions which tend to occupy large molecular domains, but in cartilage they are very concentrated and so are compressed to about 20% of their maximum molecular domain in dilute solution (1). Because of their size proteoglycans are entrapped in the collagen network, where their counter-ions exert a Donnan osmotic pressure of several atmospheres which is resisted by the collagen network even when no mechanical load is applied to the cartilage (2). The physicochemical consequences of this situation have been considered extensively by Maroudas (3) to explain the biomechanical function of articular cartilage, whose physical properties involve the interplay of

47

collagen, proteoglycans and water. The tensile strength of normal cartilage is correlated with the collagen content (4) and its 'instantaneous' deformation is inversely related to the pre-stressed tension of the collagen fibres, due to the osmotic pressure exerted by the proteoglycans within the collagen network. The instantaneous deformation is anisotropic, and is dependent on the collagen fibre orientation (5). The 'instantaneous' deformation is therefore least in the surface zone, in the direction of the predominant fibre orientation shown by the 'prick' lines revealed by Indian ink staining. The collagen content is greatest in the surface zone where the fibres are mainly oriented tangentially to the surface, so that the surface of articular cartilage can be regarded as a constraining diaphragm or 'skin'. As the collagen content of normal human knee cartilage varies considerably between individuals, particularly in the surface zone, irrespective of age or sex (4) the mechanical properties of the articular cartilage could differ markedly between one individual and another.

Since collagen performs the prime structural role, integrity of the collagen network is crucial. Osteoarthritic cartilage is abnormally hydrated (6) so that the tension on the collagen network will, in the absence of an external load, be greater than normal. As the collagen network is weaker than normal (4), it may not withstand the stress of cyclical loading of normal movement. The result would be rupture of the collagenous network (particularly in the surface zone) which, if progressive, would eventually lead to fibrillation. This loss of tensile strength of articular cartilage in experimental canine osteoarthritis has been shown to be progressive in degree and in extent (7) (*see* below).

Broom (8) has proposed that although collagen fibres are generally aligned radially, short segments along the fibres might be randomly deflected away from the primary orientation, and could be cross-linked in some way to provide a 3-dimensional network. Broom and Marra (9) have constructed an analogue model of cartilage incorporating this idea, consisting of small balloons held in place by a 3-dimensional nylon network. This model behaves somewhat like cartilage under compression and tension. From studies using interference contrast microscopy of hydrated cartilage, Broom (10) has suggested that the way the collagenous framework of osteoarthritic cartilage deforms under compressive load, and the way it tears, is consistent with the loss of some kind of cross-linking between interlacing collagen fibres, which would explain the softening of osteoarthritic cartilage (11, 12) and the development of vertical and tangential splits (12). Mizrahi *et al.* (5) have evidence to suggest that some collagen fibres may be continuous, spanning the full thickness of cartilage from the underlying bone to the articular surface, because the 'instantaneous' deformation of cartilage was much less when tested with underlying bone in place than when the bone had been removed. In osteoarthritis, damage to such a reinforcing collagenous structure would have severe adverse mechanical consequences.

Cartilage collagen is principally Type II; however, there are other minor collagens which represent a few % of the total collagen. The function of these minor collagens is not known, but it has been suggested (13, 14) that Type IX collagen which, like Type II collagen, is specific to cartilage, may stabilize the fine network of collagen fibres in cartilage by interacting with Type II collagen and so prevent the formation of thicker fibres. Type IX collagen may also mediate contact between proteoglycans and Type II collagen. If Type IX collagen has these functions, it could be the cross-link for the collagenous framework proposed by Broom, and its degradation might then produce the softening of osteoarthritic cartilage and the changes in the collagenous framework noted by Broom (8, 10). Type IX collagen has some non-helical regions in the molecule that are particularly susceptible to proteolytic attack. Thus pepsin, to which most collagens are resistant, cleaves Type IX collagen into 2 large fragments (15, 16). Type IX collagen is also remarkable in possessing covalently attached glycosaminoglycan (13), and immunolocalization shows it is present in the pericellular region (17) but also distributed throughout the matrix of avian cartilage (14).

The synthesis of Type II collagen in adult articular cartilage is normally very low, but as yet nothing is known about the synthesis of Type IX collagen, or whether or not it is co-ordinated with Type II collagen synthesis. Increased synthesis of Type IX collagen would be required if the loss of the postulated cross-linking of the collagenous framework by Type IX collagen in osteoarthritis is to be made good.

The importance of exercise and normal load-bearing movement has been demonstrated by Brandt and his colleagues using dogs. They found that immobilization by placing the leg in a cast leads to cartilage atrophy, loss of Safranin O staining, and decrease in its uronic acid content (18). These changes were reversible on remobilization unless the dog was exercised on treadmills immediately after the cast was removed. In contrast, movement without load bearing did not maintain normal cartilage (19). That cartilage responds directly to mechanical stress was shown by applying cyclic or static compressive stresses to articular cartilage in vitro. Proteoglycan synthesis was increased by cyclic stresses but reduced by static stress (20).

Joint instability which produces abnormal stresses in the joint has been widely used in experimental models of osteoarthritis in rabbits and dogs, enabling early changes in morphology and metabolism to be studied. In man the early stages of osteoarthritis can be deduced only retrospectively, as it is a slowly progressive disease which does not become symptomatic until it is well advanced. However, certain questions can usefully be examined in experimental models of the disease in which the mechanics of the joint are altered by a surgical procedure [see review by Troyer, 1982 (21)].

The following are some examples of questions that may be examined in experimental models. Is osteoarthritis initially a degradative process or does the initial metabolic response of tissues of the joint represent an attempt at repair? Which tissues respond first, or is the response uniform? Are there changes in the composition of joint tissues and, if so, when do these occur? Are there changes in the structure of important constituents or in the organization of the extracellular matrix? Which changes are detrimental and which are not, and can eventual mechanical failure be attributed to any of these changes? Are the changes reversible and, if so, which, and at what stage, and would progression of the disease be arrested?

Only by addressing such questions will it be possible to identify the aims of treatment. However, the usefulness of experimental models depends entirely on how closely they resemble human osteoarthritis.

EXPERIMENTAL CANINE OSTEOARTHRITIS: PATHOLOGY

Severing the anterior cruciate ligament of the knee of mature dogs (22) has been used by a number of independent groups (12, 18, 23, 24, 25). Our experience over a decade of use of this experimental model of osteoarthritis is summarized here.

Joint instability that results from operation leads to changes in cartilage, bone, synovial membrane, and menisci, and in order to accommodate the considerable variation between individual animals the contralateral unoperated knee is used as a control. The pathological changes closely resemble those that follow natural rupture of the anterior cruciate ligament, which is not an uncommon occurrence in dogs (26). Since immobilization of the joint after sectioning the anterior cruciate ligament prevents the pathological changes that normally follow (27), joint instability must underlie the pathology of this experimental model of osteoarthritis. The operation produces noticeable anterior drawer in extension ($\sim$2 mm) and at $90°$ of flexion ($\sim$ 9·5 mm) in addition to an increase in internal rotation ($\sim$ 150%) (28, 29), which would increase shearing forces on the articular cartilage. The majority of investigations employ arthrotomy when sectioning the ligament, whereas we have always used a procedure involving a stab incision (30), which requires skill and practice. Both procedures, however, cause some inflammation and joint effusion. After the stab incision the inflammation subsides within about a month, and sham operations where the stab incision was made but the ligament left intact never resulted in the pathological changes that were seen in joints where anterior cruciate ligament was severed (29, 31), even when considerable inflammation had been induced deliberately while leaving the ligament intact.

Although most other groups have used dogs of different breeds and various ages, in most of our work we have used only mature beagles 6–8 years old. We have to date operated on almost 300 dogs from the same colony. We find that the lesions occur reproducibly in the operated knee and appear first in the area of the tibial plateau (designated A in *Fig.* 2.1) that is not covered by the meniscus (31, 32). Judging by the results from other laboratories, the particular breed of dog is not important, however.

Cartilage

The appearance of the cartilage in area A (*Fig.* 2.1) of the tibial plateau is affected first and deteriorates progressively. The deterioration then spreads to other tibial and femoral cartilage surfaces. Surface fibrillation may be visualized by painting the articular surface with Indian ink as used by Meachim to grade fibrillation in human osteoarthritic cartilage (33). After rinsing the joint surface, the ink is retained where there are surface imperfections. The degree of retention of Indian ink first seen in area A increases progressively with time after the operation, and subsequently spreads to other areas of the joint surface (31). Surface fibrillation with erosion of the articular surface and deep clefts can be seen 4 months after the operation. Vertical and tangential splits have also been noted in different regions of the cartilage surface (12).

Histology

Histological changes also occur first in area A (*Fig.* 2.1) and then spread to other areas of the tibial and femoral condyles. Loss of glycosaminoglycan staining is first seen in the superficial zone of area A at 3–4 weeks after the operation. At 7–14 days, however, although total alcian blue staining was unchanged, there was a loss of birefringence to a depth of 88 μm below the articular surface when the alcian blue-stained cartilage was viewed in polarized light (34). The normal ordered orientation of collagen fibres, particularly in the upper zones of cartilage, would impose a general degree of orientation on the interfibrillar proteoglycans. Increase in water content in the superficial zone of area A and disorganization of the collagen network which occurred within a week of the operation (34) might explain the loss of birefringence in the superficial zone of osteoarthritic cartilage.

Another important change in area A was loss of most of the superficial chondrocytes down to a depth of 50 μm below the articular surface within 7 days of the operation (34), whereas elsewhere the number of cells increased

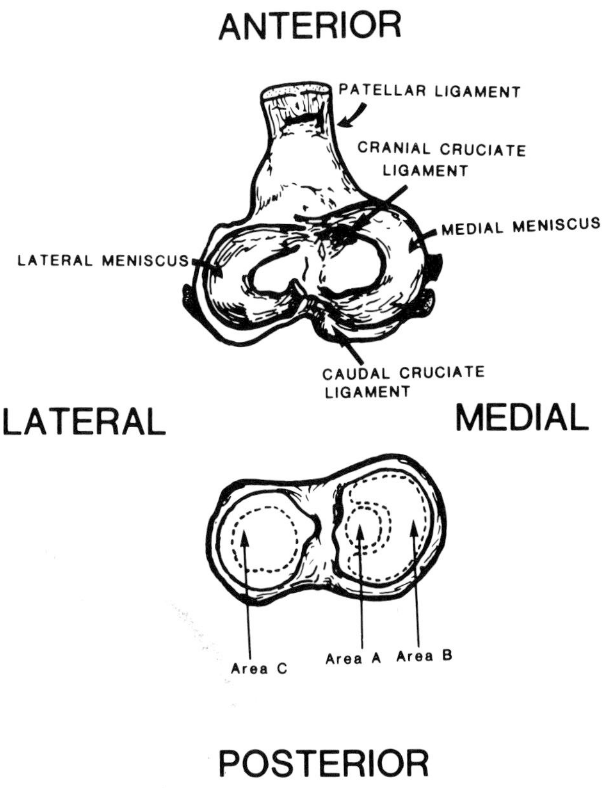

Fig. 2.1. A diagrammatic representation of the beagle tibial condyle. *Top figure* shows the position of the menisci and the attachment sites of the cranial (anterior) and caudal (posterior) cruciate ligaments. *Lower figure* shows the condyle with the menisci removed and the areas used for sampling cartilage. Area A is that part of the medial tibial plateau not covered by the meniscus; area B is the part of the medial tibial plateau which is normally protected by the meniscus. Area C represents the extent of the lateral tibial plateau used for sampling of the articular cartilage.

somewhat *over periods of 3–4 months* (31, 35, 36) with 2 or more cells in a *lacuna*. The *lacunae* appeared enlarged, particularly in regions showing decreased proteoglycan content. At later times after operation, necrosis of superficial cells has been observed (31) in other surface areas (37).

Ultrastructure

At the ultrastructural level there were changes in both matrix and cells. At the articular surface collagen fibres are normally closely packed and oriented tangential to the surface. However, in area A 4 weeks after the operation this orientation was lost, the fibres becoming separated and random in orientation (35). This change, which could result from increased hydration of the surface zone in area A even 1 week after the surgery (34), would adversely affect the tensile properties of the surface zone in area A at a very early stage in this experimentally induced osteoarthritis.

Changes in the ultrastructural morphology of the chondrocytes also occurred as early as one week after surgery. The endoplasmic reticulum and Golgi vacuoles increased, becoming most pronounced at 1–3 months, while glycogen deposits were reduced. These changes were first detected and most pronounced in cells of the mid-zone (35). They suggest increased biosynthetic activity in agreement with results of biochemical studies (*see* below).

Amorphous electron-dense material of unknown composition, absent from control cartilage, accumulated and infiltrated the articular surface. These ultrastructural changes in the matrix and in chondrocyte morphology in this experimental canine osteoarthritis model have been noted by others (24, 25). They resemble those seen in human osteoarthritic cartilage (38, 39). Cartilage of sham operated joints, however, showed no ultrastructural changes (25, 35).

Bone

A prominent feature of the experimental canine osteoarthritis was the development of exuberant osteophytes (30). Fluorochrome uptake studies showed that osteophyte development and changes in cartilage were concurrent processes (30, 31). The formation of osteophytes was first detected at the proximal limit of the femoral trochlea 2 weeks after cruciate section. They developed progressively to form early trabecular structures within the osteophyte at 8 weeks. Resorption of the femoral cortex established communication with bone marrow spaces of the femoral epiphysis (31). By 16 weeks the osteophytes were protuberant and composed largely of trabecular bone, while at 48 weeks the osteophytes had widened, the new bone consisting of mature trabeculae that were confluent with the trabeculae of the ephiphysis.

Vascular proliferation was associated with new bone development at each stage. The formation of osteophytes together with thickening of the joint capsule, particularly on the medial aspect (31), tends to re-stabilize the joint and reduce laxity, so that osteoarthritic changes never advance in this experimental model of osteoarthritis to the stage of eburnation of bone, as often occurs in advanced human osteoarthritis.

Menisci

The semilunar menisci of the knee of vertebrates increase the congruence of the joint and bear 40-70% of the load across the joint (40). They contain Type I collagen and not Type II as in cartilage (41), but the majority of proteoglycans in canine menisci are able to interact specifically with hyaluronate (shown by competition with hyaluronate oligosaccharides) and further resemble cartilage proteoglycans in containing some keratan sulphate (42). When the anterior cruciate ligament is severed, damage particularly to the medial meniscus results, beginning with slight surface splitting, going on to severe splitting and tearing and even complete disintegration (31). When graded by Indian ink staining there was moderate to severe fibrillation of the medial menisci 1 week after sectioning the ligament, whereas the lateral menisci appeared the same as controls (43). Ultrastructural changes in the menisci were somewhat like those seen in articular cartilage (44). Near the surface, collagen fibres became abnormally widely spaced 1 month after surgery and by 2 months after surgery this change had spread to deeper layers. Slight fibre disorientation at 1 week became obvious at 1 month and by 2 months there was complete loss of fibre orientation to a depth of about 20 μm (44). Considerable recovery however took place by 15 months and some degree of orientation was restored. The cells of the menisci resembled chondrocytes morphologically and underwent similar changes after cruciate ligament section, acquiring abundant Golgi and endoplasmic reticulum and thus suggesting increased biosynthetic activity. Deeper cells showed similar changes but at later times than superficial cells. By 15 months, however, all the cells looked like those in the menisci of control knees (44), unlike the situation in articular cartilage where the ultrastructural appearance of the chondrocytes had not returned to normal 15 months after the operation (35). Thus cells of the semilunar menisci appear to have a far greater capacity for recovery than those of articular cartilage.

Synovium

There was increased cellularity of the synovial membrane due to proliferation of lining cells and infiltration by mononuclear cells (31). This change, detectable by 1 week, was progressive, with small villous folds developing later in some animals and fibrosis of the subintimal layer that was especially pronounced 3–6 months after operation. Vascularity of the synovium, which was noted early, increased progressively up to 2 months but subsided after 6 months. None of these changes were seen in sham operated joints, whereas synovitis following anterior cruciate surgery has also been noted by Gardner *et al.* (45). It would thus appear that the joint instability contributes to the synovitis.

In many respects the pathology of this experimental canine osteoarthritis has resemblances to the so-called hypertrophic form of human osteoarthritis. The short time of onset of osteoarthritis after cruciate section may partly be due to the much shorter life span of the dog and perhaps to the fact that dogs are a physically active species.

EXPERIMENTAL CANINE OSTEOARTHRITIS: CARTILAGE CHANGES

Hydration

Increases in the water content of cartilage is a general finding in human osteoarthritis (2, 46). We have found that the increase in hydration occurs very early before the histological appearance of the cartilage changes (32). It does not progress with time after surgery, but appears to be irreversible.

The water content of the menisci of operated knees was also elevated, particularly the medial menisci which responded within 1 week. The lateral menisci responded later and to a lesser extent. The hydration of both menisci, however, remained elevated and did not decline over 15–18 months (43).

Increase in water content of articular cartilage and menisci, which is probably irreversible, must affect their load-bearing performance. Increased hydration may well be a crucial event in osteoarthritis. Not only will it affect the biomechanical properties of joint tissues but it will also alter the micro-environment of cells in cartilage and menisci.

Biomechanics

The tensile properties of human cartilage are directly correlated with the collagen content (4) and, as there is no significant difference in collagen content between osteoarthritis and normal human cartilage (47), increased hydration of cartilage would only result if the fibrillar network became weakened in some way. Increased latent collagenolytic activity has been detected in human (48) and experimental canine osteoarthritic cartilage (25). Whether this is responsible for reducing the tensile strength of osteoarthritic cartilage is not certain, however. Other degradative enzymes such as metalloproteinase (mainly latent) have been found in and near lesions of osteoarthritic human cartilage (49). It is likely that Type IX collagen would be degraded by metalloproteinase, which would weaken the collagenous framework if Type IX collagen indeed functions in stabilizing and cross-linking Type II collagen fibres.

Soon after sectioning the anterior cruciate ligament, we have found a marked reduction in tensile stiffness of the superficial tibial cartilage at 3 weeks, which was progressive. Loss of tensile stiffness of cartilage was apparent at 12 weeks and reached the deep zone by 23 weeks (7). This loss of tensile stiffness is analogous to that observed in human osteoarthritic cartilage (4).

Composition and Metabolism

Composition

Cartilage proteoglycans contain chondroitin sulphate and keratan sulphate, which are glycosaminoglycans containing galactosamine and glucosamine respectively. The relative proportions of chondroitin sulphate and keratan sulphate vary with development, age, anatomical site and between individuals. By measuring the molar ratios of galactosamine/glucosamine in isolated proteoglycans, or even in whole cartilage, the relative proportion of chondroitin sulphate to keratan sulphate may be estimated. Using this ratio, a general finding in osteoarthritic cartilage is that the relative proportion of chondroitin sulphate increases. In experimental canine osteoarthritis this change occurred even within 3 weeks in tibial cartilage, but was seen in all areas of cartilage 6–9 weeks after cruciate section, although there was no change in sham operated joints (31, 32). Likewise in the menisci of operated joints the content of keratan sulphate decreased (43). Similar changes were found in cartilage (32) and menisci (43) in natural canine osteoarthritis. This suggests that proteoglycans richer in chondroitin sulphate were being produced in osteoarthritic cartilage. As there was, however, no consistent change in proteoglycan content (23, 32, 36, 37), it suggests that much of the proteoglycan of the tissue was replaced by molecules richer in chondroitin sulphate.

Biosynthesis

Proteoglycans

Proteoglycan synthesis, which is generally measured by the incorporation of $^{35}SO_4$, was considerably increased in the cartilage of operated joints in vivo (36), although cell numbers were increased by less than 15% (36). This increased metabolic activity of chondrocytes in osteoarthritic cartilage is reflected in changes in their ultrastructure, with prominent Golgi organelles and rough endoplasmic reticulum (35). Similarly, increased synthesis of proteoglycans in the menisci in vivo (36) is reflected in ultrastructural changes (44). However, in sham operated joints, chondrocytes did not show ultrastructural changes (24, 35), or increased biosynthetic activity (48). Normal canine articular cartilage exhibits heterogeneity with depth from the articular surface in the activities of oxidative enzymes (50). A narrow band just below the superficial zone had the highest activities, particularly in the area unprotected by the meniscus on the tibial plateau, where osteoarthritic changes appear first.

Stimulated synthesis of proteoglycans was also seen in vitro in cartilage explants from operated knees (*Fig.* 2.2), where autoradiography using $^{35}SO_4$ uptake showed that all cells were abnormally active, rather than there being a few very active cells amongst relatively quiescent ones (36). Since these results were obtained with cartilage cultures in vitro, the enhanced metabolic activity of osteoarthritic cartilage persisted in the absence of any potential stimulating humoral factors that might have been present in vivo. Moreover, the metabolic response was not uniform in all areas of cartilage or in lateral and medial menisci of the operated knee either in vivo or in vitro (36), whereas humoral factors should produce uniform rather than regional responses. Hence, the metabolic response must be principally to mechanical stimuli in the unstable joint, particularly since 2–3 weeks post-operatively sham operations did not much stimulate proteoglycan biosynthesis in cartilage or menisci (36). In keeping with these results, increased incorporation of $^{35}SO_4$ and ^3H-glucosamine into proteoglycans of human osteoarthritic cartil-

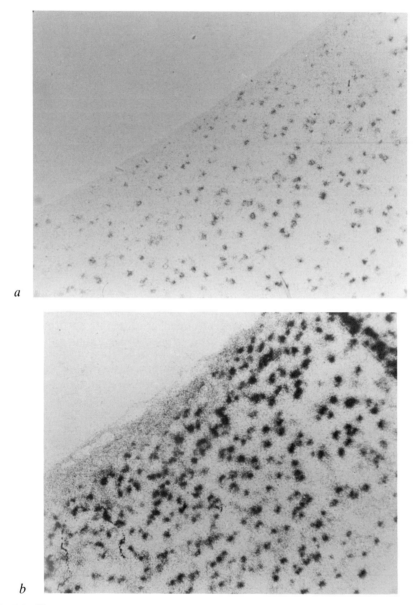

Fig. 2.2. [35]S Autoradiography of cartilage from the lateral tibial plateau of *a* control cartilage, and *b* corresponding arthritic cartilage obtained 3 months after surgery. *Note* the higher grain density of arthritic compared with control tissue, indicative of an elevated rate of ^{35}S incorporation.

age was several-fold greater than normal (51). In experimental canine osteoarthritis, however, despite increased synthesis, there was no consistent change in proteoglycan content measured as uronic acid (23, 36, 52) or fixed charge density (37) within the first 3 months after cruciate section.

Collagen

Increased metabolic activity of osteoarthritic cartilage is shown by increase in the rate of collagen synthesis. Systemic labelling with ^{3}H-proline showed that radioactivity in collagen was 10 times higher in the operated than in the unoperated control knee 2 weeks after cruciate section (53). The relative rate of collagen to non-collagenous protein synthesis was considerably elevated. Thus 80% of the radioactivity of ^{3}H-proline injected intra-articularly was in collagen of the cartilage of the operated knee, compared with 20% of that of the control knee. However, there was no change in the principal type of collagen synthesized in osteoarthritic cartilage, as the label was present only in CNBr-derived peptides of Type II collagen. No synthesis of Type I collagen was detected (53), although synthesis of more recently discovered minor collagens would not have been detected by the procedure used in this investigation.

Structural Differences in Newly Synthesized Proteoglycans from Normal and Osteoarthritic Cartilage

In experimental canine osteoarthritis an unexpected finding was that all fractions of newly formed proteoglycans, those extracted and those remaining in the cartilage residue, possessed chondroitin sulphate chains that were considerably longer than those of proteoglycans from unoperated joints, with the result that the newly formed proteoglycans were larger than those of control cartilage. This difference was maintained for at least 6 months after cruciate section and affected all anatomical sites, but was not observed in proteoglycans from sham operated joints (54). Why longer chains should be formed is not known. It might affect the interaction of proteoglycans with other constituents of the matrix, although interaction with hyaluronic acid was essentially unaffected. Longer chondroitin sulphate chains could perhaps account in part for higher galactosamine/glucosamine molar ratios of proteo-glycans from operated joints (32). Attachment of chondroitin sulphate chains to protein takes place in the Golgi cisternae immediately before secretion and prolongation of this stage produces longer chains (55), which may happen in osteoarthritic cartilage. In turn, cellular proteoglycans are not extracted by 4M guanidine HCl and the proportion of newly synthesized proteoglycans remaining in the residue of osteoarthritic cartilage was significantly higher than normal (54), supporting the possibility that proteoglycan secretion is delayed.

Catabolism of Newly Synthesized Proteoglycans by Normal and Osteoarthritic Cartilage

The fate of newly formed proteoglycans in normal and osteoarthritic cartilage explants has been examined *in vitro* using pulse-chase experiments (29). A greater proportion of labelled proteoglycans appeared in the culture medium of explants of normal cartilage over a period of 2–8 days. In both cases the loss into the medium was cell mediated, since it was greatly reduced and the difference between normal and osteoarthritic cartilage abolished when the cartilage was subjected to freeze-thawing (*Fig.* 2.3).

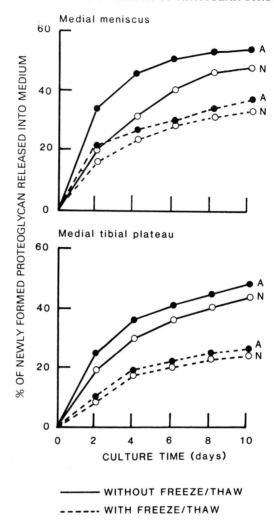

Fig. 2.3. The rate of release of ^{35}S-labelled macromolecules from cultures of (*top*) medial meniscus and (*bottom*) medial tibial plateau obtained 3 weeks after surgery. The cultures were pulse-labelled for 4 h with ^{35}S then maintained in non-radioactive medium for a chase period of 10 days, with medium changes every 48 h. The amount of ^{35}S-labelled macromolecules found in the medium was determined by liquid scintillation spectrometry. The dotted lines represent the release profiles from explant cultures which had been subjected to 3 freeze-thaw cycles after pulse-labelling in order to kill the chondrocytes. N, control cultures; A, arthritic cultures.

The medium of control cartilage explants contained some labelled proteoglycans that appeared to be undegraded and able to interact with hyaluronate, whereas almost none of the labelled proteoglycan in the medium of osteoarthritic cartilage could do so. These proteoglycans were smaller and more polydisperse than those in the medium of control cartilage, and showed a prominent highly labelled band on mixed bed gel electrophoresis (56) that was absent from the medium of control cartilage (*Fig.* 2.4). In neither case, however, were the proteoglycans extensively degraded as they migrated as discrete bands. There appears to be no difference in the catabolism of newly

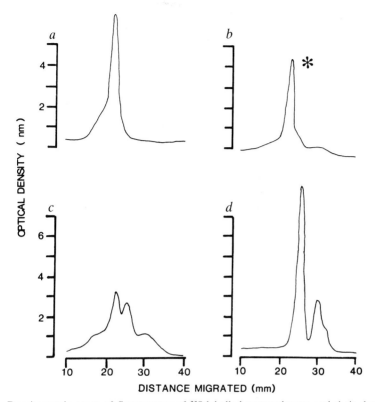

Fig. 2.4. Densitometric scans of fluorograms of ^{35}S-labelled proteoglycans and their degradation products following composite polyacrylamide–agarose gel electrophoresis (56). *a*, proteoglycans extracted from control tissue with 4M guanidine–HCl after 48 h maintenance culture. *b*, proteoglycans extracted from arthritic tissue with 4M guanidine–HCl after 48 h maintenance culture; this trace has been reduced to one half of its original value for optical density to allow all the traces to be shown on the same axes. *c*, proteoglycans released from control tissue into the maintenance medium during 48 h culture. *d*, proteoglycans released from arthritic tissue into the maintenance medium during 48 h culture. Fluorograms were scanned at 520 nm using a Shimadzu CS-930 scanning densitometer. Traces *a* and *c*, *b* and *d* represent complementary pairs of data from individual cultures.

formed and total proteoglycan, since the bands stained for proteoglycan using toluidine blue and bands visualized by autoradiography were superimposable (S L Carney, unpublished results). Although the degradative process in osteoarthritic cartilage was accelerated and more extensive, newly formed proteoglycans extracted with 4M guanidine HCl from osteoarthritic cartilage did not appear to be degraded compared with proteoglycans extracted from control cartilage. The labelled core protein from which glycosaminoglycan chains had been removed by digestion with chondroitinase and keratanase (S L Carney, unpublished results) were identical in size and remained unchanged during a 48 hour chase in both control and osteoarthritic cartilage. This indicates that proteoglycans which remain intact are retained in cartilage matrix but that once minimal degradation has occurred, even in normal turnover, they rapidly diffuse out of the cartilage.

Despite the increase in proteoglycan synthesis of about 2-fold, this does not keep up with the degradative process which gradually accelerates with time after cruciate section (*Fig.* 2.5) leading eventually to a net loss of proteoglycan. A neutral protease capable of degrading proteoglycans has been found to be raised in human osteoarthritic cartilage (49). Proteoglycan breakdown need only be minimal for them to be lost from the tissue as shown here. Whether the degradative process in osteoarthritis represents accelerated normal turnover due to activation of enzymes that are normally present, or whether mechanical instability resulting from cruciate section induces abnormal destructive enzymes to be released by chondrocytes, is not clear. The latter possibility is suggested by the appearance of a major breakdown product on gel electrophoresis that was absent from the medium of control cartilage (*Fig.* 2.4). If so, intervention to arrest the destructive process of osteoarthritis with specific enzyme inhibitors might eventually be a possibility.

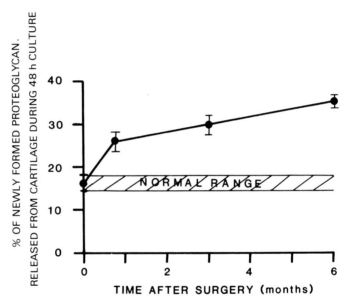

Fig. 2.5. The rate of release of ^{35}S-labelled proteoglycans from cultures of arthritic tissue examined at various times after surgery. The extent of the rate of release of ^{35}S-proteoglycans from corresponding normal tissue is indicated by the hatched area. The data points shown represent the mean ± 1 standard error.

CLINICAL SIGNIFICANCE

In its earliest stages, osteoarthritic cartilage shows considerable potential for repair and remodelling. In most cases, however, the increase in biosynthetic activity is accompanied by a progressively increasing biodegradative activity. Reports by Carney *et al.* (29) suggest that the increase in biosynthetic activity can be uncoupled from the elevated catabolic activity. Such an uncoupling of these two activities could provide a means by which therapeutic intervention could perhaps be used to arrest the progression of the disease process.

Unfortunately, it is impossible at present to diagnose osteoarthritis in humans at such early stages. When the structural integrity of cartilage has been disturbed to such an extent that it may be detected radiographically, it seems unlikely that the tissue can be restored to normal function by pharmacological means. Therefore it is of great importance to identify specific markers for osteoarthritis in the early stages in order to develop effective therapy. Although the breakdown products of proteoglycans could perhaps be used as disease markers, they have a very short half-life in serum and therefore may be of limited clinical use. Perhaps more useful markers may be proteins synthesized by the hypermetabolic chondrocytes of osteoarthritic cartilage which may have a longer serum half-life, and due to their smaller molecular size may diffuse more readily from the cartilage than proteoglycan fragments.

ACKNOWLEDGEMENTS

We thank the Arthritis and Rheumatism Council (UK), the Medical Research Council (UK), and ICI plc (Pharmaceuticals Division) for continued financial support.

REFERENCES

1. Hascall V C and Hascall G K (1981) Proteoglycans. *In*: *Cell Biology of Extracellular Matrix* (E O Hay, ed) pp. 39–63. New York: Plenum.
2. Maroudas A (1976) Balance between swelling pressure and collagen tension in normal and degenerate cartilage. *Nature* **260**: 808–9.
3. Maroudas A (1979) Physicochemical properties of articular cartilage. *In*: *Adult Articular Cartilage* (M A R Freeman, ed) pp. 215–90. Tunbridge Wells: Pitman Medical.
4. Kempson G E, Muir H, Pollard C and Tuke M A (1973) The tensile properties of the cartilage of human femoral condyles related to the content of collagen and glycosaminoglycans. *Biochim Biophys Acta* **297**: 456–72.
5. Mizrahi J, Maroudas A, Lanzir Y, Ziv I and Webber T J (1986) The 'instantaneous' deformation of cartilage; effects of collagen fibre orientation and osmotic stress. *Biorheology* **23**: 311–33.
6. Maroudas A and Venn M (1977) Chemical composition and swelling of normal and osteoarthritic femoral head cartilage. *Ann Rheum Dis* **36**: 399–406.
7. Myers E, Hardingham T E, Billingham M E J and Muir H (1986) Changes in the tensile and compressive properties of articular cartilage in a canine model of osteoarthritis. *Trans 32nd ORS* **11**: 231.
8. Broom N (1982) Abnormal softening in articular cartilage; its relationship to the collagen framework. *Arthritis Rheum* **25**: 1209–16.
9. Broom N D and Marra D L (1985) New structural concepts of articular cartilage demonstrated with a physical model. *Connect Tissue Res* **14**: 1–8.
10. Broom N (1984) The altered biomechanical state of human femoral head osteoarthritic articular cartilage. *Arthritis Rheum* **27**: 1028–39.
11. Broom N D and Poole C A (1983) Articular cartilage collagen and proteoglycans: their functional interdependency. *Arthritis Rheum* **26**: 1111–9.
12. Vignon E, Hartmann J D, Vignon G, Moyen B, Arlot M and Ville G (1984) Cartilage destruction in experimentally induced osteoarthritis. *J Rheumatol* **11**: 202–7.
13. Bruckner P, Vaughan L and Winterhalter K H (1985) Type IX collagen from sternal cartilage of chicken embryo contains covalently bound glycosaminoglycans. *Proc Natl Acad Sci USA* **82**: 2608–12.
14. Irwin M H, Silvers S H and Mayne R (1985) Monoclonal antibody against chicken Type IX collagen: preparation, characterization and recognition of the intact form of Type IX collagen secreted by chondrocytes. *J Cell Biol* **101**: 814–23.
15. Reese C A and Mayne R (1981) Minor collagens of chicken hyaline cartilage. *Biochemistry* **20**: 5443–8.
16. Von der Mark K, van Menxel M and Wiedemann H (1982) Isolation and characterization of

new collagens from chicken cartilage. *Eur J Biochem* **124**: 57–62.

17. Hartmann D J, Magloire H, Ricard-Blum S, Joffre A, Couble M L, Ville G and Herbage D (1983) Light and electron immunoperoxidase localisation of minor disulfide-bonded collagens in fetal calf epiphyseal cartilage. *Collagen Rel Res* **3**: 349–57.

18. Palmoski M J, Perricone E and Brandt K D (1979) Development and reversal of a proteoglycan aggregation defect in normal canine knee cartilage after immobilisation. *Arthritis Rheum* **22**: 508–17.

19. Palmoski M J, Colyer R A and Brandt K D (1980) Joint motion in the absence of normal loading does not maintain normal articular cartilage. *Arthritis Rheum* **23**: 325–34.

20. Palmoski M J and Brandt K D (1984) Effects of static and cyclic compressive loading on articular cartilage plugs *in vitro. Arthritis Rheum* **27**: 675–81.

21. Troyer H (1982) Experimental models of osteoarthritis: a review. *Semin Arthritis Rheum* **11**: 362–74.

22. Pond M J and Nuki G (1973) Experimentally induced osteoarthritis in the dog. *Ann Rheum Dis* **32**: 387–8.

23. Altman R D, Tenenbaum J, Latta L, Riskin W, Blanco L N and Howell D S (1984) Biomechanical and biochemical properties of dog cartilage in experimentally induced osteoarthritis. *Ann Rheum Dis* **43**: 83–90.

24. Orford C R, Gardner D L and O'Connor P (1983) Ultrastructural changes in dog femoral condylar cartilage following anterior cruciate ligament section. *J Anat* **137**: 653–63.

25. Pelletier J P, Martel-Pelletier J, Altman R D, Ghandur-Mnaymneh L, Howell D S and Woessner J (1983) Collagenolytic activity and collagen matrix breakdown of the articular cartilage in the Pond-Nuki dog model of osteoarthritis. *Arthritis Rheum* **26**: 63–8.

26. Tirgari M and Vaughan L C (1975) Arthritis of the canine stifle joint. *Vet Record* **96**: 394–9.

27. Palmoski M J and Brandt K D (1982) Immobilisation of the knee prevents osteoarthritis after anterior cruciate ligament transection. *Arthritis Rheum* **25**: 1201–8.

28. Arnoczky S P and Marshall J L (1977) The cruciate ligaments of the canine stifle: an anatomical and functional analysis. *Am J Vet Res* **38**: 1807–14.

29. Carney S L, Billingham M E J, Muir H and Sandy J D (1984) Demonstration of increased proteoglycan turnover in cartilage explants from dogs with experimental osteoarthritis. *J Orthop Res* **2**: 201–6.

30. Gilbertson E M M (1975) Development of periarticular osteophytes in experimentally induced osteoarthritis in the dog. *Ann Rheum Dis* **34**: 12–25.

31. McDevitt C A, Gilbertson E and Muir H (1977) An experimental model of osteoarthritis: early morphological and biochemical changes. *J Bone Joint Surg [Br]* **59**: 24–35.

32. McDevitt C A and Muir H (1976) Biochemical changes in the cartilage of the knee in experimental and natural osteoarthritis in the dog. *J Bone Joint Surg [Br]* **58**: 94–101.

33. Meachim G (1976) Cartilage fibrillation on the lateral tibial plateau in Liverpool necropsies. *J Anat* **121**: 97–106.

34. Dunham J, Shackleton D, Nahir A M, Billingham M E J, Bitensky L, Chayen J and Muir H (1985) Altered orientation of glycosaminoglycans and cellular changes in the tibial cartilage in the first two weeks of experimental canine osteoarthritis. *J Orthop Res* **3**: 258–68.

35. Stockwell R A, Billingham M E J and Muir H (1983) Ultrastructural changes in articular cartilage after experimental section of the anterior cruciate ligament of the dog knee. *J Anat* **136**: 425–39.

36. Sandy J D, Adams M E, Billingham M E J, Plaas A and Muir H (1984) *In vivo* and *in vitro* stimulation of chondrocyte biosynthetic activity in early experimental osteoarthritis. *Arthritis Rheum* **27**: 388–97.

37. Vignon E, Arlot M, Hartmann D, Moyen B and Ville G (1983) Hypertrophic repair of articular cartilage in experimental osteoarthrosis. *Ann Rheum Dis* **42**: 82–8.

38. Meachim G and Roy S (1969) Surface ultrastructure of mature adult human cartilage. *J Bone Joint Surg [Br]* **51**: 529–39.

39. Weiss C and Mirow S (1972) An ultrastructural study of osteoarthritic changes in the articular cartilage of human knees. *J Bone Joint Surg [Am]* **54**: 954–72.

40. Krause W R, Pope M H, Johnson R J and Wilter D J (1976) Mechanical changes in the knee after meniscectomy. *J Bone Joint Surg [Am]* **58**: 599–604.

41. Eyre D R and Muir H (1975) The distribution of different molecular species of collagen in fibrous, elastic and hyaline cartilages of the pig. *Biochem J* **151**: 595–602.

42. Adams M E, McDevitt C A, Ho A and Muir H (1986) Isolation and characterization of high-buoyant-density proteoglycans from semilunar menisci. *J Bone Joint Surg [Am]* **68**: 55–64.

43. Adams M E, Billingham M E J and Muir H (1983) The glycosaminoglycans in menisci in experimental and natural osteoarthritis. *Arthritis Rheum* **26**: 69–76.
44. Stockwell R A and Billingham M E J (1984) Early response of cartilage to abnormal factors as seen in the meniscus of the dog knee after cruciate ligament section. *Acta Biol Hung* **35**: 281–91.
45. Gardner D L, Bradley W A, O'Connor P, Orford C R and Brereton J D (1984) Synovitis after surgical division of the anterior cruciate ligament of the dog. *Clin Exp Rheumatol* **2**: 11–5.
46. Mankin H J and Thrasher A Z (1975) Water content and binding in normal and osteoarthritic human cartilage. *J Bone Joint Surg [Am]* **57**: 76–80.
47. Mankin H J and Lippiello L (1970) Biochemical and metabolic abnormalities in articular cartilage from osteoarthritic human hips. *J Bone Joint Surg [Am]* **52**: 424–34.
48. Pelletier J P, Martel-Pelletier J, Howell D S, Ghandur-Mnaymneh L, Enis J E and Woessner J (1983) Collagenase and collagenolytic activity in human osteoarthritic cartilage. *Arthritis Rheum* **26**: 63–8.
49. Martel-Pelletier J, Pelletier J P, Cloutier J M, Howell D S, Ghandur-Mnaymneh L and Woessner J F (1984) Neutral proteases capable of proteoglycan digesting activity in osteoarthritic and normal human articular cartilage. *Arthritis Rheum* **27**: 305–12.
50. Dunham J, Shackleton D R, Bitensky L, Chayen J, Billingham M E J and Muir H (1986) Enzymic heterogeneity of normal canine articular cartilage. *Cell Biochem Funct* **4**: 43–6.
51. Ryu J, Treadwell B V and Mankin H J (1984) Biochemical and metabolic abnormalities in normal and osteoarthritic human cartilage. *Arthritis Rheum* **27**: 49–57.
52. McDevitt C A, Billingham M E J and Muir H (1981) *In vivo* metabolism of proteoglycans in experimental osteoarthritic and normal canine articular cartilage and the intervertebral disc. *Semin Arthritis Rheum (Suppl 1)* **11**: 17–8.
53. Eyre D R, McDevitt C A, Billingham M E J and Muir H (1980) Biosynthesis of collagen and other matrix proteins by articular cartilage in expermental osteoarthritis. *Biochem J* **188**: 823–37.
54. Carney S L, Billingham M E J, Muir H and Sandy J D (1985) Structure of newly synthesized ^{35}S-proteoglycans and ^{35}S-proteoglycan turnover products of cartilage explant cultures from dogs with experimental osteoarthritis. *J Orthop Res* **3**: 140–7.
55. Mitchell D and Hardingham T E (1981) The effects of cycloheximide on the biosynthesis and secretion of proteoglycans by chondrocytes in culture. *Biochem J* **196**: 521–9.
56. Carney S L, Bayliss M T, Norman J M and Muir H (1986) Electrophoresis of ^{35}S-labelled proteoglycans on polyacrylamide–agarose composite gels and their visualization by fluorography. *Anal Biochem* **156**: 38–44.

Chapter 3

Joint Loading-Induced Alterations in Articular Cartilage

M. Tammi, K. Paukkonen, I. Kiviranta, J. Jurvelin, A.-M. Säämänen and H. J. Helminen

INTRODUCTION

Articular cartilage has a specialized function among animal tissues: to provide a lubricated surface for moving bones, and to serve as a cushion softening the impact loads generated between the bones. The evolutionary process has favoured species having freely moving joints with structurally delicate and complex articular cartilages. While the structure of the proteoglycans of the cartilage matrix (1), and the mechanism of how they work with absorbed water and collagen for elasticity and lubrication are known to a certain extent (2) (*see* Mow, Holmes and Lai, Chapter 11), the rules governing the differentiation of the tissue and its maintenance by the embedded chondrocytes remain to be elucidated. The problem of regulation of large matrix volumes by sparsely distributed chondrocytes is particularly challenging.

Several experiments have demonstrated that the type and magnitude of physical stress influence chondrocyte metabolism and matrix structure (*see* Helminen *et al.*, Chapter 1). It is currently considered that the stresses generated in joint loading are among the most significant factors affecting articular cartilage health. However, most current studies have been designed as models for human joint degeneration or injury and therefore do not directly characterize the physiological regulatory pattern of articular cartilage matrix. Understanding cartilage matrix regulation is important not only for scientific interest, but also for the prevention and therapy of degenerative joint disease. Information about normal cartilage behaviour will help to avoid matrix reactions that predispose the tissue to injuries in everyday life.

The experiments and analyses reviewed in this chapter aim at describing the changes that occur in articular cartilage matrix, especially in its proteoglycans, due to altered joint loading. The possible mechanisms behind the matrix regulation by loading are discussed.

REDUCED LOADING

Experimental Models

Several experimental procedures have been utilized as models for reduced weight bearing for articular cartilage matrix studies in experimental animals. Splinting the knee, which restricts both movement and weight bearing of the leg, has been used in young (3, 4) and adult rabbits (3, 4, 5, 6), young dogs (7, 8), adult dogs (3, 7, 9), adult guinea pigs (10) and rats (11, 12, 13). Unloading effects on sheep 'ankle' joint cartilages were studied following plaster cast application on one foreleg (14).

Experimental procedures have included operation on the tibial shaft in dogs, which lead to spontaneous sparing of the leg from weight bearing (15, 16, 17). An analogous arrangement was obtained by transection of the hind leg above the ankle joint in dogs, which retained movements of the knee but greatly reduced joint loading (18).

It has been difficult to obtain a comprehensive view of the consequences of immobilization. To a large extent, this is due to the obvious species differences, but also to parameters such as position of the limb (extension/flexion) (5, 6), possible cartilage compression (11, 19, 20), the rigidity of the immobilization (21, 22), and age of the animals during the experiment (23) which modify the response of the tissues.

One major technical difficulty limits the full exploitation of the *in vivo* experiments designed to analyse the influence of altered joint loading. This is the lack of a practical, direct method to quantify the *in vivo* stresses created between cartilage surfaces at different sites of the joint. Although attempts to measure stresses between cartilage surfaces have been made (24, 25), information about the change in distribution, intensity and frequency of the load on articular cartilage during experimental intervention of normal joint function is still qualitative and indirect.

Unloading and Cartilage Injury

It is now clear that joint unloading by immobilization is more or less deleterious to the articular cartilage. Rabbits seem to be particularly susceptible, since cartilage matrix staining is weakened after 2 days (26) and surface alterations are evident within 1 week after applying the splint (27, 28). This is in contrast to canine articular cartilage which does not show gross or microscopic deterioration after casting the hind limb in flexion position for up to 11 weeks (29).

The lesions that develop in rabbit knee cartilages are more pronounced when the leg is immobilized in extension (6) than in flexion (5). This may be due to the continuous compression which may develop between the tibia and femur of the extended knee due to ligament and joint capsule contraction (30). In contrast to adult animals, very young rabbits do not seem to develop cartilage lesions after plaster cast immobilization (23).

Matrix Response to Unloading

Articular cartilage glycosaminoglycans decreased due to reduced loading in all species studied so far (10, 14, 17, 31). Reduction in proteoglycans seems to be reversible, at least in the dog (9). However, complete restoration of proteoglycan concentration after immobilization varied locally (*Fig.* 3.1). The reduction in cyclic compressive forces appeared to be more important than restricted joint movement in the depletion of proteoglycans, as indicated by studies on amputated legs with complete mobility of the knee joint (18).

Elevated water content was found in the unloaded cartilages of dogs (9, 18) and rabbits (32). The proteoglycans were also more readily extracted with dissociative solvents from the articular cartilage of rabbits (32, 33), and dogs (9, 18). Both enhanced extractability of proteoglycans and high water content characterize young articular cartilage (34, 35), and adult cartilage subject to experimental joint disease (36, 37) or natural degeneration (35, 38, 39). The importance of these 2 alterations is far from understood, but it is reasonable to assume that they reflect the stability of the matrix in terms of interactions between collagen, proteoglycans and possibly other matrix proteins. Recent studies have demonstrated the presence of several non-collagenous proteins in articular cartilage, the functions of which are largely unknown as yet (40), but which are present in substantial amounts and alter in quantity in experimental joint disease (41, 42).

The magnitude of glycosaminoglycan loss during immobilization varied according to location along the cartilage surface. In cast-immobilized dogs the depletion was strongest in the peripheral areas of the femoral condyle, while the central parts, which remained in contact with the opposite joint surface, showed glycosaminoglycan levels closer to those of the control samples (29). Contact, even within the cast, apparently sufficed to better maintain normal cartilage matrix, a finding suggesting direct, local influences of compressive forces on matrix metabolism.

The matrix alterations varied according to the distance from the cartilage surface; most of the unloading-induced proteoglycan loss occurred in the superficial zone, and the calcified cartilage remained intact (29), (*Fig.* 3.1). Why the superficial zone was more affected is not known but, if catabolic messengers (43, 44) or lytic enzymes (45, 46, 47) from the synovial fluid are involved, they would have easier access to the cells and matrix close to the surface. Diffusion of proteoglycans, or partly degraded proteoglycans (48), should also have a more

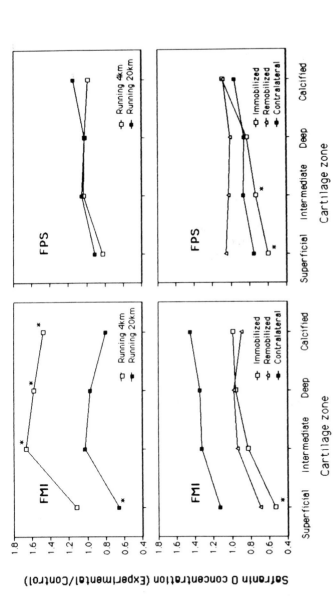

Fig. 3.1. Proteoglycan concentration of the canine distal femur in different cartilage zones from the surface to the bone, measured by a microspectrophotometer from safranin O stained sections.
Top panels: Influence of 15 weeks' moderate (4 km/day) and strenuous (20 km/day) running. Lower panels: Immobilized leg (11 weeks) and its contralateral side. The lower panels also show the effect of 15 weeks' remobilization following 11 weeks' immobilization. Two femoral sites were selected to represent samples from high weight bearing (FMI, left panels) and other areas (FPS, right panels); see Fig. 3.4 for site locations. The values represent the ratios of safranin O concentration in different cartilage zones (superficial, intermediate, deep and calcified) between experimental and control groups. Number of animals per group = 6–8; (*P < 0.05 as compared with controls, 2-tailed Mann-Whitney U-test). Note the accumulation of glycosaminoglycans in the weight-bearing site (FMI) following moderate, but not following strenuous, running. In the superficial cartilage no increase of glycosaminoglycans occurred after moderate training. Strenuous training decreased glycosaminoglycans in the superficial zone. Due to immobiliza-tion, the zones close to the cartilage surface were depleted of glycosaminoglycans, both in weight-bearing (FMI) and other areas (FPS). Also note the increase of glycosaminoglycans in the weight-bearing area of the contralateral side. Remobilization restored glycosaminoglycan content in the non-weight-bearing site (FPS), but failed to do so in the superficial zone of the weight-bearing site (FMI).

direct route out of the superficial matrix. Rough endoplasmic reticulum (RER) was specifically reduced in the superficial zone of immobilized cartilage chondrocytes, and the number of cells in this area increased. These findings suggest stimulated chondrocyte proliferation at the expense of matrix synthesis (49) (*Fig.* 3.2).

In contrast to the prominent changes in proteoglycan concentrations due to reduced loading, collagen content appeared to remain unchanged (14, 16, 32, 33, 50). This does not exclude possible rearrangements in the collagen types and fibre assembly (51). It would be particularly interesting to know whether or not unloading influences the minor collagens of articular cartilage (52, 53, 54, 55, 56). Altered collagen metabolism after cast immobilization (despite unchanged total content) was suggested by the findings of enhanced labelling of hydroxyproline in rabbits (50) and stimulation in the activity of prolyl hydroxylase in dogs (57).

Changes in Proteoglycan Structure and Metabolism

Immobilization of a limb in adult dogs and sheep reduced the content of galactosamine in the articular cartilage (14, 17). This implies that chondroitin sulphates were affected more than keratan sulphate. Histochemical analyses of dog tissues support the idea of diminished chondroitin sulphate content from the articular cartilage (29). Proteoglycan monomers from immobilized sheep and dog had a lower average molecular weight than controls (9, 14). The reduced content of proteoglycans from the unloaded joints was associated with a lower synthesis rate of glycosaminoglycans, demonstrated by $^{35}SO_4$ incorporation studies (9, 14, 18), but the contribution of facilitated degradation cannot be excluded. A lowered synthesis rate of proteoglycans in a grossly normal tissue suggested that the alteration should be classified as atrophy (9).

In contrast to sheep and dogs, immobilized rabbits showed enhanced incorporation of $^{35}SO_4$ into articular cartilage glycosaminoglycans (58). Since surface defects are present in the cartilages of this immobilization model, the result may be more comparable to injured cartilages, e.g. those in spontaneous (59) and experimental (60) osteoarthrosis, where the coexistent high synthesis rate and low content of glycosaminoglycans indicates an abnormally rapid loss of proteoglycans (61). Also, in contrast to dogs and sheep, the synthesis of chondroitin sulphate was stimulated in immobilized adult rabbits (58), while keratan sulphate synthesis seemed to be decreased (62), and the content of both glycosaminoglycans was reduced (50). In young rabbits a relative decrease of glucosamine was observed without significant loss of total glycosaminoglycans (32). It thus appears that in this species immobilization specifically increases the synthesis and turnover of chondroitin sulphate-rich proteoglycans.

The high chondroitin/keratan sulphate ratio observed in young rabbits following immobilization can be regarded as a sign of retarded maturation (33, 63), while in adult animals it may reflect regression to a more immature pattern of proteoglycan synthesis, or an attempt to repair the matrix.

After immobilization, the average degree of sulphation of chondroitin sulphates was increased in young rabbits, indicating that the matrix proteoglycans were gradually replaced by molecules of a different type as a response to

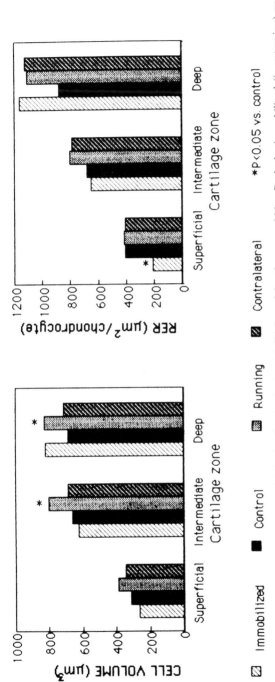

Fig. 3.2. Chondrocyte reactions to alterations of joint loading in the lateral tibial condyle of young rabbits. Both the immobilized (in extension) and the contralateral knee were analysed after 8 weeks of treatment. Non-strenuous running training (600 m/day) was conducted for 8 weeks. Age-matched animals served as controls. Each group consisted of 8 animals. *Left panel* shows the morphometrically determined volume of chondrocytes. *Right panel* depicts the surface area of rough endoplasmic reticulum (RER)/chondrocyte in the various cartilage zones ($*P < 0.05$ as compared to controls). *Note* the enlargement of chondrocytes following running training (*left panel*). There was a significant loss of RER from the superficial chondrocytes in immobilized legs, while RER appeared to be augmented by enhanced loading in the intermediate and deep layers, though not significantly so (*right panel*).

reduced mobility and weight bearing (33). Whether this increased suphation was regulation just at the level of synthesis of the glycosaminoglycan chains, or also involved synthesis of another type of proteoglycan core protein (64, 65), must await the results of further studies. The molecular weights of articular cartilage proteoglycans seemed not to be clearly altered by immobilization (32), although a greater diameter of the matrix granules in ruthenium red-stained thin sections of the tissue indicated that the properties of the proteoglycan subunits had been altered somehow (*Fig.* 3.3).

A gross functional failure emerged in the matrix following unloading, since extracted proteoglycans lost their capacity to reform hyaluronic acid-dependent aggregates in associative solutions (9, 18, 32, 66). This seems to be due to a defect – excision or lack of the hyaluronic acid-binding region in the proteoglycans – since adding high molecular weight hyaluronate did not promote aggregation (18), and the content of hyaluronic acid was not reduced in the unloaded cartilage samples (33).

That enhanced degradation contributes to the proteoglycan loss due to unloading is suggested by the high speed of the reduction which occurs in a few days (9, 26). Articular cartilage chondrocytes are capable of rapid matrix catabolism (48), which can be stimulated by extracartilaginous cells (67, 68). Since catabolin (interleukin 1 (44)), originally detected in synovial tissue (43), is capable of stimulating the proteoglycan-degrading activity of chondrocytes, it might account for the loss after immobilization. Rabbit (but not canine) joints sometimes show signs of inflammation after immobilization (Tammi *et al.* unpublished); accumulated leucocytes could be the source of extra catabolin in the joint (69). Catabolin induced an increase of high molecular weight proteoglycans, which had lost their ability to aggregate (48), also a characteristic feature of unloaded cartilage (9, 18, 32, 66).

Functional Properties of Unloaded Articular Cartilage

Due to the interdependence of proteoglycan content and the stiffness of cartilage (69, 70), it is predictable that proteoglycan loss following unloading would soften the tissue. This was confirmed in recent indentation tests of 20 different cartilage locations of immobilized canine knee joints (8). It was concluded that cartilage lost stiffness in all locations except those remaining in contact with the opposing articular surfaces. It is noteworthy that normal proteoglycan content was retained in the very same areas (29), obviously due to the residual loading at these sites.

Chondrocytes are probably vulnerable to injuries when the softened matrix encounters heavy joint loading (71). The same holds true for collagen fibres, the loss of which is considered an irreversible damage to the tissue. The damage to the softened tissue may be physically mediated through increased energy absorbtion, with the consequence of heat formation (72). Continuous maintenance of normal proteoglycan content is therefore vital to the articular cartilage, and reduced loading risks articular cartilage health through impairment of the proteoglycan matrix.

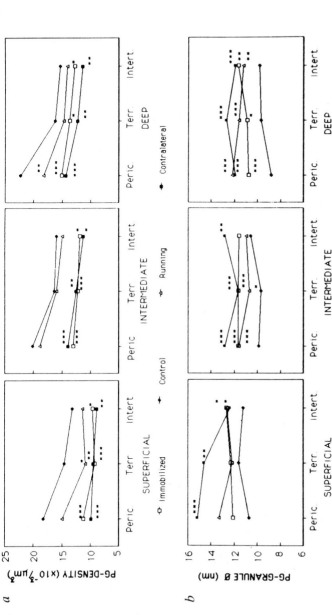

Fig. 3.3. Numerical density and diameter of proteoglycan granules in ruthenium red-stained thin sections of tibial lateral condyle of young rabbits: effects of moderate running training, immobilization and enhanced weight bearing (in contralateral to the immobilized knee). The animal material is the same as described in Fig. 3.2. The analyses were performed in the superficial, intermediate and deep zones of the cartilages, and separately from the pericellular (Peric.), territorial (Terr.) and interterritorial (Intert.) matrix. The density of granules (a) is expressed as granules/μm^3, and their average diameter (b) in nm (*$P < 0.05$; **$P < 0.01$; ***$P < 0.001$, as compared to the corresponding control with a t-test). Note the apparent higher density but smaller diameter of the granules in the pericellular vs. interterritorial matrix in controls. The deeper zones of cartilage had, on average, a higher density of smaller diameter granules. In the immobilized animals, granule density was reduced both in the immobilized and in the contralateral leg in all cartilage zones and matrix compartments. The difference in granule density between the contralateral and immobilized leg came from the apparently compensatory enlargement of the granules, which was more pronounced in the contralateral side, particularly in the superficial zone. Moderate running training slightly reduced the numerical density of the granules, but it increased granule diameters, with the most significant enhancement occurring in the intermediate and deep zones.

ELEVATED WEIGHT BEARING

Models

Data on the influence of elevated weight bearing, distinct from enhanced motion load such as running exercise, has been obtained from experiments in which the use of one limb has been eliminated by operation (15), amputation (18) or casting (14, 32). The contralateral limb then carries an increased load. A possible drawback of this technique is that the gait is also slightly changed, shifting different areas under load. The result does not, therefore, represent a pure increase of load but also an altered pattern of load bearing. This is avoided in recently described experiments where animals were made to live in centrifuge buckets, subjecting their joints to elevated weight bearing (73). A similar effect could probably be arranged by simply providing the animals with a suitable extra weight in the form of a 'back-pack'.

Elevated weight-bearing, as it occurs in the joints contralateral to the splinted leg, has not been reported to cause macroscopic damage to the articular cartilage (9, 14, 29, 32) although, in rabbits, there were minor alterations in the cartilage surface (27) and light microscopic evidence for local spots of injury (49).

Studies on the side opposite to the splinted limb have clearly indicated that this contralateral side cannot be regarded as a control tissue. The results also exclude the possibility that the cartilage changes observed after reduced loading are only due to systemic factors (e.g. hormonal regulation) induced by the treatment, because each side exhibits a different response.

Matrix Alterations

The overall concentration of glycosaminoglycans in the matrix was unchanged or slightly increased due to increased loading in dogs (17, 18) with local variation in the degree of the response (29) (*Fig.* 3.1). In rabbits glycosaminoglycan content in articular cartilage was unchanged or slightly decreased in the contralateral to the splinted limb (32, 58, 66). Sheep showed an increase of glycosaminoglycans in this type of loading (14).

Enhanced weight bearing did not change the ability of articular cartilage proteoglycans to form hyaluronic acid-dependent aggregates in rabbits (32, 66) or dogs (18). The type of proteoglycans present was changed, however, due to elevated weight bearing as suggested by the galactosamine/glucosamine ratios in proteoglycan extracts (32), in protease-solubilized extraction residues (33) and in total cartilage hydrolysates (17). These changes in the aminosugar ratios suggest that keratan sulphate increased relative to chondroitin sulphate in the dog and rabbit (17, 32, 33), but chondroitin sulphate was enhanced in the sheep (14). Results compatible with the biochemically detected increase of keratan sulphate were obtained with quantitative histochemical techniques in the dog (29). Proteoglycan monomers (granules) in the ruthenium red-stained thin sections of the contralateral cartilages of rabbits appeared larger than those in controls (*Fig.* 3.3), supporting the idea of an alteration in proteoglycan structures.

It is suggested that the interactions between proteoglycans, collagen and possibly other matrix proteins are strengthened by enhanced weight bearing, since the fraction of residual glycosaminoglycans not extracted with 4 mol/l guanidinium chloride (GuCl) was increased, an alteration opposite to that occurring in reduced loading (32, 33, 66). The contribution of collagen to the tight binding of the non-extractable proteoglycans is suggested by a trend towards greater collagen fibre diameters in these joints (51), although total collagen content was not markedly increased (32, 33, 66).

Why a certain proportion of proteoglycans resist GuCl extraction is not known. Spatial entrapment in the collagenous network may be involved (74, 75, 76, 77), while covalent bonding to the collagenous network is another possibility. A collagenous polypeptide with 1–2 covalently bound chondroitin sulphate chains has been recently described and named either Type IX collagen (55) or proteoglycan Lt (78). Because articular cartilage collagen is virtually insoluble in GuCl, this hybrid molecule could mediate the insolubility of the glycosaminoglycan chains. However, Type IX collagen was soluble, at least in the embryonic cartilage (55, 78).

Further studies in rabbits revealed that hyaluronic acid content was increased in the more loaded (contralateral) joint cartilages (33). This was not associated with any alteration in the proportion of aggregated proteoglycan monomers when the GuCl extract was chromatographed in an associative buffer (32). Neither did hyaluronic acid seem to contribute to the elevated level of non-extractable proteoglycans, since the extraction residue was almost devoid of it (33). The nature of the influence of a higher quantity of hyaluronic acid in terms of matrix structure and function remains obscure, but it has been known for a long time that, *in vitro*, hyaluronic acid strongly depresses the synthesis of proteoglycans by chondrocytes (79, 80, 81).

The content of hyaluronic acid was particularly high in adult human articular cartilage (82), and probably exceeded the amount necessary for aggregation of the proteoglycans present. It was recently demonstrated that adult cartilage contains proteins able to compete with proteoglycans for binding to hyaluronic acid (83). The high content of hyaluronic acid may therefore serve to compensate for its relative unavailability to proteoglycans in old cartilages (83).

Species differences between the reactions of contralateral articular cartilages of rabbits and dogs appear considerable, since no general increase of hyaluronic acid, non-extractable glycosaminoglycans, nor the proportion of glucosamine in extracted or non-extracted proteoglycans was noted in joints contralateral to the splinted limb of dogs (Säämänen *et al.*, unpublished). One of the contributing factors may be that the metabolic regulation of the matrix is different in rabbit tissue, an explanation consistent with the ease with which rabbit articular cartilage is injured by immobilization. Another factor may be that, because front legs take a larger proportion of the body weight in the dog than in the rabbit, the shift in the load to the contralateral hind leg is less pronouced in the dog, and does not induce significant responses. In accordance with this concept, canine articular cartilage from the contralateral side showed very local reactions, limited to the sites most loaded by the surplus of weight bearing (29), (*Fig.* 3.1).

EFFECTS OF RUNNING

General Considerations

Relatively few experiments have been published about the influences on joint cartilage of running, probably the most physiological way of enhancing articular cartilage load. The importance of these studies is stressed by the greatly increased popularity of free-time jogging; its long-term effects on articular cartilage health are not known.

Enhanced weight bearing acts as a long-lasting, static weight imposed on cartilage during all the active hours of the animal. Running programmes, on the other hand, have been applied in the form of daily training for just a few hours, subjecting the joint to intensified cyclic loading, and probably an enlarged range of motion too.

Running and Cartilage Integrity

Experimental running exercise may injure articular cartilage (84, 85, 86, 87, 88), but there are several examples supporting the opposite view (89, 90, 91, 92). It is conceivable that one of the factors that injures cartilage in running experiments is the rapid and forced beginning of the training programme. This is particularly applicable to the naturally sedentary rabbit (85, 88). Even gradual beginning of a running programme caused a transient loss of ground substance proteoglycans and exposed collagen fibres on the cartilage surfaces of rabbits (28). Articular cartilage which had atrophied due to previous unloading suffered from running exercise but not from reloading by free walking (71). The age of the animals at the beginning of the training programme may influence the vulnerability of the cartilage and its response to running. Intact tissue was found in young rabbits and dogs after running programmes (28, 92).

The shear forces between opposite cartilage surfaces, when they exist in excess, may be responsible for the surface lesions observed after strenuous running. It is suggested that these lesions develop along the same pathway as experimental osteoarthrosis in dogs (Muir and Carney, Chapter 2), where the transection of the anterior cruciate ligament is followed by joint laxity and an abnormally wide shearing movement (93).

Influence on Matrix Structure

Glycosaminoglycan content in articular cartilage has been reported to decrease after running training in dogs (86), guinea pigs and mice (84), to be unchanged in rabbits (85), or to increase in rabbits (32, 95) and dogs (96, 97). The variation between the results is probably accounted for by the initial and final intensities of the training, and possibly by the age of the animals at the beginning of the experiment.

Gradually-started, low-intensity training of young rabbits enhances proteoglycan content in knee articular cartilages, as deduced by uronic acid assays of proteoglycan extracts (32, 95). Similar stimulation occurred in young dogs, detectable both by uronic acid (97) and quantitative histochemical assays (96). Adult rabbits made to run without a reported conditioning period showed no significant change in total glycosaminoglycan concentration, measured as hexosamines or uronic acid (98).

Proteoglycan content was reduced at the spontaneous lesions developed in the femoral head cartilage of adult dogs after an 8-month-long programme of strenuous running (86). The lesions were aggravated by running in knee joints of previously immobilized dogs (71), as measured by uronic acid content or estimated after safranin O staining. This shows that enhanced loading in the form of running does not allow the restoration of the proteoglycan matrix if it was atrophic before training. On the other hand, extremely strenuous and long-lasting running exercise (1·5 km/h, 3 h daily for 63 days), was necessary to depress staining for glycosaminoglycans of initially healthy matrix in the mouse (84). No change in the normal organization of the tissue was reported even then (84).

The effect of training intensity on the response of healthy young cartilage has been studied in dogs by comparing non-strenuous and strenuous exercise. While non-strenuous running (4 km/day) increased glycosaminoglycan levels in most sites of the knee cartilages, strenuous training (20 km/day) attenuated the increase and even decreased proteoglycans at some locations (96, 97) (*Figs.* 3.1, 3.4). The strenuous training did not cause macroscopic or microscopic damage to the general structure of the tissue within this time interval (96), but longer periods of high intensity running have been reported to cause cartilage fibrillation (86).

The structure of the extractable proteoglycans was slightly changed after non-strenuous training in young rabbits, i.e. chondroitin sulphate chains were more completely sulphated and the keratan/chondroitin sulphate ratio was elevated (95). The ability of extracted proteoglycans to re-form hyaluronic acid-dependent aggregates was not altered (32), although the concentration of hyaluronic acid showed a tendency to diminish (95). The elevated keratan sulphate/chondroitin sulphate ratio resembled that found in normal maturation in this age period (33, 63). Another feature of normal maturation, enhanced by the running programme, was an augmentation of non-extractable glycosamino-glycans after 2 months' running (33).

Both enhanced weight bearing and running training of young rabbits thus modified matrix proteoglycans in the same way as maturation of the individual does: the keratan/chondroitin sulphate ratio was elevated and non-extractable proteoglycans increased (33, 63). However, the response to running partly differed from that of elevated weight bearing, since it enhanced total glycosaminoglycan content but depressed hyaluronic acid, these alterations not being a part of the maturation process (33, 63, 95).

The molecular weight distributions of proteoglycan monomers of canine knee articular cartilages were not significantly altered by moderate running exercise. Formation of aggregates was not altered by running either. On the other hand, both the molecular weight distribution of monomers and their ability to form aggregates varied slightly according to the anatomical site of the cartilage sample (Säämänen *et al.* 1987, unpublished).

The ability of proteoglycans to form aggregates is reduced, however, if cartilages are damaged during running training (71, 86), and the average size of proteoglycan monomers is reduced (86); findings common to experimental (37) and spontaneous joint disease (35, 99, 100). In the dog, the relative proportion of 4-sulphated disaccharides in chondroitin sulphates of running dogs is enhanced whether lesions were present (86) or not (97).

Running training does not significantly affect the content of collagen in articular cartilages of rabbits (32, 95) or dogs (97). The synthesis of collagen was not significantly stimulated after non-strenuous running, as indicated by the activity of prolyl hydroxylase in the articular cartilage of young dogs (57).

Chondrocyte Activity and Matrix Metabolism

The voluminous matrix of articular cartilage is synthesized and controlled by relatively sparsely distributed chondrocytes. The turnover of both proteoglycans and collagen in adult articular cartilage is slow but significant (101). Since a fairly constant proteoglycan content is maintained, it is reasonable to assume that some kind of signalling system from matrix to chondrocytes exists to regulate their synthetic activity (102). Whatever mechanisms are involved, it is evident from studies *in vitro* that cartilage responds to a depletion of proteoglycans by enhanced synthesis (103, 104, 105, 106, 107), probably as an attempt at repair.

The effect of joint loading on articular cartilage matrix degradation has not been established. Cartilage lesions developed under heavy running exercise are depleted of proteoglycans despite stimulated synthesis, indicating facilitated loss (86), but no direct data in the form of metabolic labelling is available on non-destructive training.

Another way to examine matrix metabolism is to use quantitative morphological probes to examine the activity of chondrocytes and their synthetic products. The number and size of chondrocytes were reported to increase after running training in guinea pigs and rabbits, suggesting activation of the cell and its matrix synthesis (91, 108). The hypertrophy of chondrocytes in rabbit articular cartilage as a response to running exercise has been recently confirmed using stereological techniques (109) (*Fig.* 3.2), but no increase in cell number was observed (109). The enlargement of the cells was most conspicuous in the intermediate and deep zones. Enhanced synthesis of proteins for export in the same zones was suggested by the increase of rough endoplasmic reticulum (RER) (*Fig.* 3.2), concomitant with the enhancement of matrix glycosaminoglycan concentration (96) (*Fig.* 3.1). The numerical density of proteoglycan granules was slightly smaller in ruthenium red-stained thin sections, but their size was significantly increased after moderate running (*Fig.* 3.4).

Running and Cartilage Biomechanical Properties

The thickness of non-calcified cartilage was augmented in dogs after moderate running (92, 96). This should improve the properties of articular cartilage as a shock-absorbing cushion. Thickening of articular cartilage after running training has been reported earlier in young rabbits (108), but this was not later confirmed (109).

Proteoglycans form a hydrophilic and viscous gel, embedded in the

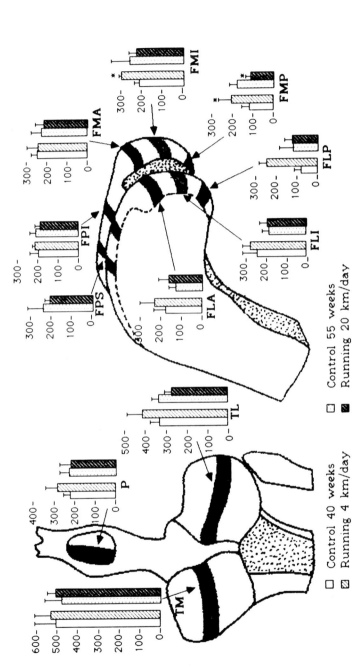

Fig. 3.4. Concentration distribution of proteoglycans in canine knee articular surfaces following moderate and strenuous running training. From the age of 15 weeks the experimental groups were accustomed to the gradually increasing training distances. The training period lasted 15 weeks at the final intensities (moderate: 4 km/day, 4 km/h; strenuous: 20 km/day, 6·1 km/h). The ages of the dogs were 40 and 55 weeks at the end of the moderate and strenuous training respectively. Tibia with attached patella is shown on the left side, the distal femur to the right. TM and TL denote medial and lateral condyles of tibia, respectively. P = patella. FPS and FPI = patellar surface of femur, superior and inferior part respectively. FMA, FMI and FMP represent anterior, intermediate and posterior parts of the medial condyle of femur, respectively, while FLA, FLI and FLP are the corresponding parts of the lateral femoral condyle. The results are expressed as uronic acid/hydroxyproline (nmol/μmol, mean ± SD, n = 5–7/group; *$P < 0.05$ as compared with controls, 2-tailed Mann-Whitney U-test). *Note* the enhanced uronic acid concentration in most sites following moderate training, and the lack of high values after strenuous running. No consistent trend in uronic acid concentration was present between the control groups at 40 and 55 weeks.

collagenous network. They efficiently retard the displacement of water from articular cartilage under load (2): proteoglycan concentrations thus play a major role in determining the biomechanical properties of articular cartilage. The increase of glycosaminoglycan concentration after moderate running training (*Figs*. 3.1, 3.4), was predicted to stiffen articular cartilage and thus make it more resistant to heavy loading (69). Analysis by a standardized indentation method proved that there was a general stiffening of several femoral and tibial articular cartilage sites of the dog knee after moderate running (92). Except for a few sites, an increase in the elastic modulus and a decrease in the deformation rate were correlated with a stimulation in total glycosaminoglycan concentration (92, 96). This indicates that the enhanced glycosaminoglycan concentration indeed decreased the bulk flow of water through the matrix, thus improving its biomechanical properties.

The influence of reduced and increased joint loading on the biomechanical properties of knee articular cartilages in young beagle dogs is summarized in *Fig*. 3.5. It is evident that the basic response to stress is stimulatory, and a new homeostatic balance settles on a higher level until the magnitude of the stress exceeds the capacity of the tissue.

COMPARISON OF *IN VIVO* AND *IN VITRO* LOADING

The studies described above have clearly demonstrated that alterations in the grade of joint loading and the type of loading have specific effects on matrix structure and chondrocyte metabolism *in vivo*. Nevertheless, studies utilizing *in vivo* models cannot give definitive answers to questions concerning the exact relationship between the local magnitude of stress and its metabolic response. The influence of systemic factors, such as hormone concentrations and nutrient supply in joints, is difficult to control *in vivo*. Furthermore, the monitoring of rapid intracellular events during loading, to reveal the mechanisms by which chondrocytes sense the stress changes, is not possible in *in vivo* experiments.

A small continuous force on the cultured mandibular condyles of newborn rats reduced synthesis of proteoglycans and collagen, but stimulated cell proliferation. On the other hand, a cyclic force (0·7 Hz) stimulated matrix synthesis while inhibiting proliferation (110). An intermittent compressive force inhibited the serum-stimulated synthesis of DNA in cultured chick and rat chondrocytes (111). A stimulation of proteoglycan synthesis by intermittent stress (4 s on/11 s off) was also observed in femoral condyle plugs of dogs; continuous stress resulted in inhibition (112). Chick embryonic chondrocytes and explants of epiphyseal cartilage reacted by enhanced proteoglycan synthesis to an intermittent force generated by compressing the gas phase of the tissue cultures (113).

The above *in vitro* studies are fully compatible with the increase of cartilage matrix proteoglycans following running exercise in rabbits (32, 33) and dogs (96, 97) (*Figs*. 3.1, 3.2). The analogy can be extended to the increased numbers of chondrocytes found in unloaded cartilages of young rabbits (49), and the concomitant reduction of the synthesis apparatus for exported proteins (*Fig*. 3.3). Furthermore, the failure of proteoglycans from unloaded cartilages to aggregate with hyaluronic acid (9, 18, 32, 66) may be comparable to the *in vitro* observation that proteoglycans from chondrocyte cultures subjected to intermittent compressive forces aggregated better with hyaluronic acid (113). The

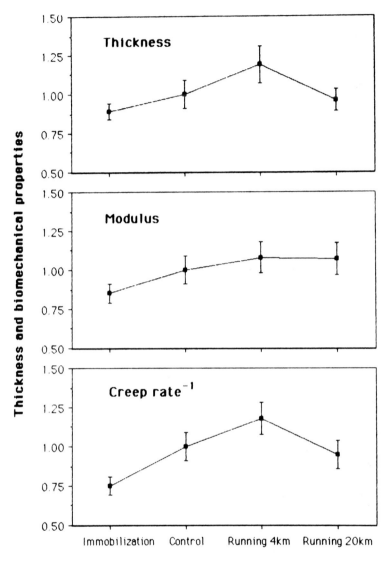

Physical training

Fig. 3.5. Biomechanical properties of canine knee articular cartilages following various degrees of joint loading. The *Figs.* include combined data from measurements of 6 surface sites of femoral, tibial and patellar cartilages (mean ± SD, 6–8 animals/group), expressed as a ratio between experimental and control animals. The treatments are the same as described in *Figs.* 3.1 and 3.4. Modulus and creep rate were calculated as in references (8, 92). In all three parameters, reduced loading (immobilization) produced values inferior to those of the controls, while moderately increased intermittent loading (running 4 km/day) induced a response leading to elevated values. Strenuous loading (20 km/day) restored the parameter values to the control level, or even below.

increased coherence between proteoglycans and other matrix components, as indicated by the increase of non-extractable proteoglycans following loading (32, 33), was also reproducible *in vitro* (113).

LOADING AND ARTICULAR CARTILAGE MATURATION

Age Changes in Articular Cartilage Matrix

Articular cartilage matrix undergoes considerable structural alteration during ageing, particularly before adulthood. The content of hydroxyproline increased in rabbits (33, 63), pigs (34) and dogs (*Table* 3.1), indicating accumulation of collagen. A larger proportion of proteoglycans remained non-extractable with 4M GuCl (33, 34, 35, 63, 114, 115). Water content of articular cartilage was lowered with ageing (34, 115).

Table 3.1. Cartilage thickness distribution and collagen concentration in maturing beagle knee articular cartilages. Thickness is expressed as μm, collagen as hydroxyproline/tissue wet weight (nmol/mg). The figures show mean ± SD from 4–8 samples/group. For localization of the sampling sites, *see Fig.* 3.4. The figures show values at the age of 40 and 55 weeks, and the relative increase between the time points (55/40 weeks ratio). * $P < 0.05$, two-tailed Mann–Whitney U-test.

Site	Thickness			Collagen		
	40 weeks	55 weeks	55/40	40 weeks	55 weeks	55/40
FPS	385±50	410±45	1·06	—	—	—
FPI	305±40	355±40	1·16	141±19	155±11	1·10
P	485±80	545±85	1·12	140±10	163±49	1·16
FMA	455±45	450±80	0·99	133±19	153±23	1·15
FMI	600±85	795±90*	1·33	132±9	141±25	1·07
FMP	445±135	365±80	0·82	167±58	146±25	0·87
FLA	370±75	370±55	1·00	137±36	182±18	1·33
FLI	405±50	485±80	1·20	108±35	167±20*	1·55
FLP	275±50	275±65	1·00	127±33	140±26	1·10
TM	950±75	1140±170	1·20	93±9	108±23	1·16
TL	645±115	915±195*	1·42	127±16	151±17	1·19

The extracted proteoglycan monomers became smaller in aged tissues (35, 74, 114, 116, 117, 118), at least partly due to shortening of the chondroitin sulphate chains (116, 117). Chondroitin-6-sulphate was increased, while 4-sulphated disaccharides were proportionally reduced in older cartilage samples (114, 116, 117, 119). Relatively more keratan sulphate existed on proteoglycans of older cartilages (35, 63, 74, 114, 117), while their oligosaccharide content was reportedly reduced (116).

The ability of purified proteoglycans of older cartilages to form hyaluronic acid-dependent aggregates was not changed despite their reduced size (35, 116). However, adult human articular cartilage extracts failed to form proteoglycan aggregates of high buoyant density (120). This seemed to be accounted for by the accumulation in aged cartilage of proteins competing with proteoglycan subunits for the limited amount of binding sites on hyaluronic acid (83). The observed increase of hyaluronic acid in aged cartilage (63, 82, 115, 121) was suggested to be a compensatory reaction to the reduced availability of binding sites on hyaluronic acid (83). In the rabbit, reduction in the synthesis of link proteins may retard aggregation of proteoglycans in old cartilage (122), and the reaction with link protein may be a limiting step for stable aggregate formation in human cartilage also (123).

Loading-related Differences between Articular Cartilage Surface Sites

Certain surface sites on the articular cartilages are more often and more heavily loaded than others. There is a tendency for the regions of frequent and heavy load bearing at the summits of femoral condyles to show thicker cartilages than the more peripheral regions (8, 92). It is interesting that the more loaded regions grew in thickness as a function of age in young dogs, while those under relatively less load did not (*Table* 3.1). The loaded regions also seemed to contain more proteoglycans (*Fig.* 3.4).

Bovine femoral condyles showed a higher absolute and relative content of keratan sulphate in surface sites subject to frequent contact and load (115). This difference between minimally and maximally loaded sites existed from early foetal periods to maturity (115). Hyaluronic acid accumulated in highly loaded sites too, but only after birth (115). Proteoglycan monomers were of similar size, but water content was lower in more loaded sites of calves.

Similar matrix alterations were thus associated with maturation of articular cartilage in general, and to the sites of high loading in particular. It was therefore hypothesized that joint loading, beginning from foetal movements, was involved in inducing the maturation of articular cartilage matrix (124, 125). However, the keratan sulphate/chondroitin sulphate ratio also increased with age in cartilages not subjected to loading (126). Comparison of age changes in proteoglycans from shoulder and knee cartilages did not demonstrate the anticipated enhancement of maturation-associated alterations in the presumably more loaded knee joint (116).

Effects of Loading on Cartilage Maturation

Direct evidence about the influence of joint loading on the maturation process in articular cartilage matrix has been obtained from young animals subjected to increased and decreased joint loading. Moderate running training of young dogs increased the thickness of articular cartilage (92). Increased loading accelerated, while decreased loading retarded, the accumulation of non-extractable proteoglycans (32, 33). In this experimental model (immobilized hind leg of the rabbit and the weight-bearing contralateral leg), the normal deposition of keratan sulphate was also reduced in the immobilized leg and enhanced in the weight-bearing leg (32, 33). Furthermore, elevated loading promoted a trend toward an increase in hyaluronic acid and collagen contents, findings compatible with accelerated maturation (32, 33, 63).

CONCLUSIONS

Unloading of the joint causes articular cartilage atrophy or injury, as indicated by the reduced content of proteoglycans in superficial zones, and in alterations of proteoglycan structures and their interaction with other matrix constituents. Atrophy was probably mediated through the lack of stimulation to chondrocytes by normal joint loading, but catabolic mediators from extracartilaginous tissues may be involved. The articular cartilage injuries observed in certain species following immobilization probably included compressive damage to contact sites due to joint contraction, invasion of mesenchymal tissue, inflammation, and nutritional factors, mixed with the basic disuse atrophy.

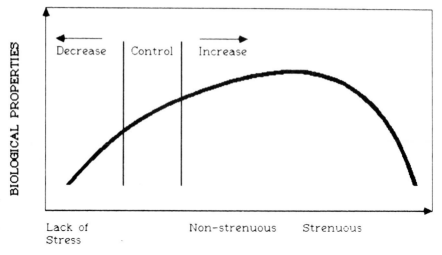

INTERMITTENT PHYSICAL STRESS

Fig. 3.6. Our hypothesis of the effect of intermittent physical stress on the biological properties of articular cartilage. We suggest that atrophy or injury occurs in articular cartilage due to sub-optimal physical stresses, while stresses within physiological limits stimulate the tissue to develop improved biological properties. Increasing the stress beyond this physiological boundary causes a progressive deterioration of its biological properties. This same rule may also be applicable to other connective tissues of the locomotory system (*see* Woo and Akeson, Chapter 12).

As a consequence of unloading, the tissue loses its stiffness, a prerequisite for its ability to shield chondrocytes and collagenous fibres from irreversible damage from newly started heavy loading. Atrophy and softening were slowly reversible under gentle reloading, but the achievement of complete restoration is not certain.

Elevated weight bearing induces a reaction in chondrocytes which either tends to increase tissue proteoglycans or, in young animals, mimics structural alterations in proteoglycans normally found with maturation or ageing.

Enhanced loading in the form of moderate running training activated chondrocytes, which responded by augmented matrix proteoglycan content in the intermediate and deep zones of articular cartilage. The structure of the proteoglycan matrix also changed in young animals, representative of normal ageing. Cartilage was thickened in some surface sites by moderate running, and there was a general trend to greater stiffness, both indicative of improved biomechanical properties.

Strenuous running largely reversed the beneficial effects found in the matrix after moderate training, including enhancements in proteoglycan concentration, thickness and stiffness. Proteoglycans were particularly depleted in the superficial zones. No visible damage in the cartilage surface nor in the general organization of the tissue were required for these matrix changes, but these kinds of alterations may well precede the overt fibrillation of articular cartilage. Large variations among different cartilage surface sites in response to increased loading were obviously due to the uneven distribution of the augmented load, supporting the idea of local, direct effects of joint loading on chondrocyte metabolism (*Fig.* 3.6).

CLINICAL SIGNIFICANCE

The present results suggest that, in clinical practice, the benefits of unloading of joints, e.g. by bed rest and cast, should be carefully considered against the possible atrophy developing during long-term treatment. It is also suggested that when unloading has occurred for a long period, care should be taken at reloading to avoid irreparable damage: gradual increase of loading up to full joint use is advisable.

Moderate physical training of normal joints in young animals improved the biomechanical properties of articular cartilage, while strenuous training reversed the benefit back to the normal level. Whether or not the influence of non-strenuous exercise on young athletes is analogous to that in animals remains an open question. Answers must be found to the key questions; where is the borderline to too strenuous exercise?–and what is the response in adult tissues? The development of non-invasive methods for the evaluation of living human articular cartilage is particularly important. These issues should be considered in the future among physicians in clinical practice, and among those responsible for the planning of human sports activities and working conditions.

ACKNOWLEDGEMENTS

This work has been supported by the Academy of Finland, Finnish Research Council for Physical Education and Sports, Ministry of Education, Finnish Cultural Foundation, the North Savo Regional Fund of Finnish Cultural Foundation, Heikki and Hilma Honkanen Foundation, and Paulo Foundation.

REFERENCES

1. Muir H (1980) The chemistry of the ground substance of joint cartilage. *In: The Joints and Synovial Fluid Vol II*, (*L Sokoloff, ed*) pp. 27–94. New York: Academic Press.
2. Maroudas A (1979) Physicochemical properties of articular cartilage. *In: Adult Articular Cartilage*, 2nd Ed (M A R Freeman, ed) pp. 215–90. Tunbridge Wells: Pitman.
3. Menzel A (1871) Ueber die Erkrankung der Gelenke bei dauernder Ruhe derselben. Ein experimentelle Studie. *Arch Klin Chir* **12**: 990–1009.
4. Moll A (1886) Experimentelle Untersuchungen über den anatomischen Zustand der Gelenke bei andauernder Immobilisation derselben. *Virchow's Arch* **105**: 466–85.
5. Sood S C (1971) A study of the effects of experimental immobilization on rabbit articular cartilage. *J Anat* **108**: 497–507.
6. Langenskiöld A, Michelsson J E and Videman T (1979) Osteoarthritis of the knee in the rabbit produced by immobilization. *Acta Orthop Scand* **50**: 1–14.
7. Reyher C (1873) Ueber die Veränderungen der Gelenke bei dauernder Ruhe. *Dtsch Z Chir* **3**: 189–255.
8. Jurvelin J, Kiviranta I, Tammi M and Helminen H J (1986) Softening of canine articular cartilage after immobilization of the knee joint. *Clin Orthop* **207**: 246–52.
9. Palmoski M, Perricone E and Brandt K D (1979) Development and reversal of a proteoglycan aggregation defect in normal canine knee cartilage after immobilization. *Arthritis Rheum* **22**: 508–17.
10. Williams J and Brandt K D (1984) Immobilization ameliorates chemically-induced articular cartilage damage. *Arthritis Rheum* **27**: 208–16.
11. Evans E B, Eggers G W N, Butler J K and Blumel J (1960) Experimental immobilization and remobilization of rat knee joints. *J Bone Joint Surg [Am]* **42**: 737–58.
12. Hall M C (1964) Articular changes in the knee of the adult rat after prolonged immobilization in extension. *Clin Orthop* **34**: 184–95.
13. Thaxter T H, Mann R A and Anderson C E (1965) Degeneration of immobilized knee joints in rats. *J Bone Joint Surg [Am]* **47**: 567–85.

14. Caterson B and Lowther D A (1978) Changes in the metabolism of the proteoglycans from sheep articular cartilage in response to mechanical stress. *Biochim Biophys Acta* **540**: 412–22.
15. Oláh E H and Kostenszky K S (1972) Effect of altered functional demand on the glycosaminoglycan content of the articular cartilage of dogs. *Acta Biol Acad Sci Hung* **23**: 195–200.
16. Kostenszky K S and Oláh E H (1975) Functional adaptation of the articular cartilage. *Acta Biol Acad Sci Hung* **26**: 157–64.
17. Oláh E H and Kostenszky K S (1976) Effect of loading and prednisolone treatment on the glycosaminoglycan content of articular cartilage in dogs. *Scand J Rheumatol* **5**: 49–52.
18. Palmoski M J, Colyer R A and Brandt K D (1980) Joint motion in the absence of normal loading does not maintain normal articular cartilage. *Arthritis Rheum* **23**: 325–34.
19. Ely L W and Mensor M C (1933) Studies on the immobilization of the normal joints. *Surg Gynecol Obstet* **37**: 212–5.
20. Salter R B and Field P (1960) The effects of continuous compression on living articular cartilage. *J Bone Joint Surg [Am]* **42**: 31–49.
21. Müller W (1924) Experimentelle Untersuchungen über die Wirkung langdauernder Immobilisierung auf die Gelenke. *Z Orthop Chir* **44**: 478–88.
22. Behrens F, Oegema T R and Kraft E L (1983) Biochemical cartilage alterations after rigid and semirigid joint immobilization. *Orthop Trans* **7**: 369.
23. Ohta N, Kawai N, Kawaji W and Hirano H (1981) Morphological changes in rabbit articular cartilages experimentally induced by joint contracture - in association with ageing. *Okajimas Folia Anat Jpn* **58**: 205–20.
24. Seedhom B B and Hargreaves D J (1979) Transmission of the load in the knee joint with special reference to the role of the menisci. Part II: experimental results, discussion and conclusions. *Engineering Med* **8**: 220–8.
25. Ahmed A M and Burke D L (1983) *In vitro* measurement of static pressure distribution in synovial joints. Part I: Tibial surface of the knee. *J Biomech Eng* **105**: 216–25.
26. Troyer H (1975) The effect of short-term immobilization on the rabbit knee joint cartilage. *Clin Orthop* **107**: 249–57.
27. Helminen H J, Jurvelin J, Kuusela T, Heikkilä R, Kiviranta I and Tammi M (1983) Effect of immobilization for 6 weeks on rabbit knee articular surfaces as assessed by the semiquantitative stereomicroscopic method. *Acta Anat (Basel)* **115**: 327–35.
28. Jurvelin J, Helminen H J, Lauritsalo S, Kiviranta I, Säämänen A-M, Paukkonen K and Tammi M (1985) Influences of joint immobilization and running exercise on articular cartilage surfaces of young rabbits. *Acta Anat (Basel)* **122**: 62–8.
29. Kiviranta I, Jurvelin J, Tammi M, Säämänen A-M and Helminen H J (1987) Weight-bearing controls glycosaminoglycan concentration and thickness of articular cartilage in the knee joint of young beagle dogs. *Arthritis Rheum* (in press).
30. Videman T (1981) Changes in compression and distances between tibial and femoral condyles during immobilization of rabbit knee. *Arch Orthop Trauma Surg* **98**: 289–91.
31. Eronen I, Videman T, Friman C and Michelsson J-E (1978) Glycosaminoglycan metabolism in experimental osteoarthrosis caused by immobilization. *Acta Orthop Scand* **49**: 329–34.
32. Tammi M, Säämänen A-M, Jauhiainen A, Malminen O, Kiviranta I and Helminen H J (1983) Proteoglycan alterations in rabbit knee articular cartilage following physical exercise and immobilization. *Connect Tissue Res* **11**: 45–55.
33. Säämänen A-M, Tammi M, Kiviranta I, Jurvelin J and Helminen H J (1987) Maturation of proteoglycan matrix in articular cartilage under increased and decreased joint loading. A study in young rabbits. *Connect Tissue Res* **16**: 163–75.
34. Simunek Z and Muir H (1972) Changes in the protein–polysaccharides of pig articular cartilage during prenatal life, development and old age. *Biochem J* **126**: 515–23.
35. Inerot S, Heinegård D, Audell L and Olsson S-E (1978) Articular cartilage proteoglycans in ageing and osteoarthritis. *Biochem J* **169**: 143–56.
36. McDevitt C A, Gilbertson E and Muir H (1977) An experimental model of osteoarthritis, early morphological and biochemical changes. *J Bone Joint Surg [Br]* **59**: 24–35.
37. Moskovitz R W, Howell D S, Goldberg V M, Muniz O and Pita J C (1979) Cartilage proteoglycan alterations in an experimentally induced model of rabbit osteoarthritis. *Arthritis Rheum* **22**: 155–63.
38. Brandt K D (1974) Enhanced extractability of articular cartilage proteoglycans in osteoarthrosis. *Biochem J* **143**: 475–8.

39. McDevitt C A and Muir H (1976) Biochemical changes in the cartilage of the knee in experimental and natural osteoarthritis in the dog. *J Bone Joint Surg [Br]* **58**: 94–101.
40. Paulsson M and Heinegård D (1984) Non-collagenous cartilage proteins. Current status of an emerging research field. *Collagen Relat Res* **4**: 219–29.
41. Fife R S (1985) Idenification of link proteins and a 116000-dalton matrix protein in canine meniscus. *Arch Biochem Biophys* **240**: 682–8.
42. Fife R S (1986) Changes in a matrix protein in canine osteoarthritis. *Scand J Rheumatol (Suppl)* **60**: 8
43. Dingle J T (1983) The role of catabolin in the control of cartilage matrix integrity. *J Rheumatol (Suppl 11)* **10**: 38–42.
44. Saklatvala J, Pilsworth L M C, Sarsfield S J, Gavrilovic J and Heath J K (1984) Pig catabolin is a form of interleukin 1. Cartilage and bone resorb, fibroblasts make prostaglandin and collagenase, and thymocyte proliferation is augmented in response to one protein. *Biochem J* **224**: 461–6.
45. Werb Z, Mainardi C L, Vater C A and Harris E D Jr (1977) Endogenous activation of latent collagenase by rheumatoid synovial cells: evidence for a role of plasminogen activator. *N Engl J Med* **296**: 1017–23.
46. Vater C A, Nagase H and Harris E D Jr (1983) Purification of an endogenous activator of procollagenase from rabbit synovial fibroblast culture medium. *J Biol Chem* **258**: 9374–82.
47. McGuire M B, Murphy G, Reynolds J J and Russel R G G (1981) Production of collagenase and inhibitor (TIMP) by normal, rheumatoid and osteoarthritic synovium *in vitro*: effects of hydrocortisone and indomethacin. *J Clin Sci* **61**: 703–10.
48. Tyler J A (1985) Chondrocyte-mediated depletion of articular cartilage proteoglycans *in vitro*. *Biochem J* **225**: 493–507.
49. Paukkonen K, Jurvelin J and Helminen H J (1986) Effects of immobilization on the articular cartilage in young rabbits. A quantitative light microscopic stereological study. *Clin Orthop* **206**: 270–80.
50. Videman T, Eronen I and Candolin T (1981) [³H]Proline incorporation and hydroxyproline concentration in articular cartilage during the development of osteoarthritis caused by immobilization. A study *in vivo* with rabbits. *Biochem J* **200**: 435–40.
51. Paukkonen K and Helminen H J (1987) Decrease of proteoglycan granule number, but increase of their size in articular cartilage of young rabbits after physical exercise and immobilization by splinting. *Anat Rec.* (In press.)
52. Sussman M D, Ogle R C and Balian G (1984) Biosynthesis and processing of collagens in different cartilaginous tissues. *J Orthop Res* **2**: 134–42.
53. Smith G N, Williams J M and Brandt K D (1985) Interaction of proteoglycans with the pericellular (1α, 2α, 3α) collagens of cartilage. *J Biol Chem* **260**: 10761–7.
54. Schmid T M, Mayne R, Bruns R R and Linsenmayer T F (1984) Molecular structure of short-chain (SC) cartilage collagen by electron microscopy. *J Ultrastruct Res* **86**: 186–91.
55. Vaughan L, Winterhalter K H and Bruckner P (1985) Proteoglycan Lt from chicken embryo sternum identified as type IX collagen. *J Biol Chem* **260**: 4758–63.
56. Wu J J and Eyre D R (1984) Cartilage type IX collagen is cross-linked by hydroxypyridinium residues. *Biochem Biophys Res Commun* **123**: 1033–9.
57. Tammi M, Kiviranta I, Peltonen L, Jurvelin J and Helminen H J (1987) Effects of joint loading on articular cartilage metabolism: assay of procollagen prolyl 4-hydroxylase and galactosylhydroxylysyl glucosyltransferase. *Connect Tissue Res.* (In press.)
58. Videman T, Eronen I and Friman C (1981) Glycosaminoglycan metabolism in experimental osteoarthrosis caused by immobilization. *Acta Orthop Scand* **52**: 11–21.
59. Ruy J, Treadwell B V and Mankin H J (1984) Biochemical and metabolic abnormalities in normal and osteoarthrotic human articular cartilage. *Arthritis Rheum* **27**: 49–57.
60. Sandy J D, Adams M E, Billingham M E J, Plaas A and Muir H (1984) Stimulation of chondrocyte biosynthetic activity in early experimental osteoarthritis as determined *in vivo* and *in vitro*. *Arthritis Rheum* **27**: 388–97.
61. Carney S L, Billingham M E J, Muir H and Sandy J D (1984) Demonstration of increased proteoglycan turnover in cartilage explants from dogs with experimental osteoarthritis. *J Orthop Res* **2**: 201–6.
62. Eronen I and Videman T (1986) Keratan sulphate metabolism during development of experimental osteoarthrosis. *Scand J Rheumatol (Suppl)* **60**: 17.
63. Zirn J R, Schurman D J and Smith R L (1984) Keratan sulfate content and articular cartilage

maturation during postnatal rabbit growth. *J Orthop Res* **2**: 143–50.
64. Heinegård D, Wieslander J, Sheehan J, Paulsson M and Sommarin Y (1985) Separation and characterization of two populations of aggregating proteoglycans from cartilage. *Biochem J* **225**: 95–106.
65. Sommarin Y and Heinegård D (1986) Four classes of cell-associated proteoglycans in suspension cultures of articular cartilage chondrocytes. *Biochem J* **233**: 809–18.
66. Golding J and Ghosh P (1983) Drugs for osteoarthrosis. II: The effects of a glycosaminoglycan polysulphate ester (Arteparon) on proteoglycan aggregation and loss from articular cartilage of immobilized rabbit knee joints. *Curr Ther Res Clin Exp* **34**: 67–80.
67. Pelletier J-P and Martel-Pelletier J (1985) Cartilage degradation by neutral proteoglycanases in experimental osteoarthritis. *Arthritis Rheum* **28**: 1393–401.
68. Pettipher E R, Higgs G A and Henderson B (1987) Interleukin 1 induces leukyte infiltration and proteoglycan degradation in the synovial joint. Proc Natl Acad Sci USA **83**: 8749–53.
69. Kempson G E (1970) *Mechanical properties of human cartilage*. Ph.D. dissertation, University of London.
70. Armstrong C G and Mow V C (1982) Variations in the intrinsic mechanical properties of human articular cartilage with age, degeneration, and water content. *J Bone Joint Surg [Am]* **64**: 88–94.
71. Palmoski M J and Brandt K D (1981) Running inhibits the reversal of atrophic changes in canine knee cartilage after removal of cast. *Arthritis Rheum* **24**: 1329–37.
72. Lee R C, Frank E H, Grodzinsky A J and Roylance D K (1981) Oscillatory compressional behaviour of articular cartilage and its associated electromechanical properties. *J Biomech Eng* **103**: 280–92.
73. Simon M R, Holmes K R and Olsen A M (1985) Effects of simulated increases in body weight on the growth of limb bones in hypophysectomized rats. *Acta Anat (Basel)* **121**: 1–6.
74. Bayliss M T and Ali S Y (1978) Age-related changes in the composition and structure of human articular cartilage proteoglycans. *Biochem J* **176**: 683–93.
75. Bayliss M T, Venn M, Maroudas A and Ali S Y (1983) Structure of proteoglycans from different layers of human articular cartilage. *Biochem J* **209**: 387–400.
76. Pottenger L A, Lyon N B, Hecht J D, Neustadt P M and Robinson R A (1982) Influence of cartilage particle size and proteoglycan aggregation on immobilization of proteoglycans. *J Biol Chem* **257**: 11479–85.
77. Pottenger L A, Webb J E and Lyon N B (1985) Kinetics of extraction of proteoglycans from human articular cartilage. *Arthritis Rheum* **28**: 323–30.
78. Noro A, Kimata K, Oike Y, Shinomura T, Maeda N, Yano S, Takahashi N and Suzuki S (1983) Isolation and characterization of a third proteoglycan (PG-Lt) from chick embryo cartilage which contains disulfide-bonded collagenous polypeptide. *J Biol Chem* **258**: 9323–31.
79. Wiebkin O and Muir H (1973) The inhibition of sulfate incorporation in isolated adult chondrocytes by hyaluronic acid. *FEBS Lett* **37**: 42–6.
80. Solursh M, Hardingham T E, Hascall V C and Kimura J H (1980) Separate effects of exogenous hyaluronic acid on proteoglycan synthesis and deposition in pericellular matrix by cultured chick embryo limb chondrocytes. *Dev Biol* **75**: 121–9.
81. Sommarin Y and Heinegård D (1983) Specific interaction between cartilage proteoglycans and hyaluronic acid at the chondrocyte cell surface. *Biochem J* **214**: 777–84.
82. Elliott R J and Gardner D L (1979) Changes with age in the glycosaminoglycans of human articular cartilage. *Ann Rheum Dis* **38**: 371–7.
83. Roughley P J, White R J and Poole A R (1985) Identification of a hyaluronic acid binding protein that interferes with the preparation of high-buoyant-density proteoglycan aggregates from adult human cartilage. *Biochem J* **231**: 129–38.
84. Krause, W-D (1969) *Mikroskopische Untersuchungen am Gelenkknorpel extrem funktionell belasteter Mäuse–Ein Beitrag Zur Aetiopathogenese degenerativer Gelenkveränderungen*. Dissertation, Köln: Gouder and Hansen.
85. Videman T, Eronen I and Candolin T (1979) Effects of motion load changes on tendon tissues and articular cartilage: a biochemical and scanning electron microscopic study in rabbits. *Scand J Work Environ Health (Suppl 3)* **5**: 56–67.
86. Vasan N (1983) Effects of physical stress on the synthesis and degradation of cartilage matrix. *Connect Tissue Res* **12**: 49–58.
87. Stofft E and Graf J (1983) Rasterelektronmikroskopische Untersuchung des hyalinen Gelenkknorpels. *Acta Anat (Basel)* **116**: 114–25.
88. Ender A and Lessel W (1983) Stadien im Arthroseprozess–eine Rasterelektronmikroskopishe Studie am Kaninchenkniegelenk. *Beitr Orthop Traumatol* **30**: 662–7.

89. Lanier R R (1946) The effects of exercise on the knee-joints of inbred mice. *Anat Rec* **94**: 311–21.

90. Holmdahl D E and Ingelmark B E (1947) Hauptresultate einer experimentellen, morpho-physiologischen Gelenkuntersuchung. *Zool Bidr Uppsala* **25**: 91–101.

91. Sääf J (1950) Effects of exercise on adult cartilage. An experimental study on guinea-pigs with relevance to the continuous regeneration of adult cartilage. *Acta Orthop Scand (Suppl)* **7**: 1–86.

92. Jurvelin J, Kiviranta I, Tammi M and Helminen H J (1986) Effect of physical exercise on indentation stiffness of articular cartilage in the canine knee. *Int J Sports Med* **7**: 106–10.

93. Gilbertson E M M (1975) Development of periarticular osteophytes in experimentally induced osteoarthritis in the dog. *Ann Rheum Dis* **34**: 12–25.

94. Kemppinen T, Kiviranta I, Tammi M and Helminen H J (1986) Both heavy loading and immobilization of the joint decrease proteoglycan concentration in the articular cartilage of young adult guinea pigs. *Scand J Rheumatol (Suppl)* **60**: 42.

95. Säämänen A-M, Tammi M, Kiviranta I, Jurvelin J and Helminen H J (1987) Long term running exercise as a modulator of proteoglycan matrix in the articular cartilage of young rabbits. (Submitted for publication.)

96. Kiviranta I, Tammi M, Jurvelin J, Säämänen A-M and Helminen H J (1986) Moderate running exercise augments glycosaminoglycans and thickness of articular cartilage in the knee joints of young beagle dogs. *J Orthop Res*. (In press.)

97. Säämänen A-M, Tammi M, Kiviranta I, Jurvelin J and Helminen H J (1986) Moderate running increased but strenuous running prevented elevation of proteoglycan content in the canine articular cartilage. *Scand J Rheumatol (Suppl)* **60**: 45.

98. Videman T and Eronen I (1984) Effects of treadmill running on glycosaminoglycans in articular cartilage of rabbits. *Int J Sports Med* **5**: 320–4.

99. Brandt K D and Palmoski M (1976) Organization of ground substance proteoglycans in normal and osteoarthritic knee cartilage. *Arthritis Rheum* **19**: 209–15.

100. Sweet M B E, Thonar E J-M A, Immelman A R and Solomon L (1977) Biochemical changes in progressive osteoarthrosis. *Ann Rheum Dis* **36**: 387–98.

101. Maroudas A (1980) Metabolism of cartilaginous tissues: a quantitative approach. *In: Studies in joint disease Vol 1* (A Maroudas and E J Holborow, eds), pp. 59–68. Tunbridge Wells: Pitman Medical.

102. Poole C A, Flint M H and Beaumont B W (1985) Analysis of the morphology and function of primary cilia in connective tissues: a cellular cybernetic probe? *Cell Motil* **5**: 175–63.

103. Bosman H B (1968) Cellular control of macromolecular synthesis: rates of synthesis of extracellular macromolecules during and after depletion by papain. *Proc R Soc London [Biol]* **169**: 399–425.

104. Milroy S J and Poole A R (1974) Pig articular cartilage in organ culture. Effect of enzymatic depletion of the matrix on response of chondrocytes to complement-sufficient antiserum against pig erythrocytes. *Ann Rheum Dis* **33**: 500–8.

105. Sandy J D, Brown H L G and Lowther D A (1980) Control of proteoglycan synthesis. Studies on the activation of synthesis observed during cultures of articular cartilages. *Biochem J* **188**: 119–30.

106. Hascall V C, Morales T I, Hascall G K, Handley C J and McQuillan D J (1983) Biosynthesis and turnover of proteoglycans in organ culture of bovine articular cartilage. *J Rheumatol (Suppl 11)* **10**: 45–52.

107. Bartholomew J S, Handley C J and Lowther D A (1985) The effects of trypsin on proteoglycan biosynthesis by bovine articular cartilage. *Biochem J* **227**: 429–37.

108. Holmdahl D E and Ingelmark B E (1948) Der Bau des Gelenkknorpels unter verschiedenen funktionellen Verhältnissen. Experimentelle Untersuchung an wachsenden Kaninchen. *Acta Anat (Basel)* **6**: 309–75.

109. Paukkonen K, Selkäinaho K, Jurvelin J, Kiviranta I and Helminen H J (1985) Cells and nuclei of articular cartilage chondrocytes in young rabbits enlarged after non-strenuous physical exercise. *J Anat* **142**: 13–20.

110. Copray J C V M, Jansen H W B and Duterloo H S (1985) Effects of compressive forces on proliferation and matrix synthesis in mandibular condylar cartilage of the rat *in vitro*. *Arch Oral Biol* **30**: 299–304.

111. Veldhuijzen J P, Bourret L A and Rodan G A (1979) *In vitro* studies of the effect of intermittent compressive forces on cartilage cell proliferation. *J Cell Physiol* **98**: 299–306.

112. Palmoski M J and Brandt K D (1984) Effects of static and cyclic compressive loading on

articular cartilage plugs *in vitro*. *Arthritis Rheum* **27**: 675–81.
113. van Kampen G P J, Veldhuijzen J P, Kuijer R, van de Stadt R J and Schipper C A (1985) Cartilage response to mechanical force in high-density chondrocyte cultures. *Arthritis Rheum* **28**: 419–24.
114. Roughley P J and White R J (1980) Age-related changes in the structure of the proteoglycan subunits from human articular cartilage. *J Biol Chem* **255**: 217–24.
115. Thonar E J-M A and Sweet M B E (1981) Maturation-related changes in proteoglycans of fetal articular cartilage. *Arch Biochem Biophys* **208**: 535–47.
116. Roughley P J, White R J and Santer V (1981) Comparison of proteoglycans extracted from high and low weight-bearing human articular cartilage, with particular reference to sialic acid content. *J Biol Chem* **256**: 12699–704.
117. Garg H G and Swann D A (1981) Age-related changes in the chemical composition of bovine articular cartilage. The structure of high-density proteoglycans. *Biochem J* **193**: 459–68.
118. Buckwalter J A, Kuettner K E and Thonar E J-M A (1985) Age-related changes in articular cartilage proteoglycans: electron microscopic studies. *J Orthop Res* **3**: 251–7.
119. Lemperg R, Larsson S-E and Hjertquist S-O (1974) The glycosaminoglycans of bovine articular cartilage. 1. Concentration and distribution in different layers in relation to age. *Calcif Tissue Res* **15**: 237–51.
120. Bayliss M T and Roughley P J (1985) The properties of proteoglycan prepared from human articular cartilage by using associative caesium chloride gradients of high and low starting densities. *Biochem J* **232**: 111–7.
121. Murata K and Bjelle A (1980) Constitutional variations of acidic glycosaminoglycans in normal and arthritic bovine articular cartilage proteoglycans at different ages. *Connect Tissue Res* **7**: 143–56.
122. Plaas A H K and Sandy J D (1984) Age-related decrease in the link stability of proteoglycan aggregates formed by articular chondrocytes. *Biochem J* **220**: 337–40.
123. Melching L I and Roughley P J (1985) The role of link protein in mediating the interaction between hyaluronic acid and newly secreted proteoglycan subunits from adult human articular cartilage. *J Biol Chem* **260**: 16279–85.
124. Bjelle A (1975) Content and composition of glycosaminoglycans in human knee joint cartilage. Variation with site and age in adults. *Connect Tissue Res* **3**: 141–7.
125. Sweet M B E, Thonar E J-M A and Immelman A R (1977) Regional distribution of water and glycosaminoglycan in immature articular cartilage. *Biochim Biophys Acta* **500**: 173–86.
126. Theocharis D A and Tsiganos C P (1985) Age-related changes of proteoglycan subunits from sheep nasal cartilage. *Int J Biochem* **17**: 479–84.

Chapter 4

Natural Ageing and Exercise Effects on Joints

J. M. Walker and S. Bernick

CONTENTS

INTRODUCTION

Arthritis, in some form, affects the daily lives of more than half the individuals in Western populations and accounts for a considerable component of the rising health care costs in those countries. Increased interest and participation, by individuals of all ages in many countries, in physical activity or formal exercise programmes make it essential to establish the interaction between natural ageing of joint tissues and exercise.

Exercise such as jogging, and often aerobic exercise routines, subjects lower limb joints to repetitive rapid loading and unloading. Such exercise is often performed on non-ideal surfaces, such as pavement, non-resilient wooden floors or even concrete floors where minimal shock absorption exists, thus increasing the potential for repetitive microtrauma to joint tissues, in particular the load-bearing surface, articular cartilage. The long-term effects of such exercise await the passage of time to determine whether these effects are beneficial or harmful to joint tissues, if any effect exists. Currently, little scientific evidence exists to support the hypothesis that repetitive rapid loading is harmful to human joint tissues, although some results from studies using animal models suggest that exercise may be harmful to at least the articular cartilage (1–4). Other investigators have shown, without consideration of age, that physical exercise did not significantly alter the articular cartilage (5–11).

Few studies have been reported that focused on the interaction between exercise and ageing of joint tissues with the exercise continued for the majority of the life span or, in fact, for periods greater than 6–10 weeks. It is not established whether exercise can prevent, retard or reverse the progressive age changes reported to occur in human weight-bearing joints, commencing between the third and fourth decades.

Our current knowledge of the interaction between natural ageing and exercise is especially limited in humans, with the difficulty of studying changes in joint tissues *in vivo* throughout the life span. Our knowledge as it exists for man is derived from autopsy and cadaver studies, as well as observations made during surgical procedures. Such populations may not represent an unbiased sample of the total population. In most studies, the health record and physical activity during life is unknown. In animal studies, environmental factors such as temperature, diet and activity, as well as genetic composition can be known. It is unclear, however, whether data obtained from animal models can be extrapolated to humans. Animals are *quadrupedal*; man is *bipedal*. Although strong similarities in joint morphology may exist, differences in joint structure and function are present between the joints of man and animals.

Our knowledge of natural ageing and the interaction with exercise has also been affected by methodological limitations in investigations conducted. Particularly early reports (12–14) were descriptive, i.e. qualitative rather than quantitative. Many other studies on ageing of articular cartilage have been based on small samples from a limited area of the total joint surface; the latter may not be representative of the overall ageing process. Biochemical studies provide quantitative information on the components of cartilage but require tissue in amounts that may necessitate pooling of cartilage samples from all subjects or animals studied (15, 16). Again, these results may not accurately reflect the within-joint and between-joint variation in ageing changes and exercise effects.

In this chapter we will briefly address the development of joints, a component of the ageing process, review the knowledge of natural ageing of joint tissues and examine the effect, if any, of exercise on joint tissues.

DEVELOPMENT OF ARTICULAR STRUCTURES AND ARTICULATIONS

In humans, the major events in joint development occur in the second half of the embryonic period, at the end of which joint cavities have appeared in most large synovial joints. Limb development is a prior event so that faulty limb development, as associated with the drug thalidomide, influences both the presence of a limb joint and its morphology (17, 18).

The only structures that invade the developing limbs from the axial embryo are vessels and nerves: articular tissues all develop *in situ*. The apical epidermal ridge exerts a major influence on the normal development of limbs (19). The first event in synovial joint formation is chondrification, which begins in the blastema and proceeds until the characteristic form of the skeletal elements is achieved. Perichondrium develops, except at the sites of future articulating surfaces.

At the zones of future joints the blastema remains as a chondrogenic homogeneous interzone. Cellular activities in the interzone result in the development of a 3-layered interzone that consists of 2 chondrogenic layers, each continuous at the future joint periphery with the perichondrium, and a middle loose layer which will form the joint cavity. *Fig.* 4.1 illustrates this

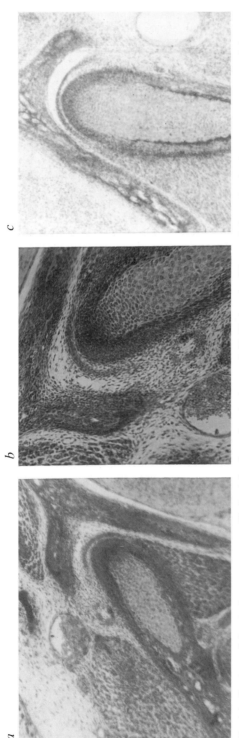

Fig. 4.1. Sections of developing temporomandibular joint from foetal mice aged 15–17 days (× 28). *a*, 15-day-old animal; *note* the presence of dense bands of collagen fibres between the mesenchymal tissue over the condyle and under the future temporal fossa. *b*, *Note* the break in the upper compartment. *c*, An articular space now present in the upper compartment; the same process will occur in the lower compartment.

process. After the appearance of the 3-layered interzone, synovial mesenchyme begins to form in the peripheral part of the interzone, becomes vascularized and gives rise to synovial membrane, fibrous capsule and intra-articular structures such as menisci and ligaments.

Cavity Formation

Cavitation, formation of the joint capsule, and development of the synovial membrane all begin about the same time for any given synovial joint (18). Although the precise nature of cavitation is not well established, it seems the process begins centrally, multiple small openings coalescing to form one cavity which then increases in absolute size while retaining its relative size (18). Hydrolytic enzymes may act on mesenchymal tissue to produce cavitation which usually commences by Stage 23 (20) in the larger joints. Some of the small joints, however, may show considerable delay between differentiation and cavitation; e.g. the joints of the foot and hand may not develop a 3-layered interzone until early in the foetal period.

Sacroiliac joint

For most joints cavitation is complete in the early foetal period, but the sacroiliac joint, which starts cavitation in the 10th week, does not appear to complete this process until the 7th month (21–23). Variability in early achievement of adult-like morphology in a joint may influence the natural ageing of the joint. Studies of the late foetal period have shown that the sacroiliac joint cavity may be interrupted by fibrous bands spanning the two surfaces (*Fig.* 4.2a) (22, 23). It is unknown whether these bands disappear with increased movement postnatally. Should these bands be retained, their presence may contribute to hypomobility in young adults and to the reported early fusion of this joint; by the fourth decade in males and the fifth in females (22–30) (*Fig.* 4.2b, *Table* 4.1).

Other joints show differences in the normal joint developmental sequence. The acromioclavicular joint does not demonstrate the usual homogeneous then 3-layered interzone; the sternochondral joints show cartilaginous continuity in the early stages, with subsequent cavitation uncertain (18) and the temporomandibular joint develops where a continuous blastema never existed (18, 31).

Temporomandibular joint

Cavity formation in the temporomandibular joint is visualized in *Fig.* 4.1. A split occurs in the mesenchymal tissue below the temporal fossa and future connective tissue disc. Soon after, a similar tearing process occurs in the mesenchymal tissue between the condylar surface and the future disc; two spaces are formed, the upper and lower compartments.

Similar to the iliac surface of the sacroiliac joint, the condylar head of the mandible consists of a thin connective tissue covering at the disc surface (*Fig.* 4.3). Perhaps because of the habitual use of this joint, the age changes

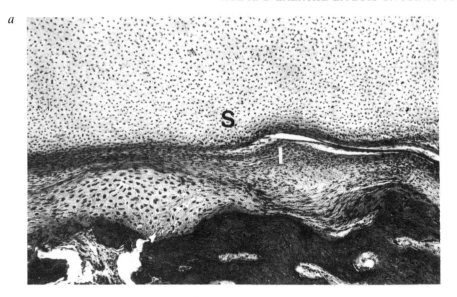

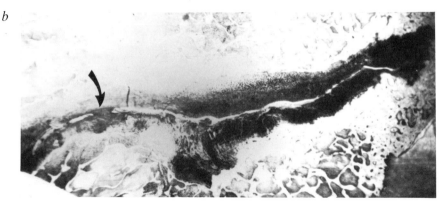

Fig. 4.2. Human sacroiliac joint. S, sacrum; I, ilium. *a*, Section from a 16-week-old foetus, CR = 15·2 cm; *note* the proximity of the iliac bone to the joint surface, partial cavitation, a fibrous band connecting the 2 surfaces, presence of the 3-layered interzone on the left, and the more fibrous iliac surface (haematoxylin, × 22). *b*, Section from an 81-year-old female; *note* the variability in the two surfaces, especially the iliac. *Arrow* indicates an area of fibrous ankylosis with chondroid cells. [From Walker, 1986 (22), with permission.]

observed are similar to those which occur in other joints studied by the authors. The temporomandibular joint, despite the fibrous mandibular surface, does not seem prone to early fusion as occurs in the sacroiliac joint (31).

The sequence of developmental events may thus vary slightly within specific joints. It is not established whether variability in early development influences the natural ageing of the joint. Detailed analyses of the development of individual joints have been provided by many investigators (31–48).

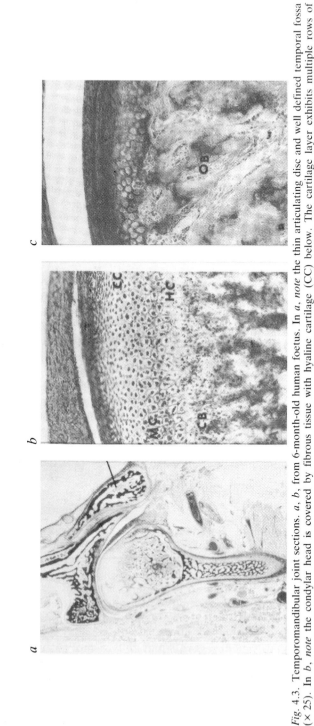

Fig. 4.3. Temporomandibular joint sections. *a*, *b*, from 6-month-old human foetus. In *a*, *note* the thin articulating disc and well defined temporal fossa (× 25). In *b*, *note* the condylar head is covered by fibrous tissue with hyaline cartilage (CC) below. The cartilage layer exhibits multiple rows of dividing chondrocytes (MC), and a hypertrophy zone made up of larger cells (HC). Bone is present below the cartilage (CB). *c*, Head of the condyle from an old marmoset; *note* the fibrous proliferation (OB) and bone sealing off the cartilage (× 50).

Table 4.1 Partial and complete ankylosis of the human sacroiliac joint, by age and percentage of sample.

Author	Number in sample	Age (years)	% of sample
Brooke, 1924 (30)	210	> 50	76 M*
Saskin, 1930 (26)	257	31–59	51 M, 5 F**
	103	> 60	82 M, 30 F
MacDonald &			
Hunt, 1952 (24)	57	20–70+	20
Resnick *et al.*, 1975 (25)	46	24–80	6.5
Stewart 1984 (27)	1417	> 50	14 M, 4 F
Walker 1986 (22)	15	49–84	33

* M = male
** F = female

Foetal Development

From the end of the 7th post-ovulatory week, foetal development of joints proceeds, most noticeably involving an increase in the size of formed structures, maturation of those structures, an increase in the amount of collagenous tissue which results in clear definition of fibrous tissue structures, and extension of the joint cavity. In certain joints such as the sacroiliac, cavitation is completed. Synovial villae and bursae appear and increase in number, fat cells are noted around the 4th–5th month, marking the sites of future fat pads, and some elastic fibres are present in the fibrous capsule. Ligaments and tendons become increasingly avascular (18). Nerve fibres begin to enter joint cavities in the foetal period but specialized neural elements, such as Ruffini and Pacini endings, only occur late in the foetal period (49).

Role of Movement in Joint Development and Maturation

Experimental studies of amphibian, avian, and mammalian joints indicate that neither growth pressure nor movement are essential to either the primary development or the initial form of joints. Experiments on avian joints, however, indicate that movement is required for the initiation and maintenance of cavitation in avians. Induced paralysis resulted in a decrease in size and often fusion of joint surface occurred, with loss of previously present 3-layered interzone (50–55).

This important role of movement in the development of avian joints is not clearly demonstrated for mammalian joints, although it is known that movement is important in maintaining and in moulding the articular form of human joints once the form is established. This process continues in the postnatal period and may be very influential in the production of normal morphology in adulthood. This may be more important in those joints whose movement excursion is increasingly restricted in the later foetal period by the finite expansion potential of the uterus with the often almost fixed posture of joints, especially those of the lower limbs. The human hip joint appears particularly affected by the late *in utero* conditions.

Studies on human foetal hip joints have demonstrated disparity between the growth rates of the hip socket and the head of femur (47). At birth, less of the femoral head is encompassed by the acetabulum than at any other life period, pre- or postnatal. Fell and Canti's studies showed the important influence of pressure on the development of the normal contour of spherical surfaces such as the acetabulum (50). It is well established that the human hip joint is frequently involved either as part of an isolated dislocation or as part of a complex of congenital malformations (56, 57). The congenital anomalies of joints, such as the shallow socket of congenital hip dysplasia, occur during the foetal period and are especially characterized by growth retardation. Dunn has termed these congenital postural deformities 'pathology which develops in the foetal period'. Many of these resolve spontaneously or respond to early postural correction. They are probably produced by mechanical factors *in utero*, related to foetal position, the amount of amniotic fluid and tightness of the uterine wall; they are essentially non-structural (58–60).

It is evident that moulding of joint surfaces by movement and pressure stimuli are important aspects of the postnatal development and maturation of joints. These factors may account for the apparent spontaneous remission of congenital hip subluxation and/or dislocation that has been reported (61, 62).

The neonatal hip joint is cartilaginous and thus is poorly visualized on radiographs before 3 months of postnatal age. Consequently many cases of simple dysplasia or shallow socket may be undetected. Osteoarthrosis frequently involves larger joints such as the hip joint. The contribution of imperfect early formation of appropriate joint morphology to early incidence of joint problems with ageing is not yet clearly established, but theoretically a contribution is likely. The so-called 'normal' hip joint of individuals with unilateral congenital hip dislocation (CHD), who were placed in hip spicas as part of the treatment procedure, also may develop ischaemic necrosis (63, 64) and present with earlier signs and symptoms of osteoarthrosis than in the non-CHD adult population. Such cases suggest that restriction of motion in the early postnatal period is not beneficial to normal development and maturation of the joint, and may influence the ageing process.

NATURAL AGEING

Studies on the ageing of articulations have been made on samples of human autopsy and cadaver materials, while most studies employing animal models have used cage-confined laboratory animals. Use of the term 'natural ageing' herein is thus limited to these populations and the findings may not be truly representative of the ageing process in free-ranging wild animals or humans. Autopsies are performed on less than 40% of Western populations, while those who donated their remains to science form an even smaller group.

Changes attributed to ageing are reported at all levels of examination, from gross appearance to cellular changes with ultramicroscopy, as well as biochemical and mechanical changes (1, 12–14, 16, 22–24, 65–84). Many of these changes lie on a continuum with those reported in pathologies such as osteoarthrosis. The distinction between changes that are physiological alterations with ageing, and pathological alterations from environmentally produced microtrauma in the absence of disease or frank injury, is unclear.

More studies have been conducted on samples of articular cartilage than examination of whole joints, so that our knowledge of the ageing process in joints is largely limited to articular cartilage and its underlying subchondral bone. Bennett *et al.* reported the first comprehensive study of the ageing process in joints (12). These investigators studied knee joints from autopsies. Other investigators have substantiated their findings (13, 14, 22, 65–81, 83, 85). The numerous changes in cartilage concomitant with ageing in human material are similar in animals (68, 71, 72, 85).

Morphological and Histological Observations

Articular cartilage undergoes a gross alteration from a bluish, transparent structure to a yellowish opaque structure. The joint surfaces exhibit variable degrees of surface cracking, fraying and fibrillation (68). Fibrillation is regarded as an age-related process (73); its presence has been noted from the third decade of life in human autopsy material (12). It was not observed in any of the knee joints we examined from 12 marmosets between 8 and 12 years of age (Walker *et al.*, unpublished data). Goodfellow and Bullough (81), however, related fibrillation seen in the human elbow joint primarily to joint mechanics, since they observed greater changes by joint type than age; i.e. the changes were greater in multiaxial joint surfaces than in uniaxial joint surfaces.

Cartilage depth may be reduced, involving changes in both the uncalcified and calcified zones, as well as the presence of multiple tidemarks. Results from several studies support the decrease in matrix components such as glycosaminoglycans and chondroitin-4- and 6-sulphates, while keratan sulphate is reported to increase with age; chondrocyte frequencies may decrease (3, 69–71, 85). There is, however, variability in the changes reported by investigators as to whether components of articular cartilage matrix increased or decreased. Biochemical studies provide better quantitative data than histochemical studies whose analysis has frequently been only qualitative. However, the pooling of samples required in biochemical studies to obtain adequate amounts of tissue for analysis obscures variability in changes that non-biochemical studies have described.

We have recently examined the histochemical changes in articular cartilage with ageing in knee joints from 38 female Wistar rats used in a study of the effects of exercise and ageing on muscle (86). Fourteen animals were obtained at 5 months of age and 24 at 10 months of age. Animals were sacrificed at 3 month intervals up to 24 months of age, which is roughly equivalent to early old age, or 65 years, in humans. The changes in joint tissues other than cartilage were unremarkable; classification of animals into age groups based on age changes in joint tissues could not be reliably made (3).

In young animals, as also observed in mouse, non-human primates and man, the articular cartilage reacts intensely to alcian blue and light pink to the PAS reaction, indicating a higher proteoglycan content. With silver nitrate impregnation the matrix was homogeneous in structure (*Fig. 4.4a*). This appearance is due to the presence of Type II collagen instead of Type I, seen in skin and bone. On the other hand, the matrices of the aged animals and man were strongly positive with Schiff's reagent and showed a loss of alcian blue staining. In the articular cartilage of the knee joint, lumbar vertebrae, and the temporomandibular joint from the above animals, there were argyrophilic fibres demonstrable in the matrices of the various joints (*Fig. 4.4c*).

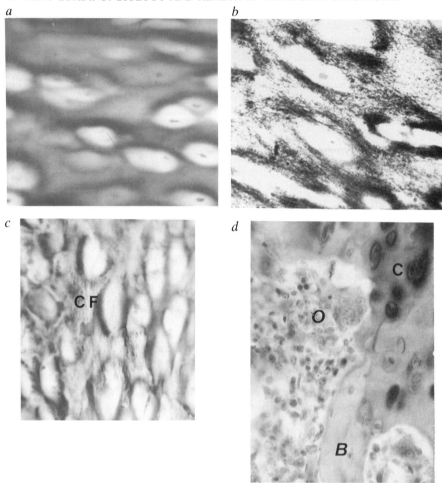

Fig. 4.4. Articular cartilage (silver nitrate impregnation; × 250). *a*, Section from a newborn marmoset; the intercellular matrix appears homogeneous and exhibits no argyrophilic collagen fibres. *b*, Section of end plate cartilage from a 17-year-old human; *note* the appearance of argyrophilic fine fibres in the matrix. *c, d*, Lumbar vertebral end plate cartilage from a female in the middle 30s; in *c*, *note* the appearance of small silver granules associated with the collagen fibres (CF) and intercellular matrix; in *d*, an osteoclast (O) is seen adjacent to the calcified cartilage (C) of the articular layer: *note* the presence of bone (B) adjacent to the calcified cartilage. [*c*: From Bernick and Cailliet, 1982 (74), with permission.]

The grainy or fibrillar appearance in the cartilage matrix of older animals is indicative of an unmasking of collagen fibres; this change can be visible even with haematoxylin and eosin staining. Silver impregnation demonstrates argyrophilic collagen fibres as well as fine black granules that are suggestive of calcification. The changes in both the ground substance and collagen fibres predisposes the cartilaginous matrix to calcification which then is susceptible to osteoclastic resorption. The loss of calcified cartilage leads to the deposition of bone adjacent to the resorbed cartilage (*Fig.* 4.4*d*).

In the rat study osteoporotic changes were evident in the subchondral bone which, in many sections, abutted the tidemark. These changes were similar to our findings in old marmosets (*Fig.* 4.5*d*, unpublished data) and to reports by other investigators (14, 24, 65–67, 71, 72, 83). Freeman and Meachim (73), however, did not find changes in the total amount of cartilage with age, although they stated this need not preclude alteration in the morphology of collagen

a   *b*

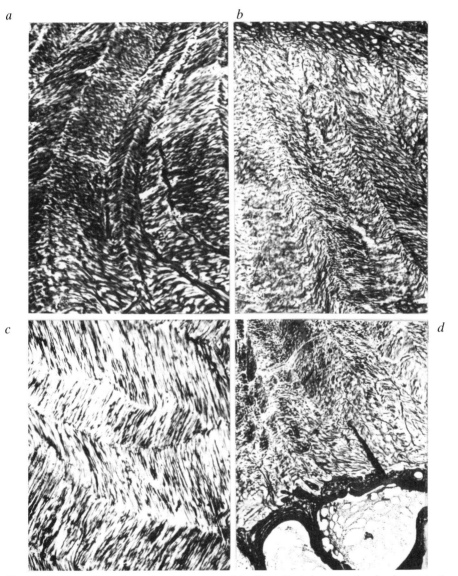

c   *d*

Fig. 4.5. Sections of annulus and vertebra exposed to silver nitrate impregnation for demonstration of argyrophilic collagen fibres ($\times$ 45). *a*, The laminae are well oriented and fibres are distinct in section from a young human adult. *b*, In a 65-year-old individual the laminae are still regularly arranged, but there is disruption and fragmentation of the collagen elements. *c*, *Note* the marked loss of collagenous fibres, and the presence of chondroid cells in section from an individual over 70 years. *d*, *Note* the thin layer of bone adjacent to the annulus and the severe osteoporosis in section from a 83-year-old female. [From Bernick and Cailliet, 1982 (74), with permission.]

fibres. Argyrophilic and large diameter fibres in Sokoloff's experience were not characteristic of human ageing or osteoarthrotic cartilage (87).

Thicker, less resilient collagen fibres within cartilage, together with calcification of the deeper layers, would alter the biomechanical properties of the load-bearing surfaces and theoretically impair normal nutrition to the deeper layers, further promoting adverse changes. In several studies, on both human material (intervertebral discs) and in animal models (marmosets, rats), many capillaries showed a thick basement membrane, staining deep red with PAS, although lymphatic vessels of the same calibre were still thin walled in older specimens (*Fig.* 4.6). (74, 75, 88). While these changes within capillaries would impair cartilage nutrition through interference with synovial fluid production, the lack of change in lymphatic vessels of the subsynovial tissues should allow removal of waste products.

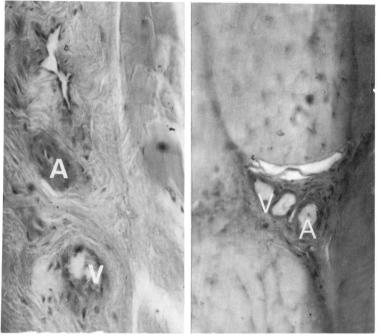

a   *b*

Fig. 4.6. Sections of microvasculature in the lateral surface of the annulus (× 150). *a*, Young human adult; the walls of the arteriole (A) and venule (V) are lightly stained by the PAS reaction. In contrast, in *b*, from an individual over 65 years of age, these vessels and the interstitial connective tissue stained intensely red by PAS–haematoxylin, and the lumina also were occluded.

With ageing, several investigators have reported fibrosis of the synovial membrane and subsynovial tissues, as well as chondroid-like changes in ligaments. Such changes in ligaments may account for increased stiffness and tensile strength (89, 90). Viidik considered this related to increase in collagen with increased amounts of inter- and intramolecular cross-links. He, however, concluded that as deleterious effects had not been demonstrated with such changes, they should be characterized as a maturing rather than an ageing process (89).

Stress/strain studies are probably more likely to reveal age changes than histological or histochemical studies, as such studies would assess the major fibrous component of these tissues, collagen. Hall (76) commented that age changes in cellular components of connective tissues are similar to those of cells in other organs and that it is in the intercellular components that most ageing changes occur. Old collagen loses its ability to return to the resting state and remains in the extended state for longer periods than young collagen. These are changes which alter the resilience and compliance of the structure (76). The altered solubility of collagen with age is due to formation of cross-bridges, first demonstrated by Verzar (91). Particularly in skin and vessels, but also in the intervertebral disc, a change in collagen type is reported to occur with ageing. Eyre (92) demonstrated increased amounts of Type II collagen in the annulus with ageing which, because Type II predominates in the nucleus, obscures the demarcation between these two disc areas as age progresses. The change in clear demarcation between the annulus and nucleus can be demonstrated histochemically, as shown in *Fig.* 4.7.

The Intervertebral Disc

Distinction of natural age-associated changes in the intervertebral disc is complicated by the high incidence of low back and cervical pathology in most populations (93), as well as the common presence of osteoporosis in vertebrae. Many investigators have reported ageing changes within the disc, ranging from decreases in chondroitin-4- and 6-sulphates (94, 95), glycoprotein content (96), and water content (97–99), as well as fibrosis, chondroid changes and calcification (Bernick, unpublished data; *Figs.* 4.5, 4.7). The ratio of chondroitin-4- and 6-sulphates to keratan sulphate decreases and this change, with the dehydration of the disc, will cause the disc to be a less resilient structure which is less capable of absorbing shock, and potentially increase microfractures within the osteoporotic vertebral bodies.

Several of these changes have considerable import to the nutrition of the disc. Vertebral end plate changes include a gradual calcification of the articular cartilage, followed by resorption of the cartilage and replacement by bone (74) (*Fig.* 4.7). Bernick and Cailliet also observed vascular changes in the bone adjacent to the articular cartilage and disc in specimens from individuals older than 45 years (74). Nutrient canals and spaces in bone adjacent to cartilage were partially or completely occluded with material which stained intensely PAS-positive, indicative of neutral polysaccharides and sialic acid. In comparison, the same canals and spaces from younger individuals were patent and filled with either loose connective tissue or myeloid elements (*Fig.* 4.6).

Similar age changes have been observed in marmoset vertebrae (75). Changes in the microvasculature, as well as obliteration of nutrient channels, in addition to the presence of calcified cartilage, would produce interference with the normal flow of nutrients through end plates to the disc. Other investigators have shown a decrease in diffusion through vertebral end plates (100–102). Holm and Rosenqvist, in a non-ageing study on female rats, showed that both transport

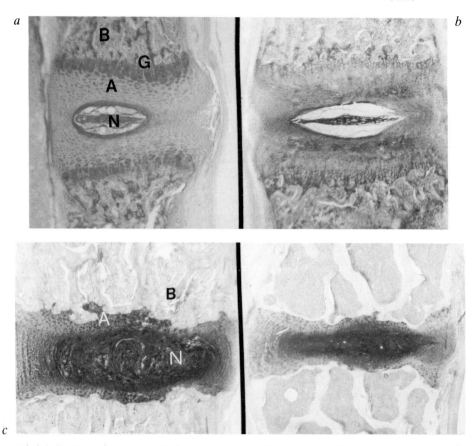

Fig. 4.7. Sections of marmoset lumbar verterbrae. *a*, Newborn; *note* the presence of growth (G) and articular (A) cartilage making up the end plates of the vertebra (N, nucleus pulposus) (× 38). *b*, At 5 months of age there are still 2 layers of cartilage in the end plates, and a decrease in the width of the growth layer (× 38). *c*, At 4 years of age there is a disappearance of the growth cartilage and a marked decrease in the width of the articulating layer; *note* that the nucleus pulposus appears fibrotic in nature (× 35). *d*, At 8 years of age there is only a thin zone of articular cartilage remaining and in certain areas bone (B) is adjacent to the disc (× 35).

and metabolism of the disc unit were 'severely affected' after 10 weeks of treadmill exercise (103). It is not established whether exercise in older animals augments or retards nutrition to the disc.

We recently examined lumbar vertebrae with the intervening intervertebral disc at autopsies, from 49 individuals of both sexes between birth and 83 years of age. The distinct organization of laminae within the annulus decreased with age, becoming disrupted and replaced with chondroid tissue; these changes were more noticeable in specimens from individuals over 65 years of age (*Fig.* 4.5) (unpublished data).

Concomitant with the changes in laminae was an apparent weakening of the anchorage of the annulus to the bony end plate as collagen fibres were embedded more superficially into the bone. Naylor (77) and Happey *et al.* (104)

showed, with roentgenographic crystallography in young adults, that annular collagen was made up of well ordered fibrils of medium thickness which should convey high tensile strength to the annulus. With increasing age, however, they demonstrated fibres with increased crystalline precipitation and fibrillation. These collagen fibre changes, together with matrix changes, may theoretically prevent normal damping and dissipation of forces from the nucleus to the annulus. The annulus is also less able to absorb uniformly the forces exerted upon it. Further negative alterations then may occur, eventually resulting in frank pathology.

Use of laboratory animals

Although minor variability exists between descriptions of age-related changes in various joints from human and animals, similarity in the overall changes in subchondral bone, articular cartilage, and other joint tissues, when included in the study, is apparent. DeRousseau (105, 106) has compared musculoskeletal ageing in both caged and free-ranging Rhesus monkeys. Both sexes, in both colonies, demonstrated similar rates of age-related decline in joint mobility. The free-ranging animals, however, developed spinal and hip degeneration some-what earlier and faster than the caged animals. Earlier onset (second decade) of degeneration was also noted in comparison with reports on humans. These studies suggest that, if there is a bias in the use of caged laboratory animals in ageing studies, it may be to underestimate the degree of change. Further, these studies indicate the need of caution in extrapolating findings from different animal species to humans.

INTERACTION BETWEEN EXERCISE AND AGEING

Few investigators have examined the interaction between exercise and ageing of articular tissues; even fewer researchers have reported studies in which exercise was performed for the majority of the animal's life span. It is not established whether exercise can prevent, retard or reverse any of the progressive age-related changes reported to commence between the second and third decades in humans and different animal species. Few data exist on this topic for joint tissues other than articular cartilage.

Without consideration of age, in studies employing young and adult animals, investigators have demonstrated that physical exercise did not significantly alter articular cartilage (5–10, 107). Many studies also have involved immobilization or continuous passive motion; these topics, as well as interaction between immobilization and physical exercise studies, will not be addressed here because they are covered by other authors within this text (108, 109).

Microtrauma (defined as undetected specific events) during the life span may theoretically result in eventual wear-and-tear changes to articular tissues, and accelerate cartilage destruction. Such microtraumas are most likely to result from high impact loading and unloading activities such as jogging, running, skipping and the jumping-type exercises which are often part of aerobic exercise programmes. Few studies employing animal models duplicate the above types of stresses to which human beings may subject their joints during a lifetime. Most animal studies have involved treadmill running of various intensities, using some type of track with a surface which is more resilient and shock absorbing than pavement or concrete surfaces. It is therefore, perhaps, not surprising that more studies have demonstrated a lack of significant effect of physical exercise on articular cartilage (5–11).

Observations on Articular Cartilage

There is, however, some evidence that exercise may be harmful to articular cartilage. Excessive stress-induced cartilage destruction has been associated with occupation and participation in professional sport (110). Recently Candolin and Videman, in a non-ageing study, showed fewer degenerative surface changes in the femoral heads of rabbits with submaximal compared to 'sudden maximal' running. These investigators noted fewer changes in wild hares compared with laboratory rabbits (111).

Vasan (2) reported greater wear-and-tear type changes in the articular area of femoral heads from dogs exercised on a treadmill compared with control animals. Detection of changes in any articular tissue, either positive or negative, may be dependent on the type of investigation conducted. Paukkonen *et al.* detected no qualitative differences between exercised and control groups of young rabbits in non-strenuous horizontal treadmill exercise for 8 weeks (112); however, an increase in cell size in articular cartilage of the exercised group was demonstrated. Sääf (113) also observed an increase in chondrocyte size in his exercised (running) group of adult guinea pigs, while Helminen and co-workers demonstrated an increase in number but a decrease in volume and volume density of chondrocytes after 'strenuous' running in beagles (114).

Although changes such as altered stainability of histological sections of cartilage from exercised animals may be observed, either fewer histological lesions (7) or no structural changes (115) were reported. Paukkonen and associates have developed a quantitative stereological method to detect small histological changes in articular tissues. As previously stated, even with this technique no such changes were observed (112). The Finnish workers have shown a positive change in articular cartilage proteoglycans following moderate but not strenuous running in young Beagles (116) with no signs of surface degeneration after a 15-week programme of running (117).

Effect of Exercise of 6 Months and Greater Duration in Rats

From a recent light microscopy study of female rats, Walker reported an inability to reliably distinguish animals by age group or exercise/sedentary groups using histochemistry (3). Animals were moderately exercised (75% of heart rate maximum) on a level treadmill 5 days/week, for periods of 6–12 months, between the ages of 6 and 24 months (86).

In contrast to other studies, however, distinct structural changes were observed in the form of defects in the articular cartilage (*Fig.* 4.8). The frequency of such defects was significantly greater in the exercised group of animals, although not between animals exercised for 6 months and those exercised for 12 months. The majority of defects observed were located immediately superficial to the tidemark in the uncalcified layer of cartilage.

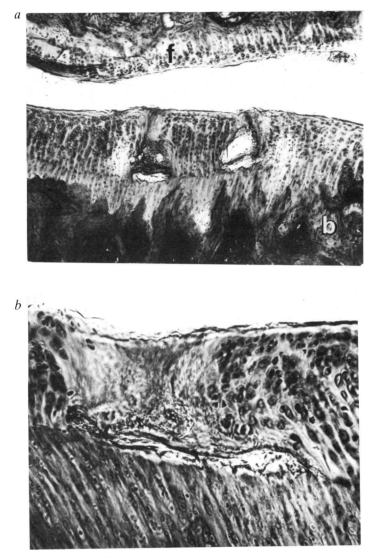

Fig. 4.8. Defects in the uncalcified articular cartilage layer of the lateral tibial condyle in *a*, an 18-month-old rat exercised for 6 months (× 30); *b*, 18-month-old animal exercised for 12 months: *note* the proximity to the tidemark, and the acellular areas superficial to the defects, as well as (in *a*) the depth difference in the femoral and tibial cartilages. f, femoral; b, subchondral bone (× 235). [From Walker, 1986 (3), with permission.]

Table 4.2 demonstrates that control animals, at all ages, also exhibited similar defects, although fewer and smaller in size than observed in the exercised animals. Fifteen months old control animals showed more sections with defects than older control animals, and had similar percentages to the exercised group. Control animals were presumed to be sedentary. All animals were housed in pairs in standard (21 × 34 cm) cages. It is unlikely that the unobserved activity of caged animals could approach that of the running group. As other conditions were held constant between groups, two conclusions may be derived from this study. Firstly, it would seem that defects in the uncalcified layer of articular cartilage occur naturally in rats and may not be related to age, since the percentage of involved sections from control animals did not increase with age. In fact, 2 old control animals (24 months) showed no defects. Secondly, the higher frequency and greater severity of defects in the exercised group suggests that exercise of the intensity used aggravated changes and may have been harmful to articular cartilage. These results differed from those of Williams *et al.* (4) who concluded, from a study of treadmill exercise by rats, that the exercise may have contributed to the frequency but not the severity of lesions. A tidemark-located lesion, similar to that reported by Walker (3), has also been observed by Van Sickle in dogs exercised in a step-up/step-down activity (personal communication, 1986).

Table 4.2 Mean percentage of defects in the articular cartilage of rats, by exercise and control groups, and age.[#]

Groups	Number in sample	Exercise duration (months)	Age at death (months)	Mean % in tissue sections
*Exercised**	13		18–24	24.0
Older	3	12	24	27.6
Younger**	4	6	18	18.9
Control	6	12	18	25.7
Older**	11		18–24	11.6
Old	4		24	12.6
	3		21	4.7
Younger	4		18	15.8
Young	13		6–15	13.3
	3		15	25.2
	3		12	14.0
	3		9	6.0
	3		6	7.9

[#] Adapted from Walker, 1986 (3).
* Significant differences in mean % between exercised animals and the older control group.
** Nonsignificant differences between animals exercised for 6 or 12 months, and between the older and young control subgroups.

Osteophyte formation at the joint margin is a frequent observation in osteoarthrotic joints. Williams and Brandt (11) recently reported acclerated osteophyte formation in joints of guinea pigs given daily treadmill exercise following a chemically induced injury to the articular cartilage. They also observed some protective effects to cartilage in the exercised animals. No osteophytes were observed in Walker's study.

CONCLUSIONS

The evidence for interaction between natural ageing (as defined) and exercise is meagre and substantive data do not exist to either support or refute a positive or negative effect of exercise over time. There is a great need for longitudinal rather than cross-sectional studies. There also is a need for investigators to achieve some standardization with respect to exercise programmes and descriptive terms applied to those programmes. Few investigators assess the maximum heart rate and develop an exercise programme which is a percentage of the maximum heart rate, a common practice in humans. Strenuous exercise for animals is usually exercise to exhaustion. In submaximal exercise, however, motivation to exercise may vary between animals; not all animals may be stressed to the same degree. More importantly, interspecies differences in joint morphology, pedalism, joint and limb mechanics make extrapolation from animal studies to man questionable. More studies are needed on humans. Inexpensive, non-invasive methodology requires development to enable *in vivo* study of the age-related changes in joint tissues and the role of exercise in the ageing process.

CLINICAL SIGNIFICANCE

The long-term effects of exercise are less well known in humans than in the laboratory animals. Many studies have shown that repetitive loading may be harmful to human joints, but a lot of evidence supports the view that physical exercise does not cause untoward effects on the articular cartilage. In this chapter potential consequences of the treatment of congenital hip disease was discussed.

Non-invasive methods are needed to examine the interaction between exercise and natural ageing *in vivo* in human joints.

REFERENCES

1. Tonna E A (1981) Electron microscopy of skeletal aging. *In*: *Aging and Cell Structure, Vol 1* (J E Johnson Jr, ed) pp. 251–304. New York: Plenum.
2. Vasan N (1983) Effects of physical stress on the synthesis and degradation of cartilage matrix. *Connect Tissue Res* **12**: 49– 58.
3. Walker J M (1986) Exercise and its influence on aging in rat knee joints. *J Orthop Sports Phys Ther* **8**(6): 310–19.
4. Williams J M, Felten D L, Peterson R G and O'Connor B L (1982) Effects of surgically induced instability on rat knee articular cartilage. *J Anat* **134**: 103–9.
5. Dekel S and Weissman S L (1978) Joint changes after overuse and peak overloading of rabbit knees *in vivo*. *Acta Orthop Scand* **49**: 519–28.
6. Jurvelin J, Kuusela T, Heikkilä R, Pelttari A, Kiviranta I, Tammi M and Helminen H J (1983) Investigation of articular cartilage surface morphology with semi-quantitative scanning electron microscopic method. *Acta Anat* **116**: 302–11.
7. Lanier R R (1946) The effects of exercise on the knee joints of inbred mice. *Anat Rec* **94**: 311–21.
8. Salter R B, Simmonds D F, Malcom B W, Rumble E J, MacMichael D and Clements N D (1980) The biological effects of continuous passive motion on the healing of full-thickness defects in articular cartilage. *J Bone Joint Surg [Am]* **62**: 1232–51.
9. Videman T (1982) The effect of running on the osteoarthritic joint: an experimental matched-pair study with rabbits. *Rheumatol Rehabil* **21**: 1–8.
10. Videman T, Eronen I and Candolin T (1979) Effects of motion load changes on tendon tissues and articular cartilage. A biochemical and scanning electron microscopic study. *Scand J Work Environ Health* **5** (Suppl 3): 56–67.
11. Williams J M and Brandt K D (1984) Exercise increases osteophyte formation and diminishes fibrillation following chemically induced articular cartilage injury. *J Anat* **139**: 599–611.

12. Bennett G A, Waine E and Bauer W (1942) *Changes in the knee joint at various ages; with particular reference to the nature and development of degenerative joint disease.* New York: Commonwealth Fund.
13. Jeffrey M R (1960) The waning joint. *Am J Med Sci* **239**: 104–24.
14. Davies D V (1961) Aging changes in joints. *In*: *Structural Aspects of Aging* (G H Bourne, ed). New York: Hafner.
15. Paquin J D, Rest M, Marie P J, Mort J S, Pidoux I, Poole A R and Roughley P J (1983) Biochemical and morphologic studies of cartilage from the adult human sacroiliac joint. *Arthritis Rheum* **26**: 887–95.
16. Buckwalter J A, Kuettner K E and Thonar E J-M (1985) Age-related changes in articular cartilage proteoglycans: electron microscopic studies. *J Orthop Res* **3**: 251–7.
17. Moore K L (1982) *The Developing Human*, 3rd Ed, p. 158. Philadelphia: Saunders.
18. O'Rahilly R and Gardner E (1978) The embryology of movable joints. *In*: *The Joints and Synovial Fluid. Vol 1* (L Sokoloff, ed.), pp. 49–103. New York: Academic Press.
19. Krey A K, Dayton D H and Goetinck P F (1984) NICHD Research workshop: normal and abnormal development of the limb. *Teratology* **29**: 315–23.
20. O'Rahilly R (1973) Developmental stages in human embryos, including a survey of the Carnegie collection. Part A: Embryos of the first three weeks (Stages 1 to 9). Washington, D.C.: Carnegie Institution of Washington (Publication 631).
21. Schunke G B (1938) The anatomy and development of the sacro-iliac joint in man. *Anat Rec* **72**: 313–31.
22. Walker J M (1986) Age-related differences in the human sacroiliac joint: a histological study; implications for therapy. *J Orthop Sports Phys Ther* **7**: 325–34.
23. Bowen V and Cassidy J D (1981) Macroscopic and microscopic anatomy of the sacroiliac joint from embryonic life until the eighth decade. *Spine* **6**: 620–8.
24. MacDonald G R and Hunt T E (1952) Sacroiliac joints. Observations on the gross and histological changes in the various age groups. *Can Med Assoc J* **66**: 157–63.
25. Resnick D, Niwayama G and Georgen T G (1975) Degenerative disease of the sacroiliac joint. *Invest Radiol* **10**: 608–21.
26. Saskin D (1930) Critical analysis of the anatomy and the pathological changes of the sacroiliac joints. *J Bone Joint Surg [Am]* **12**: 891–910.
27. Stewart T D (1984) Pathological changes in aging sacroiliac joints. A study of dissecting-room skeletons. *Clin Orthop* **183**: 188–96.
28. Volger J B, Brown W H, Helms C A and Genant H K (1984) The normal sacroiliac joint: a CT study of asymptomatic patients. *Radiology* **151**: 433–7.
29. Weisl H (1954) The articular surfaces of the sacroiliac joint and their relation to the movements of the sacrum. *Acta Anat* **22**: 1–14.
30. Brooke R (1924) The sacroiliac joint. *J Anat* **58**: 299–305.
31. Furstman L (1963) The early development of the human temporomandibular joint. *Am J Orthod* **49**: 672–82.
32. Strayer L W Jr (1943) Embryology of the human hip joint. *Yale J Biol Med* **16**: 13–26.
33. Scarpa G G P, Marchini M and Nicoletti P (1977) Osservazioni sullo sviluppo dell'articolazione scapulo-omerale nell'Uarno, con particolare riferimento al suoi rapporti con il tendine de capa lungo del musculo bicipite del braccio. *Arch Ital Anat Embriol* **82**: 85–98.
34. Rooker G (1975) The embryology of the human hip joint. *J Anat* **119**: 398.
35. Andersen H (1962) Histochemical studies of the development of the human hip joint. *Acta Anat (Basel)* **48**: 258–92.
36. Andersen H (1963) Histochemistry and development of the human shoulder and acromioclavicular joint with particular reference to the early development of the clavicle. *Acta Anat (Basel)* **55**: 124–65.
37. Andersen H and Bro-Rasmussen F (1961) Histochemical studies on the histogenesis of the joints in human foetuses with special reference to the development of joint cavities in the hand and foot. *Am J Anat* **108**: 111–22.
38. Gardner E (1972) Prenatal development of the human hip joint, femur, and hip bone. *AAOS Instruct Course Lect* **21**: 138–54.
39. Gardner E and Gray D J (1953) Prenatal development of the human shoulder and acromioclavicular joints. *Am J Anat* **92**: 219–76.
40. Gray D J, Gardner E and O'Rahilly R (1957) The prenatal development of the skeleton and joints of the human hand. *Am J Anat* **101**: 169–224.
41. Gardner E, Gray D J, and O'Rahilly R (1959) The prenatal development of the skeleton and joints of the human foot. *J Bone Joint Surg [Am]* **41**: 847–76.

42. Lewis O J (1980) The joints of the evolving foot. Part I. The ankle joint. *J Anat* **130**: 527–43.
43. O'Rahilly R, Muller F and Meyer D B (1980) The human vertebral column at the end of the embryonic period proper. 1. The column as a whole. *J Anat* **131**: 565–75.
44. Gardner E and O'Rahilly R (1968) The early development of the knee joint in staged embryos. *J Anat* **102**: 289–99.
45. Gardner E and O'Rahilly R (1972) The early development of the hip joint in staged human embryos. *Anat Rec* **172**: 451–2.
46. Gray D J and Gardner E (1951) Prenatal development of the human elbow joint. *Am J Anat* **88**: 429–69.
47. Walker J M and Goldsmith C (1982) Morphometric study of the fetal development of the human hip joint: significance for congenital hip disease. *Yale J Biol Med* **55**: 411–37.
48. Sensenig E C (1949) The early development of the human vertebral column. *Contrib Embryol Carnegie Inst* **33**: 23–41.
49. Dee R (1978) The innervation of joints, *In: The Joints and Synovial Fluid, Vol 1* (L Sokoloff, ed), pp. 177–204. New York: Academic Press.
50. Fell H B and Canti R G (1934) Experiments on the development *in vitro* of the avian knee joint. *Proc R Soc Lond* [Biol] **116**: 316–51.
51. Drachman D B and Sokoloff L (1966) The role of movement in embryonic joint development. *Dev Biol* **14**: 401–20.
52. Murray P D F and Drachman D B (1977) The role of movement in the development of joints and the related structures: the head and neck in the chick embryo. *J Embryol Exp Morphol* **22**: 349–71.
53. Holder N (1977) An experimental investigation into the early development of the chick elbow joint. *J Embryol Exp Morphol* **39**: 115–27.
54. Ruano-Gil D, Nardi-Vilardaga J and Tejedo-Mateu A (1978) Influence of extrinsic factors on the development of the articular system. *Acta Anat (Basel)* **101**: 36–44.
55. Beckman C, Dimond R and Greenlee Jr T K (1977) The role of movement in the development of a digital flexor tendon. *Am J Anat* **150**: 443–60.
56. Dunn P M (1976) Congential postural deformities. *Br Med Bull* **32**: 71–6.
57. Leck I (1976) Descriptive epidemiology of common malformations. *Br Med Bull* **32**: 42–52.
58. Smith D W (1981) *Recognisable Patterns of Human Deformation*. Philadephia: Saunders.
59. Warkany J (1971) *Congenital Malformations; Notes and Comments*. Chicago: Year Book Medical Publishers.
60. Dunn P M (1972) Congenital postural deformities: perinatal associations. *Proc Roy Soc Med* **65**: 735–8.
61. Rabin D L, Barnett C R, Arnold W D, Freiberger R H and Brooks G (1965) Untreated congenital hip disease. A study of the epidemiology, natural history, and social aspects of the disease in a Navajo population. *Am J Public Health* **55** (Suppl): 44.
62. Walker J M (1977) Congenital hip disease in a Cree-Ojibwa population: a retrospective study. *Can Med Assoc J* **116**: 501–4.
63. Salter R B, Kostuik J and Dallas S (1969) Avascular necrosis of the femoral head as a complication of treatment for congenital dislocation of the hip in young children. A clinical and experimental investigation. *Can J Surg* **12**: 44–61.
64. Visser J D (1984) Functional treatment of congenital dislocation of the hip. *Acta Orthop Scand (Suppl 206)* **55**: 1–112.
65. Tonna E A and Hatzel G (1967) Age changes in the distribution of connective tissue elements in human material studied with polarized light microscopy. *J Gerontol* **22**: 281–9.
66. Kopp S, Carlsson G E, Harisson T and Oberg T (1976) Degenerative disease in the temporomandibular, metatarsophalangeal and sternoclavicular joints. *Acta Odontol Scand* **34**: 23–32.
67. Shitama K (1979) Calcification of aging articular cartilage in man. *Acta Orthop Scand* **50**: 613–19.
68. Sokoloff L (1969) *The Biology of Degenerative Joint Disease*. Chicago: University of Chicago Press.
69. Mankin H J (1963) Localization of tritiated thymidine in articular cartilage of rabbits. III. Mature articular cartilage. *J Bone Joint Surg [Am]* **45**: 529–40.
70. Stockwell R A (1967) The cell density of human articular and costal cartilage. *J Anat* **101**: 753–63.
71. Tonna E A (1977) Aging of skeletal-dental systems and supporting tissues. *In: Handbook of Aging* (C E Finch and L Hayflick, eds), pp. 470–95. New York: Van Nostrand-Reinhold.
72. Silberberg M and Silberberg R (1961) Ageing changes in cartilage and bone. *In: Structural*

Aspects of Ageing (G H Bourne, ed), pp. 85–110. New York: Hafner.

73. Freeman M A R and Meachim G (1979) Ageing, degeneration and remodelling of articular cartilage. *In*: *Adult Articular Cartilage, 2nd Ed* (M A R Freeman, ed), pp. 487–543. Tunbridge Wells: Pitman.
74. Bernick S and Cailliet R (1982) Vertebral end-plate changes with aging of human vertebrae. *Spine* **7**: 97–102.
75. Bernick S, Cailliet R and Levy B M (1980) The maturation and aging of the vertebrae of marmosets. *Spine* **5**: 519–24.
76. Hall D A (1984) *A Biomedical Basis of Gerontology*. Bristol: Wright.
77. Naylor A (1958) Changes in the human intervertebral disc with age. *Proc Roy Soc Med* **51**: 573–6.
78. Armstrong C G and Mow V C (1982) Variations in the intrinsic mechanical properties of human articular cartilage with age, degeneration, and water content. *J Bone Joint Surg [Am]* **64**: 88–94.
79. Bonner W M, Jonsson H, Malanos C and Bryant M (1975) Changes in the lipids of human articular cartilage with age. *Arthritis Rheum* **18**: 461–73.
80. Bonucci E and Dearden L C (1976) Matrix vesicles in aging cartilage. *Fed Proc* **35**: 163–8.
81. Goodfellow J W and Bullough P G (1967) The pattern of ageing of the articular cartilage of the elbow joint. *J Bone Joint Surg [Br]* **49**: 175–81.
82. Kempson G E (1982) Relationship between the tensile properties of articular cartilage from the human knee and age. *Ann Rheum Dis* **41**: 508–11.
83. Kiss I, Morocz I and Herczeg L (1984) Localization and frequency of degenerative changes in the knee joint: evaluation of 200 necropsies. *Acta Morphol Hung* **32**: 155–63.
84. Lane L B and Bullough P G (1980) Age-related changes in the thickness of the calcified zone and the number of tidemarks in adult human articular cartilage. *J Bone Joint Surg [Br]* **62**: 372–5.
85. Silbermann M and Livne E (1979) Age-related degenerative changes in the mouse mandibular joint. *J Anat* **129**: 507–20.
86. Brown M (1984) Effects of exercise on aging in rat skeletal muscle. Unpublished doctoral dissertation. Los Angeles: University of Southern California.
87. Sokoloff L (1978) Osteoarthrosis. *In*: *The Human Joint in Health and Disease* (W H Simon, ed), pp. 91–95. Philadelphia: University of Pennsylvania Press.
88. Ballard K W, Bernick S and Soben S S (1979) Changes in the human microcirculation with age. *Microvasc Res* **17**: 511.
89. Viidik A (1973) Functional properties of collagenous tissues. *Int Rev Connect Tissue Res* **6**: 127–215.
90. Hubbard R P and Soutas-Little R W (1984) Mechanical properties of human tendon and their age dependence. *J Biomech Eng* **106**: 144–50.
91. Verzar F (1963) *Lectures on Experimental Gerontology*. Springfield, Ill: Thomas.
92. Eyre D R (1979) Biochemistry of the intervertebral disc. *Int Rev Connect Tissue Res* **8**: 275–79.
93. Vernon-Roberts B and Pirie C J (1977) Degenerative changes in the intervertebral discs of the lumbar spine and their sequelae. *Rheumatol Rehabil* **16**: 13–21.
94. Adams P and Muir H (1976) Qualitative changes with proteoglycans of human lumbar discs. *Ann Rheum Dis* **35**: 289–96.
95. Cole T C, Ghosh P and Taylor T K F (1986) Variations of the proteoglycans of the canine intervertebral disc with ageing. *Biochim Biophys Acta* **880**: 209–19.
96. Happey F, Naylor A, Palframan J, Pearson C, Reinder R N and Turner R L (1974) Variations in the diameter of collagen fibrils, bound hexose and associated glycoproteins in the intervertebral disc. *In*: *Connective Tissues: Biochemistry and Pathophysiology* (R Fricke and F Hartmann, eds), pp. 67–72. Berlin: Springer Verlag.
97. Hendry N G C (1958) The hydration of the nucleus pulposus and its relation to intervertebral disc derangement. *J Bone Joint Surg [Br]* **40**: 132–44.
98. Coventry M B (1969) Anatomy of the intervertebral disk. *Clin Orthop* **67**: 9–15.
99. Naylor A (1980) The design and function of the human intervertebral disc. *In*: *Scientific Foundations of Orthopaedics and Traumatology* (R Owen, J Goodfellow and P Bullough, eds), pp. 97–105. Philadelphia: Saunders.
100. Maroudas A, London P, Bullough P, Swanson S A V and Freeman M A R (1968) The permeability of articular cartilage. *J Bone Joint Surg [Br]* **50**: 166–76.
101. Maroudas A, Muir H and Wingham J (1969) The correlation of fixed negative charges with glycosaminoglycans content of human articular cartilage. *Biochim Biophys Acta* **177**: 492–500.

102. Brown M D and Tsaltas T T (1976) Studies on the permeability of the intervertebral disc during skeletal maturation. *Spine* **1**: 240–4.
103. Holm S and Rosenqvist A-L (1986) Morphological and nutritional changes in the intervertebral disc after spinal motion. *Scand J Rheumatol* (Suppl) **60**: 41.
104. Happey F, Pearson C H, Naylor L and Turner R L (1969) The aging of the human intervertebral disc. *Gerontologia* **15**: 174–88.
105. DeRousseau C J (1985) Aging in the musculoskeletal system of rhesus monkeys. II. Degenerative joint disease. *Amer J Phys Anthropol* **67**: 177–84.
106. DeRousseau C J, Rawlins R G and Denlinger J L (1983) Aging in the musculoskeletal system of rhesus monkeys. 1. Passive joint excursion. *Am J Phys Anthropol* **61**: 483–94.
107. Calandruccio R A and Gilmer W S Jr (1962) Proliferation, regeneration and repair of articular cartilage in immature animals. *J Bone Joint Surg [Am]* **44**: 431–55.
108. Tammi M, Paukkonen K, Kiviranta I, Jurvelin J, Säämänen A-M and Helminen H J (1987) Joint loading-induced alterations in articular cartilage. *In: Joint Loading–Biology and Health of Articular Structures* (H J Helminen, I Kiviranta, A-M Säämänen, M Tammi, K Paukkonen and J Jurvelin, eds), pp. 64–88 Bristol: Wright.
109. Akeson W H, Amiel D and Woo S L-Y (1987) Physiology and therapeutic value of passive motion. *In: Joint Loading–Biology and Health of Articular Structures* (H J Helminen, I Kiviranta, A-M Säämänen, M Tammi, K Paukkonen and J Jurvelin, eds), pp. 375–94 Bristol: Wright.
110. Lee P, Rooney P J, Sturrock R D, Kennedy A C and Dick W C (1974) The etiology and pathogenesis of osteoarthrosis: a review. *Semin Arthritis Rheum* **3**: 189–218.
111. Candolin T and Videman T (1986) Effects of running on the scanning electron microscopic appearance of joint surfaces of rabbits. *Scand J Rheumatol (Suppl)* **60**: 39.
112. Paukkonen K, Selkäinaho K, Jurvelin J, Kiviranta I and Helminen H (1985) Cells and nuclei of articular cartilage chondrocytes in young rabbits enlarged after non-strenuous physical exercise. *J Anat* **142**: 13–20.
113. Sääf J (1950) Effects of exercise on adult articular cartilage. *Acta Orthop Scand (Suppl)* **VII** (7): 1–86.
114. Helminen H J, Paukkonen K, Kiviranta I, Jurvelin J, Säämänen A-M, Parkkinen J and Lapveteläinen T (1986) Decrease of chondrocyte volume and volume density but increase of their number in the canine articular cartilage after strenuous training programme. *Scand J Rheumatol (Suppl)* **60**: 114.
115. Krause W D (1969) Mikroskopische Untersuchungen am Gelenkknorpel extrem funktionell belasteter Mäuse. *Spezialdruckerei für Dissertationen (Köln)* **26**: 1–69.
116. Säämänen A-M, Tammi M, Kiviranta I, Jurvelin J and Helminen H J (1986) Moderate running increases but strenuous running prevents elevation of proteoglycan content in the canine articular cartilage. *Scand J Rheumatol (Suppl)* **60**: 45.
117. Kiviranta I, Jurvelin J, Säämänen A-M, Arokoski J, Tammi M and Helminen H J (1986) Strenuous running exercise attenuates the increase of articular cartilage proteoglycans observed after moderate running programme of young beagle dogs. *Scand J Rheumatol (Suppl)* **60**: 43.

Chapter 5

Cartilage and Chondrocyte Responses to Mechanical Loading *In Vitro*

G. P. J. van Kampen and R. J. van de Stadt

CONTENTS

INTRODUCTION

The synovial joint is a mechanical system which allows relative movement of two body segments under load while large forces are transmitted from one body segment to another. The articular cartilage provides a surface with the lowest possible friction and supplies resistance to compressive forces.

The cartilage matrix is secreted by chondrocytes, the cellular activity of which is controlled by genetic and environmental factors. Changes in environmental factors can influence the metabolism of the cells, which ultimately will result in an altered cartilage matrix. The mechanism by which cells sense changes in their immediate environment remains one of the fundamental and important questions of biophysical science. The capacity to do so is essential to species adaptation and survival.

A number of *in vivo* studies have investigated the effects of immobilization and altered mechanical stress on joints. A decreased content of chondroitin sulphate is found in paralysis due to poliomyelitis (1) and experimental denervation (2). Absence of mechanical force leads not only to a loss of hexuronate from the articular cartilage but also to a decrease of synthesis of glycosaminoglycans (3–6).

Increased mechanical loading caused an increase in both hexuronate content and rate of proteoglycan synthesis (7). However, high impact loads (8) or abnormal loading (9), exceeding 'physiological levels', of synovial joints resulted in loss of proteoglycan from articular cartilage, fibrillation of the tissue, and cell death (10–13). These *in vivo* studies indicate that mechanical forces appear to modulate chondrocyte metabolism in such a way that articular cartilage becomes adapted to the altered mechanical needs.

Absence of mechanical stress and stresses considerably lower in magnitude than 'physiological' generally result in a loss of articular cartilage, increased catabolic activity and decreased anabolic activity of the chondrocytes. 'Physiological' stresses enhance anabolic activity and presumably reduce catabolism, resulting in maintenance or increase in the amount of articular cartilage. Higher stresses induce pathological changes in cartilage and tissue degeneration, which can be seen as loss of matrix components, fibrillation, and eventually cell death.

Articular cartilage and chondrocytes can easily be grown *in vitro* (14, 15). The *in vitro* models for the study of the effects of mechanical forces on cultured articular cartilage and chondrocytes are extensively reviewed in the next section of this chapter, although in the interests of clarity no results are given or discussed.

Later in this chapter (pp. 115–22) the response of cultured chondrocytes is described, using the perception of the stimulus, the cellular events elicited, and the response of the cells as guidelines. It is argued that when exposed to mechanical stress, cultured chondrocytes respond in a comparable way to that of articular cartilage *in vitro*.

Subsequently (pp. 122–23) the present knowledge is summarized and a hypothetical model for the response presented. It will become clear that the research performed so far lacks much important data. Much future research is needed to complete the picture.

IN VITRO MODELS USED FOR THE STUDY OF THE EFFECTS OF MECHANICAL FORCES ON CHONDROCYTES

Connective Tissue and Mechanical Forces

The significance of biomechanical forces for the development, growth and functioning of connective tissue has been extensively studied (16), but the mechanisms by which these factors exert their influence at the cellular level in bone, tendon or cartilage are still not understood. Investigation of these processes requires experimental systems which allow quantitative reproducible application of forces to skeletal tissues under controlled near-physiological conditions.

Living bone responds to the presence or absence of mechanical forces by adaptive changes in internal architecture (17). Glucksman demonstrated that many of the structural effects are due to the direct action of physical stimuli on the skeleton, since bone tissue cultures *in vitro* respond directly to physical strain (18–20). In tissue culture models, the role of electrical currents produced by piezoelectric effects and/or streaming potentials and electrets induced by mechanical forces has been investigated (21, 22). Intermittent tension was applied to rat femurs to study the effects of mechanical stress on bone remodelling (23).

An organ culture system to apply mechanical stress to cranial sutures of newborn rabbits has been developed by Meikle *et al.* (24) to study the response of fibrous joints to tensile mechanical stress.

The effects of a range of continuous and intermittent compressive forces on the proliferation and matrix synthesis of chondrocytes and on the architecture of mandibular condylar cartilage of the rat has been studied by Copray *et al.* (25, 26) in a serum-free culture system (27).

Chondrocytes and Mechanical Forces

Rodan *et al.* (28) modified the tensile force apparatus of Solomons *et al.* (23) and was the first to build an apparatus for the application of compressive forces to long bones in culture. The apparatus for the application of pressure was made from glass tuberculin syringes with individually matched polished pistons. In this apparatus it was possible to culture tibiae of 16 day old chick embryos for 5 days and study the effects of a constant pressure of $7 \cdot 89$ kPa (80 g/cm^2) on glucose consumption and DNA synthesis. The effect of a continuous compressive force of physiological magnitude $5 \cdot 9$ kPa (60 g/cm^2) on cyclic nucleotide accumulation in chick tibial epiphyses and in the cells of the different zones of the epiphyses was reported by Rodan *et al.* (29) and Norton *et al.* (30). The latter author compared the observed changes with the effects of oscillating electric fields.

Based on these ideas, Veldhuijzen *et al.* (31) constructed an apparatus that made it possible to expose chondrocytes, cultured in monolayer on the walls of tissue culture tubes, to intermittent compressive forces of $12 \cdot 8$ kPa (96 mmHg) for 6 h at a frequency of $0 \cdot 3$ Hz. The compressive force was applied to the cultures by compressing the gas phase above the culture medium. The use of sterile tubes containing culture medium allowed study of the effects of intermittent compressive forces on high density cultures of chick embryonic chondrocytes floating in the culture medium (32, 33). The highest pressure differential was 13 kPa (130 mbar) with a frequency of $0 \cdot 3$ Hz, and the cultures were exposed to this regimen for 24 and 48 h. Induced changes in proteoglycan synthesis and aggregation capacity of proteoglycan monomers with hyaluronic acid were studied in high density cultures of chondrocytes from the epiphyseal growth plate of 15 day old chick embryo tibiae (34); morphometric observations were also made (35).

Lippiello *et al.* (36) exposed bovine and human articular cartilage segments to hydrostatic pressure in a plexiglass pressure chamber. An air-driven piston produced a hydrostatic pressure ranging from $516 \cdot 75$ to $2583 \cdot 75$ kPa (75–375 lbf/in^2). The influence of hydrostatic pressure for 24 h (in the presence or absence of serum) on the metabolism was investigated. Slices of bovine articular cartilage, cultured in a nutrient medium in flexible bags and placed in hyperbaric chambers for 24 h, were studied by Kimura *et al.* (37). The ability of the cartilage to synthesize proteoglycan under increasing hydrostatic pressures up to 2750 kPa ($2 \cdot 75$ MPa) was monitored by determination of the incorporation of radioactive sulphate into proteoglycans.

A different approach was used by Jones *et al.* (38), who cultured cartilage pieces (articular surface upwards in a Petri dish) from the intercondylar region of the distal femur of 9 month old calves. The fragments were exposed to continuous mechanical pressure by lowering a second smaller Petri dish, which contained lead weights producing pressures of 735·8, 1471·5 or 2943 kPa (7·5, 15 or 30 kgf/cm²), on to the pieces for 2 and 4 days. Proteoglycan breakdown and synthesis were studied. Using the same apparatus, Klamfeldt (39) studied the effect of synovial membrane products in combination with continuous mechanical pressure on proteoglycan turnover in articular cartilage.

The influence of compressive loading on full-thickness cartilage plugs from femoral condyles of normal adult dogs was studied by Palmoski and Brandt (40). The plugs were placed between a movable glass piston and a fixed base, and cultured while static or cyclic stresses, ranging between 1·1, 5·5 and 11·0 kPa (11–110 N × 10⁻⁴/mm²), were applied for 2 h. The effect of continuous compression was compared with that of 2 duty cycles of compressive forces, 60 s on/60 s off and 4 s on/11 s off. By subsequent incubation under atmospheric pressure in a medium containing radioactive label, the net synthesis of glycosaminoglycans and protein, as well as the tissue content of DNA, uronic acid and water were monitored.

The *in vitro* system developed by Leung *et al.* (41, 42) for studying cell responses to mechanical stimulation was used by Lee and co-workers (43) to compare the effects of mechanical stess and time-varying electric fields on chondrocytes. Chondrocytes from 15 day chick embryo sternae were cultured on elastin membranes. Following 5 days of growth the membranes underwent a cyclic mechanical strain of up to 10% of the original length (1 Hz) or electrical stimulation for an 8 h culture period. Protein and collagen synthesis as well as glycosaminoglycan synthesis were studied. DeWitt *et al.* (44) studied the effect of short-term mechanical tension on chick epiphyseal chondrocytes grown in high density cultures for 14 days in a similar apparatus. Cyclical stretching with a strain of 5·5% at a frequency of 0·2 Hz was applied to the cultures for 24 h. The incorporation of radioactive sulphate in cultures subjected to mechanical loading was compared to control cultures, and the hydrodynamic size of the proteoglycans synthesized by chondrocytes exposed to stress was determined. Changes in the cellular levels of cAMP in experimental cultures were reported. Magnitudes and types of mechanical forces studied *in vitro*, and culture systems used, are summarized in *Tables* 5.1 and 5.2.

CHONDROCYTE RESPONSE TO MECHANICAL FORCES *IN VITRO*

Cartilage Matrix and Diffusion of Nutrients

Articular cartilage is approximately 65–85% interstitial water, of which a large portion is freely exchangeable with the synovial fluid bathing the tissue. The remainder of the tissue is composed of three major organic components, namely collagen fibres surrounding and intertwined among proteoglycan macromolecules and chondrocytes. It is believed that at equilibrium the collagen is in tension in order to constrain the swelling behaviour of the hydrophilic proteoglycan macromolecule, which consists of many negatively charged glycosaminoglycan chains attached to a protein core. As the tissue is deformed the interstitial fluid is exuded, causing the proteoglycan repulsive force to

Table 5.1 MAGNITUDES OF MECHANICAL FORCES

CONTINUOUS (kPa)			
Orientated		*Hydrostatic*	
8.1	Rodan *et al.*, 1975 (28)	516.8	Lippiello *et al.*, 1985 (36)
6.1	Norton *et al.*, 1977 (30)	2066.0	Lippiello *et al.*, 1985 (36)
1.1	Palmoski and Brandt 1984 (40)	2583.8	Lippiello *et al.*, 1985 (36)
11.0	Palmoski and Brandt 1984 (40)	350.0	Kimura *et al.*, 1985 (37)
759.8	Jones *et al.*, 1982 (38)	2750.0	Kimura *et al.*, 1985 (37)
3039.0	Klämfeldt, 1985 (39)		

INTERMITTENT (kPa)			
Orientated		*Hydrostatic*	
Duty cycle: 60/60 4/11		3/3	
1.1	Palmoski and Brandt, 1984 (40)	13.0	Veldhuijzen *et al.*, 1979 (31)
11.1	Palmoski and Brandt, 1984 (40)	13.0	Van Kampen *et al.*, 1985 (34)

TENSION (% strain)		
10.0	Lee *et al*, 1982 (43)	1.0 Hz
5.5	DeWitt *et al.*, 1984 (44)	0.2 Hz

Magnitude and nature of forces to which cultured chondrocytes or cartilage are exposed in the reviewed studies. Numbers, expressed in kPa, indicate the magnitude of the stimuli. In the upper and middle panels continuous and intermittent forces are separated into orientated and hydrostatic forces. In the lower part tension in percentage strain is shown.

Table 5.2 CHONDROCYTE CULTURES STUDIED

CHICK EMBRYO CARTILAGE:		
Tibia	16 days old (5 days)	Rodan *et al.*, 1975 (28).
Epiphyses	16 days old (20–48 h)	Rodan *et al.*, 1975 (29); Veldhuijzen *et al.*, 1979 (31); Van Kampen *et al.*, 1985 (34)
Epiphyseal cells	13 days old (14 days)	DeWitt *et al.*, 1984 (44)
Distal cells	16 days old (20 h)	Rodan *et al.*, 1975 (28)
Middle cells	16 days old (20–48 h)	Rodan *et al.*, 1975 (29); Veldhuijzen *et al.*, 1979 (31); Van Kampen *et al.*, 1985 (34)
Proximal cells	16 days old (20 h)	Rodan *et al.*, 1975 (28)
Sternal cells	15 days old (5 days)	Lee *et al.*, 1982 (43)
BOVINE ARTICULAR CARTILAGE:		
Fragments	9 months old (2–4 days)	Jones *et al.*, 1982 (38)
Segments	7 weeks old (24 h)	Lippiello *et al.*, 1985 (36)
CANINE ARTICULAR CARTILAGE:		
Full depth plugs	Adult (2 h)	Palmoski and Brandt, 1984 (40)

Sources of chondrocytes and tissues (donor animal and age) used in the reviewed studies. The time of exposure of the cells to mechanical stress is given in parentheses.

increase as the chains are squeezed together. This further restricts fluid flow and tissue deformation. Load removal will cause the tissue to swell, imbibing interstitial fluid. During the recovery phase both diffusion and convection will be directed into the tissue.

Nutrition of articular cartilage is accomplished by the transfer of solutes, e.g. glucose, from the synovial fluid into the tissue in 3 possible ways: solute diffusion in unloaded tissue; solute transport by fluid convection in loaded tissue; and active cellular transport. Experimental evidence suggests that active cellular transport is insignificant. Solute transport was found to be equal in whole body and cultured tissue (45), despite the fact that metabolic cell activity *in vitro* proved to be an order of magnitude greater than *in vivo*.

In unloaded tissue small solutes are transported by simple diffusion, the rate of transport decreasing with increasing solute size (46) and anionic charge density (47). Molecules of the size of haemoglobin (69 000 mol.wt) or larger are effectively 'excluded' from the tissue fluid space (48). 'Mechanical pumping', on the other hand, generated considerable interstitial fluid volume exchange (49). Tomlinson and Maroudas (50) have demonstrated a significant increase in the partition coefficient of serum albumin (69 000 mol. wt) with cyclic loading. This indicates that molecules which do not enter the matrix by passive diffusion due to size or charge enter the matrix when the tissue is exposed to cyclic loading, emphasizing the importance of tissue deformation and forced fluid permeation. However, Maroudas asserts that 'the physiological pump could under no likely circumstances be expected to increase the rate of transport of small molecular weight nutrients above that which can be achieved by diffusion'. Using this line of reasoning, conditions such as atrophy caused by joint immobilization are presumably not due to malnutrition but to the absence of a mechanical stimulus which can be sensed by the chondrocytes. Further evidence for this hypothesis comes from experiments where changes in metabolic activity (as measured by the changes in glycosaminoglycan synthesis of full depth cartilage plugs exposed to cyclic loading) were not paralleled by changes in diffusion of nutrient molecules through the cartilage during loading, as determined by uptake of ^{14}C-aminoisobutyric acid and ^{14}C-xylose (40).

These data indicate that diffusion of nutrients is the most important mode for transport through the cartilage matrix, with mechanical pumping playing a less significant role. Therefore, the metabolic changes that occur when chondrocytes are exposed to mechanical stress are very likely due to the mechanical stimulus alone.

Cartilage Matrix and Transduction of Stimuli

The investigations undertaken to study the effects of mechanical forces on chondrocytes *in vitro* have been described earlier (pp. 13–15). A wide range of machines and apparatus has been developed to expose cells (with or without surrounding matrix), pieces of articular cartilage, and even long bones, to mechanical stress. The effects of the presence of pericellular matrix on the response of the chondrocytes to mechanical forces has been studied and discussed in several reports.

In his study performed with segments of tibial epiphyses of 16 day old chick embryos, Rodan *et al.* (29) compared the changes in cAMP and cGMP in different segments of the epiphyses with the response of cells isolated from those regions. He observed that small pressures applied directly to the cells altered the amounts of cyclic nucleotides in cells but differed from those produced in intact tissue. Norton *et al.* (30) reported similar differences in the response of whole tissue compared to isolated cells, and suggested that the matrix and the arrangement of the cells within it modulate the continuous mechanical stimulus.

Intermittent compression, however, stimulated both cartilage explants and isolated cells from chick epiphyseal growth plates to significantly increase cAMP levels (31). These data indicate a less prominent role of the matrix in the transmission of intermittent hydrostatic forces. In our opinion it cannot be concluded from these data that continuously applied stress is modulated by a matrix, and that this is not the case when intermittent mechanical forces are used. It is more likely that the above-mentioned *in vitro* models are less well suited for extrapolation of data concerning the role of cyclic nucleotides as second messengers in chondrocytes to the *in vivo* situation.

Mechanoreceptor Mechanisms

In view of the aneural, alymphatic and avascular nature of cartilage, it is reasonable to speculate that mechanical deformation may be of special significance in regulatory processes of chondrocytes other than enhancement of nutrient accessibility. The mechanism by which cells sense changes in their immediate environment remains one of the fundamental and important questions of biophysical science.

From the fact that cartilage responds to mechanical forces, Kaye *et al.* (51) concludes that the cell membrane must be pressure sensitive. Rodan *et al.* (29) sees the tissue as a stimulus-receptor system in which the distortion of the cell membrane produces a mechanical, electrical (52) or chemical (53) perturbation, which initiates specific events through cyclic nucleotide modulation as second messengers. Bourret *et al.* (54) suggested that molecular changes in certain membrane components under pressure lead to an increased calcium uptake, which is believed to be a regulatory process in the chondrocyte response. Recently Poole *et al.* described a cilium on connective tissue cells (55). Perhaps this cilium functions as a baroreceptor for chondrocytes. It is obvious that the data required to formulate a mechanoreceptor mechanism are still lacking.

Intracellular Events

There are several reasons for considering cyclic nucleotides as potential second messengers in the transduction of physical stimuli into biochemical responses. Cyclic nucleotides might play a central role in development and cytodifferentiation in general (56). Carbohydrate metabolism is known to be subject to the control of cyclic nucleotides. In fibroblast cultures low levels of cAMP are correlated with growth stimulation, whereas addition of cAMP inhibits growth.

In the 1970s the role of cAMP and cGMP as second messengers in chondrocytes received much attention. Rodan and co-workers published a number of papers on this subject. Pressure significantly decreased accumulation of cAMP and cGMP in cartilage segments of chick tibial epiphyses. In cells isolated from that segment an increased amount of cAMP and cGMP was found (29, 30). The concurrent drop of cGMP does not support the hypothesis of reciprocal changes in the 2 cyclic nucleotides (56). Epiphyses and proliferative cartilage cells of 16 day old chicks have been found to respond to intermittent increases in ambient hydrostatic pressures by increasing intracellular cAMP

(31). A 2·2-fold increase in the intracellular levels of cAMP was measured when the chondrocyte cultures were subjected to mechanical tension for 24 h (44). Membranes are relatively impermeable to cations, such as Ca^{++} and K^+, which are involved in the transduction of physical perturbation at the cell–matrix interface (57). The role of Ca^{++} was studied by Bourret and Rodan (54), who found that pressure enhanced the cellular uptake of radiocalcium. The molecular changes in the membrane responsible for the increased calcium uptake are not obvious. Certain membrane components could however change their structure under pressure.

Reviewing the large body of data concerning the role of cyclic nucleotides as second messengers in cartilage, one is forced to conclude that a uniform working hypothesis accommodating most of the results cannot be formulated. Therefore, the role of cyclic nucleotides in the transduction of mechanical stimuli to metabolic events in chondrocytes remains obscure.

The role of prostaglandins in the translation of a physical stimulus into a biological message is very doubtful. Bindermann showed that increased DNA synthesis is not mediated by prostaglandin-E_2 (58). Also, the inhibition of cartilage degradation exerted by continuous mechanical pressure is not prostaglandin mediated, because indomethacin had no effect (39).

The increased metabolic activity of chondrocytes in high density cultures under load was shown by Veldhuijzen et al. using histomorphometric techniques (35). Cells in cultures exposed to intermittent compressive forces had increased cell volumes and nuclear sizes.

Cellular Proliferation

Continuous compressive force stimulates ^{14}C-thymidine incorporation into DNA of chick embryonic chondrocytes (28). Two parameters related to proliferation were investigated by Veldhuijzen et al. (31): ^{3}H-thymidine incorporation into DNA and ornithine decarboxylase activity induction. A causal relationship between ornithine decarboxylase activity and DNA synthesis has not been established. The change in ornithine decarboxylase activity could be part of a pleiotropic response (31).

Studying the effects of intermittent compressive forces on high density cultures of chick embryo chondrocytes, a significant decrease of thymidine incorporation into DNA was reported by Van Kampen et al. (33, 34). However, autoradiography of the cultures revealed that only 2–3% of the chondrocytes in the cultures had incorporated thymidine. Mitotic figures were not observed in this study (35). These results strongly suggest that proliferation of cells is of minor importance in high density cultures of chondrocytes under stress regimens.

Synthesis of Matrix Components

Nature of the mechanical forces applied *in vitro*

Articular cartilage is exposed to large mechanical forces during joint movement. During normal walking, peak resultant forces across human hip and knee have been shown to reach 4 and 7 times the body weight, respectively. *In vivo* mechanical forces are applied cyclically and chondrocytes are exposed to a composite of radial, tangential and shear stresses. Unfortunately chondrocytes *in vitro* can be exposed only to forces that partially mimic the forces to which tissue may be subjected *in vivo*. Since a large body of evidence indicates that chondrocytes *in vitro* respond to several kinds of mechanical stress, it is worthwhile studying these effects to gain more insight into the cellular processes evoked by such stimuli.

Hydrodynamic forces

A 4 h continuous hydrostatic pressure ranging from 516·8 kPa to 2066·0 kPa (75–300 lbf/in^2, which is at the lower limit of 'physiological levels') on bovine articular cartilage, resulted in a 50% decreased proteoglycan synthesis, as measured by radiosulphate uptake compared to control cultures. A higher pressure of 2583·8 kPa (375 lbf/in^2) on chondrocytes cultured in the presence of undialysed serum increased sulphate incorporation into proteoglycans by only 10–15% (36). The use of dialysed serum increased this response to 55%. Apparently a low molecular weight serum factor plays an inhibiting role in the response of cartilage to mechanical stress. Conflicting data were reported by Kimura *et al.* (37). He found no change in the amount of incorporated ^{35}S-sulphate when cartilage pieces were exposed to continuous hydrostatic pressure ranging from 350 kPa to 2750 kPa (0·35 MPa–2·75 MPa) in a compression chamber. The lack of stimulation may possibly be explained by the fact that undialysed serum was used.

The intriguing question of the existence of a threshold stimulation was studied by Veldhuijzen *et al.* (31). He studied the dose-response pattern of cells isolated from the proliferative zone of the epiphyses, cultured in monolayer, and exposed to intermittent hydrostatic forces. He reported an all-or-none response for ornithine decarboxylase activity in the cells with a threshold of 10·8 kPa (80 mmHg), accompanied by a reduction of DNA synthesis. In the future it will be important to establish that this observed phenomenon can be repeated using radiosulphate incorporation into proteoglycans in other culture systems, including explants. The switch from inhibition to stimulation of proteoglycan synthesis reported by Lippiello *et al.* (36) also indicates that some kind of threshold exists near the lower limits of physiological load levels. By exposing chick epiphyseal chondrocytes in high density cultures to intermittent hydrostatic forces of 13 kPa (100 mmHg) for 24 and 48 h, Van Kampen *et al.* (34) reported an increase in proteoglycan production determined by the incorporation of radiosulphate. This result indicated that proteoglycan synthesis is increased by a (presumably) supra-threshold stimulus. Unfortunately, experiments using lower pressures were not performed.

Release of pressure studied by Lippiello *et al.* (36) induced a burst of metabolic activity in the relaxation phase. This rebound phenomenon suggests that relaxation may be an important component of the mechanical regulatory system.

Orientated forces

Human articular cartilage pieces were exposed to unidirectional continuous pressure by Jones *et al.* (38) and Klämfeldt (39). Increasing the pressure from approximately 759·8 to 3039 kPa (7·5–30 kgf/cm^2) proportionally decreased the breakdown of proteoglycan as measured by the release of ^{35}S-sulphate from pre-labelled cartilage. The decrease was observed as early as 24 h after culture. After removal of a 3039 kPa (30 kgf/cm^2) pressure, ^{35}S release was slightly greater than that of non-weight-bearing controls, but within 48 h the ^{35}S release returned to the level of the controls. Proteoglycan synthesis during application of the same mechanical pressure to calf articular cartilage was reduced to about half the level of non-weight-bearing controls. A lower pressure of 1519·5 kPa (15 kgf/cm^2) had no significant effect on sulphate incorporation. The pressure-induced reduction of proteoglycan synthesis conflicts with the concept of stimulation by a mechanical stress of physiological magnitude. It is our opinion that in this experimental set-up, the existence of severely diminished contact areas between cartilage surface and culture medium cannot be excluded, and might explain the results obtained.

The influence of compressive loading on full-thickness cartilage plugs from femoral condyles of normal adult dogs was studied by Palmoski and Brandt (40). The plugs were cultured while static or cyclic stresses were applied, ranging from 1·1 to 11·0 kPa (11–110 N × 10^{-4}/mm^2), equivalent to 1.5 times the body weight. The effects of continuous compression and those of 2 duty cycles of compressive forces, 60 s on/60 s off and 4 s on/11 s off were compared with control cultures. A duty cycle of 60 s on/60 s off suppressed net glycosaminogly-can synthesis to 30–60% of that of control cultures under atmospheric pressure. However, glycosaminoglycan synthesis was increased by 34% when a duty cycle of 4 s on/11 s off was used. The duty cycle which increased glycosaminoglycan synthesis did not affect protein synthesis or tissue DNA, uronic acid or water content. Protein synthesis and uronic acid content were decreased in the regime which suppressed glycosaminoglycan synthesis. The 2 h stress-induced changes in proteoglycan synthesis were reversible within a subsequent 18 h culture period, during which the cartilage plugs were cultured under atmospheric pressure. Uronic acid and water content of plugs returned to control levels after 72 h. Unfortunately the authors (40) determined the metabolic activity of the cells by incubating the tissue in a medium containing radioactive precursors after removal of the pressure. This introduced a complicating factor since Lippiello *et al.* (36) reported a burst of metabolic activity after removal of the pressure.

Stretching

Lee *et al.* (43) applied a mechanical force to chondrocytes *in vitro* by stretching a supportive elastin membrane on which chondrocytes were cultured. The nature of the adherence was such that it was very doubtful that the cytoskeleton could have been deformed by stretching the membrane. However, a cyclic 10% mechanical stretch of the supporting elastin membranes for 8 h stimulated 15 day old chick embryo sternal chondrocytes to a 2–3-fold increase of glycosaminoglycan synthesis and a depression of protein and collagen synthesis.

Increased radiosulphate or ^{14}C-glucosamine incorporation into glycosamino-glycans by chick epiphyseal chondrocytes in high density cultures subjected to a strain of 5·5% at a frequency of 0·2 Hz was reported by DeWitt *et al.* (44). In cultures subjected to mechanical strain for 24 h, protein synthesis remained unchanged. Longer periods of exposure to mechanical strain increased protein(including collagen) synthesis by these cultures. When cultures are envisaged as being made up of chondrocytes entrapped in a 3-dimensional network of collagen fibres, and a tensional force is applied to the culture, one might assume that the chondrocytes are compressed by the distortion of the collagen network.

Interaction of Matrix Components

Most studies of the effects of mechanical forces on matrix production of chondrocytes *in vitro* are limited to those cell responses which can be determined by the incorporation of radioactive precursors into components of the intercellular matrix. However, not only the amount of newly synthesized proteoglycans but also the quality of the cartilage matrix is of importance for the mechanical properties of the cartilage.

The quality of the newly synthesized proteoglycans has received very little attention so far. By the application of mechanical stress to high density cultures a slightly larger proteoglycan monomer size on Sepharose 2B was found by DeWitt *et al.* (44). Van Kampen *et al.* (34) reported an increased capacity of the monomers to aggregate with hyaluronic acid when chondrocyte cultures were exposed to intermittent hydrodynamic forces. DeWitt *et al.* (44) suggests changes in the organization of the collagen fibres after cyclic stretching of high density cultures of articular chondrocytes, as revealed by microscopy. Van Kampen *et al.* (34) reported that proteoglycans deposited in the intercellular matrix of the cultures exposed to intermittent compression were less extractable, suggesting firmer anchoring in the matrix.

Clearly the rate of matrix synthesis, as well as the composition of matrix components, is affected as a result of mechanical forces. Future investigations are needed to understand these changes, which are very important for the mechanical behaviour of the cartilage matrix.

Turnover of Proteoglycans

Articular cartilage pieces were exposed to unidirectional continuous pressure by Jones *et al.* (38) and Klämfeldt (39). The main findings of these studies were that a continuous load of 3039 kPa (30 kgf/cm^2) significantly reduced the synthesis and release of prelabelled proteoglycans in both calf and human articular cartilage *in vitro*. Another observation was that the appreciable degradation of articular cartilage caused by the products of synovial tissue in this culture system was inhibited by continuous mechanical pressure (39). The limitations of applying continuous mechanical stress in this culture system for longer periods has been discussed above. All reported phenomena could possibly be explained by reduction of the contact area of the tissue with the culture medium.

CONCLUSIONS

Cultured chondrocytes and cartilage segments respond to both hydrostatic forces and tissue deforming stresses (orientated and stretch), applied to the cells for relatively short periods. *In vitro* experiments allow the study of cellular events involved in the perception of the stimulus, the intracellular events evoked by mechanical stimuli, and a detailed analysis of the newly synthesized matrix components.

In most studies, the forces to which cartilage or chondrocytes have been exposed *in vitro* only partially mimic those to which articular chondrocytes are exposed *in vivo*. The *in vitro* forces are at the lower levels of 'physiological magnitude', but 'physiological magnitude' apparently varies with the source of the tissue.

In general the response of the cells to mechanical stress *in vitro* seems to fit the proposed model, namely enhanced catabolic activity in the lower range of forces leading to atrophy of the tissue, and maintenance of the tissue or increased anabolic activity when stresses are in the physiological range. When exposed to still higher stresses the chondrocytes are no longer able to adapt the tissue to the mechanical requirements, which leads to destruction of the articular cartilage. Nutrition of the tissue plays only a minor role in these processes.

Many experiments provide no clue to the mechanism through which pressure induces metabolic events in articular cartilage. A detailed analysis of the metabolism of chondrocytes cultured under several mechanical force regimens will be needed to further investigate the regulating role of the chondrocyte in maintaining the proper cartilage matrix which is necessary for the normal functioning of the joint.

CLINICAL SIGNIFICANCE

The evidence from the *in vitro* experiments with cartilage tissue and chondrocytes strongly suggests that pressures occurring in joint loading may be a major factor in control of articular cartilage matrix synthesis, and perhaps overall cartilage homeostasis. These results should be borne in mind in all situations of clinical practice where disease or treatment interferes with the physiological range of joint loading.

ACKNOWLEDGEMENTS

The authors wish to thank Dr E C Firth for discussing and critically reading the manuscript. This study was supported by the Dutch League against Rheumatism.

REFERENCES

1. Eichelberger L, Miles J S and Roma M (1952) The histochemical characterization of articular cartilages of poliomyelitis patients. *J Lab Clin Med* **40**: 284–96.
2. Akeson W H, Eichelberger L and Roma M (1958) Biochemical studies of articular cartilage. II. Values following the denervation of an extremity. *J Bone Joint Surg [Am]* **40**: 153–62.
3. Eichelberger L, Roma M and Moulder P V (1959) Biochemical studies of articular cartilage. III. Values following the immobilization of an extremity. *J Bone Joint Surg [Am]* **41**: 1127–42.
4. Akeson W H, Woo S L-Y, Amiel D, Coutts R D and Daniel D (1973) The connective tissue response to immobility: biochemical changes in periarticular connective tissue of the immobilized rabbit knee. *Clin Orthop* **93**: 356–62.
5. Palmoski M J, Perricone E and Brandt K D (1979) Development and reversal of a proteoglycan aggregation defect in normal canine knee after immobilization. *Arthritis Rheum* **22**: 508–17.

6. Palmoski M J, Colyer R A and Brandt K D (1980) Joint motion in the absence of normal loading does not maintain normal articular cartilage. *Arthritis Rheum* **23**: 325–34.
7. Caterson B and Lowther D A (1978) Changes in the metabolism of the proteoglycans from sheep articular cartilage in response to mechanical stress. *Biochim Biophys Acta* **540**: 412–22.
8. Radin E L, Ehrlich M G M, Chernack R, Abernathy P, Paul I L and Rose R M (1978) Effect of repetitive impulsive loading on the knee joints of rabbits. *Clin Orthop* **131**: 288–93.
9. McDevitt C, Gilbertson E and Muir H (1977) An experimental model of osteoarthritis, early morphological and biochemical changes. *J Bone Joint Surg [Br]* **59**: 24–35.
10. Salter R B and Field P (1960) The effect of continuous compression on living articular cartilage. An experimental investigation. *J Bone Joint Surg [Am]* **42**: 31–49.
11. McDevitt C A and Muir H (1976) Biochemical changes in the cartilage of the knee in experimental and natural osteoarthritis in the dog. *J Bone Joint Surg [Br]* **58**: 94–101.
12. Moskowitz R W, Howell D S, Goldberg V M, Muniz O and Pita J C (1979) Cartilage proteoglycan alterations in an experimentally induced model of rabbit osteoarthritis. *Arthritis Rheum* **22**: 155–63.
13. Tammi M, Säämänen A-M, Jauhiainen A, Malminen O, Kiviranta I and Helminen H (1983) Proteoglycan alterations in rabbit knee articular cartilage following physical exercise and immobilization. *Connect Tissue Res* **11**: 45–55.
14. Green W T (1971) Behaviour of articular chondrocytes in cell culture. *Clin Orthop* **75**: 248–60.
15. Hascall V C, Handley C J, McQuillan D J, Hascall G K, Robinson H C and Lowther D A (1983) The effect of serum on biosynthesis of proteoglycans by bovine articular cartilage in culture. *Arch Biochem Biophys* **224**: 206–23.
16. Hall B K (1978) *Development and Cellular Skeletal Biology.* London: Academic Press.
17. Wolff J (1892) *Das Gesetz der Transformation der Knochen.* Berlin: Hirschwald.
18. Glucksman A (1938) Studies on bone mechanics *in vitro.* I. Influence of pressure on orientation of structure. *Anat Rec* **72**: 97–115.
19. Glucksman A (1939) Studies on bone mechanics *in vitro.* II. The role of tension and pressure on chondrogenesis. *Anat Rec* **73**: 39–55.
20. Glucksman A (1942) The role of mechanical stress in bone formation *in vitro. J Anat* **76**: 231–39.
21. Bassett C A L and Herrmann I (1961) Influence of oxygen concentration and mechanical factors on differentiation of connective tissue *in vitro. Nature* **190**: 460–1.
22. Bassett C A L and Becker R O (1962) Generation of electric potentials by bone in response to mechanical stress. *Science* **137**: 1063–4.
23. Solomons C C, Shuster D and Kwan A (1965) Biochemical effects of mechanical stress. I. Control of ^{32}P release from rat femur *in vitro. Aerospace Med* **36**: 33–4.
24. Meikle M C, Heath J K and Reynolds J J (1984) The use of *in vitro* models for investigating fibrous joints to tensile mechanical stress. *Am J Orthod* **85**: 141–53.
25. Copray J C V M, Jansen H W B and Duterloo H S (1985) Effects of compressive forces on proliferation and matrix synthesis in mandibular condylar cartilage of the rat *in vitro. Arch Oral Biol* **30**: 299–304.
26. Copray J C V M, Jansen H W B and Duterloo H S (1985) An *in vitro* system for studying the effect of variable compressive forces on the mandibular condylar cartilage of the rat. *Arch Oral Biol* **30**: 305–11.
27. Copray J C V M, Jansen H W B and Duterloo H S (1983) Growth of the mandibular condylar cartilage of the rat in serum-free organ culture. *Arch Oral Biol* **28**: 967–74.
28. Rodan G A, Mensi T and Harvey A (1975) A quantitative method for the application of compressive forces to bone in tissue culture. *Calcif Tissue Res* **18**: 125–31.
29. Rodan G A, Bourret L A, Harvey A and Mensi T (1975) Cyclic AMP and cyclic GMP. Mediators of the mechanical effects on bone remodelling. *Science* **189**: 467–9.
30. Norton L A, Rodan G A and Bourret L A (1977) Epiphyseal cartilage cAMP changes produced by electrical and mechanical perturbations. *Clin Orthop* **124**:59–68.
31. Veldhuijzen J P, Bourret L A and Rodan G A (1979) *In vitro* studies of the effect of intermittent compressive forces on cartilage cell proliferation. *J Cell Physiol* **98**: 299–306.
32. Van Kampen G P J and Veldhuijzen J P (1982) Aggregated chondrocytes as a model system to study cartilage metabolism. *Exp Cell Res* **140**: 440–3.
33. Van Kampen G P J and Veldhuijzen J P (1982) An *in vitro* model to study factors affecting matrix production and cell proliferation of chondrocytes. *In: Current Advances in Skeletogenesis* (M Silbermann and H C Slavkin, eds). Amsterdam: Excerpta Medica.
34. Van Kampen G P J, Veldhuijzen J P, Kuijer R, van de Stadt R J and Schipper C A (1985)

Cartilage response to mechanical forces studied in high density cultures. *Arthritis Rheum* **28**: 419–24.

35. Veldhuijzen J P, Huisman A H, Vermeiden J P W and Prahl-Andersen B (1987) The growth of cartilage cells *in vitro* and the effect of intermittent compressive force. A histological evaluation. *Connect Tissue Res* **16**: 107–196.

36. Lippiello L, Kaye C, Neumata T and Mankin H J (1985) *In vitro* metabolic response of articular cartilage segments to low levels of hydrostatic pressure. *Connect Tissue Res* **13**: 99–107.

37. Kimura J H, Schipplein O D, Kuettner K E and Andriacchi T P (1985) Effects of hydrostatic loading on extracellular matrix formation. *Trans Orthop Res Soc* **10**: 365.

38. Jones I L, Klämfeldt A and Sandström T (1982) The effect of continuous mechanical pressure upon the turnover of articular cartilage proteoglycans *in vitro*. *Clin Orthop* **165**: 283–9.

39. Klämfeldt A (1985) Continuous mechanical pressure and joint tissue. *Scand J Rheumatol* **14**: 431–7.

40. Palmoski M J and Brandt K D (1984) Effects of static and cyclic compressive loading on articular cartilage plugs *in vitro*. *Arthritis Rheum* **27**: 675–81.

41. Leung D V M, Glagov S and Mathews M B (1976) Cyclic stretching stimulated synthesis of matrix components by arterial smooth muscle cells *in vitro*. *Science* **191**: 475.

42. Leung D V M, Glagov S and Mathews M B (1977) A new *in vitro* system for studying cell response to mechanical stimulation. *Exp Cell Res* **109**: 285–9.

43. Lee R C, Rich J B, Kelley K M, Weiman D S and Mathews M B (1982) A comparison of *in vitro* cellular responses to mechanical and electrical stimulation. *Am Surg* **48**: 567–74.

44. DeWitt M T, Handley C J, Oakes B W and Lowther D A (1984) *In vitro* response of chondrocytes to mechanical loading. The effect of short term mechanical tension. *Connect Tissue Res* **12**: 97–109.

45. McKibbin B and Maroudas A (1979) Nutrition and metabolism. *In*: *Adult Articular Cartilage* (M A R Freeman, ed), pp. 461–86. London: Pitman Medical.

46. Maroudas A (1970) Distribution and diffusion of solutes in articular cartilage. *Biophys J* **10**: 365–79.

47. Schalkwijk J, van den Berg W B, van de Putte L B A, Joosten L A B and van den Bersselaar L (1985) Cationization of catalase, perioxidase, and superoxide dismutase. Effect of improved intraarticular retention on experimental arthritis in mice. *J Clin Invest* **76**: 1850–9.

48. Maroudas A (1976) Transport of solutes through cartilage: permeability to large molecules. *J Anat* **122**: 335–47.

49. Edwards J and Smith A (1965) The uptake of fluid by living cartilage after compression. *Proc Physiol Soc* **6**: 5–6.

50. Tomlinson N and Maroudas A (1980) The effect of cyclic and continuous compression on the penetration of large molecules into articular cartilage. *J Bone Joint Surg [Br]* **62**: 251.

51. Kaye C F, Lippiello L, Mankin H and Numata T (1980) Evidence for a pressure sensitive stimulus receptor system in articular cartilage. *Trans Orthop Res Soc* **5**: 1.

52. Bassett C A L (1968) Biological significance of piezoelectricity. *Calcif Tissue Res* **1**: 252–72.

53. Justus R and Luft J H (1970) Mechanochemical hypothesis for bone remodelling induced by mechanical stress. *Calcif Tissue Res* **5**: 222–35.

54. Bourret L A and Rodan G A (1976) The role of calcium in the inhibition of cAMP accumulation in epiphyseal cartilage cells exposed to physiological pressure. *J Cell Physiol* **88**: 353–62.

55. Poole C A, Flint M H and Beaumont B W (1985) Analysis of the morphology and function of primary cilia in connective tissues. A cellular cybernetic probe? *Cell Motility* **5**: 175–93.

56. Goldberg N D, Haddox M K, Nicol S E, Glass D B, Sanford C H, Kuehl F A and Estensen R (1975) Biologic regulation through opposing influences of cyclic GMP and cyclic AMP. The Yin Yang Hypothesis. *Adv Cyclic Nucleotide Res* **5**: 307–30.

57. Rodan G A (1981) Mechanical and electrical effects on bone and cartilage cells: translation of the physical signal into a biological message. *In*: *Orthodontics. The State of the Art* (H G Barrer, ed), pp. 315–22. Philadelphia: University of Pennsylvania Press.

58. Bindermann I, Shimshoni Z and Somjen D (1984) Biochemical pathways involved in the translation of physical stimulus into biological message. *Calcif Tissue Int* (Suppl 1) **36**: 82–85.

Chapter 6

Structure and Function of the Chondrocyte under Mechanical Stress

R. A. Stockwell

CONTENTS

INTRODUCTION

Cartilage is resilient and deformable. It forms strengthening bars in the walls of the respiratory air tubes to prevent collapse while permitting moderate changes in calibre. In the skeletal system, most developing bones are formed from cartilage, while in the vertebral column it provides cushioning, load-distributing discs; in synovial joints, articular cartilage protects the underlying bone ends, resisting compressive, tensile and shearing forces. This mechanical property resides in the matrix, a fibre-reinforced gel (formed by proteoglycan molecules which attract and bind water), the amount of matrix largely reflecting the activity of the cartilage cells (chondrocytes) which synthesize (and degrade) its macromolecules.

In the case of articular cartilage which flattens as it deforms, so increasing the contact area between the two articular surfaces and spreading the load on the underlying bone, its thickness is directly related to the species size although its cell density (cells/mm^3) is approximately inversely proportional to its thickness (1). The stress (i.e. load per unit area) on the cartilage surface is of the same order in joints of widely differing size (2) and this is probably related to the greater deformation which thicker cartilages can undergo, thereby achieving greater congruency and so spreading the greater load. Thus cartilage thickness

126

or, looking at it another way, the amount of matrix maintained per cell, reflects the total load transmitted by the joint, suggesting that in some way cartilage cells are sensitive to mechanical stimuli.

Studies of denervated and immobilized joints substantiate this concept. Cartilage becomes thinner in joints that have ceased to function due to paraplegia or poliomyelitis (3), or after experimental denervation (4). Investigations of joint immobilization with or without pressure applied to the cartilage (5, 6) similarly demonstrate areas of cartilage atrophy and often cell death. Chondrocytes (7) can sustain and survive 30% compressive strain (*Fig.* 6.1) but in 'droptower' studies, stress levels greater than 25 MN/m^2 producing strains

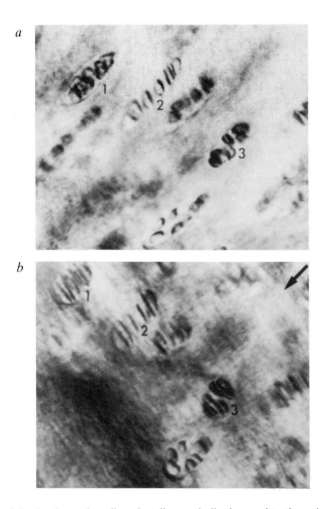

Fig. 6.1. Fresh bovine femoral cartilage (patellar area) sliced normal to the articular surface and viewed by Nomarski interference optics. *a*, cell groups (1–3) under zero compression stress applied to articular surface, 0% strain in cells; *b*, same cell groups, stress 265 g/mm^2 (approximately 2·6 MN/m^2), 28–30% strain in cells and matrix; arrow shows direction of compression (× 380). [From Broom and Myers, 1980 (7), with permission.]

greater than 40% cause tissue death (8). However, even simple immobilization applied without pressure causes atrophy. Reduced nutritional supply to the cartilage cells, due to either occlusion of the articular surface through which nutrients diffuse from the synovial fluid or lack of 'stirring' of the fluid in the immobile joint (9), probably contributes to the effects of changed mechanical stress, but the cells in the cartilage remain numerous despite the matrix loss and cartilage thinning (10). In contrast to disuse atrophy, new formation of cartilage occurs in the false joint which results from movement and stress in faulty fracture healing, and in situations where a tendon plays over a stress point. Experimentally, the use of continuous passive motion assists the healing of full thickness cartilage defects in experimental animals (11). These observations support the view that cartilage requires the optimal stimuli of movement and pressure to maintain its normal healthy structure.

Such considerations undoubtedly inspired early experimental work on cartilage expression. It was believed that mechanical forces act primarily by displacing the connective tissue fibre mesh to induce the cartilage matrix. Glucksmann (12) cultured embryonic chick bone rudiments subject to either compressive or tensile stress. He concluded that compressive forces acting on connective tissue cells enhance matrix formation, although pressure is not essential in chondrogenesis. Tension produces fibrous tissue. Confirmation of these results (13) showed that embryonic chick cells produce cartilage when placed under compressive stress, especially if the oxygen supply is kept low. To some extent these conclusions reflect what happens in articular cartilage, where the superficial cells are predominantly subject to tensile forces and have a low rate of glycosaminoglycan synthesis (14) compared with the deeper cells which are subject to compression.

EFFECTS OF MECHANICAL STRESS ON METABOLISM

Work has concentrated mainly on measuring changes in glycosaminoglycan concentration and synthesis in cartilage, although some other parameters have been investigated.

Whole Animal Experiments

In the whole animal it is rather more difficult to demonstrate the effects of additional (non-lethal) than of reduced load. Thus, after partial amputation or immobilization of one hind limb in dogs (15) or fore limb in sheep (16) glycosaminoglycan (predominantly chondroitin sulphate) is diminished in articular cartilage of the unloaded (operated side) limb compared with the contralateral loaded (intact) limb or with normal controls. The cartilage of the loaded limb may have more glycosaminoglycan, particularly glucosamine (keratan sulphate), compared with normal adequate controls (15). Keratan sulphate is also increased in cartilage in exercised dogs (17) and rabbits (18); increased weight bearing rather than merely an increase in exercise (running) is required. This is in accord with biochemical analyses showing that the weight-bearing regions of articular cartilage have more keratan sulphate than do more lightly loaded regions (19, 20). Histochemically, this is also seen in the dog humeral head (21) and in the human femoral head where the weight-bearing zenith shows denser staining due to keratan sulphate than the infra-foveal region.

Conversely, changes may be predominantly related to chondroitin sulphate. In most cases (16, 22–26) glycosaminoglycan synthesis increases, although this rather uncommonly yields a net rise in chondroitin sulphate content compared with normal controls (16, 26). Usually signs are found that the integrity of the matrix is impaired. Much of the increased activity with respect to chondroitin sulphate may result from cell multiplication and early overhydration of the matrix. The young cells formed would produce chondroitin sulphate-rich proteoglycans. If the stress applied is not great enough to initiate damage and cell proliferation, the increased synthetic activity comes predominantly from existing older cells which produce keratan sulphate-rich proteoglycans (27).

In vitro Experiments

It is easier to control experimental conditions *in vitro*. In calf articular cartilage, a continuous compressive force of 30 Kg/cm^2 (2·9 MN/m^2 or about 400 lbf/in^2, equivalent to the contact presssure in the human hip) applied for 4 days, reduces sulphate incorporation by 50% (28). This was attributed to elimination of water from the tissue under load, so concentrating the proteoglycans; raised concentrations of proteoglycans inhibit synthesis. This may have been the explanation since sulphate incorporation is stimulated by 15% using a continuous pressure of 375 lbf/in^2 for 4 h under conditions where dehydration could not occur (29).

Investigations on DNA synthesis in epiphyseal cartilage have been particularly significant. Continuous compression (60–80 g/cm^2 or about 6–8 $\times$ 10^3 N/m^2) results in stimulation of DNA synthesis and depression of glucose utilization. Levels of adenosine 3'5'-cyclic monophosphate (cAMP) are reduced in proliferative cells but not in hypertrophic cells (30). Intermittent (0.3 Hz) compression (96 mmHg; about 10^4 N/m^2) rather than continuous compression increases intracellular cAMP while changes in ornithine decarboxylase activity indicate that DNA synthesis is reduced (31).

The effects of continuous and intermittent compression on glycosaminoglycan synthesis have since been compared. There is considerable agreement that while continuous compression reduces glycosaminoglycan synthesis, intermittent compression increases synthesis and the glycosaminoglycan content of cartilage fragments, whether embryonic chick epiphyseal (32), adult dog articular (33), or immature mandibular condylar cartilage (34) is used. Cyclical stretching also enhances glycosaminoglycan synthesis and elevates cAMP (35): the authors postulate that the tensile stress might be causing a pressure effect on the cells within the tissue. In epiphyseal cartilage and the growth plate (36) intermittent but apparently not continuous pressure increases alkaline phosphatase activity (*Fig.* 6.2).

Hence there is experimental evidence that chondrocytes detect and transduce into biochemical activity quite small pressures and/or changes of pressure. Rates of glycosaminoglycan synthesis monitored only under atmospheric pressure may not reflect rates achieved *in vivo* under the loads and stresses experienced *in situ* (37).

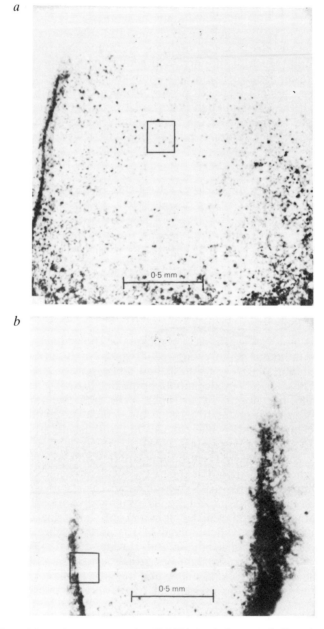

Fig. 6.2. Effect of intermittent compression (0·7 Hz) for 3 days on alkaline phosphatase activity in 4-day-old rat mandibular condyle. Enzyme activity is widespread in the chondrocytes in (*a*) compared with the control (*b*) (× 44). [From Copray *et al.*, 1985 (36), with permission.]

Role of cAMP

The effects of mechanical stress involve cAMP. The role of cAMP in cartilage cell differentiation is relevant to the problem although initial studies were confusing. Nevertheless, it was found that cAMP derivatives stimulate cartilage growth and sulphate uptake (38). Later investigations by Solursh and colleagues (39, 40) and by Kosher and colleagues (41) demonstrated conclusively that cAMP is a potent second messenger in chondrogenesis. The nucleotide is capable of bringing about precocious differentiation of the early limb bud mesenchyme, in particular of the mesenchyme beneath the apical epidermal ridge.

Endogenous cAMP increases progressively during chondrogenesis in the chick wing bud (42) and in chick pelvic chondrogenesis (43) which also responds to cAMP analogues. It is suggested that prostaglandin PGE_2 modulates cAMP levels in limb mesenchyme and peak production of PGE_2 in limb buds corresponds with the onset of chondrogenesis (44). Post-chondrogenesis, cAMP derivatives continue to stimulate cartilage growth in mice (45) and glycosaminoglycan synthesis in rats (46). In rabbit costal cartilage, parathyroid hormone stimulates cAMP and glycosaminoglycan synthesis, cAMP derivatives enhancing glycosaminoglycan synthesis (47). In adult dog articular cartilage, however, cAMP derivatives preferentially stimulate hyaluronic acid synthesis and proteoglycans are released from the cartilage slices into the medium (48).

Hence, on the whole, cAMP favours cartilage expression and, as indicated earlier, is one of the mediators in the changes of synthetic activity induced by mechanical stress. Thus, continuous compression is associated with low levels of cAMP and glycosaminoglycan synthesis and with enhanced DNA synthesis, while the reverse is true of intermittent compression (31–34, 36). Cyclical stretching also produces increased glycosaminoglycan synthesis, associated with raised levels of cAMP (35). It is of interest that intermittent compression also produces a raised level of cAMP in nanomelic mutant chick cartilage, suggesting that proteoglycans (minimal or absent in nanomelia) do not have a role in transducing the signal for cAMP synthesis (49).

Such conclusions are in accord with the general effects of cAMP. Reduced levels signal DNA synthesis, while elevated levels signal cytodifferentiation (50) via arrest of cell proliferation in the early G1 phase of the cell cycle (51). The well known stimulation of phosphorylating enzymes and in particular of the glycogenolytic cascade would be conducive to glycosaminoglycan synthesis, especially in chondrocytes.

Role of Calcium Ions

It is well known that cAMP levels are affected by Ca^{2+} concentrations. In embryonic chick epiphyses (30) the calcium ionophore A23187 mimics the effects of continuous compression by reducing the levels of cAMP in proliferative cells although not in hypertrophic cells. Pressure by itself increases Ca^{2+} uptake both in proliferative and hypertrophic cells. This indicates that adenylate cyclase in the latter cells is not susceptible to inhibition by Ca^{2+}, confirmed by analysis of fractionated plasma membranes. This suggests that pressure effects are associated with penetration of Ca^{2+} into cells.

Investigations of chondrocytes in suspension culture (following prior monolayer culture) indicated that Ca^{2+} elevates cAMP but stimulates Type I (non-cartilage) collagen synthesis; cells cultured without Ca^{2+} in the medium produce Type II collagen (52). With hindsight, it is possible that fibronectin, known to alter the phenotype (53), and which might have been produced by the cells while in monolayer, could have been responsible for this finding. Certainly, in fragments of chick vertebral cartilage, Ca^{2+} at physiological levels stimulates ^{35}S-sulphate uptake (54) while calcipenia reduces proteoglycan synthesis (and does not affect degradation) in slices of adult dog articular cartilage; the newly synthesized proteoglycans were similar both in calcipenic and normal media (55).

CELL SHAPE

The freshly isolated, living chondrocyte constantly changes its shape, putting out and withdrawing pseudopodic processes. The characteristic feature of numerous projecting cell processes is maintained in the tissues, whether the general shape of the cell is ovoid, discoid or truly spherical as in suspension culture (39). In articular cartilage, the superficial cells are flattened but become more rounded (like the deeper cells) if a slice of the cartilage is transplanted to soft tissues, originally attributed to the change in mechanical environment.

Effect of Mechanical Stress

The superficial cells in rabbit joints become more spherical for a short time immediately after brief exercise (56); this was associated with the concurrent 10% increase in cartilage thickness attributed to imbibition of fluid. Such results imply that the superficial cells are constantly changing their shape and volume in habitual joint usage. Possibly the increased extracellular lipid found in the superficial zone in a 20 years old soldier dying immediately after a route march (57) reflected cell shape change during exercise just prior to death, since such lipid is derived at least partially from the tips of cell processes shed during cell movement (58).

Such transient swelling of chondrocytes seems to be distinct from the more lasting enlargement found after long-term exercise or loading. The chondrocyte in its metabolism does more than synthesize matrix macromolecules, but the quantity of its cytoplasmic organelles such as the granular endoplasmic reticulum, the Golgi complex and mitochondria, reflect this primary function carried out in an avascular environment. In situations of altered loading, hypertrophy of the granular endoplasmic reticulum and Golgi is commonly observed, particularly in the deeper chondrocytes (59). Stereological measurements (60) of articular cartilage following long-term non-strenuous exercise disclose that the deeper cells become larger, rich in granular endoplasmic reticulum and other cytoplasmic organelles. In contrast to the immediate and transient effects of exercise, there is no change in cell size in the superficial zone but the volume of the nucleus is increased. The authors note the existence of a separate population of small nuclei in all zones in exercised and control rabbits.

Role of Cell Shape in Cartilage Expression

A third aspect of the relationship of cell shape to cell function is potentially more significant. Important progress was made when it was shown (61) that phenotypic expression by chondrocytes *in vitro* occurs in spinner (suspension) culture rather than in monolayer culture. Sokoloff (62) attributes this to the anchorage of isolated chondrocytes to the vessel wall in monolayer culture, which predisposes against the chondrogenic expression found in suspension culture. Later experiments with the adhesivity of plastic surfaces (63) demonstrated that on going from a very flat to a more rounded shape, fewer and fewer cells incorporate ^{3}H-thymidine, until finally when almost completely spherical cells fail to enter S phase.

Factors affecting chondrocyte differentiation are again relevant. Solursh *et al.* (40) propose that there is an integral relationship between cell shape, cell cycle and the differentiation process. Chondrogenesis can be obtained from a single cell clone if the cells are induced to become spherical in collagen or agarose gels (64). Prechondroblastic chick limb bud mesenchyme culture on semi-adhesive polymethacrylate (HEMA), which maintains the cells in a rounded configuration, is conducive to synthesis of a sulphated matrix (65) and cartilage formation.

More recently, it has been shown that subconfluent cultures of chick limb bud mesenchyme will secrete Type II collagen and Alcian blue-positive matrix if treated with cytochalasin D (66). The actin 'cables' of the filamentous cytoskeleton are disrupted by cytochalasin and this allows the cells to become spherical. Cytochalasin also blocks the anti-chondrogenic effect of fibronectin; fibronectin detaches from the cell surface of fibroblasts if their actin content is disrupted (67) The anti-chondrogenic action of limb ectodermal factors is also blocked by cytochalasin (68), although agents that elevate intracellular cAMP (which itself can induce chondrogenesis) are ineffective in this respect.

Thus cells which become spherical are enabled to express the cartilage phenotype, but their rounded shape may merely be a structural consequence of changes within the cytoplasm and at the cell membrane which simultaneously produce functional consequences in metabolism.

MECHANOTRANSDUCTION

We do not know how the chondrocyte detects mechanical forces or transduces them into a biochemical response. The chondrocyte responds quickly and sensitively to compressive (and tensile) forces of quite low magnitude, e.g. 60 g/cm^2 (approximately $6 \times 10^3 \text{ N/m}^2$). While this may seem impressive, many small marine animals (without a swim bladder or other gas-filled organ) can adjust their habitual depth in water (69), exhibiting a pressure sensitivity with a threshold of only about 10 g/cm^2 (10^3 N/m^2). The extreme threshold for mechanical deformation must be shown by the hair cells of the internal ear (70) which in the turtle respond to small fractions of 1 N/m^2. There are few indisputable facts about the ultimate biochemical response of chondrocytes to mechanical forces. Overloading with traumatic forces, e.g. 25 MN/m^2, can kill the cells. In the physiological range of mechanical stimuli, synthesis of the major matrix macromolecules increases particularly with intermittent compression, while on the whole DNA synthesis is reduced. Little is known about the chondrocyte response as regards the metabolism of degradative enzymes, proteinase inhibitors and so on. However, in general, enhanced macromolecular synthesis is associated with an increase in cAMP both in response to mechanical stress and in chondrogenesis. Ca^{2+} uptake is closely linked with pressure effects and with cAMP elevation. Cell shape is affected by mechanical stress and conversely a change in cell shape to a more spherical form, related to modifications of the cytoskeleton, is conducive to cartilage expression in chondrogenesis. What, therefore, can we infer about the problem of mechano-transduction in the chondrocyte?

Mechanosensitive Cells

It may be helpful to consider types of cell which can detect and respond to pressure or mechanical deformation, often with a very high sensitivity.

Bone

In the case of bone, the relationship of stress to tissue architecture has long been recognized. Although the electrical activity induced by mechanical stress has been ascribed to the piezoelectric nature of bone (71), there is now reasonable agreement that it is due to streaming potentials, i.e. the movement of ions through mechanically distorted channels (72). Both piezoelectric activity and streaming potentials have been described in cartilage and possible effects on metabolism have been reviewed by Hall (73). Results vary depending *inter alia* on the precise stimulus applied, but intermittent, pulsed voltages appear to modulate the calcium-handling ability of chondrocytes, inducing Ca^{2+} uptake and calcification. DNA synthesis can be stimulated, possibly mediated by causing ion flux across the plasma membrane, with secondary effects on cytoplasmic Ca^{2+} concentration (74). While mechanical stress on whole cartilage might be mediated by electrical activity induced through matrix components, thereby affecting the cells, it is unlikely that proteoglycans are the molecules concerned. Thus nanomelic chick cartilage, in which proteoglycan is nearly or completely absent, gives responses to mechanical stimuli which are similar to those obtained from normal cartilage (49). As a rigorous requirement for transduction, electrical effects mediated via any matrix macromolecule would seem to be eliminated by the results obtained on isolated cells in culture (31, 32).

Baroreceptors

Studies on avian aortic wall (75) show that the terminal axon runs in connective tissue matrix not unlike a cartilage lacuna (*Fig.* 6.3). The authors consider that this is a low-grade, primitive form of the lamellated Pacinian corpuscle seen in the skin and elsewhere. Collagen fibres run longitudinally along the exterior of the axon and attach to it. As the arterial wall stretches due to luminal pressure, the collagen is postulated to exert a tensile force on the axolemma, which is cushioned from other mechanical stimulation by the extracellular substance. The precise mechanism of transduction at the level of the cell membrane is unknown.

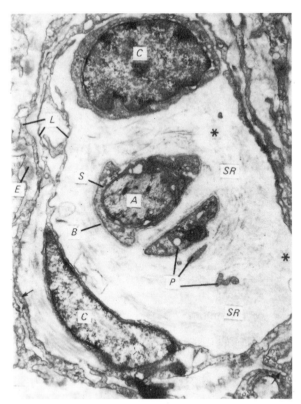

Fig. 6.3. Baroreceptor in aortic wall of domestic fowl. The near-terminal axon (A) is embedded in a Schwann cell (S) covered by a basal lamina (B). This is enclosed by capsular cells (C) forming lamellae (L) which surround a region (SR) consisting of longitudinally and a few obliquely running collagen fibrils in fluid-filled spaces (asterisks). E, elastic fibre; P, processes of Schwann cell; arrows, pinocytotic vesicles ($\times$ 9500). [From Taha *et al.*, 1983 (75), with permission.]

Skin mechanoreceptors

The Merkel cell and the Ruffini end organ may be considered. Merkel cells are found in little domes at the base of the epidermis. The base of each Merkel cell which contains neuropeptide granules is in close proximity to a flattened nerve ending, the Merkel disc. The whole complex is very sensitive to tactile stimuli, such as stroking the skin. The superficial aspect of the Merkel cell is studded with short blunt processes invaginating into, but not between, the deepest cells of the epidermis (*Fig.* 6.4). The plasma membrane between the projecting processes, but not that of the processes themselves, is attached by desmosomes to the epidermal cells (76). Mechanical perturbation of the epidermal cells would therefore cause deformation of the Merkel cell membrane, perhaps most effectively where the cell process joins the main part of the cell. The actual mechanism of transduction at the membrane is not known.

The Ruffini end organ is directionally sensitive to skin stretch and to vertical displacement. The terminal axon runs in an encapsulated space filled with 'fluid substances' (77) and exhibits thorn-like processes in contact with longitudinally

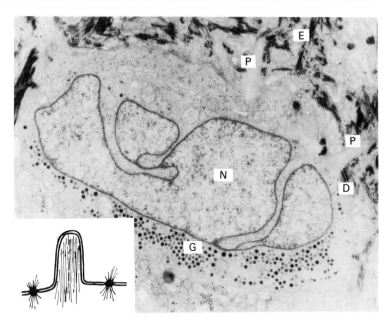

Fig. 6.4. Merkel cell (tactile receptor) in normal rat skin. Blunt cell processes (P) containing longitudinal filaments project into the basal epidermal cells (E) to which it is attached by desmosomes (D) (*see* inset diagram). The cell contains a completely folded nucleus (N) and neuropeptide granules (G) in the basal cytoplasm (× 11 500). [Reproduced by kind permission of Dr G S Findlater.]

orientated collagen (*Fig.* 6.5). Like the baroreceptor, it is suggested that the axon in its protective water cushion is sensitized to deformation in a specific direction by the suspending collagen fibres. Although the exact mechanism of transduction is not known, it is evident that when the skin is stretched, the axolemma will sustain tensile deformation, especially near the thorn-like processes.

Hair cells of internal ear

The 'hairs' of these sensitive cells (70) are stiff stereocilia (long, cylindrical processes) of varying but highly ordered lengths, containing a core of longitudinal, interconnected filaments (including actin) connected to the stereocilium membrane by other filaments. A single kinocilium (motile), with the usual 9 + 2 array of microtubules, is present but is lost in mammalian cochleae soon after birth. The tips of the hairs, or stereocilia, are partly embedded in rigid structures such as the membrana tectoria. Relative movement between the stereocilia tips and the tectorial membrane of less than 100 pm is sufficient to initiate a membrane potential in the hair cell.

It is thought that mechanoelectrical transduction is too rapid (response time of a few microseconds) to involve second messengers. Instead, Hudspeth (78) believes that ion channels at the tip of the stereocilium are opened directly. A filament is attached at one end to the tip of the stereocilium and by its other end to the side of the shaft of the neighbouring stereocilium (*Fig.* 6.6). As the

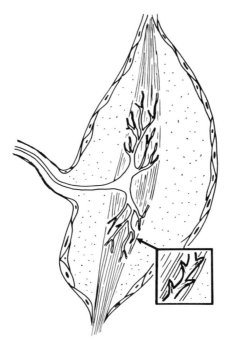

Fig. 6.5. Diagram of a Ruffini ending, a tactile receptor of skin. The axon branches in a complex way within an encapsulated organ containing hydrated material. Longitudinally running collagen fibrils pass between and close to the nerve branches, attaching to thorn-like processes on the axon (*see* inset).

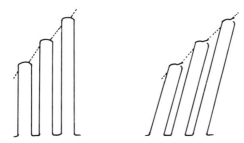

Fig. 6.6. Diagram of hairs (stereocilia) on a hair cell in the organ of Corti in the cochlea. A filament (pecked line) runs from the side of each hair to the tip of the next. When the hairs are deflected sideways (by soundwave-induced movement of the hair cells against the rigid tectorial membrane) as in the diagram to the right, the pull of the filament distorts the hairtip membrane, opening up an ion channel.

stereocilium is deflected, the filament pulls on the tip membrane carrying the transduction channels. This opens the channel and ions enter the cell, depolarizing the membrane. Voltage-dependent Ca^{2+} channels are activated, allowing Ca^{2+} to pass into the cell. The high intracellular Ca^{2+} concentration brings Ca^{2+}-sensitive K^+ channels into operation and K^+ passes out of the cell, repolarizing the membrane. Resonance is due to alternation of Ca^{2+} and K^+ channel patency.

Chondrocytes

With the possible exception of the hair cell, none of these mechanoreceptors shows a cytological configuration which is unique to detection of mechanical stress, in the same way that, for example, a synapse denotes transmission of a nerve impulse. However, a common factor seems to be that the microanatomical arrangement ultimately produces tensile or related distortions of the cell membrane. Could this apply to the chondrocyte? This cell has many projecting processes, a structural feature present in nearly all mechanoreceptors described, which include a monocilium of the non-motile $(9 + 0)$ variety.

According to Wilsman (79) there is a monocilium on every chondrocyte and he has commented *inter alia* on the possibility of a mechanotransductory function. In invertebrate animals, very small deflections of a cilium can be shown to evoke a response; although there is no direct evidence, this might occur in chondrocytes. In *Paramecium* (80) the mechanosensitive channels for Ca^{2+} are on the somatic membrane rather than on the ciliary membrane which carries the voltage-dependent Ca^{2+} channels. However, the ordinary cell processes of the chondrocyte, many of which protrude into the fibrous matrix beyond the lacuna, could like the rest of the plasma membrane give attachment to collagen via chondronectin or anchorin CII (81). Deformation of cartilage could by this means produce distortions in the plasma membrane. Directionality might be obtained in the superficial zone of articular cartilage where the cell processes are concentrated at the 'poles' of the 'flattened' cells rather than evenly distributed around the perimeter as in the midzone cells. The 'pericellular channels' and lacunar structure described by Poole *et al.* (82) might complicate the organization and possibly lend directionality in the case of the midzone cells but would not affect the fundamental mechanism.

However, as with electrical effects, it is difficult to see how such mechanisms could apply to cells in culture with no matrix. Here, it seems that mechanisms involving only the cell membrane are implicated, particularly relating to cAMP and Ca^{2+}.

Membrane Mechanisms

Pressure effects seem to be mediated ultimately by cAMP and Ca^{2+}. Normally, elevation of these second messengers within the cytoplasm is initiated by hormones (agonists) which bind to receptors on the cell surface or also, in the case of Ca^{2+}, by voltage-dependent channels in the membrane. It is worth considering the trans-membrane enzymatic mechanisms and pathways involved.

Adenylate cyclase

cAMP is synthesized from ATP by adenylate cyclase situated in the membrane and is hydrolysed by phosphodiesterase in the cytosol. Adenylate cyclase consists of three separate units – the hormone-specific receptor (H unit) in the outer leaflet of the membrane, a catalytic (C) unit in the inner leaflet, and a guanyl nucleotide-dependent protein regulator complex (N unit). The C unit is activated when complexed to the agonist-occupied H unit, also dependent on the N unit binding to GTP. Dephosphorylation to GDP in the N unit causes decoupling and hence deactivation of the C unit (*Fig.* 6.7). Ca^{2+} concentrations

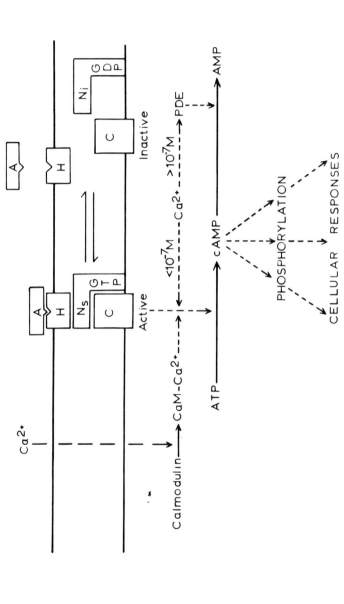

Fig. 6.7. Schematic diagram of membrane organization of adenylate cyclase with some controlling factors and effects in the cytoplasm. A, agonist; H, hormone-receptor unit; C, enzyme catalytic unit; Ns, regulator unit stimulated by binding to GTP; Ni, regulator unit inhibited by GDP; CaM, calmodulin; PDE, phosphodiesterase. Movement of subunits of cyclase occurs within the plane of the membrane. *See* text for full explanation.

of $10^{-8}-10^{-7}$ M (as exist in the resting cell) activate adenylate cyclase while higher levels ($10^{-6}-10^{-5}$ M) inhibit it but activate the diesterase (83), providing a basis for a time-dependent sequence of activation of the two enzymes as Ca^{2+} concentration rises in the cell. Calmodulin, a calcium-binding protein, activates adenylate cyclase and other enzymes (84). In the cell cycle, calmodulin is reduced by 50% at the end of the M phase and is not restored to normal levels until just before S phase. Hence, cAMP levels might be expected to be low during early G1 phase, so diminishing its inhibitory effects on cell proliferation which are greatest in early G1 (51). It is of interest that the full effect of intermittent compression on DNA synthesis, presumably induced by elevation of cAMP levels, occurs in early G1 (31). A S-100 calcium-binding protein related to calmodulin is present in human chondrocytes (85). Adenylate cyclase in foetal and adult human articular chondrocytes is stimulated by the prostaglandins and adrenalin (86).

Polyphosphoinositide system

Voltage-dependent Ca^{2+} channels in the plasma membrane are opened by membrane depolarization. Ca^{2+} levels also depend on a second biochemical trans-membrane pathway which involves the phosphoinositides (87). The appropriate agonists include growth factors which have been shown to be active on cartilage cells, e.g. platelet-derived growth factor and epidermal growth factor (88), while the action of interleukin 1, a degradative intercellular factor, involves the pathway in human chondrocytes (89). This pathway raises Ca^{2+} levels although there are other important sequelae. Agonist/receptor-mediated hydrolysis of phosphatidylinositol-(4, 5)-bisphosphate in the inner leaflet of the cell membrane by a phosphodiesterase yields diacyl glycerol and inositol trisphosphate (*Fig.* 6.8). Both products are second messengers (87). Inositol trisphosphate attaches to specific sites on the endoplasmic reticulum membrane, causing it to release Ca^{2+} into the cytosol. GTP may be involved in enhancing receptor coupling to the diesterase at the plasma membrane or may act at the endoplasmic reticulum. Putney (90) has proposed a biphasic capacitive model whereby emptying of the intracellular (i.e. endoplasmic reticulum) pool induces rapid entry of extracellular Ca^{2+} via the plasma membrane into the 'open' endoplasmic reticulum and thence into the cytosol (*Fig.* 6.8). Close association (distance not specified) of the endoplasmic reticulum with the plasma membrane is required. Qualitatively, this condition is readily fulfilled in the chondrocyte with its profuse endoplasmic reticulum; interestingly, in chondrocytes in suspension culture, endoplasmic reticulum is localized at the extreme periphery of the cytoplasm (30). Changes in Ca^{2+} concentration modulate several aspects of metabolism, including cell proliferation and adenylate cyclase activity.

The other hydrolytic product, diacyl glycerol, acts within the membrane to activate a C-kinase which induces many cellular responses, some of them (e.g. glycogenolysis) stimulated synergistically by Ca^{2+} (91). An intriguing by-product of lipase action on diacyl glycerol is arachidonic acid, the precursor of the prostaglandins. This forms part of the profuse extracellular lipid in the superficial zone of adult human cartilage (92).

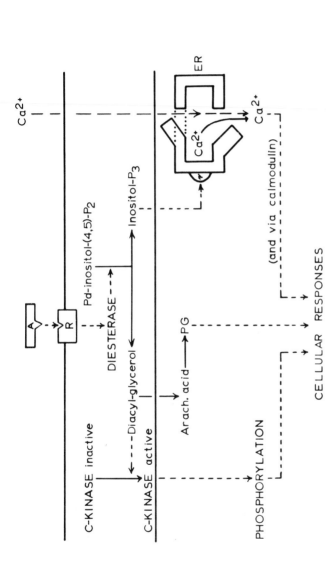

Fig. 6.8. Schematic diagram of poly(phosphoinositide) system. Trans-membrane coupling of agonist (A)-activated hormone-receptor (R) unit is required to activate diesterase which hydrolyses phosphatidylinositol-(4,5)-bisphosphate. Inositol trisphosphate binds to receptor (r) on closed endoplasmic reticulum (ER) to induce release of its Ca^{2+} pool. According to Putney (90) this in turn induces massive transfer of extracellular Ca^{2+} into cytoplasm via endoplasmic reticulum. PG, prostaglandin. *See* text for full explanation.

Membrane fluidity

The adenylate cyclase and inositol phosphate mechanisms both involve trans-membrane receptor-enzyme coupling. The concept of 'collision coupling' (93) requires molecular movement within the plane of the membrane to permit physical interaction of the components of, for example, the adenylate cyclase system to enable it to become biochemically active. The biophysical state of the membrane affects enzyme activity, perhaps via the kinetics of coupling. Investigations have been based on the concept that a membrane is essentially a mosaic phospholipid bilayer with areas which are relatively 'fluid' or 'rigid'. This is affected by such factors as temperature, the nature of the phospholipids, the proportion of cholesterol, cations and anions (including drugs) and the interactions of membrane-associated proteins with filaments of the cytoskeleton. Fluidity permits some degree of movement of embedded molecules; these might 'diffuse' laterally within the plane of the membrane or leaflet (diffusion coefficients approximately 10^{-11} cm^2/s) or have rotational motion about a relatively fixed axis perpendicular to the membrane plane.

Theoretically, increased fluidity, i.e. molecular mobility, increases the probability of coupling between receptor and catalytic unit, hence increasing enzyme activity for a given level of agonal stimulation. Thus, insertion of *cis*-vaccenic acid into erythrocyte membranes increases membrane fluidity and adenylate cyclase activity. The mode of action is not simple. The effects are more profound when the substance is inserted into the inner leaflet: large-scale diffusion is not involved, stimulation being dependent on perturbation of small distinct domains in the membrane (94). Different effects are produced before and after incubation with agonists when erythrocyte membranes are made more fluid by insertion of cationic drugs (95); drug-induced fluidity stimulates cyclase activity when the membranes are pre-incubated with effectors.

In the case of the inositol system, inositol trisphosphate produces a calcium influx which has secondary effects on cell membrane stability. Micromolar concentrations of Ca^{2+} both disrupt actin filaments (96) and reduce the interactions of cytoplasmic filaments with the membrane (97), which should permit greater membrane protein mobility. As noted earlier, similar actions by cytochalasin on mesenchymal cells induce a spheroidal shape and cartilage expression (66). Phosphatidylinositol-(4, 5)-bisphosphate itself increases lateral mobility of band 3 glycoprotein when added to erythrocyte membranes (98). Cholesterol depletion, which makes rigid domains more fluid and *vice versa*, is said to reorganize membrane domains so that the bisphosphate is no longer accessible to the diesterase (99). However, there are few data on changes in membrane fluidity relating to the inositol pathway.

Mechanolemmal considerations

Could mechanical stress cause sufficient perturbation of the membrane to bring about changes in activity of adenylate cyclase or of the inositol system? In theory, mechanical stress might provide enough energy even *in vitro*, where isolated cells respond to hydrostatic pressures of only 96 mmHg (about 10^4 N/m^2) to initiate biochemical activity. Veldhuijzen *et al.* (31) suggest that 2 kinds of membrane perturbation might occur here, either associated with progression of pressure waves across the membrane or related to cross-sectional squeezing of the membrane at the steady state. The activation energy required for fluoride-stimulated adenylate cyclase, for example, is about 84 kJ/mol (100). Hence in Veldhuijzen's experiment (31), where 2 pmol cAMP/10^6 cells were produced in 15 min of intermittent compression (0.3 Hz; 10^4 N/m^2) the energy required would have been about 17×10^{-8} J. The volume of the plasma membrane is approximately 1.9×10^{-18} m^3 (for a spheroidal chondrocyte, radius 5 μm and membrane thickness 6 nm). If the plasma membrane were a physically elastic solid and *if* it underwent cross-sectional compressive strain of 30% (i.e. equivalent to the maximum possible strain in whole cells which just permits survival), then the strain energy would be about 285×10^{-17} J/cell/ cycle. The total strain energy available (if all absorbed) to all the cells over about 300 cycles would be 85×10^{-8} J, which is of the same order as the activation energy required.

Of course, such calculations and values mean little. The membrane characteristics are not known, energy produced and absorbed from mechanical compressive or other effects on the membrane would be much less than the above figure, and 100% transformation of mechanical into chemical energy is unlikely. The pressure differential is probably much too small to provide enough energy, and cell amplification following a trigger event has to be assumed (31). In that case, perturbation might open ion channels with 'knock on' effects on Ca^{2+} concentrations, as postulated for the ear hair cells (78). This might be harnessed to stimulation of the key enzymes by calmodulin or similar calcium-binding proteins, or by relaxation of the membrane through disruption of cytoplasmic filaments. Alternatively, analogous to the effects of changing membrane fluidity, mechanical perturbation amounting to a mere 'stirring' effect on the membrane might cause a greater probability of receptor/catalytic unit interaction, leading to greater activity of key membrane enzymes for a given level of agonists and co-factors. Effects on the chondrocyte *in situ* are perhaps easier to consider in terms of membrane distortion via cell attachment to the matrix fabric (*Fig. 6.9*).

We lack data on many aspects of the effects of mechanical stress at the cellular level, even in chondrocytes. Perhaps these speculations may indicate some avenues to be explored.

CONCLUSIONS

Mechanical stress increases the synthetic activity of cartilage chondrocytes, while decreased compression lowers it. The type of compression seems to be important: intermittent rather than continuous compression is beneficial. One of the mediators of synthetic activity appears to be cAMP; high levels of cAMP in chondrocytes are associated with a high synthesis rate of matrix macromolecules. The intracellular cAMP level is affected by calcium ions. It is interesting to note that pressure increases the penetration of Ca^{2+} into the cells and the intracellular cAMP level. There are several possible mechanisms by which mechanical stress increases cAMP concentration and the penetration of Ca^{2+} ions through the cell membrane. These include voltage-dependent channels, the inositol system, and the action of adenyl cyclase. Mechanical stress also affects cell shape, making it more spherical which is conducive to chondrocyte expression.

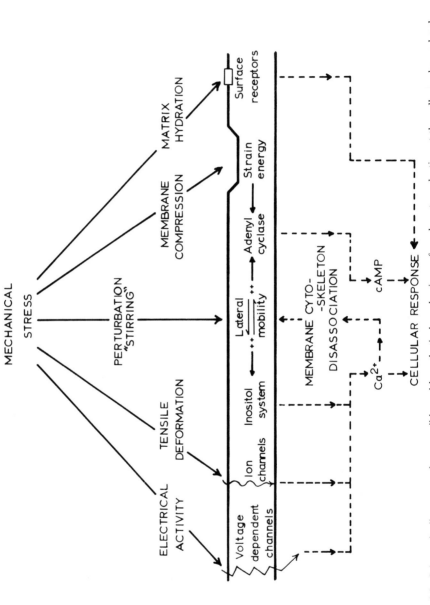

Fig. 6.9. Schematic diagram to show possible and hypothetical mechanisms of mechanotransduction at the cell membrane level.

CLINICAL SIGNIFICANCE

The degeneration and loss of cartilage in synovial and other joints leads to significant pain and disability. It is useful to gain information concerning the effects of mechanical stress, the prime stimulus which cartilage sustains. We know much about the effects on joints of immobilization and denervation, and of alteration in loading. In the laboratory, we are beginning to learn about the effects of stress under controlled conditions on cartilage and chondrocyte metabolism. The latter is of the utmost importance because it is the cells which produce and maintain the mechanically resilient matrix. Intermittent rather than continuous stress induces useful metabolic changes in the cells. Effects on the cell membrane and on cAMP and Ca^{2+} concentrations appear to be significant. Further studies may enable us to avoid mechanical factors which cause tissue damage through excessive stress, and to explore treatments utilizing controlled mechanical stress to aid cartilage regeneration and repair. It would be most useful to learn more about the site and nature of mechanotransduction in the cells, since this could lead to successful drug treatment.

ACKNOWLEDGEMENTS

I thank Dr Neil Broom, University of Auckland, Dr J V C M Copray, University of Amsterdam, Dr Gordon Findlater, University of Edinburgh and Professor Tony King, University of Liverpool, for allowing me to use their material. I am most grateful to Miss Helen Dingwall for her helpful secretarial assistance.

REFERENCES

1. Stockwell R A (1971) The interrelationship of cell density and cartilage thickness in mammalian articular cartilage. *J Anat* **109**: 411–21.
2. Simon W H (1970) Scale effects in animal joints. I. Articular cartilage thickness and compressive stress. *Arthritis Rheum* **13**: 244–56.
3. Collins D H (1949) *The Pathology of Articular and Spinal Diseases*. London: Arnold.
4. Akeson W H, Eichelberger L and Roma M (1958) Biochemical studies of articular cartilage. II. Values following the denervation of an extremity. *J Bone Joint Surg [Am]* **40**: 153–62.
5. Thompson R C and Bassett C A L (1970) Histological observations on experimentally induced degeneration of articular cartilage. *J Bone Joint Surg [Am]* **52**: 435–43.
6. Akeson W H, Woo S L-Y, Amiel D, Coutts R D and Daniel D (1973) The connective tissue response to immobility: biochemical changes in periarticular tissue of the immobilized rabbit knee. *Clin Orthop* **93**: 356–62.
7. Broom N D and Myers D B (1980) A study of the structural response of wet hyaline cartilage to various loading stresses. *Connect Tissue Res* **7**: 227–37.
8. Repo R U and Finlay J B (1977) Survival of articular cartilage after controlled impact. *J Bone Joint Surg [Am]* **59**: 1068–76.
9. Gritzka T L, Fry L R, Cheesman R L and Lavigne A (1973) Deterioration of articular cartilage caused by continuous compression in a moving rabbit joint. *J Bone Joint Surg [Am]* **55**: 1698–720.
10. Sood S C (1971) A study of the effects of experimental immobilization on rabbit articular cartilage. *J Anat* **108**: 497–507.
11. Salter R B, Simmonds D F, Malcolm B W, Rumble E J, MacMichael D and Clements N D (1980) The biological effect of continuous passive motion on the healing of full thickness defects in articular cartilage. *J Bone Joint Surg [Am]* **62**: 1232–51.
12. Glucksmann A (1939) Studies on bone mechanics *in vitro*. II. The role of tension and pressure in chondrogenesis. *Anat Rec* **73**: 39–56.
13. Bassett C A L and Herrmann I (1961) Influence of oxygen concentration and mechanical forces on differentiation of connective tissues *in vitro*. *Nature* **190**: 460–1.
14. Maroudas A and Evans H (1974) Sulphate diffusion and incorporation into human articular

cartilage. *Biochim Biophys Acta* **338**: 265–79.

15. Olah E H and Kostenszky K S (1976) Effect of loading and prednisolone treatment on the glycosaminoglycan content of articular cartilage in dogs. *Scand J Rheumatol* **5**: 49–52.
16. Caterson B and Lowther D A (1978) Changes in the metabolism of the proteoglycans from sheep articular cartilage in response to mechanical forces. *Biochim Biophys Acta* **540**: 412–22.
17. Van Sickle D C and Kincaid S A (1976) Modulability of canine articular cartilage histochemistry. *Proc V Int Congr Histochem Cytochem* **358**: (Abstr).
18. Tammi M, Säämänen A M, Jauhiainen A, Malminen O, Kiviranta I and Helminen H (1983) Proteoglycan alterations in rabbit knee articular cartilage following physical exercise and immobilization. *Connect Tissue Res* **11**: 45–55.
19. Bjelle A (1975) Content and composition of glycosaminoglycans in human knee joint cartilage. *Connect Tissue Res* **3**: 141–7.
20. Sweet M B E, Thonar E J-M A and Immelman A R (1977) Regional distribution of water and glycosaminoglycans in immature articular cartilage. *Biochim Biophys Acta* **500**: 173–86.
21. Kincaid S A and Van Sickle D C (1981) Regional histochemical and thickness variations of adult canine articular cartilage. *Am J Vet Res* **42**: 428–32.
22. McDevitt C A, Gilbertson E and Muir H (1977) An experimental model of osteoarthritis; early morphological and biochemical changes. *J Bone Joint Surg [Br]* **59**: 24–35.
23. Radin E L, Ehrlich M G, Chernack R, Abernethy P, Paul I L and Rose R M (1978) Effect of repetitive impulsive loading on the knee joints of rabbits. *Clin Orthop* **131**: 288–93.
24. Palmoski M J and Brandt K D (1981) Running inhibits the reversal of atrophic changes in canine knee cartilage after removal of a leg cast. *Arthritis Rheum* **24**: 1329–37.
25. Vasan N (1983) Effects of physical stress on the synthesis and degradation of cartilage matrix. *Connect Tissue Res* **12**: 49–58.
26. Donahue J M, Buss D, Oegema T R and Thompson R C (1983) The effects of indirect blunt trauma on adult canine articular cartilage. *J Bone Joint Surg [Am]* **65**: 948–57.
27. Shulman H J and Meyer K (1968) Cellular differentiation and the aging process in cartilaginous tissues. *J Exp Med* **128**: 1353–62.
28. Jones I L, Klämfeldt A and Sandström T (1982) The effect of continuous mechanical pressure upon the turnover of articular cartilage proteoglycans *in vitro*. *Clin Orthop* **165**: 283–9.
29. Lippiello L, Kaye C, Neumata T and Mankin H J (1985) *In vitro* metabolic response of articular cartilage segments to low levels of hydrostatic pressure. *Connect Tissue Res* **13**: 99–107.
30. Bourret L A and Rodan G A (1976) The role of calcium in the inhibition of cAMP accumulation in epiphyseal cartilage cells exposed to physiological pressure. *J Cell Physiol* **88**: 353–62.
31. Veldhuijzen J P, Bourret L A and Rodan G A (1979) *In vitro* studies of the effect of intermittent compressive forces on cartilage cell proliferation. *J Cell Physiol* **98**: 299–306.
32. Van Kampen G P J (1983) Modulation of chondrocyte metabolism *in vitro*. University of Amsterdam: Doctoral Thesis.
33. Palmoski M J and Brandt K D (1984) Effects of static and cyclic compressive loading on articular cartilage plugs *in vitro*. *Arthritis Rheum* **27**: 675–81.
34. Copray J V C M (1984) *Growth regulation of mandibular cartilage in vitro*. University of Groningen: Doctoral Thesis.
35. DeWitt M T, Handley C J, Oakes B W and Lowther D A (1984) *In vitro* response of chondrocytes to mechanical loading. The effect of short term mechanical tension. *Connect Tissue Res* **12**: 97–110.
36. Copray J V C M, Jansen H W B and Duterloo H S (1985) Effect of compressive forces on phosphatase activity in mandibular condylar cartilage of the rat *in vitro*. *J Anat* **140**: 479–89.
37. Slowman S D and Brandt K D (1986) Composition and glycosaminoglycan metabolism of articular cartilage from habitually loaded and habitually unloaded sites. *Arthritis Rheum* **29**: 88–94.
38. Drezner M K, Neelon F A and Lebovitz H E (1976) Stimulation of cartilage macromolecular synthesis by adenosine-3', 5'-monophosphate. *Biochim Biophys Acta* **425**: 521–31.
39. Ahrens P B, Solursh M and Reiter R S (1977) Stage-related capacity for limb chondrogenesis in cell culture. *Dev Biol* **60**: 69–92.
40. Solursh M, Ahrens P B and Reiter R S (1978) A tissue culture analysis of the steps in limb chondrogenesis. *In Vitro* **14**: 51–61.
41. Kosher R A and Savage M P (1980) Studies on the possible role of cyclic AMP in limb morphogenesis and differentiation. *J Embryol Exp Morphol* **56**: 91–105.
42. Solursh M, Reiter R S, Ahrens P B and Vertel B M (1981) Stage- and position-related changes in chondrogenic response of chick embryonic wing mesenchyme to treatment with dibutyryl cyclic AMP. *Dev Biol* **83**: 1–19.

43. Burch W M and Lebovitz H E (1981) Adenosine-3', 5'-monophosphate. A modulator of embryonic chick cartilage growth. *J Clin Invest* **68**: 1496–502.
44. Gay S W and Kosher R A (1985) Prostaglandin synthesis during the course of limb cartilage differentiation *in vitro*. *J Embryol Exp Morphol* **89**: 367–82.
45. Merker H-J and Gunther T (1979) The influence of insulin, cAMP and the calcium ionophore x537A on the growth of the cartilage anlagen of limb buds *in vitro*. *Experientia* **35**: 1307–8.
46. Miller R P, Husain M and Lohin S (1979) Long acting cAMP analogues enhance sulfate incorporation into matrix proteoglycans and suppress cell division of fetal rat chondrocytes in monolayer culture. *J Cell Physiol* **100**: 63–76.
47. Takigawa M, Takano T and Suzuki F (1981) Effects of parathyroid hormone and cyclic AMP analogues on the activity of ornithine decarboxylase and expression of the differential phenotype of chondrocytes in culture. *J Cell Physiol* **106**: 259–68.
48. Stack M T and Brandt K D (1980) Dibutyryl cyclic AMP affects hyaluronate synthesis and macromolecular organization in normal adult articular cartilage *in vitro*. *Biochim Biophys Acta* **631**: 264–77.
49. Bourret L A, Goetinck P F, Hintz R and Rodan G A (1979) Cyclic 3, 5-AMP changes in chondrocytes of the proteoglycan-deficient chick embryonic mutant, nanomelia. *FEBS Lett* **108**: 353–5.
50. McMahon D (1974) Chemical messengers in development: a hypothesis. *Science* **185**: 1012–21.
51. Froelich J E and Rachmeler M (1976) Inhibition of cell growth in the G1 phase by adenosine 3', 5'-cyclic monophosphate. *J Cell Biol* **60**: 249–57.
52. Deshmukh K, Kline W G and Sawyer B D (1977) Effects of calcitonin and parathyroid hormone on the metabolism of chondrocytes in culture. *Biochim Biophys Acta* **499**: 28–35.
53. Kleinmann H K, Klebe R J and Martin G R (1981) Role of collagenous matrices in the adhesion and growth of cells. *J Cell Biol* **88**: 473–85.
54. Shulman H J and Opler A (1974) The stimulating effect of calcium on the synthesis of cartilage proteoglycan. *Biochem Biophys Res Commun* **59**: 914–19.
55. Palmoski M J and Brandt K D (1979) Effect of calcipenia on proteoglycan metabolism and aggregation in normal articular cartilage *in vitro*. *Biochem J* **182**: 399–406.
56. Ekholm R and Norback B (1951) On the relationship between articular changes and function. *Acta Orthop Scand* **21**: 81–98.
57. Schallock G (1942) Untersuchungen zur Pathogenese von Aufbrauchveränderungen an der Knorpeligen Anteilen des Kniegelenkes. *Veröff Konstit Wehrpath* **49**: 1–68.
58. Ghadially F N, Meachim G and Collins D H (1965) Extracellular lipids in the matrix of human articular cartilage. *Ann Rheum Dis* **24**: 136–46.
59. Stockwell R A, Billingham M E and Muir H (1983) Ultrastructural changes in articular cartilage after experimental section of the anterior cruciate ligament of the dog knee. *J Anat* **136**: 425–39.
60. Paukkonen K, Selkäinaho K, Jurvelin J, Kiviranta I and Helminen H (1985) Cells and nuclei of articular cartilage chondrocytes in young rabbits enlarged after non-strenuous physical exercise. *J Anat* **142**: 13–20.
61. Srivastava V M, Malemud C J and Sokoloff L (1974) Chondroid expression by rabbit articular cells in spinner culture following monolayer culture. *Connect Tissue Res* **2**: 127–36.
62. Sokoloff L (1976) Articular chondrocytes in culture. *Arthritis Rheum* **19** (Suppl): 426–9.
63. Folkmann J and Moscona A (1978) Role of cell shape in growth control. *Nature* **273**: 345–9.
64. Solursh M, Linsenmeyer T F and Jensen K L (1982) Chondrogenesis from single limb mesenchymal cells. *Dev Biol* **94**: 259–64.
65. Archer C W, Rooney P and Wolpert L (1982) Cell shape and cartilage differentiation of early chick limb bud cells in culture. *Cell Differ* **11**: 245–51.
66. Zanetti N C and Solursh M (1984) Induction of chondrogenesis in limb mesenchymal cultures by disruption of the actin cytoskeleton. *J Cell Biol* **99**: 115–23.
67. Ali U I and Haynes R O (1977) Effect of cytochalasin B and colchicine on attachment of major surface protein of fibroblasts. *Biochim Biophys Acta* **471**: 16–24.
68. Zanetti N C and Solursh M (1986) Epithelial effects on limb chondrogenesis involves extracellular matrix and cell shape. *Dev Biol* **113**: 110–8.
69. Knight-Jones E W and Qasim S Z (1955) Response of some marine plankton animals to changes in hydrostatic pressure. *Nature* **175**: 941–2.
70. Hudspeth A J (1983) Mechanoelectrical transduction by hair cells in the acousticolateralis sensory system. *Annu Rev Neurosci* **6**: 187–215.
71. Bassett C A L (1971) Biophysical principles affecting bone structure. *In: The Biochemistry and Physiology of Bone Vol. 3* (G H Bourne, ed) pp. 1–76. London, New York: Academic Press.
72. Law H T, Annan I, McCarthy I D, Hughes S P F, Stead A C, Camburn M A and Montgomery H

(1985) The effect of induced electrical currents on bone after experimental osteotomy in sheep. *J Bone Joint Surg [Br]* **67**: 463–9.
73. Hall B K (1983) Bioelectricity and cartilage. *In: Cartilage, Vol. 3* (B K Hall, ed) pp. 309–38. London, New York: Academic Press.
74. Rodan G A, Bourret L A and Norton L A (1978) DNA synthesis in cartilage cells is stimulated by oscillating electric fields. *Science* **199**: 690–2.
75. Taha A A M, Abdel-Magied E M and King A S (1983) Ultrastructure of aortic and pulmonary baroreceptors in the domestic fowl. *J Anat* **137**: 197–207.
76. Iggo A and Muir A R (1969) The structure and function of a slowly adapting touch corpuscle in hairy skin. *J Physiol* **200**: 763–96.
77. Chambers M R, Andres K H, Duering M V and Iggo A (1972) The structure and function of the slowly adapting type II mechanoreceptor in hairy skin. *Q J Exp Physiol* **57**: 417–45.
78. Hudspeth A J (1985) The cellular basis of hearing: the biophysics of hair cells. *Science* **230**: 745–52.
79. Wilsman N J (1978) Cilia of adult canine articular chondrocytes. *J Ultrastruct Res* **64**: 270–81.
80. Machema H and Ogura A (1979) Ionic conductances of membranes in ciliated and deciliated *Paramecium*. *J Physiol* **296**: 49–60.
81. von der Mark K, Mollenhauer J, Kuhl U, Bee J and Lesot H (1984) Anchorins: a new class of membrane proteins involved in cell-matrix interactions. *In: The Role of Extracellular Matrix in Development* (R L Trelstad, ed), pp. 67–87. New York: A R Liss.
82. Poole C A, Flint M H and Beaumont B W (1984) Morphological and functional interrelationships of articular cartilage matrices. *J Anat* **138**: 113–38.
83. MacNeil S, Lakey T and Tomlinson S (1985) Calmodulin regulation of adenylate cyclase activity. *Cell Calcium* **6**: 213–26.
84. Means A R, Lagace L, Guerriero V and Chafouleas J G (1982) Calmodulin as a mediator of hormone action and cell regulation. *J Cell Biochem* **20**: 317–30.
85. Mohr W, Kuhn C, Pelster B and Wessinghage D (1985) S-100 protein in normal, osteoarthrotic and arthritic cartilage. *Rheumatol Int* **5**: 273–7.
86. Houston J P, McGuire M K B, Meats J E, Ebsworth N M, Russell R G G, Crawford A and MacNeil S (1982) Adenylate cyclase of human articular chondrocytes. *Biochem J* **208**: 35–42.
87. Berridge M J (1984) Inositol trisphosphate and diacylglycerol as second messengers. *Biochem J* **220**: 345–60.
88. Pieter A, Prins A, Lipman J M and Sokoloff L (1982) Effect of purified growth factors on rabbit articular cartilage in monolayer culture. *Arthritis Rheum* **25**: 1217–38.
89. Skjodt H, Crawford A, Dobson P R M, Brown B L and Russell R G G (1985) Effects of interleukin 1 on phosphoinositide metabolism and diacylglycerol and protein kinase C levels in connective tissue cells *in vitro*. *Proc Br Soc Rheumatol* (Abstr) **107**: 143.
90. Putney J W (1986) A model for receptor-regulated calcium entry. *Cell Calcium* **7**: 1–12.
91. Nishizuka I (1984) The role of protein kinase C in cell surface signal transduction and tumour promotion. *Nature* **308**: 693–8.
92. Bonner W M, Jonsson H, Malanos C and Bryant M (1975) Changes in the lipids of human articular cartilage with age. *Arthritis Rheum* **18**: 461–73.
93. Freedman R B (1981), Membrane-bound enzymes. *In: Membrane Structure* (J B Finean and R H Michell, eds) pp. 161–214. Amsterdam: Elsevier.
94. Henis Y, Rimon G and Felder S (1982) Lateral mobility of phospholipids in turkey erythrocytes. *J Biol Chem* **257**: 1407–11.
95. Salessi R, Garnier J and Daveloose D (1982) Modulation of adenylate cyclase activity by the physical state of pigeon erythrocyte membrane. *Biochemistry* **21**: 1587–90.
96. Bretscher A (1981) Fimbrin is a cytoskeletal protein that crosslinks F-actin *in vitro*. *Proc Natl Acad Sci USA* **78**: 6849–53.
97. Branton D, Cohen C M and Tyler J (1981) Interaction of cytoskeletal proteins on the human erythrocyte membrane. *Cell* **24**: 24–32.
98. Sheetz M P, Febbroriello P and Koppel D E (1982) Triphosphoinositide increases glycoprotein lateral mobility in erythrocyte membranes. *Nature* **296**: 91–3.
99. M'zala H and Giraud F (1986) Phosphoinositide reorganization in human erythrocyte membrane upon cholesterol depletion. *Biochem J* **234**: 13–20.
100. Dipple I and Houslay M D (1978) The activity of glucagon-stimulated adenylate cyclase from rat liver plasma membrane is modulated by the fluidity of its lipid environment. *Biochem J* **174**: 179–90.

Chapter 7

Synovial Fluid and Trans-synovial Flow in Stationary and Moving Normal Joints

J. R. Levick

CONTENTS

INTRODUCTION

Synovial fluid plays a key role in diarthrodial joint function, lubricating the moving synovial and cartilaginous surfaces and supplying nutrient to much of the avascular articular cartilage. This chapter describes recent advances in our knowledge of the volume, pressure and dynamics of synovial fluid under various physiological conditions (rest, exercise, etc.) and emphasizes the healthy (cf.

arthritic) joint, which has received increasing attention in the last decade. The diffusional exchange of nutrients, drugs, etc. is reviewed elsewhere (1, 2), as also is lubrication (3, 4). Comprehensive references to early studies of synovial fluid will be found in references (5), (6) and (7).

DEVELOPMENT OF CURRENT IDEAS

The slippery, synovial (= like egg-white) fluid within limb joints was known to Hippocrates, Galen and Paracelsus (8). In 1743 the 25-year old anatomist William Hunter, delivering his first communication to the Royal Society (9) described the periarticular vasculature, the circulus articuli (not 'articularis') vasculosus; and he speculated whether these vessels might 'pour out a dewy (i.e. synovial) Fluid' (10). In 1800 Bichat refuted Havers' erroneous opinion that the fluid was an active glandular secretion (8). The next major advance, in 1896, was on a broader front, when Starling defined the principles governing fluid exchange between plasma and interstitial spaces (11) – a process of ultrafiltration across a semipermeable membrane, the capillary wall. Bauer, Ropes and others stressed that the synovial cavity is structurally essentially a giant interstitial space (5, 12); and they showed that, chemically, synovial fluid conformed with Starling's hypothesis in resembling a plasma ultrafiltrate in many ways (5). Only in the last few years however have the *dynamic* predictions of Starling's hypothesis been tested directly for the blood–joint interface.

PROPERTIES OF SYNOVIAL FLUID

Composition & Viscosity (Table 7.1)

Normal synovial fluid contains few cells ($60–375/mm^3$; 5, 13, 14), mainly mononuclear phagocytes. Occasional tiny fragments of cartilage have been reported even in normal synovial fluid (13).

Small solutes and gases

The electrolytes and most other small solutes in synovial fluid (urea, urate, etc.) are in near equilibrium with plasma, allowing for the Gibbs–Donnan effect of protein (5) and hyaluronate (6) on charged solute distribution. Synovial and plasma glucose levels are often not in equilibrium (5, 15), although the ratio sometimes averages close to 1. The fluid's H^+ concentration and P_{CO_2} are a little higher than mixed venous levels, and increase in exercise (16); but normal P_{O_2} (cf. arthritic) seems unreported (17). In rheumatoid fluid there is evidence of a local metabolic acidosis, namely low glucose, low P_{O_2}, high H^+ concentration and high lactate (Pasteur effect: 17, 18, 19, 20) and this is at its worst each morning, coinciding with morning stiffness (21).

Lipids

Recent investigations of synovial fluid lipid indicate a fat content of 0·24 g/ 100 ml (human knee) of which $\frac{2}{3}$ is neutral fat and $\frac{1}{3}$ phospholipid (22); and it has been suggested that a surfactant-like phospholipid could play a role in joint lubrication (23).

Table 7.1 Some Characteristic Properties of Normal Synovial Fluid (SF)

	SF	Plasma	SF/Plasma	Source
Na$^+$ (mM)	145	156	0·93	Cattle ankle (5)
Cl$^-$ (mM)	111	110	1·01	Cattle ankle (5)
Urea (mg/100 ml)	8·2	8·5	0·96	Cattle ankle (5)
Urate (mg/100 ml)	1·55	1·84	0·84	Cattle ankle (5)
Glucose (mg/100 ml)	66	91	0·73 (variable)	Cattle ankle (5)
Total Lipid (g/100 ml)	0·24	~0·70	0·34	Human knee (22)
Phospholipid (g/100 ml)	0·08	0·20	0·40	Human knee (22)
Protein (g/100 ml)	1·90	6·77	0·28	Human knee (1)
Albumin (g/100 ml)	1·20	3·27	0·37	Human knee (1)
γ-Globulin (g/100 ml)	0·24	1·13	0·21	Human knee (1)
Hyaluronate (g/100 ml)	0·2–0·4	$4·2 \times 10^{-6}$	~ 70 000	Human knee (1)
Lubricating glycoprotein	?	?	?	Cattle (41, 42)
Aspiratable volume (mean, ml)	0·45–1·1	(3000)	–	Human knee (5, 13)
Hydrostatic pressure (cmH$_2$O)	−2·6	(100–11)	–	Human knee (60, 61)
Colloid osmotic pressure (cmH$_2$O)	12–15	35	0·34–0·43	Human knee (6, 24)
Intrinsic viscosity (ml/g)	$1–4 \times 10^3$	–	–	Various (28)

Macromolecules

Like leg-lymph, normal synovial fluid contains plasma protein at an average 30% (human knee)–45% (rabbit limb-joints) of plasma level. As a result, its colloid osmotic pressure is $\frac{1}{3}$–$\frac{1}{2}$ that of plasma (5, 24, 25, 26). There are significant differences between varieties of joint, protein concentration and colloid osmotic pressure being least in the ankle (hock) of cattle hindlimbs (27) and wrist of dogs (26) (see 'Gravitational Influence'; p. 173). Sadly, comparative data are not available for man. In a given kind of joint, macromolecular concentration tends to decline as fluid volume increases (25, 28) and to increase with age (29).

Numerous studies show that the ratio of synovial fluid to plasma concentration for individual proteins declines as molecular size increases (e.g. 6, 30), and this is attributed to molecular sieving mechanisms at the capillary wall and synovial interstitium (1, 31). In arthritic effusions the plasma-protein concentration reaches up to 70% of plasma levels, and the molecular selectivity of the blood–joint barrier is greatly reduced, i.e. the relative increase is most marked for the largest proteins (e.g. 30, 31, 32, 33).

Secreted macromolecules

Normal synovial fluid contains several macromolecular species actively secreted by synovium. Of these a highly polymerized hyaluronate is most abundant (70 000 times plasma level), albeit at only 0·2–0·6 g/100 ml (6, 25, 28, 34, 35). The solvated, entangled hyaluronate chains endow the fluid with a significant elasticity at oscillation frequencies > 1 Hz (36, 37, 38) and it is estimated that 77% of the energy input to the fluid during running (2·5 Hz) is stored elastically in young adults (37). Hyaluronate also accounts for the fluid's very high, shear-rate-dependent viscosity (intrinsic viscosity 10^3 to 4×10^3 ml/g; 28), which seems important for the lubrication of synovial surfaces but not cartilage. Variation in hyaluronate concentration and polymerization presumably account for the enormous variation in fluid viscosity between joints (e.g. 5, 15, 27), but the functional significance of these variations is obscure. Viscosity tends to relate inversely to synovial fluid volume (15, 28). In arthritides both the concentration and polymerization of hyaluronate decline (e.g. 28, 39).

In addition to dominating the mechanical properties of synovial fluid, hyaluronate may affect rate of solute diffusion (40). It also partly excludes macromolecules from the fluid, but not sufficiently to account fully for the low protein content of the fluid (31).

Other functionally important macromolecular constituents not derived from plasma include cartilage-lubricating glycoproteins (41, 42) and, in rheumatoid arthritis, both immunoglobulins and fibronectin (32, 43, 44, 45). (For other constituents *see* 46.)

Volume and Film Thickness

The volume of synovial fluid is important not only as a clinical sign and a source of morbidity in arthritis but also, in normal joints, as a necessary vehicle for transport of nutrients to articular cartilage (1, 47, 48). Volume has been estimated by (*1*) percutaneous aspiration (49), either *in vivo* or from opened joints post mortem (probably underestimating true volume) (36); (*2*) the indicator dilution method using indium (50), radiolabelled albumin (51) or hydroxyethyl starch (52) – underestimating volume if mixing is incomplete and overestimating volume if the indicator permeates the synovial tissue and cartilage, which indium does at a faster rate than macromolecules. The indicator method has been applied mainly to arthritic joints to date.

Aspiratable volume is very small in most normal limb joints (5, 6, 25, 26, 27, 53) – 'small', that is, in relation to the 'size' of the joint, i.e. its internal surface area. In the human adult knee, for example, aspiratable volume averages around 0·5 ml (e.g. 13). The internal surface area is stated to be 425 cm^2 (277 cm^2 synovium, 148 cm^2 cartilage†; 53). Therefore, there is

---

†Cartilage volume may therefore be underestimated in (1), leading to an underestimate of glucose concentration gradient across the blood–joint barrier required to nourish cartilage.

0·0012 ml aspiratable fluid per cm² surface. If the fluid were evenly 'sand-wiched' between the outer and inner faces of the cavity, it would form a layer only 24 μm thick, which is about the same thickness as the film of pleural fluid (54). For the rabbit knee (synovial area 16 cm², volume 0.024 cm²; 25) the mean film thickness is similar (30 μm). For the dog knee (synovial area 27–59 cm²; 55: volume 0·2– 0·4 cm³; 26) the calculation predicts a thicker film (67–270 μm). It is unlikely that the film is actually of uniform thickness, however (see below, p. 157). Unfortunately the only joint other than knee whose net internal surface area seems known is the human ankle (77 cm²; 53).

The relatively lax, poorly congruous shoulder joint consistently has larger volumes of fluid than other limb joints in small species (25, 26), about double that of the knee. In taller species, however (e.g. cattle, horse) the ankle joint is particularly voluminous (12–25 ml; 15, 27, 53, 56, 57), which may be a consequence of gravity, discussed later.

Pressure

The pressure of synovial fluid affects trans-synovial flow and hence the volume of fluid in the cavity; and pathological pressures affect the hydraulic conductance of synovium (see 'Yield phenomenon', p. 167). In 1929 Müller discovered that synovial fluid pressure is several mmHg sub-atmospheric ('negative') in human and canine limb joints at natural relaxed joint angles (58), a discovery which fits with the impression that the synovial cavity is a 'collapsed' space. A striking proof that pressures are sub-atmospheric is the simple observation that saline in the hub of a percutaneously-inserted intra-articular cannula is visibly sucked into the joint cavity when opened to the atmosphere (59). Failure to prevent this occurrence during pressure measurement (by pre-connection of cannula to transducer) can lead to falsely raised pressure measurements, especially if the joint is then flexed upon the increased volume (59). This kind of error seems to some degree inevitable when a cannula-with-stylet system is used.

Recent studies confirm sub-atmospheric pressure in the human knee (mean = −5 mmHg (60) to −1·6 mmHg (61)), cat knee (62), rabbit limb joints (25, 59, 63), and dog limb joints (29, 64, 65, 66), except wrist (+1·3 mmHg; 29). The sub-atmospheric pressures persist even during stationary load bearing, outside the areas of direct articular contact (58, 66, 67) and also persist for many hours after death (58, 66). The negativity has been attributed to trans-synovial efflux of fluid upon flexion, and the stimulation of lymph flow by movement (6).

The synovial cavity ceases to be a 'collapsed' space when effusions or haemarthroses inflate it to supra-atmospheric pressures, which are commonly 6–33 mmHg in rheumatoid knees (volume 6–190 ml; 68, 69, 70). Under these circumstances, intra-articular pressure in the human knee does increase upon weight bearing (cf. normal); and even increase with dependency (68, 71). The latter effect is probably caused by synovial vascular volume expansion (due to gravity) as demonstrated experimentally in the rabbit knee (72). Increased synovial fluid volume and pressure are a source of morbidity, giving rise to a sense of tension, or even pain if formed rapidly (73, 74); also reflex muscular weakness (61, 75, 76) impairment of synovial blood flow above a critical effusion pressure (77, 78, 79, 80), and even direct mechanical limitation of movement (55).

PROPERTIES OF THE JOINT CAVITY

Volume–Pressure Curve: Compliance and Elastance

The relation between intra-articular pressure (p_j) and volume (V), sometimes called the 'compliance' curve, depends on joint dimensions and wall compliance (stretchiness). The relation is sigmoidal over the full physiological–pathological range (*Fig.* 7.1). The physiological, sub-atmospheric part of the relationship has been described in the last few years and is very steep – i.e. small volume changes (ΔV) cause relatively large pressure swings (Δp_j) (55, 81; cf. 63). The volumetric compliance $\Delta V/\Delta p_j$ is low because of the collapsed nature of the space (81), and this low compliance presumably helps in the homestasis of volume, since a relatively large change in pressure after a small addition of trans-synovial filtrate will oppose further filtration.

At 5–10 mmHg (a pathological level for neutral angles) the curve is flattest, i.e. compliance $\Delta V/\Delta p_j$ is greatest. The cavity walls are no longer collapsed, but nor are they greatly distended, so they are at their most stretchable – and the volume-homeostatic process referred to above is at its least effective. As volume increases, the curve then steepens again, both in the knee (55, 62, 68, 73, 74, 81, 82, 83; cf. 84) and hip (85). The steepening of the relationship results from the increasing stiffness of the stretched, tense walls (capsule, muscle and ligaments; 86). Indeed, in several kinds of joint the volumetric elastance $\Delta p_j/\Delta V$ (an index of wall stiffness) increases linearly with supra-atmospheric pressure from its minimum value just above atmospheric pressure, as shown in *Fig.* 7.1b (knee, 55, 81, 82: hip, data from 85). The process(es) responsible for the increasing elastance, such as orientation of stressed collagen fibrils, are discussed in (71, 81, 82, 87).

The intrinsic stiffness of a material is indicated by Young's incremental modulus (88). The approximate magnitude of this modulus for the walls of a joint cavity can be estimated, with considerable licence, from Δp_j and ΔV in (81) (rabbit knee). Approximating the joint investment by a uniform spherical shell of mean thickness 2 mm and initial radius 0·75 cm, Young's incremental modulus for the wall is of the order $0·2 \times 10^6$ dynes/cm^2 at 5 cmH$_2$O fluid pressure, to $3·8 \times 10^6$ dynes/cm^2 at 45 cmH$_2$O. This estimate may not be too unrealistic, in spite of the grossly simplified shell geometry adopted in the calculation: for example, Young's modulus for the abdominal aorta inflated by 40 mmHg pressure is $1·2 \times 10^6$ dynes/cm^2 (89).

Flexion raises pressure (*see* p. 172) and also steepens the pressure–volume relation greatly (55, 71, 81). At very high pressures (usually > 100–200 mmHg in man; less in rabbit) the synovial lining can rupture, often posteriorly in the case of the knee. If the joint contained a pathological effusion (cf. saline) the extravasated fluid can produce a thrombophlebitis-like syndrome in the calf, similar to that of a ruptured popliteal cyst (67, 71, 83, 104, 105). Such pressures would be generated *in vivo* probably only by sudden flexion upon a considerable effusion. The sudden loss of intra-articular pressure on joint rupture (67) is of some physiological interest, for it indicates that the normal joint lining has a considerably higher hydraulic resistance than the subjacent tissue planes.

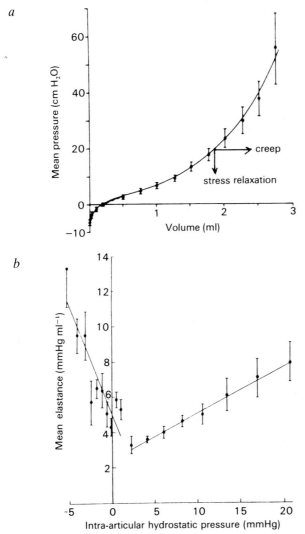

Fig. 7.1. Properties of the synovial joint cavity. *a*, Relation between mean pressure and injected volume of non-absorbable fluid in 10 rabbit knees [from Knight and Levick, 1982 (81), with permission.] *Note* the steep physiological part of the curve at sub-atmospheric pressures. Arrows show the increase in volume at constant pressure (viscous creep) or decrease in pressure at constant volume (stress relaxation) which result from the viscoelasticity of the cavity wall. *b*, The slope of the relation, dP/dV, or 'elastance' shows a minimum close to atmospheric pressure, then increases linearly with pressure (mean for 7 dog knees). [From Nade and Newbould, 1984 (55), with permission.]

Viscous Creep and Stress Relaxation

The complexity of the pressure–volume relationship at pathological pressures is being increasingly revealed. The nature of the studied infusate is important, however; saline, formerly universally employed in compliance studies, over-estimates compliance because it is absorbed from the joint cavity (55, 81, 82, 85, 90). This problem has been circumvented in animal studies by infusing a non-absorbable oil (55, 91) or, for a faster intra-articular distribution, a low-viscosity mixture of oils (81, 82, 92). With a non-absorbable fluid, the dependence of the p_J–V relation on time and previous history emerges unambiguously, and it is found that the volume of the cavity subjected to constant pressure increases slowly with time (non-linearly) over an hour or more (72, 91), indicating 'viscous creep' of the cavity wall. Conversely the pressure of a constant volume of intra-articular fluid declines with time due to loss of tension in the wall (stress relaxation), both in the knee (59, 74, 82, 90, 93) and in the hip (80, 85, 94), with a time-course of days in the hip (80). Such behaviour can be described by a simple Kelvin–Hooke model, i.e. a spring in series with parallel spring ($\equiv$ collagen network?) and dashpot ($\equiv$ interstitial fluid?) (82). The viscoelastic properties of the walls are also revealed by hysteresis of the p_J–V relationship – that is to say, pressure at a given volume during infusion exceeds that during aspiration (73, 82) – in fact, 37% of the energy injected as pressure is dissipated by viscous creep within the walls in the rabbit knee. Viscoelasticity is also evident from the greater pressures generated by fast as compared with slow infusions (82, 90). In addition the joint investment displays a degree of plasticity (82).

Viscoelasticity of the cavity's wall has a number of practical consequences:

1. It helps explain why rapidly forming effusions (e.g. infective, traumatic) can cause pain associated with high wall tension and relieved by aspiration (70, 95) whereas larger but slower-forming effusions may be less tense and relatively painless.
2. Viscoelasticity and plasticity of the wall contribute to the overall mechanical properties of the joint during motion (96, 97).
3. Viscoelasticity helps explain poor clinical correlations between pressure and aspiratable volume of an effusion (68, 70). Because of creep there can be no unique, time-independent relation between p_J and V in a given joint.
4. Viscoelasticity contributes to the adaptation and hysteresis of discharge by periarticular mechanoreceptors such as Ruffini afferents (90, 93, 98, 99, 100), which are closely related to collagen fibrils (101). The activity of these receptors is increased by effusions, causing a reflex inhibition of quadriceps motoneurones leading to extensor weakness (61, 75, 76, 102, 103).
5. Because of viscoelasticity, very high (arterial level) intra-articular pressures are most unlikely to be sustained for long periods, and this has led recently to doubts about the old 'tamponade' theory (vascular obstruction by intra-articular pressure) as the cause of Legg–Calve–Perthe syndrome (juvenile femoral-head necrosis) (85, 94; cf. 78). Nevertheless there is evidence that, above a critical pressure, raised intra-articular pressure does reduce synovial blood flow somewhat (77, 78, 79, 80).

Organization of Synovial Fluid: Collapsed Spaces, Compartments and Cysts

Synovial fluid is commonly depicted as a uniform thin sheet of fluid separating the inner and outer surfaces of the joint cavity; but the requirements of mechanical equilibrium make it more likely that the space is partially 'collapsed' (59, 81). Since atmospheric pressure exceeds intra-articular pressure, it tends to press the outer synovial lining on to the opposite, inner face of the cavity. It has been suggested that the trans-mural pressure difference is prevented from totally obliterating the space by points of contact, which act like pillars; and this, presumably, is what is meant by the popular phrase 'partially collapsed space'. Alternatively, it is conceivable that mechanical equilibrium is infrequently attained, a continuous film being maintained by occasional movements plus a very high fluid viscosity at low shear rates. The nature of the space has never yet been investigated directly, even though its nature must be relevant to inter-synovial lubrication, synovial fluid convection, and perhaps articular lubrication.

Even when fluid volume is increased to inflate the space, there remain cartilage-on-cartilage regions which infused fluids fail to penetrate. This is apparent from filling defects in acrylate casts of joint cavities (e.g. femoral–tibial cartilage contact; 92: subpatellar area; 55). These filling defects could indicate solid contacts between loaded surfaces. Alternatively they could represent a persistent, highly viscous thin film of synovial fluid coating the articular surface. An old but fascinating observation by Ogston and Stanier (38) raises this possibility; synovial fluid was shown to be capable of forming a permanent though extremely thin (30–50 nm) layer between two static surfaces, even under considerable loads, due to the voluminous trapped hyaluronate particles and/or short-range electrical repulsive forces. Roberts (106) has confirmed the existence of 10–30 nm-thick films during loads up to 10 atm for 3–6 h. *In vivo* somewhat thicker films might possibly be maintained between loaded surfaces by movement. Additional intra-articular regions where there is solid contact or negligible fluid mobility are revealed also by the phenomenon of fluid compartmentation in the knee, discovered only recently (92). The anterior region of the rabbit knee is anatomically continuous with the posterior space (as in human knees), yet fluid infused into one space fails to pass at a detectable rate into the other until a critical pressure is reached (variable, average 15 cmH$_2$O). A similar phenomenon was recently demonstrated in cat knees at 5 cmH$_2$O (62). Below these pressures, the cat or rabbit knee behaves hydraulically like 2 discrete compartments. The establishment of anterior-posterior hydraulic communication is marked by a run-off, which flattens the pressure–volume curve of the infused space provided infusion is intermittent. The cause of the compartmentation is that the channels of communication (which run around the cruciate ligaments and under the collateral ligaments) are closed at low fluid pressures by the tension of the cruciate and collateral ligaments. The possibility of compartmentation in the human knee merits further study. Fluid compart-mentation has long been recognized, however, in popliteal (Baker's) cysts, which can be in anatomical continuity, but only intermittently in hydraulic continuity, with the anterior joint space (71, 107, 108).

BULK TURNOVER OF SYNOVIAL FLUID

Rather surprisingly, estimates of the normal rate of formation of synovial fluid have appeared only in the last few years. It must be noted at once that the existence of a bulk turnover (formation and reabsorption) of normal synovial fluid has been deduced (1, 6, 59) but never yet measured directly. That synovial fluid is not a stagnant pool of fluid, but is undergoing continual absorption and reformation, has been deduced from the concentration of plasma protein in synovial fluid. This remains lower than in plasma (*Table 7.1*) despite a continuous influx of protein across the slightly permeable capillary wall. The concentration of extra-capillary plasma protein can only remain lower than plasma level, in the face of a continual protein influx (dm/dt), if there is an accompanying trans-capillary flux of water (dV/dt). The definition of extravascular protein concentration C_i in the presence of fluxes becomes:

$$C_i = \frac{(dm/dt)}{(dV/dt)} \qquad (Eqn.\ 7.1)$$

Since dm/dt is finite (109), trans-capillary flow dV/dt must be greater than zero. The thin layer of synovium overlying the capillaries is permeable to fluid, so it may be expected that some of the filtrate enters the joint cavity, especially during periods of immobility, when the removal of fluid from the subsynovial space by the lymph vessels becomes negligible (*see* 'Lymph Flow', p. 171). It also seems probable (though not proved beyond argument) that a net pressure gradient exists from synovial capillaries into the synovial cavity of the knee, shoulder and elbow in their neutral positions (25; *see* 'Balance', p. 170), which provides a second line of evidence for fluid filtration into relaxed joints.

The rate of turnover of the fluid has been estimated, with reasonable consistency, by 3 different approaches:

1. The first clue came from the observation that the negative pressure in the stationary rabbit knee rises slowly with time (1–2 cmH_2O/h; 59, rabbit: 66, dog). This slow pressure change must be due to a slow change in fluid volume in the immobile joint, since its rate and direction are sensitive to capillary pressure (72). In this event, fluid formation rate (dV/dt) is given by rate of pressure increase (dp_j/dt) multiplied by compliance at that pressure (dV/dp_j). This led to an estimated filtration rate of 20–40 $\mu l/h$ (1·3– 6·7 $\mu l/cm^2$ synovium/h) in the stationary, extended rabbit knee.

2. *Eqn.* (7.1) has been used to estimate average filtration rate into the stationary human knee, calculating dm/dt from the protein permeability of the human blood–joint barrier (data from 109, 110) and C_i from the protein concentration in normal human synovial fluid (6, 31). The estimated turnover of fluid is 0·7–1·0 ml/h, or 2·5–3·5 $\mu l/cm^2$ synovium/h. This result is close to the above estimate for the rabbit knee. It suggests that roughly the whole fluid volume of the cavity turns over in 1 h on average. In the rheumatoid knee, steady state dV/dt was calculated to be roughly double the normal rate, i.e. ~ 2 ml/h (31). This seems consistent with direct measurement of dV/dt in the rheumatoid knee in the *non*-steady state after aspiration, where dV/dt averages 5 ml/h (69).

3. Over a period of time flow of fluid and protein into the cavity (filtration) must equal their drainage out of the cavity (absorption) if volume and protein concentration are to remain in a steady state over the long term. Studies by Bauer, Short & Bennett (111) established that, in healthy joints, intra-articular protein removal is virtually entirely via the flow of synovial lymph. The time-averaged rate of absorption of fluid from human arthritic knees can therefore be estimated from the rate of removal of radiolabelled albumin

(51). The calculated drainage rate is 1·8 ml/h (osteoarthrosis) to 4·3 ml/h (rheumatoid arthritis).

Filtration Fraction

Thus 3 very different approaches (dp_j/dt, protein influx and protein efflux) lead to mutually compatible estimates of fluid turnover rate for the knee. It is likely that this fluid is elaborated mainly by a very thin, superficial layer of tissue (*see* 'Structure' *below*). It is not clear, however, what fraction of the synovial plasma flow the fluid formation represents, because blood flow through the superficial 20–40 μm of synovium is uncertain (*see* 'Blood Flow', p. 162). However, if the clearance of tritiated water from the joint cavity is adopted as a measure of synovial intimal blood flow (1 ml/min in human knees; 109, 110), then intimal plasma flow is 36·7 ml/h for a haematocrit of 0·45 and 0·9 g H_2O/ml blood. The normal filtration fraction for synovial plasma becomes 0·02–0·03 according to these data. A similar calculation for the rheumatoid knee, equating intra-articular albumin clearance with lymph flow (4·3 ml/h; 51) and iodide clearance with intimal plasma flow (115 ml/h) gives a plasma filtration fraction of 0·04. In dogs the latter approach gives a filtration fraction of 0·04 (normal knee) – 0·09 (normal wrist) (112).

STRUCTURE OF THE BLOOD–JOINT BARRIER (*Fig. 7.2*)

Synovial structure is reviewed in references (6, 113, 114). In recent years some progress has been made in a more quantitative direction, with the establishment of information about the areas, distances, capillary densities etc. involved in the exchange process. Two layers of tissue constitute the blood–joint barrier, namely the capillary wall and the synovium, and these are described next.

The Synovial Component

The synovial lining is very thin. It consists of a cellular layer, the 'intima', mostly 1–3 cells deep (20–40 μm thick, man; 116: rabbit; 117) and this layer rests on deeper loose connective tissue backed by skeletal muscle, fibrous capsule, tendon (e.g. patellar tendon), or fat. Terminology is not universally standardized, but here 'synovium' and 'synovial initima' are synonyms for the highly vascular, richly cellular superficial layer 20–40 μm thick. 80% of the intimal layer consists of cells (115), of two main kinds (118). 'A' cells, vacuolated and possessing filopodia, are phagocytic (e.g. 119). They are thought to clear necrotic debris from the fluid, and may also secrete hyaluronate (113). 'B' cells have much rough endoplasmic reticulum and probably secrete interstial collagen (120). The cells form an uneven surface (121) and in large joints can form villous protruberances, some of which are avascular (122), so a specialized exchange function for villi seems improbable. The cell layer lacks a basement membrane, and cellular junctions are scanty (113), so there is little justification for the term synovial 'membrane'.

Between the cells are spaces, 1–2 μm wide (115, 123), occupying 17–21% of

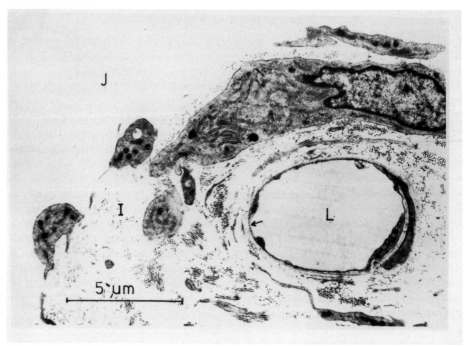

Fig. 7.2. Electron micrograph of synovium from rabbit knee, showing joint cavity (J); intimal lining cell ('B' cell) and cell processes; interstitium (I) rich in collagen fibrils and forming part of the synovial surface in places; and a synovial capillary (lumen L), whose wall is only ~5 μm below the synovial surface at its nearest point. The arrow points to a row of fenestrae, just discernible at this magnification. [From Knight and Levick, 1984 (115), with permission.]

the synovial surface area, and thus creating a substantial interstitial area for trans-synovial exchange. The intercellular regions are occupied by a material ('interstitium') permeable to quite large protein molecules (123), and it is through this matrix that most nutritional and fluid fluxes occur. The matrix is essentially a meshwork of fibrous molecules and microscopic fibrils. The composition is still not well defined, but includes proteoglycans (124), perhaps mainly dermatan-sulphate proteoglycan (125), with hyaluronate (126) probably as a minor component (127); also glycoproteins (127) including fibronectin (128, 129). These molecular fibres are interwoven between abundant collagen fibrils (20–50% of dry weight of whole tissue), of which 50% is Type III and the rest mainly Type I (129, 130, 131). Although progress is evident in identifying constituents, there remains an almost total absence of quantitative composition-al data, both for normal and rheumatoid synovium. Without such data, no link-up is yet possible with available theories describing flow and diffusive transport through fibrous matrices (e.g. 40). Relevant to fluid transport is the claim that the synovial interstitial matrix is penetrated by a system of fine proteoglycan-deficient channels of radius 71 nm (132). Their putative hydraulic effect has been calculated and found plausible (6), but the evidence for their existence (deposition of ferrocyanide in clumps) does not seem conclusive (133).

The Vascular Component

To reach synovial interstitium, nutrients, drugs and plasma water must first cross the walls of capillaries (and possibly venules). The richness and superficiality of the synovial capillary network makes it well adapted for exchange with the joint cavity (53). Some of the venules too are very superficial. Quantitative information, vital for the interpretation of solute or fluid exchange data, is confined to rabbit knee synovium (115, 117). The capillaries are concentrated in a remarkably sharp zone 6–11 μm below the surface (*Fig.* 7.3), where the peak capillary density (58–171 $\times$ 10^3/cm^2) is considerably greater even than in the nearby skeletal muscles (29 $\times$ 10^3/cm^2). These features, besides being important to transport, presumably contribute to the frequency with which haemarthroses complicate haemophilia.

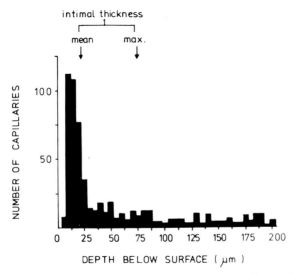

Fig. 7.3. Histogram showing distribution of capillaries with respect to distance below the surface of the synovium, in the posterior region of the rabbit knee. Capillaries are concentrated mainly in the superficial 20μm. [Data from Knight and Levick, 1983 (117).]

The extremely skewed distribution of capillaries with respect to distance from the synovial surface is suggestive of an angiogenic influence near the surface, and an angiogenic factor has very recently been identified in rheumatoid synovial fluid (134, 135, 136). Because of the skewed capillary distribution, the great majority of nutritional exchange with the joint space derives from the thin superficial layer of synovium. For example, the 'functional thickness' of synovium (defined arbitrarily as the thickness from which 80% of trans-synovial solute flux derives) is calculated to be 7–20 μm for a small lipid-insoluble solute undergoing diffusion-limited exchange, or 9–39 μm for flow-limited exchange (137). In rheumatoid synovium, where there is good evidence of a 'metabolic-perfusion imbalance' (*see* 'Composition', p. 150), it would be of considerable interest to discover whether capillary density changes, and whether the capillaries retain their extreme superficiality or become buried under hyperplastic synovium (as inspection of published sections (69) suggests).

Roughly half the profiles of sectioned intimal capillaries contain fenestrae (15/profile), which are extremely thin circular 'windows' in the endothelium, bridged by a thin diaphragm (115, 138, 139, 140). An interesting adaptation to function is the preferential occurrence of fenestrae on the side of the capillary facing the joint cavity (*Fig.* 7.2). Fenestrae are highly permeable to water and small solutes, but not to plasma proteins. Their permeability has recently been analysed in terms of pore theory and fibre-matrix theory (141), with a surprising conclusion – that the ultrastructurally obvious obstacle, the diaphragm, offers only a minor part of the pathway's resistance to water and solute exchange. The basement membrane and/or endothelial glycocalyx appear more important than the diaphragm in the fenestral pathway.

The permeability of non-fenestrated regions of endothelium in general is reviewed in (142, 143, 144), and the non-fenestrated routes are probably as follows. Lipid-soluble solutes (e.g. oxygen, carbon dioxide, xenon) diffuse straight through the whole endothelial cell membrane. Small lipid-insoluble solutes (e.g. glucose, urate) diffuse through the far less extensive endothelial intercellular junctions (123, 145), and water flows down pressure gradients via the same pathway. Plasma proteins are greatly impeded at the intercellular junctions, yet even the largest ones obtain slow access to interstitium, either via rare, wide intercellular junctions (becoming far commoner in acute inflammation; (146, 147, 148), or via a slow-transporting system of endothelial vesicles (123, 144, 149), or even via rare trans-endothelial channels formed by fused chains of vesicles (144).

The plasma-derived materials next diffuse or flow through the capillary basement membrane, which is thicker than usual in synovial capillaries (~100 nm: 115), perhaps to their mechanical advantage. In places the basement membrane encloses a pericyte; and, remarkably, a 'pericyte' and 'endothelial cell' are occasionally seen to be one and the same cell in cytoplasmic continuity (114). Deep to the capillary network is a relatively little investigated, less rich network of lymphatic vessels (114, 150) which are emptied by movement of the joint.

Synovial Blood Flow: A Critical Appraisal

Blood flow through synovium is difficult to measure, because synovium is not a discrete organ, and has a multiplicity of vessels supplying it. Moreover, the available measurements are difficult to interpret precisely because the volume of tissue through which the blood flow is recorded is unclear, and because blood flow is probably highly non-homogeneous with respect to depth (*see Fig.* 7.3).

Five methods for estimating synovial blood flow have been reviewed recently (1, 151). The most popular, being applicable to man, is a clearance method derived from that of Kety (152) (e.g. 51, 153, 154, 155). In this method, the rate of disappearance from the joint cavity of a rapidly-diffusing radioactive solute (e.g. ^{23}Na, ^{131}I, ^{132}Xe, tritiated water) is used to calculate blood flow (or, for an extracellularly-confined solute like Na^+, plasma flow) per unit volume of distribution of solute. Assumptions include (*1*) that exchange is purely flow limited (i.e. plasma equilibrates fully with the joint fluid in one transit) and (*2*) that clearance of tracer is entirely by the bloodstream, not by diffusion into the surrounding tissues. The latter assumption has some experimental justification. Simkin has stressed the importance of recognizing that the method gives blood or plasma flow per unit *volume of distribution* of solute (not just per *synovial* volume) (2, 51). In joints containing injected fluid or effusions the distribution volume exceeds the volume of vascularized tissue – by as much as two orders of magnitude in an unaspirated effusion – so this is an important 'correction' to apply.

Simkin's point is worth re-emphasizing, and indeed taking further. In a normal joint the injected solute's distribution volume must include cartilage, menisci and ligaments as well as intra-articular fluid, and so must considerably exceed synovial tissue volume. The volume of vascularized synovium involved in clearing the solute can be roughly estimated for the human knee, where the method is commonly applied. Synovial area is ~277 cm^2 (53), and the functional thickness of synovium for flow-limited exchange is 9–39 μm (115, 116, 117, 137), so the volume of tissue responsible for the observed clearance is only 0·25 cm^3–1·08 cm^3. To illustrate the importance of tissue volume, consider a clearance rate constant of 0·03 ml/min/ml distribution volume for radiosodium in a normal adult knee, a typical result (154). The distribution volume of Na^+, assuming rapid and uniform spread throughout the joint (an assumption of the method) equals (*1*) the extracellular volume of the clearing tissue (about 1/5th the synovial volume of 0·25– 1·08 cm^3); plus (*2*) injected fluid volume (e.g. 0·5 cm^3); plus (*3*) endogenous synovial fluid (0·5 cm^3); plus (*4*) a large fraction (75%) of the volume of articular cartilage (area 148 cm^2 (53)), thickness 0·2 cm conservatively, volume 30 cm^3), plus (*5*) part of the meniscal and cruciate volumes. The distribution volume adds up to roughly 28 cm^3. The absolute plasma flow was therefore 0·03 × 28 = 0·84 ml/min and the blood flow 1·53 ml/min. This blood flow passes almost solely through synovium (volume 0·25–1·08 cm^3) so synovial blood flow is 1·42–6·12 ml/min/cm^3 in human synovium. (Iodide clearance data from dog knees (112) lead to a similar result, 2·0–4·5 ml/min/cm^3 synovium, for a synovial area 27–59 cm^2 (55) by 30 μm deep.) Contrast this with an apparent blood flow two orders of magnitude smaller which might be inferred casually from the clearance rate, 0·03 ml/min/cm^3 distribution volume! This point was not adequately recognized in an earlier review (1). The worked example here demonstrates the very great care needed in interpreting the clearance method in a non-homogeneous structure like the joint; and vividly illustrates the importance of quantitative data for synovial area and thickness, and for cartilage.

A method only recently applied to measure flow in periarticular tissue (synovium and capsule) is the radiolabelled microsphere technique (64, 65, 78, 156). From the counts generated by impacted microspheres in 2 g capsular biopsies from dogs, blood flows were calculated to be 0·9 ml/min/100 g knee tissue (64) to 10 ml/min/100 g hip capsule (78). Biopsies of 'synovium' (weight 0·79 g) gave results of 2·6 ml/min/100 g (knee) to 1·9 ml/min/100 g (wrist) (157). However, judging by the sample weights, and without the benefit of histological reports on the samples, it seems likely that the highly vascularized superficial

20–40 μm of synovium constituted only a small fraction of these samples, so that true synovial intimal flow is probably grossly underestimated by these values. Nevertheless the microsphere method does offer the best potential for resolving superficial, intimal blood-flow: it should prove possible to section sphere-labelled synovium normal to its surface and, by autoradiography, obtain local tissue perfusion.

Synovial blood flow is affected by many factors (for reviews, *see* 1, 151, 158) such as intra-articular fluid pressure (*see* 'Volume–Pressure', p. 154), local temperature, joint motion (*see* pp. 171–79), sympathetic vasoconstrictor nerves and reflexes (159), and vasoactive chemicals such as prostaglandin E, which is released into rheumatoid and experimental arthritic effusions (160).

FLUID EXCHANGE ACROSS THE JOINT LINING

Theory: Application of Starling's Hypothesis

Synovial fluid is primarily an ultrafiltrate of plasma, so Starling's hypothesis of trans-capillary ultrafiltration (11) provides a valuable theoretical framework for approaching this subject. Starling's hypothesis predicts that the rate of fluid filtration (J_V) across the walls of synovial capillaries should be a linear function of capillary blood pressure (p_c) and extra-capillary colloid osmotic pressure (π_i), and a negative linear function of plasma colloid osmotic pressure (π_p) and extra-capillary hydraulic pressure (p_i);

$$J_V = L_p A \left[(p_c - p_i) - \sigma(\pi_p - \pi_i) \right] \qquad (Eqn.\ 7.2)$$

where L_p is the hydraulic conductance of unit area of capillary wall; A is total area of capillary wall; and σ, the osmotic reflection coefficient, is a measure of the semipermeability of the capillary wall to plasma protein (range from 1·0, for a perfect membrane totally retaining proteins, to 0 for a membrane offering no hindrance to protein). The product $L_p A$ may be termed the capillary filtration capacity K_c. For a review of trans-capillary flow *see* (161).

The Starling equation above, however, does not fully describe trans-*synovial* (c.f. trans-*capillary*) exchange, since additional pathways are involved in trans-synovial exchange (*Fig.* 7.4). From the pericapillary region, fluid exchanging with the joint cavity (pressure p_J) must traverse a further layer, the synovial intima (hydraulic conductance K_s). Moreover pericapillary fluid might also flow into the deeper, loose subintimal tissues (pressure p_D, conductance K_1). The simplest possible description of trans-synovial flow therefore involves 3 pathways (*Fig.* 7.4). The extracapillary pathways can be described by the law of Darcy, which describes viscous flow through a porous medium. Putting the equations for the 3 pathways together gives a single theoretical expression for trans-synovial exchange, $\dot{Q}_S$ (72, 162, 163):

$$\dot{Q}_S = \frac{K_S(K_1 + K_C)}{\Sigma K} p_J - \frac{K_S K_C}{\Sigma K}(p_C - \sigma(\pi_p - \pi_i)) - \frac{K_S K_1}{\Sigma K} p_D \qquad (Eqn.\ 7.3)$$

where $\Sigma K = K_S + K_1 + K_C$. $\dot{Q}_S$ is defined here for a direction of flow out of the

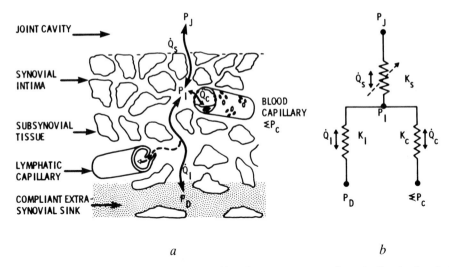

Fig. 7.4. *a*, Diagram showing pathways for fluid exchange across synovium. *b*, Simple electrical analogue of pathways to illustrate how the intimal pathway is linked in series with 2 parallel pathways, the trans-capillary route and the subsynovial route. Symbols are explained in the text; $\Sigma P_C = P_C - \sigma(\pi_p - \pi_i)$. [From Levick, 1983 (6) with permission.]

joint cavity (absorption) because this is the direction of exchange generally studied in experiments.

Some of the relations implicit in *Eqn.* 7.3 have now been examined experimentally, and some of the key parameters (K_S, K_C, σ) have been evaluated for the rabbit knee.

Effect of Capillary Pressure (p_C) and Colloid Osmotic Pressure (π_p)

The pressure of blood in the synovial microvessels (p_C) can be controlled and varied by perfusing the hindquarters of an anaesthetized rabbit with blood from an extra-corporeal circuit (72). With this technique it has been shown that raising p_C causes a slow rise in knee p_J at normal sub-atmospheric joint pressures, indicating filtration into the joint cavity. Conversely, at higher pathological joint pressures, where trans-synovial flow is out of the cavity (absorption), the rate of absorption of fluid from the cavity declines with capillary pressure ($\dot{Q}_S \alpha - p_C$) in conformity with *Eqn.* 7.3 and Starling's hypothesis (*Fig.* 7.5).

When the colloid osmotic pressure of the vascular perfusate is changed (by resuspending red cells in various albumin solutions), trans-synovial absorption rate increases with plasma colloid osmotic pressure (*Fig.* 7.5), again in conformity with *Eqns.* 7.2 and 7.3 (164). Sustained osmosis across the blood–joint interface is also demonstrated by a reduction of intra-articular pressure to a more sub-atmospheric value when plasma π_p is raised (6), and also by an inverse relation between intra-articular volume and plasma π_p in the elbow

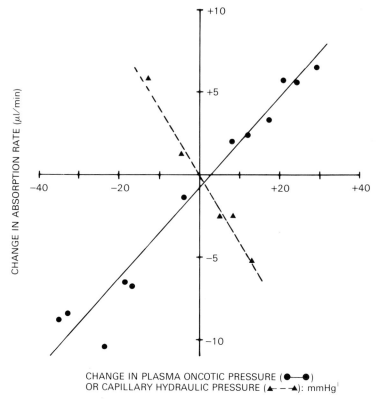

Fig. 7.5. Effect of capillary blood pressure (triangles) or plasma colloid osmotic pressure (circles) on rate of absorption of Krebs solution from the same joint cavity (rabbit knee, P_J = 18 cm H_2O, isolated perfused hindquarter preparation). *Note* that the osmotic slope is less steep (and, of course, of opposite sign) to the blood-pressure slope, indicating that the osmotic reflection coefficient to albumin is less than 1 (0·7 here). [Data from Knight and Levick, 1984 (164).]

and shoulder of anaesthetized rabbits (25). By contrast, small solutes added to plasma (e.g. sucrose; 165: glucose or NaCl; 166) cause only a transient, though marked, absorption of fluid from the joint, because they rapidly equilibrate across the capillary wall.

The Osmotic Reflection Coefficient σ: the Blood–Joint Interface as an Imperfect Semipermeable Membrane

It can be seen in *Fig.* 7.5 that a given change in perfusate colloid osmotic pressure has slightly less effect on trans-synovial flow than has the same change in plasma hydraulic pressure, i.e. absolute slope $d\dot{Q}_S/d\pi_p$ is less steep than absolute slope $d\dot{Q}_S/dp_C$. This indicates that the full osmotic potential of the plasma colloid (here plasma albumin) is not exerted across the blood–joint interface, i.e. the osmotic reflection coefficient is less than 1 – as of course must be the case, since some plasma protein normally gets into synovial fluid. From

Eqn. 7.3 it can be shown that the ratio of the observed slopes, $(d\dot{Q}_S/d\pi_p)/(d\dot{Q}_S/dp_C)$ equals the osmotic reflection coefficient. For plasma albumin across the blood–joint interface in the perfused rabbit knee, the reflection coefficient averages 0·78 (167), a value similar to that of several other capillary beds (161).

Effect of Intra-articular Hydraulic Pressure (p_J): the Yield Phenomenon

As is predicted by *Eqns.* 7.2 and 7.3, the rate of absorption of fluid from the joint cavity increases if intra-articular pressure is increased (*Fig.* 7.6a). However, after an initial fairly linear section of low slope, the relation steepens 4- to 6-fold at around 9 cmH$_2$O. The slope change is often, but not always, an abrupt one. The steepening was first discovered in skin by McMaster (168) and in synovium by Edlund (165) and was christened the 'breaking point'. The phenomenon persists when the circulation is arrested (163) or the animal is dead (163, 165), so it seems to be a physical property of the synovial component rather than vascular component. It was attributed by Edlund to an abrupt breakdown in the hydraulic resistance of the synovial tissue (i.e. increase in K_S, *Eqn.* 7.3), although not a macroscopic rupture (91, 165).

Confirmation of Edlund's seminal observations followed 30 years later (91), although the phenomenon still awaits investigation in other joints and species. But it also became clear that several features of the $\dot{Q}_S - p_J$ relation argued against the 'abrupt breakdown' explanation. Rather, the shape of the relation implies a progressive increase in synovial hydraulic conductance (K_S) above 9 cmH$_2$O, i.e. a gradual yielding of synovial resistance above 9 cmH$_2$O (162, 163). The phenomenon persists when the intra-articular fluid (saline in the original experiments) contains haemoglobin (165), plasma protein, or hyaluronate (unpublished observations). The yield-point *is* abolished, however, by acute (pyogenic) inflammation (165) and by congestive cardiac failure (169), because both conditions increase conductance even below 9 cmH$_2$O.

Testing the Yield Hypothesis

Eqn. 7.3 represents a hypothesis concerning how trans-synovial flow is governed. To it we must now add the 'yield' hypothesis, namely that K_S increases as a function of p_J above yield point ($K_S = \mathrm{f}(p_J)$) (163). This leads to an interesting prediction. *Eqn.* 7.3 shows that the slope $d\dot{Q}_S/dp_C$, relating trans-synovial flow to blood pressure (*Fig.* 7.5) equals the term $K_S K_C/\Sigma K$. If K_S increases with joint pressure, then slope $d\dot{Q}_S/dp_C$ too should increase with joint pressure. In other words, trans-synovial flow should be more sensitive to capillary pressure at high joint pressures than at lower ones.

This prediction has recently been tested by nearly 1000 changes of capillary pressure at 10 different values of p_J in perfused rabbit hindquarters (162). The prediction appears to be true; the slope relating $\dot{Q}_S$ to p_C steepens as a continuous hyperbolic function of intra-articular pressure (*Fig.* 7.6b). A further prediction of the yield hypothesis, that the sensitivity of trans-synovial flow to plasma colloid osmotic pressure (i.e. $d\dot{Q}_S/d\pi_p$) should increase with joint pressure, has also been tested and verified (167).

a

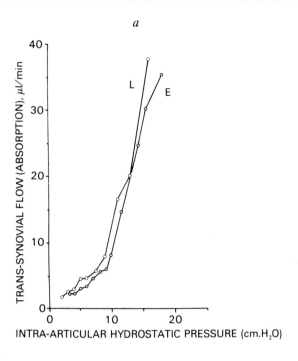

b

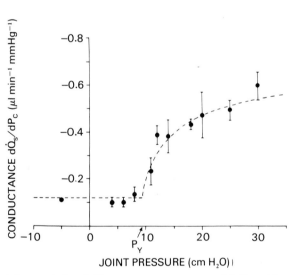

Fig. 7.6. Effect of intra-articular fluid pressure on trans-synovial flow (absorption rate) and conductance in the rabbit knee. *a*, The pressure–flow relation or 'Edlund curve'. *Note* increase in slope at ~9 cmH₂O ('break' or 'yield' point). [Redrawn from Edlund (curve E; reference 65) and Levick (curve L; reference 91).] *b*, The hydraulic conductance of the synovium–endothelium layer (slope dQ_S/dP_C from *Fig.* 7.5) plotted against intra-articular pressure: note the progressive increase in conductance above 9 cm H₂O. [From Knight and Levick, 1985 (162), with permission.]

The cause of the yield phenomenon at the ultrastructural level remains speculative (162), but preliminary histological work reveals definite changes in synovial structure. As intra-articular pressure and volume rise, the synovial intima becomes stretched and thinner, and the synovial capillaries even more superficially located than normal (McDonald & Levick, unpublished observations). The practical significance of the yield phenomenon lies in its implication for exchange kinetics in pathologically distended joints: and in the information it provides about the nature of interstitial hydraulic resistance.

Coefficients Governing Blood–Joint Exchange

The main coefficients governing flow between plasma and joint cavity are σ, K_C and K_S. The system's reflection coefficient for albumin (0·78; 167) might underestimate that for whole plasma (which includes globulins) – but probably only slightly so, in that albumin is the major colloid osmotic constituent of plasma (170). The filtration capacity of the whole synovial capillary bed, K_C, can be extrapolated from the data in *Fig.* 7.6b, and in conjunction with capillary surface area A (117) leads to L_p, the conductance of unit area of synovial endothelium. This averages $1 \cdot 1 \times 10^{-9} - 1 \cdot 4 \times 10^{-9}$ cm$^3 \cdot$ s$^{-1} \cdot$ dyne^{-1}, which is greater than the conductance of continuous endothelium and less than that of the more abundantly fenestrated renal glomerular capillaries – a logically consistent result. K_S too can be evaluated from the data in *Figs.* 7.6a and 7.6b and, in conjunction with synovial morphometric data (115), leads to a value for the hydraulic conductivity of a unit cube of synovial interstitium, viz. $2 \cdot 8 \times 10^{-12} - 7 \cdot 0 \times 10^{-12}$ cm$^4 \cdot$ s$^{-1} \cdot$ dyne^{-1} below yield pressure, (saline, 37 °C; 162). Thus synovial interstitium is more conductive than articular cartilage (conductivity $0 \cdot 7 - 0 \cdot 2 \times 10^{-12}$ cm$^4 \cdot$ s$^{-1} \cdot$ dyne^{-1}; 171) and less conductive than vitreous body ($3000-6000 \times 10^{-12}$ cm$^4 \cdot$ s$^{-1} \cdot$ dyne^{-1}; 172). It is calculated that the presence of the fibrous elements (proteoglycan, collagen) in the synovial intercellular spaces raises the hydraulic resistance of the synovial intima to several thousand times greater than that caused by the cells alone (162).

Intra-articular Colloid Osmotic Pressure

The effect of intra-articular macromolecules (proteins, hyaluronate) on trans-synovial flow are as yet little explored, but it is at present supposed that intra-articular protein exerts an osmotic effect at the capillary wall and not to a significant extent across synovial interstitium. Newbould has reported that intra-articular dextran solution of high osmolarity causes a slight osmotic flow into the joint, as indicated by a small rise in p_J (173). Conversely, replacement of a protein-rich effusion by an equal volume of saline in rheumatoid knees causes marked fluid absorption (69). Intra-articular proteins and dextran must also affect trans-synovial flows however by a second mechanism, namely by raising the viscosity of the fluid passing through synovium. Whether hyaluronate does so too depends on its ease of penetration of the synovial lining – which *a priori* seems likely to be low for such a voluminous molecule (*see* 174).

'Balance' or 'Imbalance' of Pressures and Flow across Synovial Exchange Vessels?

The relations between pressures and trans-synovial flow are becoming clear; but what are the actual magnitudes of the pressures and flows in normal joints; and do they 'balance' out i.e. summate to zero? To avoid confusion it is vital to differentiate between 3 different 'balances' (or 'imbalances'):

1. *Pressure* balance: do the four Starling pressures in *Eqn.* 7.2 balance (sum to zero) at a given point along the exchange vessel?
2. *Flow* balance: is there a balance (equality) between filtration flow and reabsorption flow (if any) across the walls of the synovial exchange vessels?
3. *Volume* balance: is synovial fluid volume held constant over the long term?

We can be confident that a 'balance' is the normal situation only for the third case, that of synovial fluid volume.

Trans-capillary pressure imbalance

In some capillary beds, filtration across the arterial portion of the exchange vessels may give way to absorption in the downstream vessels as capillary pressure falls below plasma oncotic pressure (170), although this is probably not the case in all capillary beds (e.g. 161, 175). In a microcirculation where proximal filtration gives way distally to absorption, there exists an intermediate point where the 4 Starling pressures balance (sum to zero) and fluid flux is zero. This point occurs where capillary pressure falls low enough to equal the other pressures. We can attempt to estimate this critical 'nul-flux' pressure ($p°$) in synovium. From *Eqn.* 7.2, if $J_V = 0$:

$$p° = p_C = p_i + \sigma(\pi_p - \pi_i) \qquad (Eqn.\ 7.4)$$

where σ is roughly 0·8 (167). If it is assumed (*a*) that p_i equals p_J at the point of zero transcapillary flow; (*b*) that π_i at the same point is close to equilibrium with π_J, colloid osmotic pressure in the joint cavity; and (*c*) that mixed venous colloid osmotic pressure π_V equals π_p at the nul point (i.e. filtration fraction is negligible), then:

$$p° = p_J + \sigma(\pi_v - \pi_J) \qquad (Eqn.\ 7.5)$$

This approach has been applied to rabbit knee (6, 59), and more recent data for rabbit knee, shoulder and hip give $p° = 7·6–9·7\ cmH_2O$ (25). In dog knee and shoulder the calculation gives a similar result; but dog wrist gives a higher value (15·7 mmHg; 29). But can the value of $p°$ actually be attained in the capillary *in vivo*? Venous pressure sets a lower limit to the true value of p_C *in vivo*, and is usually $\sim$11 cmH_2O in rabbit hindlimbs at heart level. Thus p_C *in vivo* ($>$11 cmH_2O) exceeds $p°$ ($\leq$9·7 cmH_2O) even at the venous end of the exchange vessels. These sums indicate that filtration dominates throughout the synovial microcirculation, except possibly in the dog wrist.

It must be noted, however, that the assumptions made in moving from the valid *Eqn.* 7.4 to the sum actually performed (*Eqn.* 7.5) reduce the security of this conclusion. Inspection of *Eqn.* 7.3 shows that, owing to the existence of the third (subintimal) pathway, the equation $p_i = p_J$ is not wholly justifiable; so the result, although suggestive, is not entirely conclusive. It must be stressed also that even if the above assumptions are valid, the value of $p°$ does *NOT* tell us the average pressure which exists *in vivo* in the capillary bed, because we know (from the flow of synovial lymph) that on average J_V is *NOT* zero *in vivo*.

An imbalance of pressures is especially likely in the dependent joints of large animals (e.g. human ankle) because gravity greatly increases arterial, capillary and venous pressures (*see* 'Gravitational Influence, p. 173). Indeed it is possible that, as a result of greater filtration in dependent joints, considerable haemoconcentration may occur by the end of the highly permeable fenestrated vessels, as occurs even in continuous capillaries in the foot (176).

In the case of arthritic knees the sum $p_J + \Delta\pi$ is increased (RA = 30 mmHg, OA = 22 mmHg; 177); but σ is unknown and presumably lower than normal.

Trans-capillary flow imbalance

It seems reasonably certain that filtration across the synovial capillary bed exceeds any reabsorption by venous capillaries or venules (if any occurs at all; *see* p. 158), when averaged over a reasonable period of normal usage (say 24 h). The evidence for this statement is primarily that synovial fluid is not stagnant but is constantly being elaborated, then removed as lymph (*see* 'Turnover', p. 157).

Lymph Flow and Volume Homeostasis

If there is a net filtration of fluid from plasma into the normal joint cavity (*see* 'Turnover', p. 157), volume can only be maintained constant in the long term by lymphatic drainage of the cavity. Moreover, lymphatic vessels are the only effective way of removing plasma protein from the joint cavity (111), so they are equally vital for protein level homeostasis, preventing a rise in π_J. Early work established that subintimal lymph vessels drain the cavity and are activated by joint motion, which pumps lymph along the vessels (49, 111, 150, 163, 178). Flexion may also help volume homeostasis by raising p_J, which drives fluid out across the permeable synovial lining towards the subintimal lymphatic vessels (6, 59). It seems probable that flexion is important in producing volume homeostasis in the long term, since the stationary joint in extension is *not* in a state of volume balance, judging by the slow rise in p_J with time (*see* 'Turnover', p. 157).

There is, sadly, very little recent work on synovial lymph flow. However, Simkin and his colleagues have recently studied the clearance of radiolabelled albumin from arthritic human joints (51), which estimates lymph flow provided that labelled-albumin clearance is exclusively by lymph vessels (as in healthy joints). High clearance rates were found in arthritic knees (4 ml/h, rheumatoid; 2 ml/h, osteoarthrosis, patients ambulant), an important result because it indicates that arthritic effusions are *not* primarily due to 'lymphatic insufficiency' but rather to increased trans-capillary filtration rates.

INFLUENCE OF PHYSIOLOGICAL STATE OF JOINT ON FLUID EXCHANGE

Most of the work described so far has involved joints in their simplest state – stationary, in a neutral position, close to heart level. The primary function of a joint, however, is to move. Normal movement is intermittent; periods of cyclical movement (minutes–hours), usually in an upright posture, normally alternate with periods of immobility. During the latter periods the joints are at varying angles, and at varying distances below heart level. All of these circumstances are likely to affect fluid exchange. The effect of arthritis on fluid exchange is discussed elsewhere (6).

Effect of Angle of Stationary Joint

When a joint contains an effusion, it has a neutral position in which the surrounding tissues are least tense (179). As a result of the operation of LaPlace's law intra-articular pressure is minimal in that position (95, 180) (*Fig.* 7.7). For predominantly hinge joints this neutral position is ~ 30° from full extension (59, 60, 66, 95, 180), and corresponds to the 'position of ease' and flexion deformity in arthritis (181). Displacement in either direction from this optimal angle raises p_J (man; 95) and acute flexion can lead to rupture (67). Moreover, the sensitivity of pressure to angle increases with the size of an effusion (55, 59, 60, 81, 83).

It is generally considered that bulk movement of synovial fluid within the cavity is important to cartilage nutrition (e.g. 1, 48). In man Menschik has shown

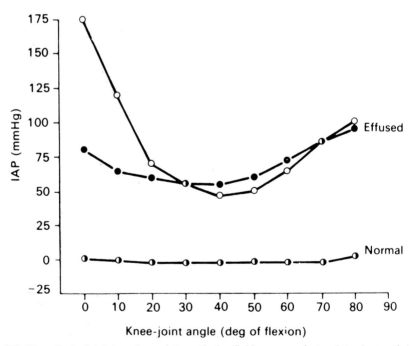

Fig. 7.7. The effect of joint angle on intra-articular fluid pressure (anterolateral aspect) in the human knee at normal fluid volume and at a raised fluid volume (10 ml dextran solution). Open symbols = active movement of limb. Closed symbols = passive movement. *Note* the relative insensitivity of the joint pressure to angle at a normal fluid volume. [From Baxendale, Ferrell and Wood, 1985 (60), with permission.]

that flexion of the human knee containing a small artificial effusion pumps fluid from the anterior compartment into the posterior compartment, presumably by setting up a pressure gradient within the joint cavity (182), and there is limited support for this in the distribution of acrylate in casts of flexed knee joints (55, 92). But Menschik's work, with a non-physiological intra-articular volume, appears to be the only direct study of intracavity flow set up by a change of angle.

The above studies relate to raised intra-articular volumes. The effect of flexion in joints containing normal, very small synovial fluid volumes is far less dramatic (rabbit, 59, 81: man, 60, 183) (*Fig.* 7.7). In these studies, in which care was taken to prevent any entry of fluid into the sub-atmospheric joint space during cannulation, pressure changed only modestly with angle, rising to only a few cmH$_2$O above atmospheric pressure even upon extreme flexion. There are some discrepancies between laboratories here, possibly related to technique. Greater changes with flexion are reported in studies where a catheter-and-stylet method was used (66, 67). This method of cannulation necessitates open contact, albeit briefly, with ambient pressure – which introduces the possibility of a slight volume influx into the cannulated space, to which the pressure–angle relationship is exceedingly sensitive (59). But whether this wholly accounts for the discrepancies between various laboratories remains unclear, especially for a joint as large as the human knee.

The pressure–angle relationship has important implications for homeostasis of synovial fluid volume. Elevation of p_J to supra-atmospheric pressures by fluid infusion causes fluid absorption from the cavity (*Fig.* 7.6), and elevation of p_J by flexion probably has the same effect (59, 66). Its importance is that this is the only physiological mechanism described to date which *reduces* intra-articular fluid volume. As noted earlier, net flow in the resting extended joint appears to be *into* the cavity; and in vigorous exercise (*see* p. 175) flow into the cavity appears to be enhanced. Thus the effect of passive sustained flexion on trans-synovial flow, coupled with the concomitant emptying of subsynovial lymph vessels, seems at present the best way of accounting for long-term homeostasis of synovial fluid volume.

Gravitational Influence: Effect of Position Relative to Heart Level

The direct effect of gravity on vertical pressure distribution within a synovial cavity has never been investigated. Many animals' joints are sufficiently small for the gravitational effect to be slight, but one wonders whether the knees of large mammals might display a pleural-like gradient (184). By contrast gravity has a major, direct effect on vascular pressures (*Fig.* 7.8). In the upright position, arterial as well as venous pressure increases linearly with vertical distance below heart level due to the gravitational force on the fluid column. In the ankle of a standing man, for example, arterial pressure is around 180 mmHg and venous pressure around 100 mmHg. As a result, capillary pressure increases with vertical distance below heart level (in spite of a compensating arteriolar vasoconstriction) and reaches ~100 mmHg in the human foot (175). There is therefore a major increase in the net filtration force into the synovial cavity in dependent joints (*Eqns.* 7.2., 7.3), especially when the limb is immobile, and also to some degree when the limb is moving, since mean venous pressure is reduced by rhythmic contraction of the calf muscles only to ~30 mmHg, while dependent arterial pressure is not reduced at all. This helps explain the particularly large synovial fluid volumes relative to joint size in the most dependent joints of sizeable mammals, and the correspondingly low hyaluronate concentrations and viscosities (15, 27, 56, 57).

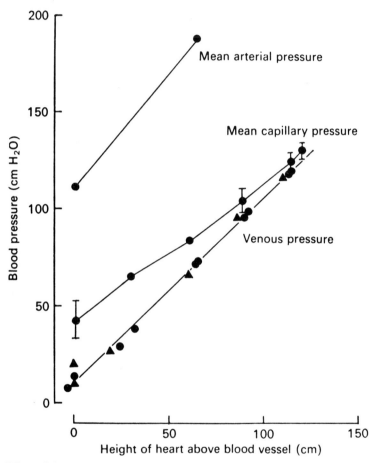

Fig. 7.8. Effect of dependency below heart level on vascular pressures. Arterial pressures were measured indirectly, by sphygmomanometry of the popliteal artery. Venous pressure was measured directly in the dorsal vein of the foot. Capillary pressure was measured by direct micropuncture in the skin at the base of the toe-nail. [From Levick and Michel, 1978 (175), with permission.]

Effect of Passive Movement of Joints

Continuous passive movement, confusingly referred to as 'exercise' in some papers, hastens the removal of injected solutions and suspensions from the cavity (49, 53, 185) and also doubles the rate of resolution of experimental haemarthroses (186). Passive movement causes intra-articular pressure to oscillate with 1 or 2 peaks per cycle (59, 60, 66, 67, 83) and the peak pressure declines progressively with repeated flexion (66), in line with the idea of a trans-synovial pumping effect (59). Stimulation of trans-synovial flow, coupled with activation of lymph flow, would account for enhanced removal of fluid by continuous passive motion. Continuous passive movement also improves the quality of healing of experimental cartilaginous defects in small animals (187).

The above evidence of an absorptive effect was obtained in joints containing enhanced fluid volumes. In contrast, Ekholm and Norback (188) found that passive movement of the normal rabbit knee caused a highly significant 2·4-fold increase in aspiratable fluid volume from the opened cavity, accompanied by dilution of the hyaluronate and protein. A possible explanation for this finding is that vigorous prolonged passive movement (90 cycles/min for 3 h) might provoke a synovial hyperaemia and therefore a rise in capillary filtration pressure. Tenuous indirect evidence for such a hyperaemia exists in the form of rise in intra-articular temperature (189) and increased rate of small-solute flux (190). It even seems conceivable that prolonged vigorous manipulation might cause a mechanically-induced synovitis, since the rate of penetration of protein-bound gold from blood into the joint cavity is increased by passive movements (90 cycles/min for 20 min; 191), and venular gaps permeable to carbon particles develop (35 cycles/min for 50–145 min; 139).

Effect of Active Movement of Joints (Exercise)

Active movement is a more complex situation than passive movement, because not only are there additional local influences on fluid exchange (e.g. the effect of contracting muscle on capsule tension and p_J), but also there are systemic influences (changes in blood pressure, venous muscle pump, vasodilator influences).

Intra-articular pressure in exercise

The intra-articular pressure changes can be more complicated during active movement than during passive movement, being determined not only by joint angle but also by the mechanical effect of muscles acting around the joint, which affect the stress in the joint capsule. Muscle contraction can either compress the capsule and raise intra-articular pressure, as occurs in the knee flexed as part of a withdrawal reflex (59), or it can pull on the capsule and reduce intra-articular pressure, as in the human knee during walking (67).

Jayson and Dixon (67) have provided one of the very few studies of pressure oscillations in the knee during normal limb usage. They found that elevation of the straight leg reduced intra-articular pressure to around −44 mmHg, and resisted attempts at elevation lowered it even further, to −107 mmHg. The suggested reason was that the quadriceps tends to distract the capsule of the relatively 'empty' normal joint. In striking contrast, when the knee contained an effusion, the same manoeuvre had the opposite effect, raising p_J to over 200 mmHg. Here the mechanics of the system are such that quadriceps contraction compresses the distended capsule, an effect noted previously by

Caughey and Bywaters (68). The large transient increases in p_J might be a factor in the generation of rheumatoid bone cysts (67).

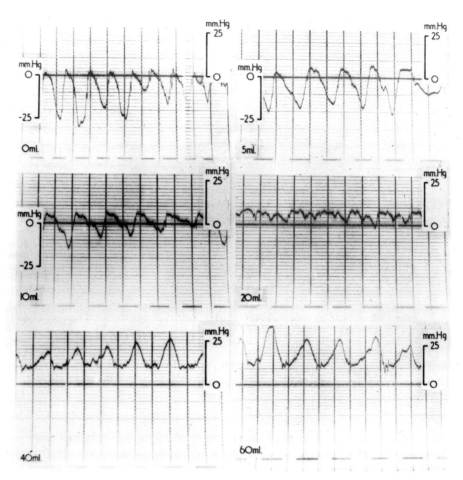

Fig. 7.9. Intra-articular pressure in the anterior region of the human knee during walking. Transducer strapped to subject's thigh and connected to cannula by short length of tubing. The period of foot stance is marked by a horizontal bar. *Note* the large swings to sub-atmospheric pressure during extension and heel-strike in the normal joint. When intra-articular volume was raised, these swings reversed sign, becoming positive. [From Jayson and Dixon, 1970 (67), with permission.]

Reflex active flexion of the knee transiently raises p_J, but only by a few cmH_2O (withdrawal reflex, rabbit knee; 59). Walking produces a more complicated cycle of fluid pressure changes in man; the dominant component (*Fig.* 7.9) is a highly negative pressure (average -15 mmHg) coinciding with foot stance, during the first half of which phase the quadriceps is known to be contracting. Reeves (183) by contrast briefly reported no major pressure changes. The presence of an effusion reverses the direction of the pressure oscillation, which becomes positive on foot stance. The dog knee probably has a cycle similar to the normal human knee, for transient pressures of around −20 mmHg have been recorded by Nade and Newbould at moments of active extension (66). Other joints seem unexplored during usage.

Volume changes

The changes in trans-synovial flow and synovial fluid volume in active movement are not well documented. Reeves, in a too-brief paper, reported that pressure in the resting human knee rose by 5 mmHg after 20–45 min of cycling, implying an accumulation of fluid (183). Recently an increase in aspiratable fluid volume was reported for 3 out of 6 human knees after running several miles (and a decrease in 1 out of 6), along with an increased number of cartilage fragments in all the joint fluids, and increases in β-glucuronidase levels (lysosome-derived enzyme) (13). The highly negative pressures in the actively extended joint (67) could create the enhanced gradient needed to explain enhanced filtration into the exercising joint. A second factor might be a raised synovial capillary pressure due to synovial arteriolar vasodilatation accompanying exercise (*see* below).

Blood-flow changes

The evidence for synovial vasodilatation in exercise is, however, conflicting. Lindström (192) asserted that synovial vasodilatation was apparent by inspection of the opened joint after exercise. A rise in intra-articular temperature could indicate synovial vasodilatation (189), but might alternatively be secondary to changes in muscle and skin blood-flow. An increased rate of clearance of Na^+ has been observed, but in only 2 out of 6 subjects (154). More recently, increased microsphere deposition has been reported in soft periarticular tissue ('synovium') after exercise, the calculated flow increasing 3 times in the knee and 7 times in the wrist (157). In contrast, however, xenon clearance is reduced by exercise (151). As xenon clearance may largely reflect the flow through articular adipose tissue (79), it seems possible that differential changes occur in blood flow to areolar synovium and articular fat.

A possible mechanism mediating synovial vasodilatation, besides reduced sympathetic vasomotor tone (159), is liberation of vasodilator substances like H^+, CO_2, K^+ by contracting muscle fibres, which lie very close to synovium in the anterior region of the knee. This possibility is supported by the interesting observation that synovial fluid pH falls markedly in the exercising dog knee (16) (*see Fig.* 7.10). Such changes in fluid composition offer a potential signal to chondrocytes (additional to stress) of the level and duration of exercise.

Exercise and the blood–joint barrier

Concerning the properties of the blood–joint interface during and after exercise, 2 interesting observations exist. First, Edlund (165) reported that the inflexion or yield point (*Fig.* 7.6) on the pressure v. absorption curve disappeared in 8 out of 13 animals after exhausting 4 min runs on a treadmill; the relationship was steeper than normal, below 9 cmH_2O even 17–18 h after the exercise. Second, vigorous passive flexion may increase the permeability of the barrier to macromolecules and particles (139, 191), as noted above (p. 174). Such observations raise the possibility that the mechanical trauma of vigorous synovial movement may enhance its hydraulic conductance and permeability to macromolecules. However, further work is needed in this poorly explored area.

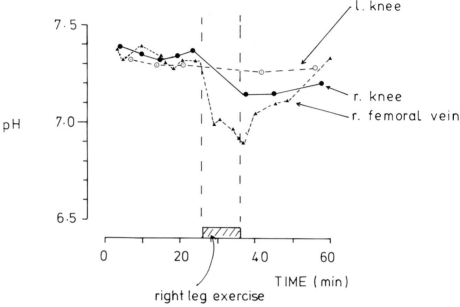

Fig. 7.10. Change in pH of synovial fluid and femoral vein blood in the exercised hind-limb of a dog. Femoral vein pH dips sharply on right leg exercise, due presumably to release of acidic metabolites by skeletal muscle. Right knee synovial fluid pH also dips, more slowly, suggesting a direct transfer of muscle metabolites across the joint lining; the left knee (unexercised control) shows no such dip. Nature of exercise not described. [Data from Joseph, Reed and Homburger, 1946 (16).]

Effect of Prolonged Immobilization of Joints

Little seems known about the effect of the converse of exercise, prolonged immobilization, upon synovial fluid exchange – which is surprising since human limbs are not infrequently immobilized in Plaster of Paris! The removal of material from the joint cavity (e.g. haemarthrosis; 186) is known to be delayed by immobilization, as one might anticipate from the dependence of synovial lymph flow upon joint movement. In the normal joint one might anticipate that fluid volume should increase slowly during immobility, since p_J increases slowly in anaesthetized laboratory animals (59) (*see* 'Bulk Turnover', p. 157). Indeed an 'increase of synovial fluid' after immobility has been reported qualitatively (193), but no quantities are available. The ill-effects of prolonged immobilization on cartilage viability (e.g. 63) and repair (187) are attributed to a lack of the internal convection of nutritive synovial fluid, which is assumed to occur normally. A contributory factor could be reduced synovial vascularity, as suggested by inspection (192), although no counts were reported, and others make no comment on changing vascularity (e.g. 63) or else report 'hyperaemia' (193) after prolonged immobilization. A hypertrophy and thickening of the synovial intima seems a generally agreed consequence, however, so trans-synovial exchange may be to some degree impaired.

FUTURE DEVELOPMENTS

This survey has revealed many areas of synovial fluid physiology and pathology where data are scanty or non-existent. Topics which seem worth further work, because of their theoretical or practical interest, include the effects of exercise and prolonged immobilization on synovial fluid volume; the effect of movement on flow within the joint cavity; the effect of movement (active and passive), immobilization and disease on the numbers and depth of intimal exchange vessels and their blood flow; the question of whether excessive usage of joints (passively in experiments, or actively in marches and sport training) might produce a mechanical synovitis; and the elucidation of the physical basis of the yield phenomenon.

CONCLUSIONS

Starling's hypothesis of fluid exchange emerges as a valuable cornerstone upon which our understanding of synovial fluid dynamics can be based. It is also now clear that the hypothesis requires elaboration to account fully for the hydraulic flow occurring between the synovial joint cavity and blood. The exact nature of these flows during joint usage remain poorly defined.

CLINICAL AND PRACTICAL SIGNIFICANCE

The analytical approach utilized above offers a basis for understanding and calculating the fluid exchanges which occur in joints under a variety of normal and abnormal conditions. The practical significance of changes in trans-synovial flow in exercise are not clear. The clinical consequences of disordered fluid exchange are more apparent, and the morbidity created by effusions has been summarized.

ACKNOWLEDGEMENTS

I should like to thank the Arthritis and Rheumatism Council of Great Britain, which has supported many of the writer's investigations of fluid phenomena in joints.

REFERENCES

1. Levick J R (1984) Blood flow and mass transport in synovial joints. The cardiovascular System IV: The Microcirculation. *In: Handbook of Physiology* (E M Renkin and C C Michel, eds), pp. 917–47. Bethesda: American Physiological Society.
2. Simkin P A and Nilson K L (1981) Trans-synovial exchange of large and small molecules. *Clin Rheum Dis* 7: 99–129.

3. McCutchen C W (1981) Joint lubrication. *Clin Rheum Dis* **7**: 241–57.
4. Swanson S A V (1979) Friction, wear and lubrication. *In: Adult Articular Cartilage*, 2nd Ed (M A R Freeman, ed), pp. 415–60. London: Pitman.
5. Bauer W, Ropes M W and Waine H (1940) The physiology of articular structures. *Physiol Rev* **20**: 272–312.
6. Levick J R (1983) Synovial fluid dynamics: the regulation of volume and pressure. *In: Studies in Joint Disease*, Vol. 2 (E J Holborow and A Maroudas, eds), pp. 153–240. London: Pitman.
7. McCarty D J (1980) The physiology of the normal synovium. *In: The Joints and Synovial Fluid*, Vol. II (L Sokoloff, ed), pp. 294–315. New York: Academic Press.
.8 Rodnan G P, Benedek T G and Panetta W C (1966) The early history of synovia (joint fluid). *Ann Int Med* **65**: 821–42.
9. Illingworth C (1967) *The Story of William Hunter*. Edinburgh: Livingstone.
10. Hunter W (1743) Of the structure and diseases of articulating cartilages. *Philos Trans R Soc Lond [Biol]* **42**: 514–21.
11. Starling E H (1896) On the absorption of fluids from connective tissue spaces. *J Physiol* **19**: 312–26.
12. Edwards J C W, Sedgwick A D and Willoughby D A (1981) The formation of a structure with the features of synovial lining by subcutaneous injection of air: an *in vivo* culture system. *J Pathol* **134**: 147–56.
13. Fawthrop F, Hornby J, Swan A, Hutton C, Doherty M and Dieppe C (1985) A comparison of normal and pathological synovial fluid. *Br J Rheumatol* **24**: 61–9.
14. Yehia S R and Duncan H (1975) Synovial fluid analysis. *Clin Orthop* **107**: 11–24.
15. Van Pelt R W (1962) Properties of equine synovial fluid. *J Am Vet Med Assoc* **141**: 1051–61.
16. Joseph N R, Reed C I and Homburger E (1946) An *in vivo* study of the pH of synovial fluid in dogs. *Am J Physiol* **146**: 1–11.
17. McCarty D J (1974) Selected aspects of synovial membrane physiology. *Arthritis Rheum* **17**: 289–96.
18. Lund-Olsen K (1970) Oxygen tension in synovial fluids. *Arthritis Rheum* **13**: 769–76.
19. Richman A I, Su E Y and Ho G (1981) Reciprocal relationship of synovial fluid volume and oxygen tension. *Arthritis Rheum* **24**: 701–5.
20. Roberts J E, McLees B D and Kerby G P (1967) Pathways of glucose metabolism in rheumatoid and non-rheumatoid synovial membrane. *J Lab Clin Med* **70**: 503–11.
21. Brothers G B and Hadler N M (1983) Diurnal variations in rheumatoid synovial effusions. *J Rheumatol* **10**: 471–74.
22. Rabinowitz J L, Gregg J R and Nixon J E (1984) Lipid composition of the tissues of human knee joints. II. Synovial fluid in trauma. *Clin Orthop* **190**: 292–8.
23. Hill B A and Butler B D (1984) Surfactants identified in synovial fluid and their ability to act as boundary lubricants. *Ann Rheum Dis* **43**: 641–8.
24. Jensen C E and Zachariae L (1959) The contributions from hyaluronic acid and from protein to the colloid osmotic pressure of human synovial fluid. *Acta Rheum Scand* **5**: 18–28.
25. McDonald J N, Levick J R and Knox P (1986) Forces governing fluid exchange in major limb joints. *Scand J Rheumatol [Suppl]* **60**: 26.
26. Simkin P A and Pickerel C C (1984) Interarticular differences in oncotic pressure of canine synovial fluid. *J Rheumatol* **11**: 14–6.
27. Davies D V (1944) Observations on the volume, viscosity and nitrogen content of synovial fluid, with a note on the histological appearance of the synovial membrane. *J Anat* **78**: 68–78.
28. Sunblad L (1953) Studies on hyaluronic acid in synovial fluids. *Acta Soc Med Upsal* **58**: 113–238.
29. Simkin P A and Benedict R S (1985) Microvascular pressures in normal canine joints. *Arthritis Rheum [Suppl]* **28**: S90.
30. Reiman M D, Arnoldi C C and Nielsen O S (1980) Permeability of synovial membrane to plasma proteins in human coxarthrosis. *Clin Orthop* **147**: 297–300.
31. Levick J R (1981) Permeability of rheumatoid and normal human synovium to specific plasma proteins. *Arthritis Rheum* **24**: 1550–60.
32. Kushner I and Somerville J A (1971) Permeability of human synovial membrane to plasma protein. *Arthritis Rheum* **14**: 560–70.
33. Wallis W J, and Simkin P A (1986) Protein traffic in human synovial effusions. *Scand J Rheumatol [Suppl]* **60**: A84.
34. Balazs E A, Watson D, Duff I F and Roseman S (1969) Hyaluronic acid in synovial fluid. I. Molecular parameters of hyaluronic acid in normal and arthritic human fluids. *Arthritis Rheum* **10**: 357–76.

35. Hamerman D and Schuster H (1958) Hyaluronate in normal human synovial fluid. *J Clin Invest* **37**: 57–64.
36. Anadere I, Chmiel H and Laschner W (1979) Viscoelasticity of 'normal' and pathological synovial fluid. *Biorheology* **16**: 179–84.
37. Balazs E A and Gibbs D A (1970) The rheological properties and biological function of hyaluronic acid. *In: Chemistry and Molecular Biology of Intercellular Matrix* (E A Balazs, ed), pp. 1241–53. New York: Academic Press.
38. Ogston A G and Stanier J E (1953) The physiological function of hyaluronic acid in synovial fluid; viscous, elastic and lubricating properties. *J Physiol* **119**: 244–52.
39. Dahl L B, Dahl I M, Engström-Laurent A and Granath K (1985) Concentration and molecular weight of sodium hyaluronate in synovial fluid from patients with rheumatoid arthritis and other arthropathies. *Ann Rheum Dis* **44**: 817–22.
40. Comper W D and Laurent T C (1978) Physiological function of connective tissue polysaccharides. *Physiol Rev* **58**: 255–315.
41. Swann D A and Mintz G (1979) The isolation and properties of a second glycoprotein (LGP-II) from the articular lubricating fraction from bovine synovial fluid. *Biochem J* **179**: 465–71.
42. Swann D A and Radin E L (1972) Purification and properties of the glycoprotein articular lubricant. *Fed Proc* **31**: 466A.
43. Carnemolla B, Cutolo M, Castellani P, Balza E, Raffanti S and Zardi L (1984) Characterization of synovial fluid fibronectin from patients with rheumatic inflammatory diseases and healthy subjects. *Arthritis Rheum* **27**: 913–21.
44. Cecere F, Lessard J, McDuffy S and Pope R M (1983) Evidence for the local production and utilization of immune reactants in rheumatoid arthritis. *Arthritis Rheum* **25**: 1307–15.
45. Patel V, Panayi G S and Unger A (1983) Spontaneous and pokeweed mitogen-induced *in vitro* immunoglobulin and IgM rheumatoid factor production by peripheral blood and synovial fluid mononuclear cells in rheumatoid arthritis. *J Rheumatol* **10**: 364–72.
46. Swann D A (1978) Macromolecules of synovial fluid. *In: The Joints and Synovial Fluid* (L Sokoloff, ed), pp. 407–37. New York: Academic Press.
47. Maroudas A, Bullough P, Swanson S A V and Freeman M A R (1968) The permeability of articular cartilage. *J Bone Joint Surg [Br]* **50**: 166–77.
48. McKibbin B and Maroudas A (1979) Nutrition and metabolism. *In: Adult Articular Cartilage*, 2nd Ed. (M A R Freeman, ed), pp. 461–86. London: Pitman.
49. Adkins E W O and Davies D V (1940) Absorption from the joint cavity. *Q J Exp Physiol* **30**: 147–54.
50. Rekonen A, Oka M and Kuikka J (1973) Measurement of synovial fluid volume by a radioisotope method. *Scand J Rheumatol* **2**: 33–5.
51. Wallis W J, Simkin P A, Nelp W B and Foster D M (1985) Intra-articular volume and clearance in human synovial effusions. *Arthritis Rheum* **28**: 441–9.
52. Heilmann H H, Engelmann L, Lindenhayn K and Haupt R (1986) The determination of the volume of synovia in the guinea pig. *Scand J Rheumatol [Suppl]* **60**: A66.
53. Davies D V (1946) Synovial membrane and synovial fluid of joints. *Lancet* **62**: 815–22.
54. Lai-Fook S J and Kaplowitz M R (1985) Pleural space thickness *in situ* by light microscopy in five mammalian species. *J Appl Physiol* **59**: 603–10.
55. Nade S and Newbould P J (1984) Pressure-volume relationships and elastance in the knee joint of the dog. *J Physiol* **357**: 417–39.
56. Ogston A G and Stanier J E (1950) On the state of hyaluronic acid in the synovial fluid. *Biochem J* **46**: 364–76.
57. Seppälä P O and Balazs E A (1969) Hyaluronic acid in synovial fluid. III. Effect of maturation and aging on the chemical properties of bovine synovial fluid of different joints. *J Gerontol* **24**: 309–14.
58. Müller W (1929) Über den negativen Luftdrück in Gelenkraum *Dtsch Z Chir* **218**: 395–401.
59. Levick J R (1979) An investigation into the validity of subatmospheric synovial pressure recordings and their dependence on joint angle. *J Physiol* **289**: 55–68.
60. Baxendale R H, Ferrel W R and Wood L (1985) Intra-articular pressures during active and passive movement of normal and distended knee joints. *J Physiol* **369**: 179P.
61. Spencer J D, Hayes K C and Alexander I J (1984) Knee joint effusion and quadriceps reflex inhibition in man. *Arch Physical Med Rehabil* **65**: 171–7.
62. Wood L and Ferrell W (1985) Fluid compartmentation and articular mechanoreceptor discharge in the cat knee. *Q J Exp Physiol* **70**: 329–35.
63. Wigren A, Wik O and Falk J (1975) Repeated intra-articular implantation of hyaluronic acid:

an experimental study in normal and immobilized adult rabbit knee joints. *Ups J Med Sci [Suppl]* **17**: 3–20.

64. Bunger C, Hjermind J and Bulow J (1983) Haemodynamics of the juvenile knee in relation to increasing intra-articular pressure. An experimental study in dogs. *Acta Orthop Scand* **54**: 80–7.

65. Bunger C, Hjermind J, Bach P, Bunger E H and Myhre-Jensen O (1984) Haemodynamics in acute arthritis of the knee in puppies. *Acta Orthop Scand* **55**: 197–202.

66. Nade S and Newbould P J (1983) Factors determining the level and changes in pressure in the knee joint of the dog. *J Physiol* **338**: 21–36.

67. Jayson M I V and Dixon A St. J (1970) Intra-articular pressure in rheumatoid arthritis of the knee. III. Pressure changes during joint use. *Ann Rheum Dis* **29**: 401–8.

68. Caughey D E and Bywaters E G L (1963) Joint fluid pressure in chronic knee effusions. *Ann Rheum Dis* **22**: 106–9.

69. Palmer D G and Myers D B (1968) Some observations of joint effusions. *Arthritis Rheum* **11**: 745–55.

70. Ropes M W and Bauer W (1953) *Synovial Fluid Changes in Joint Disease*. Cambridge Massachusetts: Harvard University Press.

71. Jayson M I V (1981) Intra-articular pressure. *Clin Rheum Dis* **7**: 149–66.

72. Knight A D and Levick J R (1984) The influence of blood pressure on trans-synovial flow in the rabbit. *J Physiol* **349**: 27–42.

73. Jayson M I V and Dixon A St. J (1970) Intra-articular pressure in rheumatoid arthritis of the knee. I. Pressure changes during passive joint distensions. *Ann Rheum Dis* **29**: 261–5.

74. Myers D B and Palmer D G (1972) Capsular compliance and pressure-volume relationships in normal and arthritic knees. *J Bone Joint Surg [Br]* **54**: 710–6.

75. Baxendale R H, Ferrell W R and Wood L (1985) Knee-joint distension and quadriceps maximal voluntary contraction in man. *J Physiol* **367**: 100P.

76. deAndrade J R, Grant C and Dixon A St. J (1965) Joint distension and reflex muscle inhibition in the knee. *J Bone Joint Surg [Am]* **47**: 313–22.

77. Jayson M I V and Dixon A St. J (1970) Intra-articular pressure in rheumatoid arthritis of the knee. II. Effect of intra-articular pressure on blood circulation to the synovium. *Ann Rheum Dis* **29**: 266–8.

78. Lucht U, Bunger C, Krebs B, Hjermind J and Bulow J (1983) Blood flow in the juvenile hip in relation to changes of the intra-articular pressure. *Acta Orthop Scand* **54**: 182–7.

79. Phelps P, Steele A D and McCarty D J (1972) Significance of Xenon-133 clearance rate from canine and human joints. *Arthritis Rheum* **15**: 360–70.

80. Tachdjian M O and Grana L (1968) Response of the hip to increased intra-articular pressure. *Clin Orthop* **61**: 199–212.

81. Knight A D and Levick J R (1982) Pressure-volume relationships above and below atmospheric pressure in the synovial cavity of the rabbit knee. *J Physiol* **328**: 403–20.

82. Knight A D and Levick J R (1983) Time-dependence of the pressure-volume relationship in the synovial cavity of the rabbit knee. *J Physiol* **335**: 139–52.

83. O'Driscoll S W, Kumar A and Salter R B (1983) The effect of volume of effusion, joint position and continuous passive motion on intra-articular pressure in the rabbit knee. *J Rheumatol* **10**: 360–3.

84. McCarty D J, Phelps P and Pyenson J (1966) Crystal-induced inflammation in canine joints. *J Exp Med* **124**: 99–114.

85. Gershuni D H, Hargens A R, Lee Y F, Greenberg E N, Zapf R and Akeson W H (1983) The questionable significance of hip-joint tamponade in producing osteonecrosis in Legg-Calve-Perthes syndrome. *J Pediatr Orthop* **3**: 280–6.

86. Crowningshield R, Pope M H and Johnson R J (1976) An analytical model of the knee. *J Biomech* **9**: 397–405.

87. Steer G, Jayson M I V, Dixon A St. J and Beighton P (1971) Joint capsule collagen: analysis by the study of intra-articular pressure during joint distension. *Ann Rheum Dis* **30**: 481–6.

88. Caro C G, Pedley T J, Schroter R C and Seed W A (1978) *The Mechanics of the Circulation*. Oxford: Oxford University Press.

89. Bergel D (1961) The static elastic properties of the arterial wall. *J Physiol* **156**: 451–61.

90. Wood L and Ferrell W (1984) Responses of slowly adapting articular mechanoreceptors in the cat knee joint to alterations in intra-articular volume. *Ann Rheum Dis* **43**: 327–32.

91. Levick J R (1979) The influence of hydrostatic pressure on trans-synovial fluid movement and on capsular expansion in the rabbit knee. *J Physiol* **289**: 69–82.

92. Knight A D and Levick J R (1982) Physiological compartmentation of fluid within the synovial cavity of the rabbit knee. *J Physiol* **331**: 1–15.

93. Grigg P and Hoffman A H (1982) Properties of Ruffini afferents revealed by stress analysis of isolated sections of cat knee capsule. *J Neurophysiol* **47**: 41–54.
94. Singleton W B and Jones E L (1979) The experimental induction of subclinical Perthes' disease in the puppy following arthrotomy and intra-capsular tamponade. *J Comp Pathol* **89**: 57–71.
95. Eyring J E and Murray W R (1964) The effect of joint position on the pressure of intra-articular effusions. *J Bone Joint Surg [Am]* **46**: 1235–41.
96. Johns R J and Wright V (1962) Relative importance of various tissues in joint stiffness. *J Appl Physiol* **17**: 824–8.
97. Johns R J and Wright V (1964) An analytical description of joint stiffness. *Biorheology* **2**: 87–95.
98. Ferrel W R, Nade S and Newbould P J (1986) The interrelation of neural discharge, intra-articular pressure and joint angle in the knee of the dog. *J Physiol* **373**: 353–65.
99. Grigg P (1975) Mechanical factors influencing response of joint afferent neurones from cat knee. *J Neurophysiol* **38**: 1473–84.
100. McCall W D, Farias W J, Williams W J and BeMent S L (1974) Static and dynamic responses of slowly-adapting joint receptors. *Brain Res* **70**: 221–43.
101. Halata Z (1977) Ultrastructure of the sensory endings in the articular capsule of the knee joint of the domestic cat (Ruffini corpuscles and Pacinian corpuscles). *J Anat* **124**: 717–24.
102. Ekholm J, Eklund G and Skoglund S (1960) On the reflex effects from the knee joint of the cat. *Acta Physiol Scand* **50**: 167–74.
103. Lundberg A, Malmgren K and Schomburg E D (1978) Role of joint afferents in motor control exemplified by effects on reflex pathways from Ib afferents. *J Physiol* **284**: 327–43.
104. Cowper R A, Jayson M I V and Dixon A St J (1970) Synovial rupture. Experiments on cadaver knees. *Ann Rheum Dis* **30**: 162–5.
105. Jayson M I V, Swannell A J, Kirk J A and Dixon A St. J (1969) Acute joint rupture. *Ann Physical Med* **10**: 175–9.
106. Roberts A D (1971) Role of electrical repulsive forces in synovial fluid. *Nature* **231**: 434–6.
107. Jayson M I V (1968) Study of a valvular mechanism in the formation of synovial cysts. *Ann Physical Med* **9**: 243–5.
108. Wigley R D (1982) Popliteal cysts: variations on a theme of Baker. *Semin Arthritis Rheum* **12**: 1–10.
109. Simkin P A and Pizzorno J E (1974) Trans-synovial exchange of small molecules in normal human subjects. *J Appl Physiol* **36**: 581–7.
110. Simkin P A and Pizzorno J E (1979) Synovial permeability in rheumatoid arthritis. *Arthritis Rheum* **22**: 689–96.
111. Bauer W, Short C L and Bennett G A (1933) The manner of removal of proteins from normal joints. *J Exp Med* **57**: 419–33.
112. Simkin P A and Benedict R S (1986) Clearance of iodide and albumin from normal canine wrists and knees. *Scand J Rheumatol [Suppl]* **60**: 77.
113. Ghadially F N (1978) Fine structure of joints. *In: The Joints and Synovial Fluid* (L Sokoloff, ed), pp. 105–76. New York: Academic Press.
114. Schumacher H R (1975) Ultrastructure of the synovial membrane. *Ann Clin Lab Sci* **5**: 489–98.
115. Knight A D and Levick J R (1984) Morphometry of the ultrastructure of the blood–joint barrier in the rabbit knee. *Q J Exp Physiol* **69**: 271–88.
116. Castor C W (1960) The microscopic structure of normal human synovial tissue. *Arthritis Rheum* **3**: 140–51.
117. Knight A D and Levick J R (1983) The density and distribution of capillaries around a synovial cavity. *Q J Exp Physiol* **68**: 629–44.
118. Barland P, Novikoff A B and Hamerman D (1962) Electron microscopy of the human synovial membrane. *J Cell Biol* **14**: 207–20.
119. Linck G and Porte A (1981) Cytophysiology of the synovial membrane: distinction of two cell types of the intima revealed by their reaction with horseradish peroxidase and iron saccharate in the mouse. *Biol Cell* **42**: 147–52.
120. Linck G and Porte A (1981) B-cells of the synovial membrane. III. Relationship with specific collagenous structure of the intimal interstitium in the mouse. *Cell Tissue Res* **218**: 117–21.
121. Wysocki G P and Brinkhous K M (1972) Scanning electron microscopy of synovial membranes. *Arch Pathol* **93**: 172–7.
122. Davies D V and Edwards D A W (1948) The blood supply of the synovial membrane and intra-articular structures. *Ann R Coll Surg Engl* **2**: 142–56.
123. Hamanshi C (1978) Ultrastructural basis of blood-synovial barrier – results with five

electron-opaque tracers. *Arch Jpn Chir* **47**: 259–79.
124. Highton T C, Myers D B and Rayns D G (1968) The intercellular spaces of synovial tissue. *N Z Med J* **67**: 315–25.
125. Castor C W, Roberts D J, Hossler P A and Bignall M C (1983) Connective tissue activation. XXV. Regulation of proteoglycan synthesis in human synovial cells. *Arthritis Rheum* **26**: 522–7.
126. Hamerman D and Ruskin J (1959) Histological studies on human synovial membranes. Metachromatic staining and the effects of streptococcal hyaluronidase. *Arthritis Rheum* **2**: 546–52.
127. Okada Y, Nakanishi I and Kajikawa K (1981) Ultrastructure of the mouse synovial membrane: development and organisation of the extracellular matrix. *Arthritis Rheum* **24**: 835–43.
128. Clemmensen I, Holund B and Andersen R B (1983) Fibrin and fibronectin in rheumatoid synovial membrane and rheumatoid synovial fluid. *Arthritis Rheum* **26**: 479–85.
129. Linck G, Stocker S, Grimauld J A and Porte A (1983) Distribution of immunoreactive fibronectin and collagen (type I, III, IV) in mouse joints. *Histochemistry* **77**: 323–8.
130. Eyre D R and Muir H (1975) Type III collagen: a major constituent of rheumatoid and normal human synovial membrane. *Connect Tissue Res* **4**: 11–6.
131. Weiss J B, Shuttleworth C A, Brown R and Hunter J A A (1975) Polymeric type-III collagen in inflammed human synovia. *Lancet* **2**: 85–7.
132. Casley-Smith J R and Vincent A H (1978) The quantitative morphology of interstitial tissue channels in some tissues of the rat and rabbit. *Tissue Cell* **10**: 571–84.
133. Aukland K and Nicolaysen G (1981) Interstitial fluid volume: local regulatory mechanisms. *Physiol Rev* **61**: 556–643.
134. Brown R A, Tomlinson I W, Hill C R, Weiss J B, Phillips P and Kumar S (1983) Relationship of angiogenesis factor in synovial fluid to various joint diseases. *Ann Rheum Dis* **42**: 301–7.
135. Davidson J M, Klagsbrun M, Hill K E, Buckley A, Sullivan A, Brewer P S and Woodward S C (1985) Accelerated wound repair, cell proliferation and collagen accumulation are produced by a cartilage-derived growth factor. *J Cell Biol* **100**: 1219–27.
136. Semble E L, Turner R A and McCrickard E L (1985) Rheumatoid arthritis and osteoarthritis synovial fluid effects on primary endothelial cell cultures. *J Rheumatol* **12**: 237–41.
137. Levick J R (1984) An analysis of the effect of synovial capillary distribution upon trans-synovial concentration profiles and exchange. *Q J Exp Physiol* **69**: 289–300.
138. Nishijima T and Yamamoto T (1978) Ultrastructure of the synovial membrane. *J Electron Microsc (Tokyo)* **27**: 72.
139. Schumacher H R (1969) The microvasculature of the synovial membrane of the monkey; ultrastructural studies. *Arthritis Rheum* **12**: 387–404.
140. Suter E R and Majno G (1964) Ultrastructure of the joint capsule in the rat: presence of two kinds of capillaries. *Nature* **202**: 920.
141. Levick J R and Smaje L H (1987) An analysis of the permeability of a fenestra. *Microvasc Res* (In press.)
142. Crone C and Levitt D G (1984) Capillary permeability to small solutes. *In: Handbook of Physiology, Cardiovascular System IV, The Microcirculation.* (EM Renkin and C C Michel, eds), pp. 411–66. Bethesda: Amer Physiol Soc.
143. Renkin E M and Curry F E (1978) Transport of water and solutes across capillary endothelium. *In: Membrane Transport in Biology.* (G Giebisch, D C Tosteson and H H Ussing, eds), pp. 1–45. Berlin: Springer-Verlag.
144. Simionescu M and Simionescu N (1984) Ultrastructure of the microvascular wall: functional correlations. *In: Handbook of Physiology, Cardiovascular System IV, The Microcirculation* (E M Renkin and C C Michel, eds), pp. 41–102. Bethesda: Amer Physiol Soc.
145. Mitnick H, Hoffstein S and Weissman G (1978) Fate of antigen after intravenous and intra-articular injection into rabbits. *Arthritis Rheum* **21**: 918–28.
146. Bignold L P and Lykke A W J (1975) Increased vascular permeability induced in synovialis of the rat by histamine, serotonin and bradykinin. *Experientia* **31**: 671–2.
147. Graham R C and Griffin R (1972) Arthus synovitis with horseradish peroxidase as antigen: sequential participation of platelets and leucocytes. *Br J Exp Path* **53**: 578–85.
148. Schumacher H R (1973) Fate of particulate material arriving at the synovium via the circulation. An ultrastructural study. *Ann Rheum Dis* **32**: 212–8.
149. Chamberlain M A, Petts V and Gollins E (1972) Transport of intravenously-injected ferritin across the guinea-pig synovium. *Ann Rheum Dis* **31**: 493–9.
150. Davies D V (1946) The lymphatics of the synovial membrane. *J Anat* **80**: 21–3.
151. Liew M and Dick W C (1981) The anatomy and physiology of blood flow in a diarthrodial joint.

Clin Rheum Dis **7**: 131–48.

152. Kety S S (1949) Measurement of regional circulation by the local clearance of radioactive sodium. *Am Heart J* **38**: 321–8.

153. Dick W C, St. Onge R A, Gillespie F C, Downie W W, Nuke G, Gordon I, Whaley K, Boyle J A and Buchanan W W (1970) Derivation of knee joint synovial perfusion using the xenon (^{133}Xe) clearance technique. *Ann Rheum Dis* **29**: 131–4.

154. Harris R and Millard J B (1956) Clearance of radioactive sodium from the knee joint. *Clin Sci* **15**: 9–15.

155. Harris R, Millard J B and Banerjee S K (1958) Radiosodium clearance from the knee joint in rheumatoid arthritis. *Ann Rheum Dis* **17**: 189–95.

156. Christensen S B, Reimann I, Henriksen O and Arnoldi C C (1982) Experimental osteoarthritis in the rabbit. A study of ^{133}Xenon washout rates from the synovial cavity. *Acta Orthop Scand* **53**: 167–74.

157. Simkin P A, Huang A and Benedict R S (1986) Exercise induces bidirectional changes in blood flow to canine articular tissues. *Scand J Rheum [Suppl]* **60**: A133.

158. Simkin P A (1979) Synovial physiology. In: *Arthritis and Allied Conditions* (D J McCartey, ed), pp. 167–78. Philadelphia: Lea & Febiger.

159. Cobbold A F and Lewis O J (1956) The nervous control of joint blood vessels. *J Physiol* **133**: 467–71.

160. Moncada S and Custodio R (1976) Prostaglandins and blood flow in the dog's knee joint. *Adv Prostaglandin Thromboxane Res* **2**: 825–8.

161. Michel C C (1984) Fluid movements through capillary walls. In: *Handbook of Physiology, Cardiovascular System IV, The Microcirculation 1.* (E M Renkin and C C Michel, eds), pp. 375–409. Bethesda: Amer Physiol Soc.

162. Knight A D and Levick J R (1985) Effect of fluid pressure on the hydraulic conductance of interstitium and fenestrated endothelium in the rabbit knee. *J Physiol* **360**: 311–32.

163. Levick J R (1980) Contributions of the lymphatic and microvascular systems to fluid absorption from the synovial cavity of the rabbit knee. *J Physiol* **306**: 445–61.

164. Knight A D and Levick J R (1984) Osmotic flows and albumin reflection coefficients across the endothelium-synovium layer in rabbit knees. *J Physiol* **351**: 47P.

165. Edlund T (1949) Studies on the absorption of colloids and fluid from rabbit knee joints. *Acta Physiol Scand [Suppl]* **18** (62): 1–108.

166. Levick J R and Knight A D (1985) Comparison of osmotic effects of large and small solutes across the blood-joint barrier. *Int J Microcirc Clin Exp* **4**: 196P.

167. Levick J R and Knight A D (1984) Osmotic flow and variable conductance across the combined interstitium-endothelium layer in rabbit knees. *Int J Microcirc Clin Exp* **3**: 512P.

168. McMaster P D (1941) An enquiry into the structural conditions affecting fluid transport in the interstitial tissue of the skin. *J Exp Med* **74**: 9–28.

169. Edlund T and Linderholm H (1952) The resistance to flow of fluid through synovial membranes in hydrops of cardiac origin. The lack of influence of mersalyl. *Acta Physiol Scand* **26**: 148–55.

170. Landis E M and Pappenheimer J R (1963) Exchange of substances through capillary walls. In: *Handbook of Physiology. Circulation*, Sect 2, Vol II (W F Hamilton, ed) pp. 961–1034. Washington DC: Am Physiol Soc.

171. Maroudas A (1980) Physical chemistry of articular cartilage and the intervertebral disc. In: *The Joints and Synovial Fluid*,Vol 2 (L Sokoloff, ed), pp. 239–91. New York: Academic Press.

172. Fatt I (1978) *Physiology of the Eye: an Introduction to the Vegetative Functions*. Boston: Butterworths.

173. Newbould P J (1983) *Some aspects of the physiology of the canine knee joint*. Ph.D. Thesis, University of Western Australia.

174. Antonas K N, Fraser J R E and Muirden K D (1973) Distribution of biologically labelled radioactive hyaluronic acid injected into joints. *Ann Rheum Dis* **32**: 103–11.

175. Levick J R and Michel C C (1978) The effects of position and skin temperature on the capillary pressures in the fingers and toes. *J Physiol* **274**: 97–109.

176. Moyses C and Michel C C (1984) Fluid balance between blood and tissues in the feet. *Int J Microcirc Clin Exp* **3**: 172.

177. Wallis W J and Simkin P A (1984) Starling forces in synovial effusions: clinical correlations. *Arthritis Rheum* **27**: 534.

178. Smith M and Campbell J R (1928) Observations on the lymphatic drainage of joint cavities. *Proc Soc Exp Biol Med* **26**: 395–7.

179. Brantigan O C and Voshell A F (1941) The mechanics of the ligaments and menisci of the knee. *J Bone Joint Surg* **23**: 44–66.

180. Favreau J C and Laurin C A (1963) Joint effusions and flexion deformities. *Can Med Assoc J* **88**: 575–6.
181. Barnett C H, Davies D V and MacConail M A (1961) *Synovial Joints – their Structure and Mechanics*. New York: Longmans.
182. Menschik A (1976) Die synoviapumpe des Kniegelenkes. *Z Orthop* **114**: 89–94.
183. Reeves B (1966) Negative pressures in knee joints. *Nature* **212**: 1046.
184. Wiener-Kronish J P, Gropper M A and Lai-Fook S J (1985) Pleural liquid pressure in dogs measured using a rib capsule. *J Appl Physiol* **59**: 597–602.
185. Gumpel J M, Williams E D and Glass H I (1973) Use of Yttrium 90 in persistent synovitis of the knee. I. Retention in the knee and spread in the body after injection. *Ann Rheum Dis* **32**: 223–7.
186. O'Driscoll S W, Kumar K and Salter R B (1983) The effect of continuous passive motion on the clearance of a hemarthrosis from the joint and synovium of the rabbit knee. *Clin Orthop* **176**: 305–11.
187. Salter R B, Simmonds D F, Malcolm B W, Rumble E J, MacMichael D and Clements N D (1980) The biological effect of continuous passive motion on the healing of full-thickness defects in articular cartilage. *J Bone Joint Surg [Am]* **62**: 1232–51.
188. Ekholm R and Norback B (1951) On the relationship between articular changes and function. *Acta Orthop Scand* **21**: 81–98.
189. Horvath S M and Hollander L (1949) Intra-articular temperature as a measure of joint reaction. *J Clin Invest* **28**: 469–73.
190. Rhinelander F W, Bennett G A and Bauer W (1939) Exchange of substances in aqueous solution between joints and the vascular system. *J Clin Invest* **18**: 1–13.
191. Ekholm R (1951) Articular cartilage nutrition. How radioactive gold reaches the cartilage in rabbit knee joints. *Acta Anat [Suppl 11]* **15**: 1–76.
192. Lindström J (1963) Microvascular anatomy of synovial tissue. *Acta Rheum Scand [Suppl]* **7**: 1–82.
193. Finsterbush A and Friedman B (1973) Early changes in immobilised rabbit knee joints. A light and electron microscopic study. *Clin Orthop* **92**: 305–19.

Chapter 8

The Intervertebral Disc: Factors Contributing to its Nutrition and Matrix Turnover

S. H. Holm and J. P. G. Urban

CONTENTS

INTRODUCTION

Low back pain is one of most common medical problems of today. About 90% of the population are likely to have at least one severe episode at some time during their lives and about 7% of these will be off work for 3 months or more. Apart from the direct drain on medical resources, the economic costs of low back pain are high. Costs of treatment and compensation are estimated as 14 billion dollars a year in the United States of America and this does not take account of the economic costs of days lost from work (1, 2, 3, 4).

A high proportion of the cases of low back pain are idiopathic, i.e. no specific lesion can be identified as being responsible for the problem. Even where a definite diagnosis has been established, the aetiology of the disorder is generally unknown, and the method of treatment is not agreed. For instance, the number of laminectomies for low back pain and sciatica is 8 times higher in the United States of America than in Great Britain (3) but the results after 4 years are no better for patients who were operated upon than those who were treated conservatively.

Much of low back pain arises from the intervertebral disc, either directly through disc herniation or indirectly because degenerate discs throw undue stresses on other spinal structures. Disc failure has usually been thought to arise from some mechanical insult to the spine. Thus there is an extensive body of work describing the mechanical properties of the disc and of the spinal segment (6, 7). Less work has been done on the biology of the disc, although it is now becoming clear that the health of the disc depends on the well-being of the cells which renew and maintain the matrix of the disc itself. Recent work suggests that the cells respond to the mechanical stresses on the disc, and in this chapter we will review present knowledge in this field. We will also review the structure and chemistry of the disc in relation to its function, and attempt to relate how changes in the disc matrix affect its behaviour.

THE STRUCTURE OF THE DISC

The intervertebral discs occupy about one third of the spine. Since they provide the spinal column with its flexibility and act as shock absorbers between the vertebrae, their behaviour has a great impact on the mechanics of the whole spine (7).

The intervertebral disc may be considered as consisting of two separate regions, the inner soft pulpy nucleus pulposus and the outer firm annulus fibrosus. The cartilaginous endplates which are interposed between the discs and the bony vertebral bodies are generally not considered to be part of the discs themselves (*Fig.* 8.1). The nucleus pulposus occupies about 30–50% of the disc volume. The nucleus in young humans and in most animal discs is highly hydrated, soft and translucent. It is surrounded by the firmer, less hydrated, annulus fibrosus. When the human disc matures, the hydration of the nucleus drops markedly, the nucleus loses its translucency and becomes firmer and the boundary between the nucleus and the annulus becomes difficult to distinguish. Similar changes are seen in some animals such as chondrodrystrophoid dogs (8), but in other animals the discs remain translucent throughout life (9, 10). The most noticeable feature of the annulus is the series of concentric lamellae which are visible to the naked eye when the disc is sectioned horizontally. The lamellae consist of bundles of collagen fibres which run obliquely between the adjacent vertebral bodies and are firmly anchored to them or the cartilaginous endplate. The resulting angle formed between the fibre bundles of the lamellae and the vertebral bodies varies between 40° and 70°, the direction of the fibres alternating in each neighbouring lamella (11, 12, 13, 14).

The human disc degenerates early; by the age of 30 years clefts and fissures are already visible in the annulus. There are also chemical changes and a loss of disc height can be seen in X-ray pictures. It is not clear, however, whether these changes may be regarded as part of a normal ageing process or whether they are degenerative (*Fig* 8.2) (15, 16).

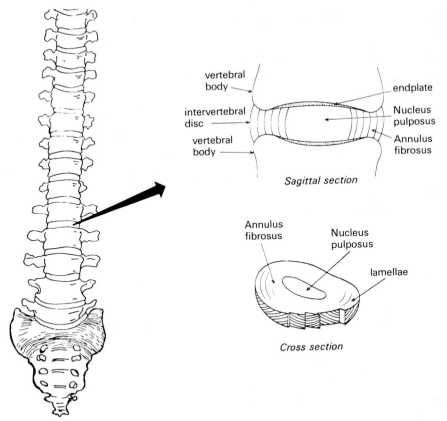

Fig. 8.1. A schematic view of the spine and the different regions in the intervertebral disc. Included also is the arrangement of the annulus lamellae, showing alternating directions of collagen bundles. [From Schultz, 1974 (110), with permission.]

CHEMICAL COMPOSITION OF THE DISC

The chemical composition of the intervertebral disc has been reviewed in detail (17, 18). The major structural macromolecules in the disc are collagen and proteoglycans. Other glycoproteins, elastin, and some serum proteins have all been reported in minor quantities. However, the disc acts mechanically as a concentrated proteoglycan solution held within a collagen network.

Proteoglycans

Proteoglycans are a family of macromolecules consisting of glycosaminoglycan chains bound to a central protein core to form a brush-like structure (Fig. 8.3). These proteoglycan monomers are large polydisperse molecules with a molecular weight of 50 000 to several million. The major glycoasaminoglycans (GAGs) in the disc are chondroitin (CS) and keratan (KS)

a

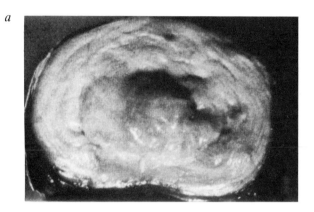

b

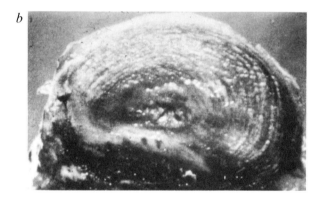

c

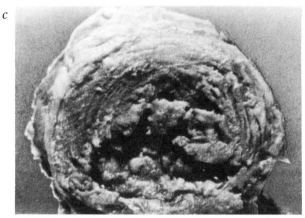

Fig. 8.2. Photographs of the intervertebral disc showing (*a*) a normal disc with translucent nucleus pulposus and collagen arrangement in the lamellae of outer annulus. As the disc becomes adult (*b*) the central nucleus area will be more fibrous and collagen fibres coarser. In the old disc (*c*) there are signs of degeneration.

sulphate. These glycosaminoglycans occupy different regions of the protein core. The keratan sulphate-rich region lies towards one end of the core, and beyond it the core ends in two globular regions, one of which is the hyaluronic acid-binding region, so called because a proportion of the proteoglycan monomers are attached to long chains of hyaluronic acid to form proteoglycan aggregates. The aggregates are stabilized by link protein. It has been suggested that aggregation helps to keep proteoglycans in tissue, but the function of aggregation is not yet understood. A recent review of proteoglycan structure is provided by Heinegård and Paulsson, 1984 (19).

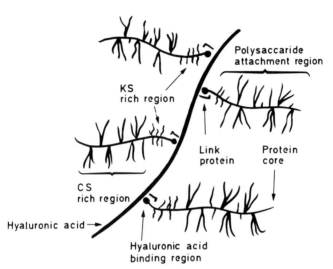

Fig. 8.3. Schematic model of the proteoglycan monomer and aggregate. [From Urban and Maroudas 1980 (56), with permission.]

The proteoglycans of the intervertebral disc are smaller than those found in most other cartilages and are richer in keratan sulphate (17, 18, 20, 22, 23, 24, 25). A large fraction of disc proteoglycans are not able to aggregate; this fraction increases with age. It has been suggested that this loss of aggregation results from enzymatic removal of the hyaluronic acid-binding region of the core protein (20, 26, 27). Enzymatic attack on the disc proteoglycans could account for their small size and polydispersity, since it is interesting to note that newly synthesized proteoglycans are much larger than those which are resident in the tissue; the majority can aggregate in the presence of hyaluronic acid and contain a much higher proportion of chondroitin sulphate. The newly synthesized proteoglycans of the disc are therefore very similar to those synthesized in other cartilages. These studies suggest that the major population of the resident small non-aggregated proteoglycans of the disc do not arise through synthesis of a separate small proteoglycan population (26, 28).

In disc degeneration there is extensive loss of proteoglycans, particularly of the small species, and thus the remaining proteoglycans are larger. Also a greater proportion is able to aggregate than in normal age-matched discs. Since these proteoglycans are more representative of those found in young discs, several authors (8, 26, 27) suggest that the change in proteoglycan structure results from faster turnover of proteoglycans as an attempt at tissue repair. However, the same tissue composition would result if the small proteoglycan population escaped from degenerate discs, leaving only the larger and aggregated population behind. So the mechanism for change in composition of these discs is still not known.

Fixed charge density

Both chondroitin sulphate and keratan sulphate contain charged acidic groups (SO_3^{2-} and $COOH^-$) which impart a fixed negative charge to the matrix. From the structural formulae of these molecules it can be seen that chondroitin sulphate has two charges per disaccharide, whereas keratan sulphate has only one (*Fig.* 8.4). The concentration of fixed negative charges, the fixed charge density (FCD), thus does not only depend on the concentration of proteoglycan in the tissue, but also on the chondroitin sulphate–keratan sulphate ratio. The fixed charge density confers important properties on the disc, as it controls the distribution of the charged solutes and hence osmotic pressure, as will be discussed later (*Fig* 8.5).

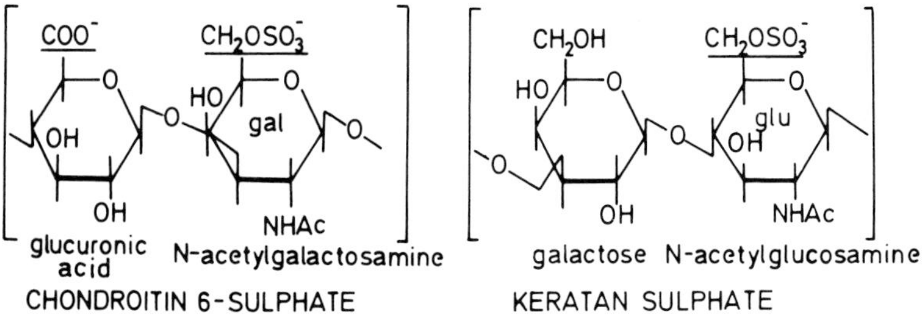

Fig. 8.4. Structural formulae of chondroitin sulphate and keratan sulphate, showing the sites of the charged groups.

Collagen

The disc contains two major collagen types. The fine fibrils of the nucleus are virtually all Type II collagen, whereas the outer annulus is predominantly Type I collagen. The proportion of Type I collagen in the annulus decreases towards the nucleus as the proportion of Type II collagen rises (18, 29). It is not known whether the fibrils of the disc are of mixed collagen types or whether each collagen type forms its own fibril. Chemical evidence from staining with specific antibodies suggests the latter (17). Minor collagens, particularly Types V, VI and IX have been found in significant quanitites in the calf disc (31).

The organization of collagen fibrils in the disc is highly specialized. The three-dimensional collagen framework has been described and illustrated by scanning electron micrographs by Inoue and Takeda, 1975 (12). In the annulus, collagen is arranged in 15–20 concentric lamellae made of parallel bundles

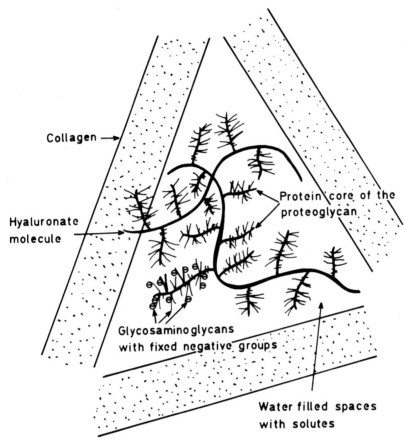

Collagen →

Hyaluronate
molecule

Protein core of the
proteoglycan

Glycosaminoglycans
with fixed negative groups

Water filled spaces
with solutes

Fig. 8.5. Diagram of the network structure of the proteoglycan–water matrix between the collagen fibres.

10–50 μm in size. Each bundle is composed of fine fibrils 0·1–0·2 μm in diameter. These lamellae are visible to the naked eye and vary from 200 to 400 μm in width, the outer lamellae being thickest. The lamellae in the posterior part of the disc are not as wide as those in the rest of the disc.

The fibre bundles of each lamella run obliquely between the adjacent vertebral bodies and are firmly anchored to them or to the cartilaginous endplate. The resulting angle formed between the fibre bundles of the lamellae and the vertebral body varies between 40° and 70°, the direction of the fibres alternating in the neighbouring lamellae (*Fig.* 8.6). Happey (1980) has described how the angle changes with position in the annulus (11).

In the nucleus the collagen fibres are much finer than in the annulus, mostly about 20–50 nm in diameter, and are arranged in a loose irregular meshwork. The nucleus fibrils are not connected to the cartilaginous endplate, however; at the boundary with the annulus these fibrils merge with those of the inner concentric lamellae.

The arrangement of the collagen network in the disc has an important influence on how load is distributed. The fibre bundles of the adjacent lamellae are only loosely interconnected. Even though collagen is only slightly extensible, the fact that the lamellae can move separately gives the structure itself considerable extensibility, especially in the vertical direction. The annulus is thus able to move and bulge outwards under the pressure evenly applied to it by the gel-like nucleus, or increase in height during extension by changing the crossing angle of its fibres (5, 12, 14, 32, 33, 34, 35, 36, 37).

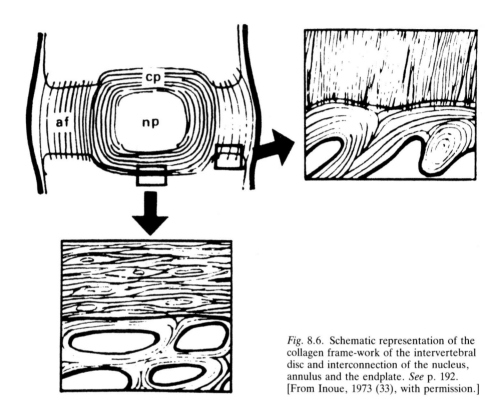

Fig. 8.6. Schematic representation of the collagen frame-work of the intervertebral disc and interconnection of the nucleus, annulus and the endplate. *See* p. 192. [From Inoue, 1973 (33), with permission.]

Water

Water is the major constituent of the disc; 90% of the young nucleus is water. Although the water content decreases with age, water is still a major constituent of the old and degenerated disc. The water content of the disc is not constant but varies with applied load, as will be discussed later (38).

Because of the low cell content the majority of this water is extracellular and is associated with the collagen and proteoglycans. About 0·8–1·4 g water/g dry collagen is associated with the collagen. Thus a significant proportion of the water in aged or degenerate discs with low proteoglycan content may be intrafibrillar (39). The intrafibrillar fraction of water is freely exchangeable, but is not available to the proteoglycans and other large macromolecules which are sterically excluded from within the collagen fibrils.

Other Tissue Components

A considerable proportion of non-collagenous proteins has been reported in the disc (8, 11). These proteins have not been characterized. Glycoproteins whose biological function is unknown have been found, as well as some serum proteins, particularly in aged and degenerated discs. A part of this fraction probably consists of proteoglycan core protein and minor collagens.

Composition of the Extracellular Matrix

In any disc the proportion of the three main components, i.e. collagen, proteoglycans and water, vary with position. Concentrations of proteoglycans and water are highest in the nucleus and fall to low values in the outer annulus. The reverse profiles are shown for collagen.

The disc composition changes with age and with spinal level (20). The concentration of proteoglycans is highest in the nucleus and falls to lower values in the outer annulus. The reversed profile occurs for the collagen. There is a corresponding fall in water content (*Fig 8.7*).

FUNCTION OF TISSUE COMPONENTS

Proteoglycans

The mechanical properties of the intervertebral disc depend to a large extent on the tissue's hydration (40, 41). It is the proteoglycans which are responsible for the maintenance of disc hydration under the high external loads placed upon it; both osmotic pressure and resistance of tissue to fluid loss under pressure are controlled by proteoglycans.

We will review briefly the effect of proteoglycan content on these properties and discuss how proteoglycan content influences the rate of fluid loss from the disc.

Proteoglycan osmotic pressure

The high osmotic pressure of proteoglycan solution results from 2 factors. Firstly, the proteoglycans themselves are polyelectrolytes, i.e. there are fixed negative charges on the glycosaminoglycans; hence the tissue acts as an 'ion-exchanger' and its ion content is high compared to that of the surrounding plasma. Ions distribute themselves between the plasma and the disc in order to maintain electrochemical equilibrium for all species. At the fixed-charge density found in the disc, there is no evidence of ion binding, and the Gibbs–Donnan equilibrium appears to describe ion partitions between the disc and plasma (42, 43, 44, 45, 46). For NaCl the equations are:

$$\bar{m}_{Na^+} = FCD + \bar{m}_{Cl^-} \qquad (Eqn.\ 8.1)$$

$$\bar{m}_{Na^+} = \frac{FCD + (FCD^2 + 4m^2\ (\gamma/z)^2)^{1/2}}{2} \qquad (Eqn.\ 8.2)$$

where $\overline{m}_{Na}^{+}$ and $\overline{m}_{Cl}^{-}$ are the molal concentrations of sodium and chloride in the tissue and γ/z is the ratio of external to internal mean ionic activity coefficient of sodium chloride; the FCD is the molal fixed-charge density of the tissue. m is the molal concentration of m_{NaCl} in the plasma. These equations show that because of the net negative charge on the disc, the total number of ions in the tissue is always greater than in the plasma; since the osmotic pressure results from a difference in the number of dissolved particles between the two phases, the excess number of ions in the tissue leads to the high osmotic pressure of the disc. The second factor which contributes to the osmotic pressure of the

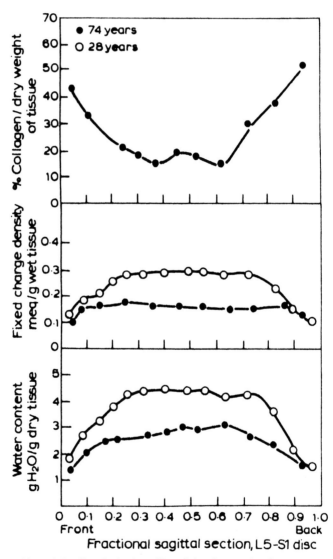

Fig. 8.7. Composition of the disc. Sagittal profiles of the glycosaminoglycan content expressed as fixed-charge density and water content in 28 and 74 year old discs and % collagen/dry weight in 74 year old disc. [From Urban, 1977 (64), with permission.]

disc depends on the excluded volume contributions of the macromolecular segments and hence on the size and shape of the proteoglycans. In cartilaginous tissues this factor is insignificant compared to that from the Donnan ionic contribution; it is thus not surprising that proteoglycan size or degree of aggregation has little influence on osmotic pressure compared with the charge density (42, 47, 48).

The variation of disc osmotic pressure with fixed charge density is shown in *Fig.* 8.8. The osmotic pressure depends on charge concentration rather than on proteoglycan size or degree of aggregation. This curve will describe the osmotic pressure of most discs, whether the discs are degenerated or normal. It can be seen that osmotic pressure increases steeply as the fixed charge density increases. In the nucleus of the adult disc the fixed charge density lies between 0·2 and 0·4 mEq/ml, depending on age. The osmotic pressure expressed by the proteoglycans of these discs is consequently 0·1–0·3 MPa (1–3 atm). The

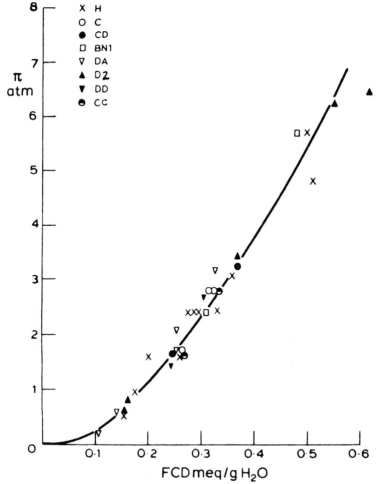

Fig. 8.8. Osmotic pressure of proteoglycans extracted from various cartilaginous tissues. [From Urban *et al.*, 1979 (47), with permission.]

fixed-charge density of the annulus, and hence its osmotic pressure, is somewhat lower but is still considerable in comparison with that of non-weight-bearing tissues. It should be noted that the values of fixed-charge density quoted here have been obtained from cadaveric discs, i.e. from discs under no external load. Discs which are loaded are considerably less hydrated than these and hence will have a higher fixed-charge density and a higher osmotic pressure.

Hydraulic permeability

In the schematic view of the disc matrix shown in *Fig.* 8.5, the matrix can be seen to consist of densely packed proteoglycans between the collagen fibrils. Because of the dense packing there is much overlap and interweaving of the glycosaminoglycan chains. The distance between the glycosaminoglycan chains is on the average only 2–4 nm, although in such a random network some of the spacings will be considerably greater than this (50). The chains effectively divide the matrix into small pores; the higher the glycosaminoglycan concentration, the more closely packed are the entangled glycosaminoglycan chains and the smaller the effective pore size. Since the collagen fibres are spaced at 30–50 nm, the fine pore structure of the matrix is thus determined by proteoglycan concentration rather than by the collagen network. The rate of which fluid can flow through the matrix is governed by the pore size and is described in terms of a hydraulic permeability coefficient. The larger the pores the higher the value of the hydraulic permeability coefficient and the faster the rate of the fluid flow.

Fluid flow in the disc

As in other interstitial tissues, bulk fluid flow in the disc is largely passive. Fluid flow can be described by Darcy's law which, for flow through an element in one direction, is given by:

$$J = - k \frac{dp}{dx}$$ (*Eqn.* 8.3)

where J is the rate of fluid flux, k is the hydraulic permeability coefficient, dp is the driving force for fluid flow and is given by $(p - \pi)$, i.e. the difference between the hydrostatic and osmotic pressure differences given by Starling's law (42), and x is the distance. To describe fluid flow between the disc and its surroundings, and the flow pattern within the disc, this equation has to be integrated over the whole disc. No solution as yet exists, so we will describe qualitatively which factors influence fluid flow in the disc. When the disc is at equilibrium and there is no fluid flow, from *Eqn.* 8.3 J = 0 and $p = \pi$. However, the intervertebral disc is under constantly changing external loads which result from changes in posture and activity. These changes in load disturb the balance between the pore pressure p and the osmotic pressure π and hence result in fluid flow. Since osmotic pressure is related to proteoglycan content and so its hydraulic permeability coefficient, the rate of fluid flow is sensitive to proteoglycan content. In most humans, during the day's activities the loads are higher than at night during rest (6, 51). Thus there is a net outflow of fluid from the disc during the day and a net influx of fluid during the night. The changes in fluid content are enough to cause a noticeable change in height of about 1–2 cm between morning and evening (52, 53). *In vitro* studies have estimated that on average the intervertebral disc, starting from a resting position, will lose about 12% of its fluid after 4 hours of loading to physiological daily levels. However, some degenerate discs can lose up to 25% of their fluid under these conditions (54). Changes in fluid content alone influence many properties of the disc. Its mechanical response to bending or compressive stress is affected by fluid content (35, 41). Creep or loss of disc height is related to fluid loss (35, 56). With the extent of fluid loss seen in degenerate discs, the loss in height may be sufficient to cause excessive loads on the apophyseal joints and explain the relationship seen between degenerate discs and osteoarthritis of the back facets (54, 57). Disc nutrition is also influenced by fluid content, since diffusivities and partitions are very dependent on proteoglycan concentration (66). Recent work *in vitro* has also shown that proteoglycan synthesis itself is influenced by the fluid content of the disc (59). Although we now have some understanding of the factors which influence fluid flow in the disc, the overall patterns of fluid flow, i.e. the directions which fluid flows and how it exchanges with external fluid, is not known. For instance, the change in the proteoglycan concentration in the annulus might determine whether most of the fluid from the disc flows through the annulus itself into the interstitium surrounding the periphery of the annulus, or else flows vertically from the disc through the nucleus into the vertebral bodies (60). Changes in the microcirculation around the disc can also drastically affect fluid flow patterns within the disc. These latter boundary conditions will of course be influenced by exercise.

Solute distributions and movement

As discussed above, the disc matrix can be thought of as a network of collagen fibres stuffed with proteoglycans and inflated by the water imbibed through the osmotic properties of the proteoglycans. The proteoglycans interpenetrate and divide the space between the collagen fibrils into small pores. The mean pore size depends on proteoglycan concentration. Not only does the pore size control the rate at which water can flow through the disc, as discussed above, but pore size also controls the distribution of large solutes in a tissue. Small solutes, such as urea or simple ions, can fit into virtually all the pores of the tissue. As the molecular size of solutes increases, the number of pores into which the solutes can fit decreases. Even glucose (200 molecular weight) is excluded from 10–15% of the pores in the dog nucleus pulposus. Large proteins, the size of serum albumin or above (60 000 molecular weight), are virtually excluded from the normal disc nucleus (49, 66). With loss of proteoglycan and increase in pore size, serum proteins may enter the disc in increasing concentrations; high concentrations of serum proteins have been reported in older discs (61, 62). The effect of this is not known.

Not only are the concentrations of large solutes determined by proteoglycan content but, through the Donnan equilibria, proteoglycan concentration (as expressed by the fixed-charge density) also determines the partitions of ions. Cations such as Na^+, Ca^{2+}, Mg^{2+}, and K^+ will have a higher concentration in the tissue than in the surrounding plasma, whereas that of anions such as Cl^- and SO_4^{2-} will be lower because they are excluded by the fixed negative charges (*Fig.* 8.9). Calcium content is of course important for both normal and pathological calcification and hence will be influenced by proteoglycan concentration. Inorganic ions, moreover, may regulate a number of cellular processes such as proteoglycan and collagen synthesis, and hence may provide a feedback mechanism for controlling the rate of matrix synthesis (63).

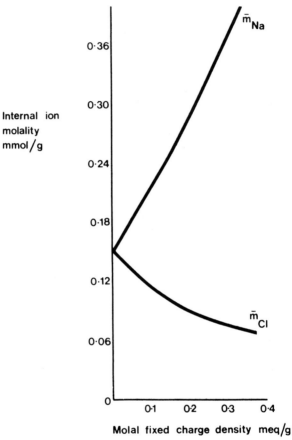

Fig. 8.9. Internal concentrations of Na⁺ and Cl⁻, vs. the molal fixed-charge density of disc and cartilage in equilibrium with 0·15 M NaCl solution. [From Urban and Maroudas, 1979 (46), with permission.]

Solute diffusivity is of course important for cellular nutrition and removal of metabolic waste products. Solute diffusivities have not been extensively studied in the intervertebral disc. However, the information that is available (49, 64) indicates that diffusivities in the disc are similar to those in articular cartilages of equivalent composition. In articular cartilage it has been shown that the diffusivity of most small solutes is approximately one third to one half of its value in free solution, and appears to depend on the tortuosity of its path rather than on matrix interactions, even for highly charged solutes such as calcium (43, 45,

65). For larger molecules such as serum albumin, the diffusion coefficient is affected by frictional considerations, but even here its value is as high as one quarter of its value in free solution (66). Hence the diffusion coefficient itself is not very sensitive to proteoglycan concentration.

Collagen

In this chapter we will not discuss the function of the collagen network in any great detail. However, it is obvious that the proteoglycans on their own would not form any coherent structure and would simply dissolve and disappear from the tissue. The strength and coherence of the intervertebral disc is provided by the specialized network of collagen fibrils. Proteoglycans are held within the tissue by the collagen fibrils, either through some specific interaction or else simply by entanglement. When the collagen network is damaged, proteoglycan loss is seen in both articular cartilage and in the intervertebral disc (67, 68). The collagen network is also essential for the mechanical functioning of the disc. Collagen is strong in tension, although it cannot withstand any compressive stress (37). When the disc is loaded the collagen fibres are placed under tension by the deformation of the disc, which bulges both radially and into the vertebral bodies (5, 34). Since collagen is barely extensible (3%) (69)) this bulge results only slightly from lengthening of the collagen fibres, but mostly from a rearrangement of the collagen network (32, 34). When the disc is subjected to torsional or shear stresses rather than straight compressive stresses, the disc deforms because the lamellae are only loosely interconnected and are able to slip past one another. Therefore, in torsion for instance, the lamellae in one direction will be slack whereas those in the alternate orientation will be placed under tension (32). The ability of the disc to act as a joint, and therefore the flexibility of the whole spine, is thus dependent on the arrangement of the collagen network. Collagen network orientation is maintained through disc hydration and hence by the proteoglycans. Loss of proteoglycan and hence of disc turgor can lead to the disarray of the collagen network seen in degenerate discs (70), and may even lead to coalescence of the fibrils.

DISC NUTRITION AND MATRIX TURNOVER

Nutrition of the Intervertebral Disc

The mechanical functioning of the intervertebral disc depends on the integrity of the disc's matrix. Until now we have discussed briefly how the material properties of the tissue relate to its function. We should not forget, however, that the matrix is produced and maintained by the cells of the disc and thus the health of the tissue depends to a large extent on the viability of these cells. Their continuing activity must depend on an adequate supply of nutrients and an efficient removal of metabolic waste products. In the remaining part of this chapter we will discuss factors associated with disc cells, their nutrition and matrix turnover.

Disc cells

The cells of the annulus, like those of other cartilaginous tissues, are thought to arise from the mesenchyme. However, those of the nucleus come from the notochord. In humans the notochordal cells have disappeared by late childhood (58), but in some animals these notochordal cells of the nucleus persist into adulthood. The cells of the adult disc may be considered as chondrocytes or chondrocyte-like cells; some authors judge the cells of the outer annulus to be more like fibrocytes (71, 72). The cells in the nucleus are rounded whereas in outer annulus they are more cigar shaped (71).

The cell density in the intervertebral disc is relatively low, as shown in *Table* 8.1. It is very uniform across the disc, except towards the disc margins and in the outer annulus. In the nucleus the normal value is $4–6\cdot000$ cells/mm^3 for the human disc and $8–14\cdot000$ cells/mm^3 for the adult canine disc (*Fig.* 8.10). Profiles of the cell density across human discs can hence be seen in *Fig.* 8.11 (71).

Table 8.1 A summary of oxygen consumption rates and cell densities for some avascular structures reported in the literature (cell density figures within brackets do not correspond to the references given in this paper). Two vascular tissues are included in the table for comparison reasons. [From Holm *et al.*, 1981 (9), with permission.]

Tissue	Oxygen uptake (μmol/g/h)	Cell density (cells/mm^3)	Reference
Cartilage			
Rat	8·93–2·95	250 ($\times 10^3$)	111
Rabbit	4·46	(250)	111
Rabbit	2·01	128	82
Rabbit	2·14–0·89	250	83
Dog	0·59	39·5	9
Bovine young	1·16	133	85
Bovine adult	0·31	47·2	85
Bovine old	0·11	34·0	85
Stroma			
Rabbit	3·08	(500)	112
Rabbit	2·81	(500)	113
Human	1·77	(500)	114
Human	3·79	(500)	115
Disc			
Annulus human	0·076	5·0	71
Nucleus human	0·063	4·3	71
Annulus dog	0·25	16·1	9
Nucleus dog	0·21	14·4	9
Liver			
Rabbit	344	620	82
Kidney			
Rabbit	482	1100	82

FACTORS INFLUENCING NUTRIENT CONCENTRATION IN THE DISC

Nutrition

The concentration of any solute or nutrient in the disc matrix will be influenced by a number of factors. For solutes which are not metabolized or only slowly metabolized relative to their rate of transport through the tissue, the

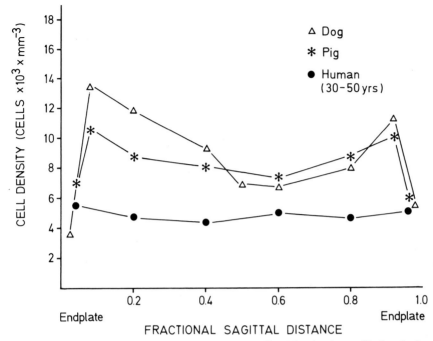

Fig. 8.10. Cell density profiles across the intervertebral disc. The density profile for the human disc is very flat, whereas for the animals the profiles tend to decrease very close to the vertebral endplate where a fluid layer is generally to be seen.

concentration will be determined purely by ionic and steric factors and the partition of the solute between disc and plasma will be at or close to its equilibrium value. For metabolites other considerations also arise. The first of these is the pattern of blood flow and architecture of the microcirculation around the tissue, since these determine the exchange area between the disc and the blood supply. The second consideration is the rate at which solutes are consumed or produced by the cells. The third consideration is the solute diffusivity and the influence of convective flow on transport of solutes through the matrix. We will discuss each of these in turn.

Exchange Area and Transport Routes

The adult human disc is avascular (16); therefore nutrients can only be supplied to these cells by transport of the necessary solutes through the matrix of the disc from the surrounding blood vessels. The existence of 2 nutritional routes into the disc was first demonstrated by Brodin, 1955 (73) and has been confirmed since then by other workers (9, 49, 64, 74, 75, 76, 77) (*Fig.* 8.12). These investigations have shown that the permeability in the peripheral part of the vertebral endplate is low, and that solute transport into the disc occurs mainly from the blood vessels surrounding the annulus, and also from the blood vessels which penetrate the calcified layer in the central region of the vertebral body and contact the

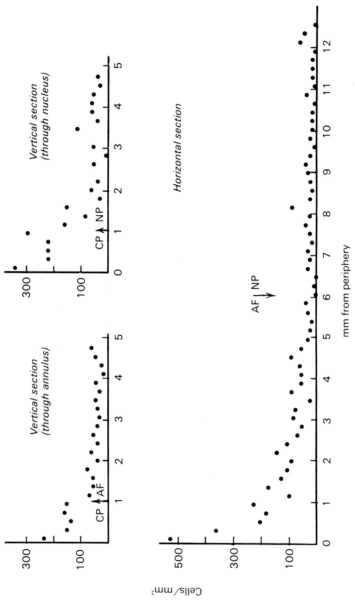

Fig. 8.11. Distribution of cells in the human intervertebral disc (18 years old). CP, cartilage endplate; AF, annulus fibrosus; NP, nucleus pulposus. Arrows indicate transitional zones. [From Maroudas *et al.* 1975 (71), with permission.]

cartilaginous endplate. There are indications that the permeability of the calcified layer decreases with age and degeneration (69, 75, 77) (*Fig.* 8.13). Blockage of this route might just be a factor which initiates or accelerates cell necrosis and hence disc degeneration.

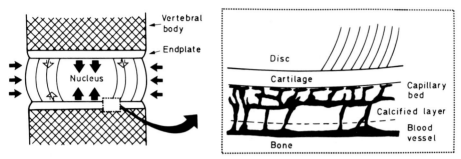

Fig. 8.12. Schematic diagram of the nutritional routes into the intervertebral disc and an enlarged view of the area underneath the hyaline cartilage. [From Holm *et al.*, 1981 (9), with permission.]

There have been some studies of the detailed arrangement of the vascular terminations in the region of the vertebral endplate. Holm (1981) visualized the contact between the blood vessels and the hyaline cartilage of the endplate by injecting a fluorescent dye into dogs before sacrifice and subsequently viewing serial sections under a fluorescent microscope (9). He showed that in the region of the nucleus the blood vessel contacts were extremely numerous and covered about 80% of the cartilage area. The contacts in the inner annulus were far less numerous and in the region of the outer annulus they virtually disappeared (*Fig.* 8.13). A similar study was performed on adult greyhounds by Crock and Goldwasser (1984) who used intra-arterial infusions of ink with barium sulphate to visualize the microvasculature (78). Their observations were similar to those of Holm, and they described the capillary terminations at the disc interface over the area of the nucleus pulposus as being like suckers on the tentacles of an octopus. They described the drainage of the capillary network in detail. Factors which decrease peripheral circulation, such as smoking and possibly vibration, have a dramatic influence on the concentration of rapidly utilized metabolites such as oxygen in the disc (79, 80). However, at present one can only speculate on the long-term effects of a decreased circulation around the disc.

Ogata *et al.* (1981) severed the blood vessel contacts in the vertebral endplate and found there was a rapid fall in concentration of tracer in the nucleus (75).

Transport of Nutrients through the Matrix

Solutes move through the disc mainly by diffusion through the matrix under gradients set up by consumption or by production of solutes by the disc's chondrocyte-like cells. The distances for diffusion are large. In adult human discs some cells may be as much as 6–8 mm from the blood supply, since a human lumbar disc is typically 10–17 mm thick and 30 mm across its shortest diameter.

a

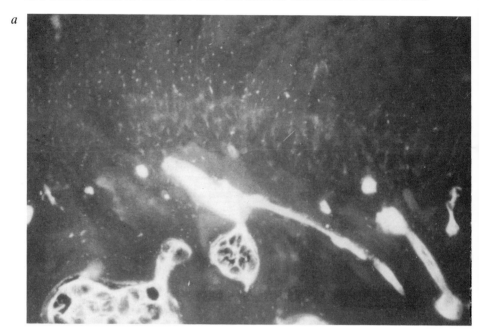

b

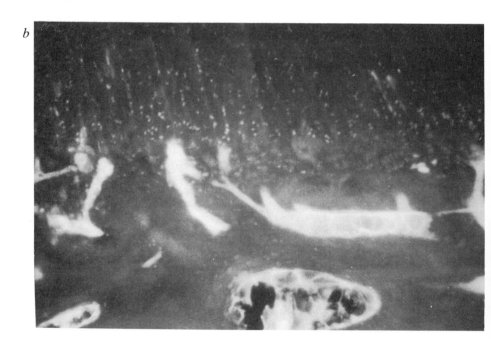

c

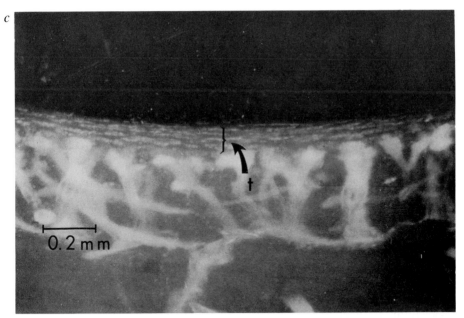

0.2 mm

Fig. 8.13. Photographs of the bone–disc interface in the region of outer annulus fibrosus (*a*), inner annulus fibrosus (*b*) and in the area of nucleus pulposus (*c*); t, hyaline cartilage thickness. Tetracycline was injected intravenously and the discs were excised. After a histological preparation disc slices were viewed in a fluorescence microscope.

It has been suggested that movement of fluid in and out of the disc, following changes of load, aids nutrition by enhancing the rate of transport of metabolites to and from the cells. However, no evidence for this has been found experimentally. Urban *et al.* (1982) examined the transport of radioactively labelled sulphate into the discs of 2 sets of labrador dogs *in vivo* (81). One set was anaesthetized between injection and death, while over the same period the other set exercised continuously. Both sets of dogs were killed at times between 1 and 6 hours after injection and the concentrations of tracer in their discs were examined. In both cases the sulphate tracer concentration profile was similar to that expected to arise from diffusion alone, and no significant difference could be seen between the 2 sets of dogs. If fluid flow was important for the transport of such a solute a difference should have been detectable, since the direction of fluid flow would be opposite in the 2 cases. The moving dogs would tend to pressurize their discs and thus to lose fluid. The dogs under anaesthesia would have low loads on their discs, and so their discs would tend to imbibe water. That diffusion is the major mechanism for the transport of nutrients into the discs is not surprising, since in humans the overall direction of fluid flow is out of the disc for about 16 h out of the 24, and it is difficult to envisage how the disc cells could rely on fluid transport to supply their basic nutrients. Calculations show that convective transport supplies not more than about 3% of the total glucose reaching the disc. However, since the distances for diffusion are large and the supply is at its limits in some regions of the disc, even this small fraction may be important for the long-term health of the disc.

Cell Metabolism

There is little information in the literature of the metabolic requirements of the cells of cartilaginous tissues. Work on articular cartilage reports 2 pathways, namely anaerobic catabolism and oxidative phosphorylation (9, 82, 83, 84, 85, 86). Holm *et al.* (1981) investigated oxygen consumption and lactic acid production in different regions of the canine disc (9). Oxygen concentration was measured in the disc using a polarographic, membrane-covered electrode. It consisted of a 5 μm platinum thread encased in a glass capillary. The reference electrode was a silver cylinder surrounding the glass capillary and leaving only the tip of it free. The electrode was incorporated into a stainless steel cannula, and hence the electrode could be introduced directly into the nucleus pulposus *in vivo*. This same electrode was used to study oxygen consumption rates by designing a cannula which enclosed a small amount of material from the nucleus pulposus around the tip of the electrode. This electrode was thus used to measure both oxygen consumptions and oxygen concentrations in the nucleus of canine discs. The intradiscal oxygen concentration was measured with the cannula in the opened position and a stable reading was usually obtained within 10 min. The probe chamber containing a known quantity of tissue was then closed. The rate of decay of oxygen concentration was recorded continuously until it fell to zero, and hence the rate of oxygen consumption by the nucleus tissue could be calculated.

The results obtained *in vivo* using the electrode were compared to those obtained *in vitro* by incubating nucleus, inner annulus and outer annulus strips in a Gilson differential respirometer (87). In this apparatus the variation of oxygen consumption rate could be followed at varying oxygen concentrations. Oxygen concentrations between 0·3% and 20·9% were tested; the low tensions correspond to those found *in vivo* in the central region of the disc, and the results at 20·9% could be compared with those quoted in the literature for other avascular tissues. Lactic acid production and carbon dioxide evolution were also measured *in vitro* at varying oxygen concentrations (9).

The variation of oxygen consumption with oxygen tension is shown in *Fig.* 8.14. When the results obtained in the Gilson respirometer were corrected for the swelling of the tissue the results obtained *in vivo* and the results obtained *in vitro* agreed well. This encouraging agreement implies that the results of *in vitro* tests on human discs are likely to represent the behaviour of the tissue *in vivo*. The mean value of the oxygen consumption rate in the nucleus pulposus ranged from 0·06 μmol/g wet weight/h at 1 mmHg oxygen tension to 0·16 μmol/g wet weight/h at 7 mmHg. At low oxygen tensions, i.e. oxygen tensions below 4 mmHg and the tensions therefore which are of interest *in vivo* in the intervertebral disc, the oxygen consumption rate is very dependent on oxygen concentration. However, above 4 mmHg the consumption rate becomes fairly independent of oxygen tension level. The results of *Fig.* 8.14 could be fitted by Michaelis–Menten type equation. When the results at high oxygen tensions were corrected for cell density the results compared well with those of other connective tissues.

The rates of carbon dioxide production and of lactic acid production measured *in vitro* are in agreement with the rates of oxygen consumption measured if the disc uses predominantly an anaerobic pathway for its energy requirements. However, even though only about 2% of the glucose used is oxidized to carbon

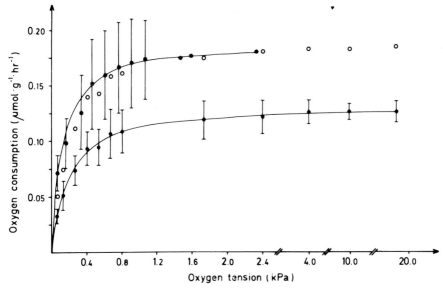

Fig. 8.14. Graphs of mean oxygen consumption *vs.* oxygen tension obtained using an oxygen electrode. The lower curve represents the raw *in vitro* results. The open circles show *in vitro* results corrected for swelling. The upper solid curve represents the *in vivo* results. [From Holm *et al.*, 1981 (9), with permission.]

dioxide, this pathway provides about 40% of the total energy produced. That is because per mol glucose, complete oxidation gives rise to 36 mol ATP, while anaerobic glycolysis produces only 2 mol ATP. Lactic acid production is also dependent on oxygen tension levels; it increases about 40% as the oxygen tension decreases from 70 to 7 mmHg. The canine nucleus pulposus has a particularly high rate of lactic acid production compared to other cartilaginous tissues. This rate becomes even more marked on a cell basis since the cell density of the intervertebral disc is extremely low. This high rate of lactic acid production could arise from the very low oxygen tensions in the centre of the disc. Rates of glycolysis and of lactic acid production for the nucleus are given in *Table* 8.2.

Table 8.2 Rates of glycolysis in the nucleus pulposus obtained after incubations at various oxygen tension levels. Included also are values of oxygen consumption rates obtained in a Gilson respirometer. [From Holm *et al.*, 1981 (9), with permission.]

Oxygen tension (kPa)	Oxygen uptake (μmol/g/h)	Glucose uptake (μmol/g/h)	Lactic acid production (μmol/g/h)	Carbon dioxide production (μmol/g/h)
0·3	0·039	3·3	6·4	0·042
0·9	0·10	3·3	6·4	0·075
1·8	0·13	2·9	6·0	0·13
3·9	0·165	2·7	5·1	0·13
9·8	0·18	2·3	4·5	0·17
19·9	0·19	2·3	4·6	0·17

Oxygen Concentration Profiles in the Intervertebral Disc

The disc is large and avascular, hence concentration gradients arise for metabolites if the rate of consumption is large compared to the rate of solute transport to the cells. Such conditions apply to oxygen. In a similar study to that outlined above, but using a different probe, Holm et al. (1981) measured the oxygen concentration profiles in vivo in different regions of the canine intervertebral disc (Fig. 8.15) (9). The oxygen concentrations were found to vary considerably with position within the intervertebral disc, being highest near the periphery of the annulus and the endplate, and lowest in the centre of the nucleus and inner annulus. In the nucleus, the oxygen tension was about 16 mmHg close to the endplate, but decreased to about 2–8 mmHg in the centre. In the outer annulus, however, the concentration profile was very flat; there was very little decrease in oxygen concentration with decreasing distance from the endplate. This confirmed previous indications that in this region the endplate is almost totally impermeable and that any solutes entering this region of the disc must enter from the blood vessels surrounding the annulus periphery. Holm et al. (1981) showed that the oxygen profiles measured in vivo could be predicted by a diffusion equation (9). The existence of this steep profile in oxygen concentration, and its agreement with the calculated concentration gradient, is further evidence that the major transport mechanism for nutrients such as oxygen is diffusion rather than convection.

Lactate Profiles in the Disc

Steep gradients in concentration across the disc also arise for lactate. Lactate concentration profiles were determined by Holm et al. (1981) in slices cut from nucleus pulposus excised from spines frozen immediately after the dogs had been killed. The lactate concentration profiles found are shown in Fig. 8.16 (9). The lactate concentration in the centre of the disc was 5–8 times higher than that in the blood, while the lactate concentration near the endplate was very similar to that found in the circulation. Thus, there is a steep rise in lactate concentration with distance from regions in contact with blood vessels, as predicted from the diffusion equations. The high lactate levels which are observed must be associated with the lowering of pH. It should be noted that values of pH as low as 5·6 have been found in human discs which were being removed at operation.

It is known that the intervertebral disc contains many proteases (17, 88). More recently collagenases, some in latent form, and elastase have also been found (89). A system of protease inhibitors has also been extracted from human intervertebral discs (90). It is evident from the degradation of newly formed proteoglycans (26, 28) that some degradative enzyme systems are present in the intervertebral disc matrix. In the healthy disc there is likely to be a delicate balance between the active and latent forms of the enzymes and of the potency of the inhibitors present; this balance could be very pH-sensitive and hence changes in the disc's metabolism which decrease pH could lead to rapidly accelerating matrix breakdown.

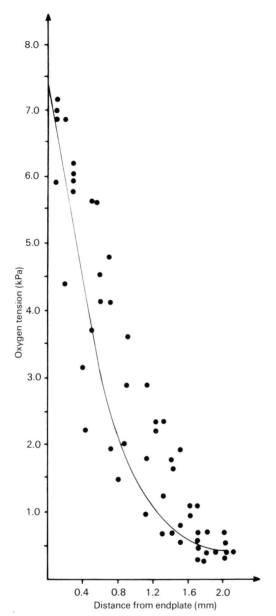

Fig. 8.15. Oxygen concentrations in the nucleus pulposus as a function of distance from the vertebral endplate. The solid curve has been theoretically calculated. [From Holm *et al.*, 1981 (9), with permission.]

EFFECT OF EXERCISE ON INTERVERTEBRAL DISC NUTRITION

During exercise several factors which are concerned with intervertebral disc nutrition may change. Firstly, during prolonged exercise the disc deforms both through bulk movement and through fluid loss under prolonged external load (35, 91, 92, 93). The change in disc dimension may affect the concentration of nutrients in the centre of the disc; the rate of diffusion is a function of the square of disc thickness. Exercise may also affect the peripheral circulation and hence alter the rate at which metabolites reach the disc interface. Finally, exercise itself changes the concentration of blood solutes such as lactic acid, and may affect pH. These changes may influence the concentration of such substances in the disc itself. The above changes would be expected to be immediate and reversible.

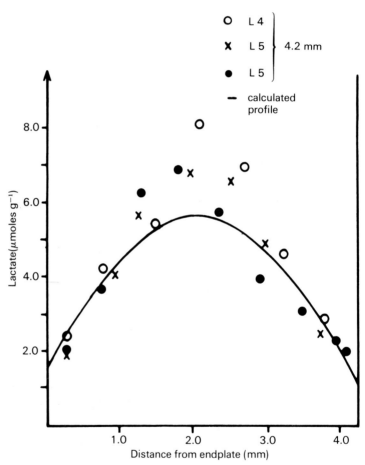

Fig. 8.16. Lactate concentration in the nucleus pulposus as a function of distance from the vertebral endplate. Experimental points correspond to 3 discs of the same thickness obtained from 3 different animals. [From Holm et al., 1981 (9), with permission.]

In contrast a prolonged period of training, or alternatively of immobilization, of disc segments appears to have a dramatic and permanent influence on the transport of nutrients into the disc. In this section we will describe some recent experimental work on these topics.

Disc Fusion

Fusion immobilizes the fused segments and changes mechanical stresses in both the fused and adjacent discs (94). Holm and Nachemson (1982) examined the effect of fusion on the nutrition of a group of mature labrador dogs 3, 5 and 8 months after thoracolumbar spinal fusion (95). They examined the concentration profiles of oxygen and rates of oxygen uptake by the cells using the electrode already described. After the dogs were killed the glucose and oxygen consumption rates and rates of lactic acid production were measured as before (*Fig.* 8.17). The oxygen consumption rate fell with time after fusion in discs of the fused segment. The degree of oxygen consumption was higher at 3 months after fusion than at 8 months after fusion. Consistent with this fall in oxygen consumption rate the oxygen tension in the disc rose (*Fig.* 8.18). These changes suggest that the metabolic activity per volume of disc decreased after fusion; possibly a proportion of the cells died. Somewhat unexpectedly, however, they found a significant increase in the lactic acid concentration in the discs of the fused segments (*Fig.* 8.19). Since the oxygen concentration was higher than normal, the disc's metabolism would be expected to be less anaerobic, consistent with the measured fall in the rate of lactic acid production. It is therefore somewhat surprising to find that lactate concentration increased. A possible mechanism for this increase could be a decreased rate of transport of lactate from the disc. Perhaps fusion gradually reduced the blood supply to the endplate of the disc, thus partially closing one route for movement of solutes out of the tissue and allowing the concentration of metabolic products to build up (*Fig.* 8.20). All their results are in fact consistent with the decreased nutritional supply to the nucleus. However, since it was not possible to examine the blood vessel contacts with the disc, we cannot be certain that this is the mechanism by which fusion influenced disc nutrition. It is of interest to note that in the discs adjacent to the fused segments, which presumably also underwent abnormal mechanical stresses, the changes seen were in an opposite direction to those seen in the fused segments, and were more akin to those seen in the discs of trained dogs which we will describe in the next section.

Effect of Training

Here we will describe two sets of experiments with differing results. In the first set of experiments 4 groups of dogs were taken through an exercise regime daily for 3 months. One group was moderately exercised for 30 min/day, a second group was made to jog over flat ground for 2 h/day, a third group was made to run as fast as possible and the fourth group was made to run over a course involving many obstacles which had to be crawled under or jumped over. This fourth set of exercises involved much flexion and extension as well as lateral bending of the spine. Full details are given by Holm and Nachemson (1983) (10). After 3 months of training the dogs were killed and their discs were analysed as described above. The changes found in the thoracolumbar region were in direct contrast to those found in discs of the fused segments. Holm and Nachemson found an increase in the rate of transport of solutes into the discs and a greater consumption rate by the cells. These changes are summarized in *Table* 8.3 and in *Fig.* 8.21. We can speculate that the differences between transport into the discs which had been fused and those of the exercised dogs could result from

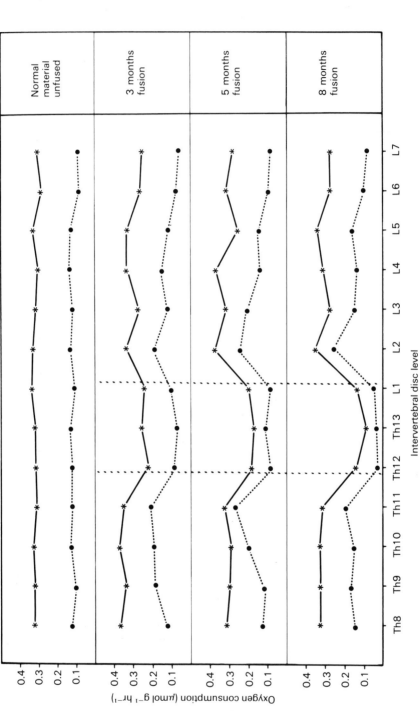

Fig. 8.17. Oxygen consumption rates in a normal (unfused) and fused canine intervertebral discs. The discs adjacent to the fusion as well as the incorporated discs were already affected after 3 months of fusion. These changes progressively increased with increasing fusion time. The results presented are means, each representing more than 8 determinations. Nucleus pulposus is indicated by use of filled circles, results of the outer annulus fibrosus determinations are marked with stars. [From Holm and Nachemson, 1982 (95), with permission.]

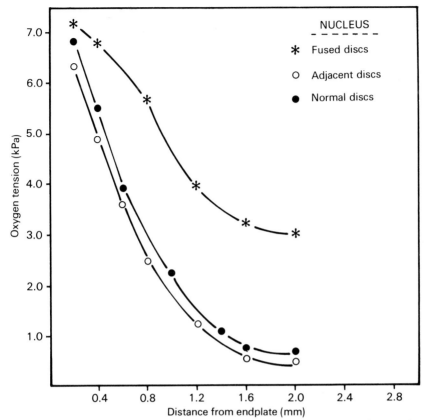

Fig. 8.18. Oxygen tension profiles in the nucleus pulposus, which were measured *in vivo* by thin needle electrodes. In the central area of the fused discs a roughly 5-fold increase of the oxygen tension was noted as compared to the normal and adjacent discs. Close to the vertebral endplate the different discs exhibited oxygen tensions of a similar order of magnitude. [From Holm and Nachemson, 1982 (95), with permission.]

long-term changes in the contact area between the disc and the blood supply; exercise increased this contact, thus improving nutrition, while fusion results in a diminution of these blood contacts. Exercise affects capillary growth in some other tissues (96).

In the second set of tests, Spraque–Dawley rats were exercised daily for 1–2 h on a horizontal treadmill (97). The rats were killed after 4–10 weeks of this exercise regime. Transport into the disc and metabolism in the central portion of the disc appeared to be adversely affected after 10 weeks of such exercise, and the disc showed indications of degeneration. The mechanism for this change is not known. However, it should be noted that the exercise undertaken by these rats was severe compared to what they would normally experience (98).

The results from these 2 sets of experiments show that the effects of exercise on the disc are at present unclear. Under some circumstances exercise may be beneficial for disc nutrition and metabolism, but under other circumstances exercise may be detrimental. At present we cannot differentiate sufficiently between the regimes to predict the effects of exercise, but results suggest moderate exercising regimes may be beneficial (*Table 8.4* and *Fig. 8.22*) (10).

Table 8.3 Transport of radioactive sulphate and methyl glucose into the intervertebral discs (Th = thoracic, L = lumbar). A daily 30 min programme including moderate exercise was used. Results are presented as a percentage of the results obtained from the control group, where the positive sign means an increase in tracer concentration. The levels of significance are indicated by stars [* = P < 0·05 and ** = P < 0·01]. Standard statistical methods were used to calculate the mean and standard deviation. The Mann–Whitney nonparametric ranking test was used for comparison between different groups. [From Holm and Nachemson, 1983 (10), with permission.]

Disc level	Outer annulus fibrosus		Central nucleus pulposus	
	Sulphate	Methyl glucose	Sulphate	Methyl glucose
Th12–L2	+19·5%*	+30·4%	+29·5%**	+35·6%
L3–L6	+13·2%	+19·1%	+17·0%*	+22·4%
L7	+5·1%	+8·8%	+10·4%	+14·7%

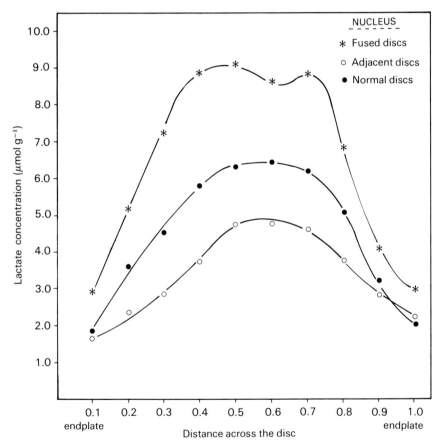

Fig. 8.19. Lactate concentration profiles across the nucleus pulposus (endplate–endplate section) for normal discs and discs being fused for 8 months. In the central nucleus of the fused disc the lactate concentration increased significantly, both with respect to the normal disc and to the adjacent discs (P < 0·01). The concentration profiles decreased towards the endplates. Standard statistical procedures were used to calculate mean and standard deviation. Wilcoxon's test was used for comparison of paired samples, and Mann-Whitney test for comparison of independent samples. [From Holm and Nachemson, 1982 (95), with permission.]

Table 8.4 Utilization of glucose, oxygen and glycogen in the outer annulus and in the central nucleus of intervertebral discs from moderately exercised spines (daily exercise for 30 min). The presented results are deviations from the results of the control group. [From Holm and Nachemson, 1983(10), with permission.]

Disc level	Outer annulus fibrosus			Central nucleus pulposus		
	Glucose	Oxygen	Glycogen	Glucose	Oxygen	Glycogen
Th12–L2	+8·6	+13·0	+6·1	+11·1	+10·7	+7·9
L3–L6	+8·0	+7·7	+4·8	+6·4	+9·5	+7·5
L7	+1·3	+4·7	+2·2	+5·0	+1·9	+3·9

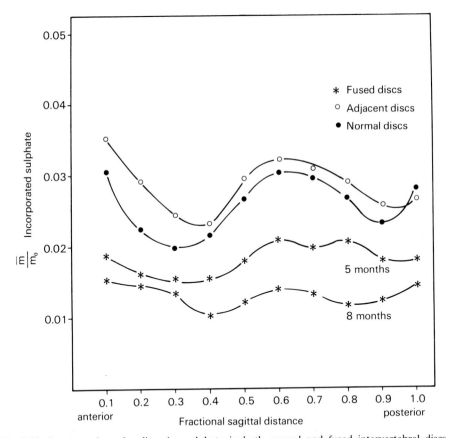

Fig. 8.20. Incorporation of radioactive sulphate in both normal and fused intervertebral discs. The adjacent discs correspond to and should be compared to the disc being fused for 8 months. In the anterior part of the annulus of the adjacent discs the incorporation was significantly increased in comparison to the normal discs ($P < 0.05$), whereas in other parts of the tissue this difference was not significant although it was higher. For statistical methods *see* Fig. 8.19. [From Holm and Nachemson, 1982 (95), with permission.]

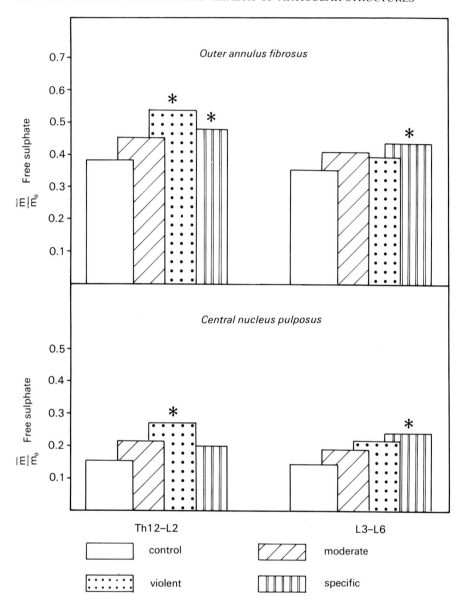

Fig. 8.21. Inorganic (free) sulphate concentration in the outer annulus fibrosus and in the central nucleus pulposus. Two spinal areas are shown, viz. Th12–L2 and L3–L6. Moderate, violent and specific spinal movements were performed daily for 30 min during a 3 months period. Significant levels compared to the control group are marked with a star ($P < 0.05$). For statistical methods *see Fig.* 8.19. [From Holm and Nachemson, 1983 (10), with permission.]

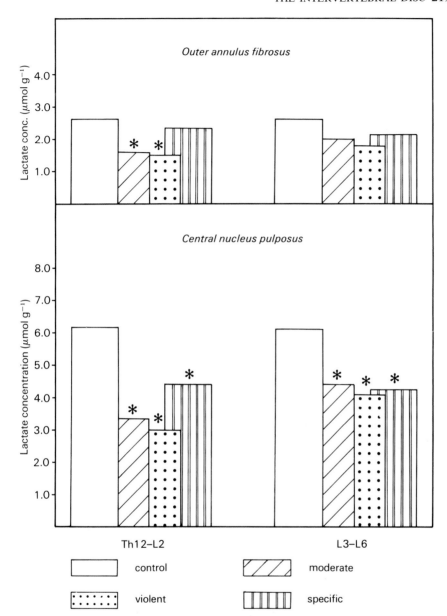

Fig. 8.22. Lactate concentration in annulus and nucleus of discs from a control group and from the 3 groups which daily used a 30 min exercising programme. Lactate concentration decreased for all different exercising regimes. The level of significance is indicated by a star ($P < 0.05$). For statistical methods *see Fig.* 8.19. [From Holm and Nachemson, 1983 (10), with permission.]

MATRIX SYNTHESIS

Although matrix synthesis and turnover has been extensively studied in articular cartilage (19), there is relatively little information on matrix synthesis in the intervertebral disc. There have been a number of *in vivo* studies which show that there is proteoglycan turnover in the intervertebral disc; hormones have been shown to influence the type of glycosaminoglycan synthesized in the disc (101). Lohmander (1973) showed that in the guinea pig nucleus pulposus there was a slow turnover of proteoglycans; he found several pools which turned over at different rates (23). The total proteoglycan turnover rate in adult dogs has been estimated to be between 2 and 4 years (49). An autoradiographic study (102) which examined the uptake of radioactive sulphate (a precursor for proteoglycan synthesis) into the disc found that the transitional zone was most active, as did a study on protein synthesis in the rabbit. Studies on dogs have also found that the rate of synthesis is not constant across the disc (49). These few *in vivo* studies indicate that proteoglycans of the disc are continuously but slowly synthesized by the disc cells; as in articular cartilage the total turnover time is many months and the capacity for repair is relatively low.

There have been few quantitative *in vitro* studies on proteoglycan synthesis in disc segments because of the problems which arise when the disc is incubated *in vitro*; i.e. the disc swells and loses proteoglycans (9, 93, 103). A method has recently been published (59) for incubating the disc *in vitro* while preventing swelling and proteoglycan loss. Hopefully, this technique will enable more information on matrix synthesis to be established. However, while there is very little quantitative information on the rates of matrix synthesis in the disc, there is increasing evidence that exercise or fusion influences the type of matrix synthesized and therefore the concentration and quality of the remaining proteoglycans in the disc.

Effect of Fusion

Holm and Nachemson (1982) examined the total proteoglycan concentration in the discs of their fused segments and found that the proteoglycan concentration fell with time after fusion. More information on proteoglycan synthesis and structure in fusion has come from the work of Ghosh and co-workers (26, 104). They found that the effect of fusion on proteoglycan composition depended on both the age and breed of the dogs. Fusion had apparently no effect on the composition of mature greyhound discs. In contrast the discs of both immature and fully grown beagles showed pronounced changes. The immature discs showed a loss of collagen and a change in proteoglycan structure. In the adult beagles there was a net loss of proteoglycans from the nucleus of the fused discs, but the most prominent feature in all discs examined from the spinal fusion segments was the decreased ability of the isolated proteoglycans to aggregate. Loss of proteoglycan aggregation occurred for both the newly synthesized and the major population of proteoglycans and suggested enhanced enzymatic cleavage of the hyaluronic acid binding region. The resident proteoglycan population was significantly larger than that of the control groups. Ghosh and co-workers interpret these findings to indicate that as the resident proteoglycan population of the fused discs was depleted because of proteoglycan degradation, biosynthesis was stimulated, and hence the proteoglycans resident in the disc were a younger population and therefore larger than those present in non-fused specimens.

The reason for the differences between the species of dogs examined is not known. However, beagles are a chondrodystrophoid canine breed susceptible to disc disorders and the discs of these dogs have much in common with their human counterparts. Like the human disc the notochordal cells are lost from the beagle nucleus early in life. On the other hand greyhounds are non-chondrodystrophoid and notochordal cells persist in adult life (21, 105, 106, 107). Since the most marked changes occurred in the nucleus, it is possible that the notochordal cells respond differently to the changes in loading and nutrition induced by fusion. Although Holm and Nachemson did not examine the proteoglycan structure in their tests on fused discs (95), they did examine the total proteoglycan content expressed as fixed-charge density and also the rate of labelled sulphate uptake. The dogs they tested were adult labradors, which are a non-chondrodystrophoid breed; they saw distinct changes in proteoglycan synthesis with time after fusion. The rate of proteoglycan synthesis fell, as did the total fixed-charge density. The results of a decreased rate of proteoglycan production should be a gradual fall in concentration of proteoglycans and hence a fixed charge in the matrix; in adult dogs proteoglycan turnover time is about 2 years and hence the loss of fixed charge would be expected to be slow if the rate of synthesis fell but did not decrease to zero. Since about half the fixed charge was lost within 8 months, the results point to an increasing rate of proteoglycan breakdown and not only a decrease in synthesis rate.

The results on fused discs appear somewhat contradictory. However, it is clear that under some circumstances fusion can drastically affect proteoglycan turnover and concentration in the fused segments. Whether this results from a change in the nutrients supplied to the disc, possibly because of a reduced blood supply in the fused segments, or whether the cells themselves are able to detect changes in loads and this influences proteoglycan synthesis rates, we are not yet able to say.

Effects of Exercise on Proteoglycan Synthesis Rates

We know of no direct experimental evidence of the effect of exercise on proteoglycan synthesis rates in the disc. In the tests on exercised dogs described above, Holm and Nachemson (1983) did not examine the proteoglycan composition of the disc; however, they did not report any evidence of disc degeneration (10). This is in contrast to the tests on rats which were exercised on a treadmill in which degeneration was seen within 10 weeks (97). Studies using bipedal mice and rats (108, 109) have found that the adoption of upright stance induced degenerative changes in nucleus of these animals. Examination of the histological sections shown in their papers suggest that the thickness of the calcified layer between the disc and the vertebral body may have increased. It is thus possible that the nutritional route through the endplate was interrupted by increased calcification and that this interruption of the nutritional supply led to disorders of the disc.

CONCLUSIONS

The studies which have been conducted on the disc show clearly that exercise or lack of exercise has long-term effects on the disc matrix and cell metabolism. The reported results are confusing, however, as exercise seems to be beneficial for dogs but harmful for over-exercised rats. In some studies it has been found that fusions have effects on beagles and labradors, but in other studies no effects were seen. This confusion probably arises because only a few series of experiments have been reported and these have been on different breeds of various ages using different regimes.

It is difficult to compare different exercising regimes; is 2 h of running for the dog equivalent to 2 h for the rat? One would think not. Our observations suggest that during treadmill exercise the animals are remarkably tense and this could be an additional exercising factor. Exercise as such is only of significance to the disc in that it imposes a loading pattern onto it, and the problem is really to normalize this loading pattern in relation to relevant factors, several of which we might not be aware of. Without such normalization it is difficult to compare studies such as those discussed above and to obtain further understanding of the effects of exercise. However, the results point to certain general trends; removal of load from the disc can lead to deleterious changes. Alternatively, moderate exercise appears to improve transport and metabolism and is probably necessary for the health of the intervertebral disc.

CLINICAL SIGNIFICANCE

Although it is firmly established that exercise influences intervertebral disc metabolism, there are still too few studies conducted in this area to allow any conclusions about its long-term effects on disc health. This concerns particularly the type and magnitude of the exercise.

REFERENCES

1. Akeson W H and Murphy R W (1977) Editorial comment: low back pain. *Clin Orthop* **129**: 2–3.
2. Nachemson A (1976) The lumbar spine. An orthopaedic challenge. *Spine* **1**: 59–71.
3. Nachemson A L and Andersson G B J (1982) Classification of low back pain. *Scand J Work Environ Health* **8**: 134–6.
4. White A A, Edwards T W, Liberman K, Hayes W C and Lewinnek G E (1982) Biomechanics of lumbar spine and sacroiliac articulation: relevance to idopathic low back pain. *In: Idiopathic Low Back Pain: Symposium, American Academy of Orthopaedic Surgeons* (A A White and S L Gordon, eds), pp. 296–322. London: C V Mosby.
5. Brinckmann P, Frobin N, Hierholzer E and Horst M (1983) Deformation of the vertebral end-plate under axial loading of the spine. *Spine* **8**: 851–56.
6. Andersson G B J (1982) Measurements of load on the lumbar spine. *In: Idiopatic low back pain: Symposium American Academy of Orthopaedic Surgeons* (A A White and S L Gordon, eds), pp. 220–51. London: C V Mosby.
7. Pope M, Wilder D and Booth J (1982) The biomechanics of low back pain. *In: Idiopathic low back pain: Symposium, American Academy of Orthopaedic Surgeons* (A A White and S L Gordon, eds), pp. 252–95. London: C V Mosby.
8. Ghosh P, Taylor T K F, Braund K G and Larsen L H (1976) The collagenous and non-collagenous proteins of the canine intervertebral disc and their variation with age, spinal level and breed. *Gerontologia* **22**: 124–32.

9. Holm S, Maroudas A, Urban J P G, Selstam G and Nachemson A (1981) Nutrition of the intervertebral disc. *Connect Tissue Res* **8**: 101–19.
10. Holm S and Nachemson A (1983) Variations in the nutrition of the canine intervertebral disc induced by motion. *Spine* **8**: 866–74.
11. Happey M (1980) Studies of the structure of the human intervertebral disc in relation to its functional and ageing processes. *In: The Joints and Synovial Fluid* (L Sokoloff, ed), pp. 95–137. London: Academic Press.
12. Inoue H and Takeda T (1975) Three dimensional observations of collagen framework of lumbar intervertebral discs. *Acta Orthop Scand* **46**: 949–56.
13. Szirmai J A (1970) Structure of the intervertebral disc. *In: Chemistry and Molecular Biology of the Intracellular Matrix* (E A Balazs, ed), pp. 1279–308 New York: Academic Press.
14. Takeda T (1975) Three-dimensional observation of collagen framework of human lumbar discs. *J Jpn Orthop Ass* **49**: 45–57.
15. Beadle O A (1931) The intervertebral disc: observations of the normal and morbid anatomy in relation to certain spinal deformations.*Report* **161,** London MRC.
16. Schmorl G and Junghanns H (1971) *The Human Spine in Health and Disease.* New York: Grune and Stratton.
17. Ayad S and Weiss J B 1986) Biochemistry of the intervertebral disc. *In: The Lumbar Spine and Back Pain (3rd Ed)* (M I V Jayson, ed), pp. 407–36. Edinburgh: Churchill Livingstone.
18. Eyre D E (1979) Biochemistry of the intervertebral disc. *Int Rev Connect Tissue Res* **8**: 227–90.
19. Heinegard D and Paulsson M (1984) Structure and metabolism of proteoglycans. *In: Extracellular Matrix Biochemistry* (K A Piez and A H Reddi, eds). New York: Elsevier.
20. Adams P and Muir H (1976) Qualitative changes with age of proteoglycans of human lumbar discs. *Ann Rheum Dis* **35**: 289–96.
21. Braund K G, Ghosh P, Taylor T K F and Larsen L H (1975) Morphological studies of the canine intervertebral disc. The assignment of the beagle to the achondroplastic classification. *Res Vet Sci* **19**: 167–72.
22. Emes J H and Pearce R H (1975) The proteoglycans of the human intervertebral disc. *Biochem J* **145**: 549–56.
23. Lohmander S, Antonopoulos C A and Friberg U (1973) Chemical and metabolic heterogeneity of chondroitin sulphate and keratan sulphate in guinea pig cartilage and nucleus pulposus. *Biochim Biophys Acta* **304**: 430–48.
24. Stevens R L, Ewans R J F, Revell P A and Muir H (1979) Proteoglycans of the intervertebral disc. *Biochem J* **179**: 561–72.
25. Stevens R L, Dondi P and Muir H (1979) Proteoglycans of the intervertebral disc. *Biochem J* **179**: 573–78.
26. Cole T C, Burkhardt D, Frost L and Ghosh P (1985) The proteoglycans of the canine intervertebral disc. *Biochim Biophys Acta* **839**: 127–38.
27. Lyons G, Eistenstein S M and Sweet M B E (1981) Biochemical changes in intervertebral disc degeneration. *Biochim Biophys Acta* **673**: 443–53.
28. Oegema T R, Bradford D S and Cooper K M (1979) Aggregated proteoglycan synthesis in organ cultures of human nucleus pulposus. *J Biol Chem* **254**: 10579–81.
29. Eyre D R and Muir H (1977) Quantitative analysis of types I and II collagens in human intervertebral disc at various ages. *Biochim Biophys Acta* **492**: 29–42.
30. Bushell G R, Ghosh P, Taylor T K F and Akeson W H (1977) Proteoglycan chemistry of the intervertebral discs. *Clin Orthop* **129**: 115–21.
31. Wu J, Eyre D R and Slayter H (1986) Type VI collagens in cartilage and intervertebral disc. Abstract Xth meeting of FECTS, Manchester, England. A388.
32. Hickey D S and Hukins D W L (1980) The relationship between the structure of the annulus fibrosus and the function and failure of the intervertebral disc. *Spine* **5**: 105–16.
33. Inoue H (1973) Three-dimensional observation of collagen framework of intervertebral discs in rats, dogs and humans. *Arch Histol Jpn* **36**: 39–56.
34. Klein J A, Hickey D S and Hukins D W (1983) Radial bulging of the annulus fibrosus during compression of the intervertebral disc. *J Biomech* **16**: 211–7.
35. Koeller W, Meier W and Hartmann F (1984) Biomechanical properties of human intervertebral discs subjected to axial dynamic compression. A comparison of lumbar and thoracic discs. *Spine* **9**: 925–33.
36. Pearcy M, Portek J and Shepherd J (1985) The effect of low back pain on lumbar spinal movements by three-dimensional X-ray analysis. *Spine* **10**: 150–3.
37. Viidik A (1973) Functional properties of collagenous tissues. *Int Rev Connect Tissue Res* **6**: 127–215.

38. Eklund J A and Corlett E N (1984) Shrinkage as a measure of the effect of load on the spine *Spine* **9**: 189–94.
39. Grynpas M D, Eyre D S and Kirschner D A (1980) Collagen of the intervertebral disc: X-ray diffraction evidence for difference in molecular packing of types I and II collagens. *Biochim Biophys Acta* **626**: 346–55.
40. Adams M A and Hutton W C (1983) The effects of posture on the fluid control of the lumbar intervertebral disc. *Spine* **8**: 665–671.
41. Andersson G B J and Schultz A B (1979) Effects of fluid injection on mechanical properties of intervertebral disc. *J Biomech* **12**: 453–58.
42. Grodzinsky A J (1983) Electromechanical and physicochemical properties of connective tissue. *Crit Rev Biomed Eng* **9**: 133–99.
43. Maroudas A (1970) Distribution and diffusion of solutes in articular cartilage. *Biophys J* **10**: 365–79.
44. Maroudas A and Evans H (1974) Sulphate diffusion and incorporation into human articular cartilage. *Biochim Biophys Acta* **338**: 265–79.
45. Parker K, Maroudas A and Winlove P (1987) Diffusivities and partitions of inorganic ions in CS and HA solutions. *Biorheology*. (In press.)
46. Urban J P G and Maroudas A (1979) Measurement of fixed charge density in the intervertebral disc. *Biochim Biophys Acta* **586**: 166–78.
47. Urban J P G, Maroudas A, Bayliss M T and Dillon J (1979) Swelling pressures of proteoglycans at the concentrations found in cartilaginous tissues. *Biorheology* **16**: 447–64.
48. Comper W D and Preston B N (1974) Model connective tissue systems: a study of polyion-mobile ion and of excluded volume interactions of proteoglycans. *Biochem J* **143**: 1–9.
49. Urban J P G, Holm S and Maroudas A (1978) Diffusion of small solutes in the intervertebral disc; an *in vivo* study. *Biorheology* **15**: 202–23.
50. Byers P, Bayliss M T, Maroudas A, Urban J and Weightman B (1983) Hypothesizing about joints. In: *Studies in Joint Diseases II* (A Maroudas and E J Holborow, eds), pp. 241–276. Tunbridge Wells: Pitman Medical.
51. Nachemson A (1960) Lumbar interdiscal pressure. *Acta Orthop Scand [Suppl.]* **43**:
52. DePuky P (1935) The physiological oscillations of the length of the body. *Acta Orthop Scand* **6**: 338–43.
53. Tyrrell A R, Reilly J and Troup J D G (1985) Circadian variation in stature and the effects of spinal loading. *Spine* **10**: 161–4.
54. Adams M A and Hutton W C (1983) The effect of fatigue on the lumbar intervertebral disc. *J Bone Joint Surg [Br]* **65**: 199–203.
55. Kazarian L E (1975) Creep characteristics of the human spinal column. *Orthop Clin North Am* **6**: 3–18.
56. Urban J P G and Maroudas A (1980) The chemistry of the intervertebral disc in relation to its physiological functions and requirements. *Clin Rheum Dis* **6**: 51–46.
57. Lewin T (1964) Osteoarthritis in lumbar synovial joints – a morphological study. *Acta Orthop Scand (Suppl)* **73**: 5–108.
58. Maroudas A (1980) Metabolism of cartilaginous tissues: a quantitative approach. In: *Studies in Joint Disease* (A Maroudas and E J Holborow, eds), pp. 59–86. London: Pitman Medical.
59. Bayliss M T, Urban J P G, Johnstone B and Holm S (1986) An *in vitro* method for measuring synthesis rates in the intervertebral disc. *J Orthop Res* **4**: 10–17.
60. Simon B R, Wu J, Carlton M W, Kazarian L E, France E P, Evans J H and Zienkiewicz O C (1985) Dynamic structural models of rhesus spinal motion segments. *Spine* **10**: 494–507.
61. Naylor A (1962) The biophysical and biomechanical aspects of intervertebral disc herniation and degeneration. *Ann R Coll Surg Engl* **31**: 91–114.
62. Naylor A (1970) The structure and function of the intervertebral disc. *Orthopaedics (Oxford)* **3**: 7–22.
63. Stockwell R A (1975) Structural and histochemical aspects of the pericellular environment in cartilage. *Philos Trans R Soc Lond [Biol]* **271**: 243–5.
64. Urban J P G (1977) *Fluid and Solute Transport in the Intervertebral Disc*. Ph D Thesis, London University.
65. Preston B N and Snowdon J (1973) Diffusional properties of model extracellular systems. In: *Biology of the Fibroblast* (E Kulonen and J Pikkarainen, eds) pp. 215–30. New York: Academic Press.

66. Maroudas A (1979) Physicochemical properties of articular cartilage. *In: Adult Articular Cartilage* (M A R Freeman, ed), pp. 131–70. London: Pitman Medical.
67. Maroudas A (1976) Balance between swelling pressure and collagen tension in normal and degenerate cartilage. *Nature* **260**: 808–9.
68. Roberts S, Beard H K and O'Brian J P (1982) Biochemical changes of intervertebral discs in patients with spondylolisthesis with tears of posterior annulus fibrosus. *Ann Rheum Dis* **41**: 78–85.
69. Brown M D and Tsaltas T T (1976) Studies on the permeability of the intervertebral disc during skeletal maturation. *Spine* **1**: 240–44.
70. Sylvest J, Hentzer B and Kobajasi T (1977) Ultrastructure of prolapsed disc. *Acta Orthop Scand* **48**: 32–40.
71. Maroudas A, Stockwell R A, Nachemson A and Urban J (1975) Factors involved in the nutrition of the human lumbar intervertebral disc: cellularity and diffusion of glucose *in vitro*. *J Anat* **120**: 113–30.
72. Postacchini F, Bellocci M and Massobrio M (1984) Morphologic changes in annulus fibrosus during ageing. *Spine* **9**: 596–603.
73. Brodin H (1955) Paths of nutrition in articular cartilage and intervertebral discs. *Acta Orthop Scand* **24**: 177–80.
74. Hansen H J and Ullberg S (1961) Uptake of ^{35}S in the intervertebral disc after injection of ^{35}S-sulphate. An autoradiographic study. *Acta Orthop Scand* **30**: 84–90.
75. Ogata K and Whiteside L A (1981) Nutritional pathways of the intervertebral disc: an experimental study using hydrogen washout technique. *Spine* **6**: 211–6.
76. Urban J, Holm S, Maroudas A and Nachemson A (1977) Nutrition of the intervertebral disc. An *in vivo* study of solute transport. *J Clin Orthop* **129**: 101–14.
77. Nachemson A, Lewin T, Maroudas A and Freeman M A R (1970) *In vitro* diffusion of dye through the end-plates and the annulus fibrosus of human lumbar intervertebral discs. *Acta Orthop Scand* **41**: 589–607.
78. Crock H W and Goldwasser M (1984) Anatomic studies of the circulation in the region of the vertebral end-plate in adult greyhound dogs. *Spine* **9**: 702–6.
79. Holm S and Nachemson A (1985) Nutrition of the intervertebral disc: effects induced by vibrations. *Orthopaedic Transactions* **9**: 451.
80. Holm S and Nachemson A (1984) Immediate effects of cigarette smoke on nutrition of the intervertebral disc of the pig. *Orthopaedic Transactions* **8**: 380.
81. Urban J P G, Holm S, Maroudas A and Nachemson A (1982) Nutrition of the invertebral disc. Effect of fluid flow on solute transport. *Clin Orthop* **170**: 296–302.
82. Bywaters E G L (1937) Metabolism of joint tissues. *J Pathol Bacteriol* **44**: 247–68.
83. Lane J M, Brighton C T and Menkowitz B J (1977) Anaerobic and aerobic metabolism in articular cartilage. *J Rheumatol* **4**: 334–42.
84. Marcus R F (1973) The effect of low oxygen concentration on growth, glycolysis and sulphate incorporation by articular chondrocytes in monolayer culture. *Arthritis Rheum* **16**: 646–56.
85. Rosenthal O, Bowie M A and Wagoner G (1940) Studies on the metabolism of articular cartilage. I. Respiration and glycolysis in relation to its age. *J Cell Physiol* **17**: 221–33.
86. Tushan F, Rodnan G P and Altman M (1969) Anaerobic glycolysis and lactate dehydrogenase (LDH) isoenzymes in articular cartilage. *J Lab Clin Med* **73**: 649–56.
87. Gilson W E (1963) Differential respirometer of simplified and improved design. *Science* **141**: 531.
88. Naylor A (1974) Late results of laminectomy for lumbar disc prolapse. A review after ten to twenty-five years. *J Bone Joint Surg [Br]* **56**: 17–29.
89. Sedowofia S K A, Tomlinson I, Jayson M I V and Weiss J B (1979) Identification of collagenase and other neutral proteinases in human intervertebral discs. *Ann Rheum Dis* **38**: 573–92.
90. Knight J A, Stephens R W, Bushell G R, Ghosh P and Taylor T K F (1979) Neutral protease inhibitors from human intervertebral disc and femoral head articular cartilage. *Biochim Biophys Acta* **584**: 304–10.
91. Krämer J (1971) Zur Biomechanik des lumbalen bewegungselements. *In: Die Wirbelsäule in Forschung und Praxis* (H Junghans, ed), pp. 19–63. Stuttgart: Hippokrates.
92. Krämer J (1977) Pressure-dependent fluid shifts in the intervertebral disc. *Orthop Clin North Am* **8**: 211–16.

93. Urban J P G and Maroudas A (1981) Swelling of the intervertebral disc *in vivo*. *Connect Tissue Res* **9**: 1–10.
94. Frymoyer J W, Hanley E N, Howe J, Kuhlman D and Matteri R E (1979) A comparison of radiographic findings in fusion and nonfusion patients ten or more years following lumbar disc surgery. *Spine* **4**: 435–40.
95. Holm S and Nachemson A (1982) Nutrition changes in the canine intervertebral disc after spinal fusion. *Clin Orthop* **169**: 243–58.
96. Hudlicka' O and Tyler K R (1984) The effect of long-term high-frequency stimulation on capillary density and fibre types in rabbit fast muscles. *J Physiol (Lond)* **353**: 435–45.
97. Holm S and Rosenqvist A-L (1986) Morphological and nutritional changes in the intervertebral disc after spinal motion. *Scand J Rheumatol [Suppl]* **60**: A117.
98. Holm S (1986) Nutritional variations in articular cartilage induced by exercise. *Scand J Rheumatol [Suppl]* **60**: A116.
99. Bayliss M T, Ridgeway G D and Ali S Y (1983) Differences in the rates of aggregation of proteoglycans from human articular cartilage and chondrosarcoma. *Biochem J* **215**: 705–8.
100. Maroudas A and Bannon C (1981) Measurements of swelling pressure in cartilage and comparison with the osmotic pressure of constituent proteoglycans. *Biorheology* **18**: 619–32.
101. Davidson E A and Small W (1963) Metabolism *in vivo* of connective tissue mucopolysaccharides. Chondroitin sulphate C and keratan sulphate of nucleus pulposus. *Biochim Biophys Acta* **69**: 445–52.
102. Souter W A and Taylor T K F (1970) Sulphated acid mucopolysaccharide metabolism in the rabbit intervertebral disc. *J Bone Joint Surg [Br]* **52**: 371–84.
103. Pousty J, Bari-Kahn M A and Butler W F (1975) Histology of the disc. *Histochem J* **7**: 361–65.
104. Taylor T K F, Ghosh P, Braund K G, Sutherland J M and Sherwood A A (1976) The effect of spinal fusion on intervertebral disc composition. An experimental study. *J Surg Res* **21**: 91–104.
105. Braund K G, Taylor T K F, Ghosh P and Sherwood A A (1977) Spinal mobility in the dog. A study in chondrodystrophoid and non-chondrodystrophoid breeds. *Res Vet Sci* **22**: 78–82.
106. Hansen H J (1959) Comparative views on the pathology of disc degeneration in animals. *Lab Invest* **8**: 1242–66.
107. Hoerlein B F (1971) *Canine Neurology – Diagnosis and Treatment*. Philadelphia: Saunders.
108. Higuchi M, Abe K and Kenada K (1983) Changes in the nucleus pulposus of the invertebral disc in bipedal mice. *Clin Orthop* **175**: 251–57.
109. Yamada K (1962) The dynamics of experimental posture. Experimental study of intervertebral disc herniation in bipedal animals. *J Exp Med* **8**: 350–61.
110. Schultz A B (1974) Mechanics of the human spine. *Appl Mech Reviews* **27**: 1487–97.
111. Laskin D M and Sernat B G (1953) Metabolism of fresh, transplanted and preserved cartilage. *Surg Gynecol and Obstet* **96**: 493–99.
112. Langham M E and Taylor I S (1956) Factors affecting the hydration of the cornea in the excised eye of the living animal, *Br J Ophth* **40**: 321–40.
113. Takahashi G H, Fatt I and Goldstick T K (1966) Oxygen consumption rate of tissue measured by a micropolarographic method. *J Gen Physiol* **50**: 317–35.
114. Fatt I and Bieber M T (1968) The steady-state distribution of oxygen and carbon dioxide in the *in vivo* cornea. I. The open eye in air and the closed eye. *Exp Eye Res* **7**: 103–12.
115. Lin S H (1976) Oxygen diffusion in a spherical cell with non-linear oxygen uptake kinetics. *J Theor Biol* **60**: 449–57.

Chapter 9

Genetical and Mechanical Features Governing the Growth of Epiphyseal Cartilage

D. R. Johnson

CONTENTS

INTRODUCTION

Cartilage is unique amongst skeletal tissues because it alone is capable of interstitial growth. Romer (1) suggested that because of this cartilage should be regarded as a specialization of the growing animal and not as a primitive skeletal tissue. A cartilaginous skeleton is able to grow *en masse* by division of chondrocytes without disturbing the structures around it or which attach to it. Bone, growing slowly by apposition and remodelled from the surface, could never grow sufficiently fast to accommodate the embryonic skeleton.

But cartilage also grows in other ways; appositionally by the division of cells on the surface of cartilage, in volume by the deposition of matrix and in cellular volume by the enlargement of cartilage cells. It is also possible that cells can be recruited from adjacent tissue. The method of growth of cartilage is also likely to vary according to the age of the specimen.

Cartilage is recognizable when the first matrix is laid down. During the subsequent life history of the cartilage interstitial growth, appositional growth, recruitment of cells from surrounding tissues, and cell and matrix enlargement will play different roles at different times. If the cartilage is destined to be replaced by bone, then hypertrophy and endochondral ossification will follow. If it is to become ligamentous (like the central part of Meckel's cartilage) then only the perichondrium survives, growing appositionally.

These 4 mechanisms of cartilage growth must be under some sort of control, either extrinsic or intrinsic, or probably a mixture of the two. Understanding intrinsic control demands that we study the genetic factors acting on a piece of

227

cartilage. Two adjacent cartilaginous blastemata of much the same size may become bones as disparate as tibia and fibula. How does this come about? Extrinsic control may depend upon hormones, deficiency of a nutrient, a surfeit of an unwanted chemical in the environment or on mechanical constraints. Chemical environmental susceptibility may be due to the unique method of nutrition in cartilage, which depends on diffusion and lacks a blood supply. I have argued elsewhere (2) that cartilage survives in a siege economy because of this.

Cartilage growth, of whatever type, has two elements. Cartilage must grow to the right size and to the right shape. Thorogood (3) has pointed out the important distinction between growth, which merely increases size, and morphogenesis, which controls shape. At a given point in development a cartilage anlage may be within the normal limits of variation, too large or too small. If it is too large or too small certain consequences follow.

Grüneberg (4) reviewed a series of mouse mutants with variously deformed limbs. He pointed out that reduction in size of the mesenchymal blastema that is to become a cartilage has certain sequelae. Histogenesis of cartilage will be delayed, apparently because a critical size is necessary in order to proceed further, and this is reached later in the smaller mutant blastemata. Small blastemata give rise to small cartilages and later small bones, and very small blastemata may fail to reach a critical size and consequently disappear through failure to chondrify. In the congenital hydrocephalus (*ch*) mouse, for example, there is a systemic effect reducing blastemal size throughout the embryo. Chondrification is delayed and smaller cartilages are found everywhere, e.g. in vertebrae and ribs. Some components, such as the arcus anterior atlantis, are absent altogether. Reduction in size may prevent the normal fusion of adjacent cartilages, e.g. the neural arches of the vertebrae tend to remain unfused posteriorly. Clearly, not being the right size may have far-reaching consequences.

The effects of growth on shape are legion. A moment's consideration will show that the femur of an achondroplastic dwarf is not only smaller than that of a 6 foot man but also an entirely different shape. Decreased growth here produces not a miniature but perfect bone, but a bone with entirely different proportions. This kind of defective growth inevitably produces transformation of shape.

METHODS OF GROWTH

Let us return to the possible methods of cartilage growth and consider them in more detail. We might expect to find an increase in mitotic rate in the developing blastema. This has been reported in some cases (5, 6) but incorporation of tritiated thymidine has failed to demonstrate any such mitotic burst in the chick limb bud (7, 8): rather, the mitotic rate tends to fall as the proportion of specialized cells increases (9, 10, 11). Although chondrocytes can both divide and secrete matrix, the latter seems to inhibit the former. The increase in cellular density in a blastema is up to 60% (12). This is not due to cell division, predates matrix secretion and is not accompanied by an increase in cell volume: it is based upon cellular recruitment around the periphery of the blastema as described by Ede *et al.* (13).

Newman (14) studied the effect of cell density in the mesodermal blastema. He found that blastemal cells raised in culture at less than confluent density became fibroblastic, and cells raised at confluence became cartilaginous.

Even precartilage cells are characteristically orientated at right angles to the long axis of the blastema (15, 16). With the appearance of the first matrix the cells gradually become separated. Hall (17) has reviewed the interesting idea that matrix components may be involved in feedback governing cartilage growth.

Interstitial cell division seems initially to be at random within developing cartilage. As the daughter cells move apart, however, they tend to form 'nests', usually consisting of an even number of chondrocytes, presumably the products of recent mitoses, occupying a single lacuna in the matrix.

Cell proliferation makes a large contribution to early cartilage growth but is gradually augmented by matrix secretion. The classical view is one of increasing secretion and decreasing division, but it should be remembered that chondrocytes can both secrete and divide: some mitoses are seen in mature cartilage and the classic picture is one of decreasing interstitial growth with increasing age. Stockwell (18), however, considers this view ill founded. Studies with radioactive thymidine show that mitoses are found in cartilages of all ages, in the bulk of the tissue and not exclusively near its surface, as would be the case were growth largely appositional (19, 20). In contrast Searls (9) has good evidence that 75% of chondrocytes in chick limb bone cartilages have dropped out of the cell cycle, whereas at the limb bud stage all cells are dividing. It is possible that the exhaustion of the potential of, for instance, the small-celled region in the epiphyseal growth plate, may be used as a growth-limiting mechanism.

Streeter (21) (*Fig.* 9.1) described a series of characteristic changes undergone by developing cartilage. Of his 5 phases the first 3 are common to all cartilage and the last 2 peculiar to cartilage undergoing endochondral ossification. Phase 1 corresponds to a process which we have already described, separation of randomly dispersed actively dividing cells by an appreciable amount of metachromatically staining matrix. This phenomenon spreads throughout the tissue until only a narrow superficial layer, the perichondrium, is excluded. Subsequent changes also develop from the centre of the cartilage mass, spreading centrifugally. In Phase 2 the dividing cells become elongated in a direction tangential to the primary growth centre. In Phase 3 there is an increase in matrix volume and the cells become larger and cuboidal. At this stage, according to Streeter, mitosis ceases. In Phase 4 cells are relatively huge and vacuolated (hypertrophied) and in Phase 5 calcified matrix surrounds the degenerating cells.

How do we explain relative growth? Hicks (22) examined the developing tibia and fibula of the embryonic chick in organ culture. Primordia were dissected free with intact perichondria at 6 days of incubation. At this stage the tibia was 4 times the volume of the fibula. After 6 days in culture it was 12 times as large. Co-culture showed that the growth of each element was independent of the other. During this period matrix synthesis (estimated by the uptake of ^{35}S) was identical, as was mitotic index (estimated by ^{3}H-thymidine incorporation). The factor responsible for differential growth here was cell volume, although mitosis and matrix secretion both contributed to the overall growth of each element.

This much, then, is common to all cartilage: we have seen that growth may occur by (*1*) cell division, (*2*) matrix deposition, (*3*) hypertrophy or

(*4*) subperiosteal appositional growth, and we have seen that Aniken, Streeter, and Ede (15, 21, 16) have all noted orientation of cartilage cells within a cartilage mass. These are the factors which govern the growth of our main object of interest, the epiphyseal plate.

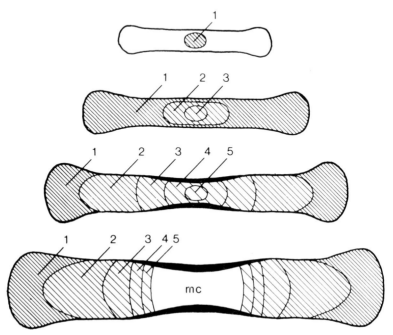

Fig. 9.1. Zones of cartilage maturation in the developing long bone. Streeter's Type 1 cartilage (21) appears first in the centre of the developing cartilaginous blastema (*top*) then spreads through the developing rudiment. At later stages (*below*) central cartilage has matured and been displaced by a marrow cavity whilst peripheral cartilage has reached stages 2–5. [From Hinchliffe and Johnson (104), with permission.]

THE EPIPHYSIS

The epiphyseal plate is a specialization peculiar to certain higher vertebrates. In cartilaginous fishes the cartilaginous elements may become partially calcified, corresponding to Streeter's Stages 4 and 5. In bony fishes we find a compound skeletal element, a rod of cartilage surrounded by a tube of periosteal bone and corresponding to the periosteal cuff stage seen in developing mammalian long bones (23). Elements such as this can increase in length only at their ends because of their periosteal collar. Haines (24) (*Fig.* 9.2) described the epiphyseal ends of such bones, a cylinder of bone capped at either end by a plug of cartilage. In *Sciaena* Haines was able to distinguish zones of unspecialized cartilage, flattened cells and hypertrophy within the epiphysis. The typical fish epiphysis thus consists of a mass of cartilage extending beyond the bony shaft and covered by a layer of articular fibrocartilage which allows appositional growth of the epiphyseal surface. Opposite the end of the bony shaft is a growth zone formed by layers of flattened cells irregularly arranged. Derived from this zone, on the side facing the shaft are randomly arranged hypertrophic cells. Resorption is very variable between species, sometimes being absent so that the epiphysis resembles an ice cream cone wedged into a tube, mechanically stable, sometimes so extensive as to leave only a narrow zone of hypertrophied cells.

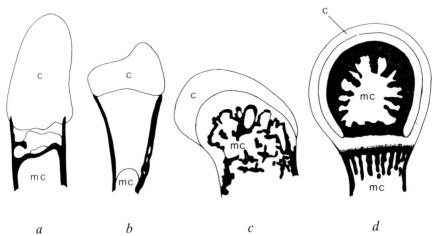

Fig. 9.2. Evolution of the vertebrate epiphysis. Forms seen here are (a) bony fish, (b) young chelonian, (c) part grown chelonian, and (d) mammal. c, cartilage; mc, marrow cavity. [From Hinchliffe and Johnson (104), with permission.]

This form of epiphysis or a modification of it survived the transition from sea to land in the early Reptilia (amphibians show many specializations). In the Chelonia young epiphyses resemble those of fish, older ones have a distinctly curved growth plate. Fossil reptilian bones have radially arranged bone trabeculae in the epiphyseal region, suggesting that they were very like the Chelonia. Change came with the postural rearrangement concerned with tucking the limbs beneath the body. Animals which do this no longer have the articular surface at the end of the long bone (think of the human femoral head) and it is very difficult to make the radial epiphysis cope with this arrangement. Specialization arose at least 5 times: in the fossil Amphibia, in *Sphenodon*, in the Lacertilia, birds and mammals (25). The new flat growth plates, which separate shaft growth and articular surface growth, were often strengthened by a secondary centre of ossification. Stronger bones were also produced in some cases by the arrangement of cartilage cells into orderly columns (26).

The mammalian long bone thus has 3 growth functions, increase in length of the diaphysis, increase in diameter or transverse expansion of the growth plate and growth of the articular surface. The first 2 of these depend upon the epiphyseal cartilage.

MECHANICAL STRUCTURE OF THE MAMMALIAN EPIPHYSIS

The characteristic structure of the mammalian epiphysis was described by Dodds (27), (*Fig.* 9.3), who noted that cartilage cells were arranged in rows parallel to the long axis of the bone and asked himself how this came about. In this classic paper Dodds noted the essential differences between hyaline cartilage and that in the epiphysis. In hyaline cartilage cells are small and rounded, and mitotic divisions take place in all planes. Division is rather slow, and after division daughter cells drift apart and become separated by matrix. In epiphyseal cartilage Dodds recognized four important changes.

1. The mitotic figures are orientated in a definite way.
2. The daughter cells resulting from a single division remain close together.
3. The daughter cells become discoidal (flattened) rather than rounded.
4. All daughter cells remain in this orientation with their diameters parallel to the long axis of the bone.

Dodds noted that each row of flattened cells is derived from a 'row mother cell'. Since the rows are mitotic products of the 'row mother', rows tend to consist of 2^n cells, i.e. 2, 4, 8 etc. This increase in the number of cells/column inevitably increases the length of the column and hence contributes to longitudinal growth. Transverse growth is produced by an increase in the number of row mother cells, and hence the number of columns. Matrix is laid down in 2 distinct regions, as longitudinal septa between rows and as thinner transverse plates between daughter cells.

The mode of division of the row mother cell is obviously crucial to this process of growth. In divisions contributing to the elongation of the column (i.e. usually) the row mother cell divides transversely, with the spindle aligned with the long axis of the cell and the metaphase plate across the short axis. The 2 daughter

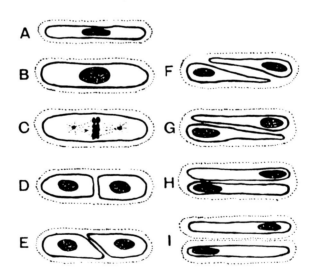

Fig. 9.3. Diagrammatic drawings to show the mode of division of the discoid cells in rows of cartilage cells in endochondral ossification. [From Dodds (27), with permission.]

cells thus initially lie side by side. Re-orientation so that the cells lie one above the other is a separate process involving the cells growing past each other, which causes them temporarily to become wedge shaped. In divisions contributing to the number of cell mothers the process must differ: either the plane of the mitotic spindle is different or, perhaps more likely, the second part of the process does not occur. Dodds notes, in fact, that the alignment of the mitotic spindles is not always perfect: 'In some other cases the divisions of the row mother cells seem to take place in other planes, but if they do, the resulting cells promptly change their orientation, so that all the flattened pairs become orientated in the same way'. Lacroix (28) suggests that the increase in the number of cell columns is more likely to happen peripherally because centrally longitudinal bars of cartilage are held in place by calcification and would tend to remain parallel. There is evidence that this growth occurs at the 'ossification groove' around the growth plate (29, 30, 31, 32).

Buckwalter et al. (33) have recently returned to the study of cartilage cell orientation in the epiphysis. They used actively growing C57BL mice aged 5–28 days and examined the tibial epiphysis. They measured the ratio of cell width: cell height and expressed this ratio as the degree of eccentricity (departure from a circular profile). A test grid of parallel lines was superimposed on electron microscope negatives to establish orientation. Saltykov (34) has argued that the number of intersections with such a grid would increase if there was a degree of non-randomness in the material studied.

Cells of the reserve zone, lower proliferative zone and upper hypertrophic zone were essentially circular in transverse sections. This was temporarily upset by mitosis. At mitosis nearly all mitotic figures were perpendicular to the long axis of the bone. Cells from the hypertrophic zone were polygonal in cross-section.

In longitudinal sections the cells had major and minor principal axes, with the major one being horizontal in all zones but the lower hypertrophic. In general cells were flatter and more strongly orientated in the faster growing regions and at the times of greatest growth. Thus the flattest and most strongly orientated cells were found in the lower proliferative zone at 7 and 15 days.

Moss-Salentijn et al. (35) have made computer reconstructions of rabbit cartilage cell columns. These showed proximal tibial growth plates 400–500 μm in height with straight regular columns, most extending from the small cell zone to the ossification zone. Some columns, however, were incomplete (not extending through the whole of the plate) or interrupted. Some showed splitting. Although most columns were straight and regular, orientated with their long axis normal to the plane of the growth plate, incomplete columns occurred which tended to cause deformation of adjacent complete ones 'to make room'. Segments of interrupted columns were also often oblique. Columns also varied widely in diameter, interrupted ones being narrowest and duplicated ones widest.

The organization of cells into columns has an effect on the surrounding matrix. Matrix structure has recently been redefined by Eggli et al. (36) (Fig. 9.4). They studied TEM and SEM specimens conventionally fixed and with the addition of cationic dyes (which prevent the loss of matrix proteoglycans, which may be as high as 70% (37) during fixation). With cationic dyes added, Eggli was able to demonstrate a pericellular matrix chiefly composed of proteoglycans, although the presence of tropocollagen molecules is also likely. Of greater interest to us at present is the arrangement of collagen. Eggli argues that, in the pericellular area, the matrix is exposed to multidirectional tension by virtue of the volume and surface increase of the growing cells and this is reflected in the random orientation of the innermost collagen fibres. Longitudinal septa, however, are exposed to predominantly longitudinal forces, stretched by the lengthening of cell columns in the direction of growth. This is reflected in the alignment of their collagen fibrils parallel to the axis of the column. The longitudinal walls of the lacunae thus have an inner layer of territorial matrix, rather like a basket, and an outer layer where longitudinal orientation predominates. This arrangement is not seen in transverse septa, where fibril orientation is random. The matrix here is made of a denser felt, perhaps due to pressure exerted on the transverse matrix by hypertrophying cells.

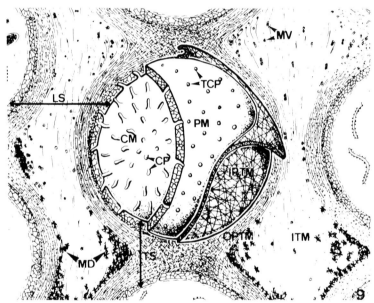

Fig. 9.4. Schematic drawing of a hypertrophic chondrocyte and its surrounding matrix. CM, cell membrane; CP, protruding cell processes; PM, pericellular matrix; TCP, tips of cell processes; IPTM, inner territorial matrix; OPTM, outer territorial matrix; ITM, interterritorial matrix; MV, matrix vesicles; MD, mineral deposits; LS, longitudinal septum; TS, transverse septum. [From Eggli (36), with permission.]

On the other hand Lacroix (29) and Speer (38) turned this argument on its head and suggested that the organization of the growth plate matrix may be responsible for the increase in height, rather than diameter, of hypertrophic cells.

This subdivision of the matrix may have chemical as well as physical consequences. Compartmentalization may provide preferential pathways for diffusion and transport of metabolites. The pericellular membrane, now revealed as a dense covering of proteoglycans around the cell, may act as a diffusion barrier for larger molecules (39, 40) and is significantly penetrated by cell processes. The longitudinal organization of matrix within columns will facilitate longitudinal diffusion, especially from the nutritive vessels on the epiphyseal surface into the cartilage. Pita and Howell (41) noted that, after micropuncture and the injection of a fluorescent dye, staining was restricted to the interterritorial matrix.

We thus have the following view of the epiphyseal plate:
1. The cells are elliptical in outline when seen in longitudinal section, the major axis of the ellipse being horizontal. The degree of eccentricity depends on the rate of growth.
2. They are formed into vertical columns.
3. Mitosis is such that the cells divide to lie side by side. Usually the cells then slide over each other so that they lie one above the other, increasing the length of the column. Column number is increased when this does not occur, probably peripherally.
4. Matrix fibrils (collagen) are longitudinally arranged in the vertical septa between columns, but not in the horizontal septa between cells.
5. The cells exhibit growth processes seen elsewhere in cartilage; mitosis, matrix synthesis and cell enlargement.

What is the relationship between these factors? The correlation between cell division rate and cell shape is well known according to Buckwalter et al. (33), who presumably seek to establish a relationship between eccentricity of a cell and the plane of the mitotic spindle. Although this seems a good argument on common sense grounds, the mitotic spindle perhaps needing the space allowed by the long axis of the cell to form, it is worth noting that, of the 6 references cited by Buckwalter et al., 5 refer to plant cells and 1 to detergent foam. Until evidence from animal cells is forthcoming it seems unsafe to rely too heavily on this demonstration in the plant cell, which is quite differently organized, although one could argue that the cellulose wall of the plant is analogous to the cartilage matrix. The argument could also be reversed: Lufti (42) has pointed out that the cytoskeletal elements forming the mitotic spindle can change cell shape. A mitotic spindle orientated in a specific direction could therefore determine the flattened shape of epiphyseal cartilage cells. There is certainly a correlation between rate of cell division and the degree of flattening of the cells (33): a similar correlation is seen in cells in culture (43, 44).

The rate of longitudinal bone growth is a product of cell growth rate and the length of the column of hypertrophied cells (45). As the latter is sensibly constant, longitudinal bone growth is a measure of the rate of cartilage cell production. Although absolute rates vary according to species (45, 46, 47) and age (48) and even within a single bone (28, 49, 50, 51), there is sufficient precision for comparisons to be made. The major elongation in the rabbit third metatarsal (28) is at the end carrying an epiphysis, but Serafini-Fracassini and Smith (49), for example, noted that one end of a bone with 2 epiphyses may grow faster than the other: this phenomenon of the 'growing end' of a bone is well known. What determines relative growth rate is unknown but, if one end of a long bone is accidentally or experimentally damaged, compensatory growth occurs at the other epiphysis of the bone (50, 51). The mechanism of this compensation is also unknown. During maturation the cell division rate declines in parallel with shaft elongation.

Column formation may be experimentally induced or suppressed. One approach to the problem is to use healthy cartilage cells and to explant them. Rigal (30) grew epiphyseal tissue from a rabbit in Duthie chambers implanted elsewhere in the rabbit. He describes the way in which a block of regular columns explanted from the central area of the epiphyseal growth plate, and hence 'released from the normal physical and mechanical factors', loses its regular columnar arrangement after 2 weeks. Johnson (52) unwittingly produced an excellent control experiment for Rigal, explanting intact mouse tail vertebrae beneath the kidney capsule of siblings. In this case the columnar architecture was preserved. Once again, however, we do not know what happens to the mitotic rate of the cells. Does it decrease after explanting?

The reverse experiment, imposing columnar arrangement on tissue where none previously existed, has also been performed. Krompecher (53) produced columns in cartilaginous callus by placing it under compression. Lacroix (28) (*Fig.* 9.5) grafted rib cartilage into the centre of the proximal tibial epiphysis in 2-week-old rabbits. After 8 days Lacroix remarks 'c'est incontestablement dans la transplant que commence à se manifester la différenciation considerée', and after 4 months the grafts were almost totally assimilated and had formed columns aligned with those of the host.

Columnar organization is also dependent upon the extracellular matrix, since disruption of the matrix also disrupts columns. The administration of papain, which affects proteoglycan complexes and decreases chondroitin sulphate levels (54, 55, 56) produces pseudo-chondrodystrophic mice with shortened limbs (57) and irregular cartilage columns.

MECHANICAL PROPERTIES OF THE MATRIX

Any change in the cartilage matrix, however brought about, is likely to affect its mechanical properties. Wirth *et al.* (58) found significant negative correlations between tensile failure stress and structure in chondromalactic human patellar cartilage (using the grading scheme of Mankin *et al.* (59) to assess degeneration). Armstrong and Mow (60) related the compressive equilibrium modulus to structural category, and found a weak negative correlation.

Rather than try to assess gradations in degeneration, Kempson *et al.* (61) compared the tensile properties of human articular cartilage close to and distant from areas of fibrillation. Tensile strength and the linear part of the stress/strain curve were both reduced near fibrillation.

Cartilage is also affected by externally applied external pressure. The ultimate effect of increasing mechanical pressure on chondrocytes is death. Many studies on joint loading (62, 63) have shown that, if areas of articular cartilage are forced into actual contact, i.e. subjected to continuous compression, a series of pathological changes ensues, starting with loss of nuclear staining and terminating in complete necrosis of the cartilage and exposure of the underlying bone.

However, some mechanical stimulation seems to be necessary for healthy cartilage growth. Where a joint is fixated (64) cartilage is replaced by connective tissue. Cartilage surfaces in contact, but not exposed to frank pressure, do not deteriorate. In areas exposed to pressure, such as between the femoral condyle and the overlying patella, fibrillation and erosion occur.

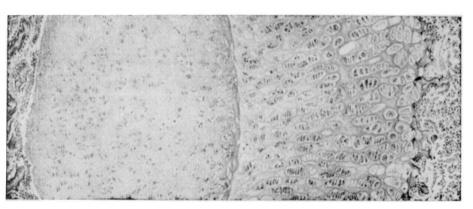

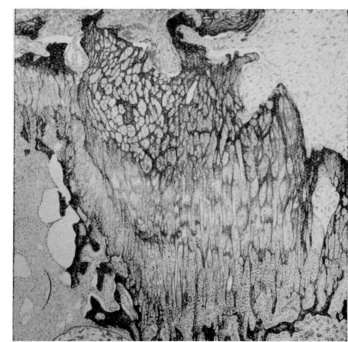

Fig. 9.5. Graft of non-columnar rib cartilage into tibial epiphysis in the rabbit. *a*, after 8 days; *b*, after 4 months. [From Lacroix (28), with permission.]

GENETIC MUTATIONS

We have seen that a number of factors could be important in the maintenance of the mammalian epiphysis. One way of investigating the interaction between these factors is to look at genetically controlled chondrodystrophies. Many of these are known, in man, laboratory and domestic animals, and all produce an effect primarily seen as the failure of limb bones to elongate (although all cartilages in the body are characteristically affected). Within the limb bones width is essentially normal (e.g. *see* 65), but length is characteristically decreased.

Since these disorders are produced by separate acts of mutation in separate genes, they supply a reservoir of possible first causes which may help us better to understand the normal development and growth of the epiphyseal plate. The growth plate cells in a range of such disorders have been variously described as bizarrely shaped (dog; 66) somewhat disorderly in arrangement (*cn* mouse; 67) and even arranged obliquely or perpendicularly to the long axis of the bone (*cho* mouse; 68). Cell columns have been described as disarranged (man; 69), collapsed and disorganized (*dw* mouse; 70: not a chondrodystrophy but decreasing growth by virtue of its effect on the pituitary gland) or absent (*cho* mouse; 68: *smc* mouse; 71). The iliac crest of achondroplastic patients grows faster than the long bones and column formation here is normal (69). Could it be that rapid cell division and columnar form of epiphyseal plates are interrelated? One is reminded of the findings of Lacroix (28) in the rabbit metatarsal. The end which grows faster has a regular epiphysis with cartilage columns, that which grows more slowly has nests of cells. Are these slower-growing nests of cells equivalent to the disturbed epiphyseal columns in the chondrodystrophies?

Cell Kinetics in Mutants

Cell kinetics have been examined autoradiographically in a number of mouse mutants. In stumpy (*stm*; 72) (*Fig.* 9.6) Thurston *et al.* found the labelling profile very irregular, with dividing cells seen right down to the onset of the zone of hypertrophy. The height of hypertrophic cells was much reduced. Johnson (73) had already described very abnormal cell division in this mutant (*Fig.* 9.7). Stumpy cells tend to stay together after cell division and to interdigitate their cell membranes. Desmosomes are also seen uniting the cell membranes of daughter cells. A similar appearance has been described by Bingel *et al.* (65) in the dwarf Alaskan malamute.

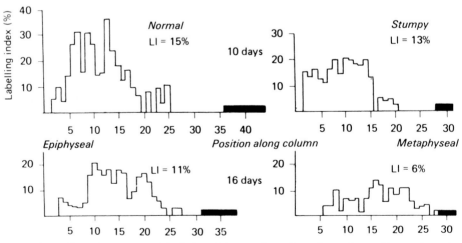

Fig. 9.6. Profiles of percentage labelled nuclei at each position down the cartilage column in normal and *stm* mice aged 10 and 16 days.

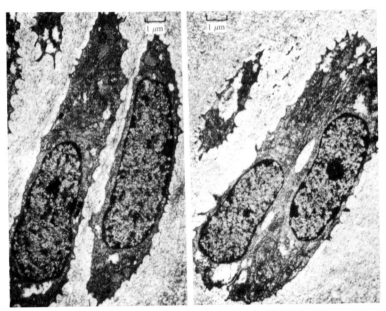

Fig. 9.7. Pairs of cartilage cells from normal (*left*) and *stm* (*right*) epiphyseal plates.

In achondroplasia (*cn*; 74), although the position was confused by the apparent presence of two distinct types of homozygote, the message was essentially clear. Mitotic rate and labelling profile were normal, but hypertropic cell height was again reduced. In spondylo-metaphyseal chondrodysplasia (*smc*; 75) the columns are so irregular that conventional cell kinetic studies are not possible. The amount of labelling with tritiated thymidine was, however, much reduced (to 25% normal at 16 days).

What do these mutants tell us about epiphyseal cartilage? In *stm* something has gone wrong with cell division. The defect seems to concern the inability of cells to move apart after mitosis. This seems to account for the presence of dividing cells anywhere in the column, and not just in the normal zone of division. This in turn upsets the normal cell maturation and hence cell height and growth. In the other mutants it looks as if a defect in cell kinetics is not primarily responsible for the abnormal cartilage. In *cn* the defect is not clear cut. The absence of abnormalities in division rate and cell profile suggest that cell division is normal: but again hypertrophic cell height is reduced. Perhaps this is a defect in the poorly understood process of hypertrophy, or is reduced cell height merely a symptom of reduced growth due to another cause? *smc* is obviously different again, as mitotic rate is grossly deficient and the cell columns are so disrupted as to have ceased to exist.

Deficiencies in the Matrix

In some mutant conditions there is a clear and specific defect in cartilage matrix. The nanomelic chick (*nm*; 76) will serve as an example of these. The true nature of the nanomelic defect has only recently become apparent, but biochemical studies of the matrix date back to 1967 when Mathews (77) found a 90% defect in matrix mucopolysaccharides. Turnover studies (78) showed a synthesis defect. Argraves et al. (79) finally located the defect as an absence of the core protein upon which mucopolysaccharides are normally arrayed. Interestingly, collagen synthesis is normal in nanomelia, suggesting that synthesis of the 2 main matrix components is not co-regulated.

The cartilage matrix deficiency mouse (cmd; 80) (Fig. 9.8) seems to suffer from a similar defect, again having reduced mucopolysaccharide synthesis. Kimata et al. (81) were able to test for mucopolysaccharide core protein by raising an antibody in the rabbit: again the protein was found to be absent. The spondylo-metaphyseal chondrodysplasia (smc) mouse, mentioned above in connection with cell kinetics, seems to resemble cmd closely in ultrastructure, and Johnson (2) suggests that these mutants may have similar first causes. In man diastrophic dysplasia (82) cartilage is very similar in ultrastructural appearance to that from cmd and smc mice.

Ultrastructural resemblance may be sufficient grounds to suspect a similar first cause *within* a species, but *between* groups as different as mammals and birds caution must be employed: although the nanomelic chick and the cmd mouse have a very similar defect at the biochemical level, their cartilage does not look at all similar at light microscopic or ultrastructural levels (Fig. 9.9).

Generalized Biochemical Defect

The nanomelic chick, cartilage matrix deficiency mouse and probably smc mouse all have a specific defect related to cartilage, i.e. the absence of a molecule usually present in the matrix. Because of the unique nutritional method of cartilage it seems that generalized metabolic deficiencies, i.e. in molecules not confined to cartilage, often show themselves as a chondrodystrophy, presumably because other tissues are better able to cope with sub-optimal conditions. The brachymorphic mouse (bm; 65) is a typical chondrodystrophy with short limbs and tail and a domed skull. Chondrocyte columns are irregular and epiphyses small (83) (Fig. 9.10). The matrix stains poorly for sulphated glycosaminoglycans and, although collagen fibres are normal, matrix granules of mucopolysaccharide are not visible or much reduced when cartilage is viewed by the transmission electron microscope.

Biochemical studies have shown that the total amount of mucopolysaccaride present in the matrix is in fact normal, but the degree of sulphation is much reduced (84). Sugahara and Schwartz (85) suggested that the under-sulphation could be due to a defect in the conversion of adenosine-5'-phosphosulphate (APS) to 3-phosphoadenosine-5'-phosphosulphate (PAPS), a sulphate donor, and demonstrated a 93% decrease in APS-kinase in newborn bm mice. More recent work (86) suggests that both APS-kinase and ATP-kinase are affected. Schwartz (86) suggests that a subunit common to both enzymes may be affected by the bm gene.

A similar situation, another generalized biochemical defect making itself evident in cartilage, is seen in the achondroplastic rabbit (ac; 87, 88, 89). Grossly this again is a typical chondrodystrophy. The cartilage shows a high concentra-

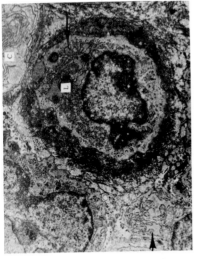

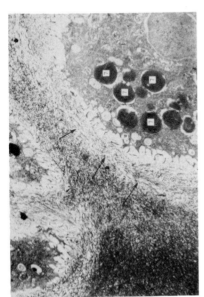

Fig. 9.8. Chondocytes from (*a*) *smc* mouse mutant: L, lipid vacuoles; arrows point to rim of collagen fibres. *b, cmd* mouse mutant: C, pycnotic chondrocyte; L lipid inclusions; arrows point to rough endoplasmic reticulum. *c,* Human diastrophic dysplasia (DD). [*smc* from Johnson (71). *cmd* from Rittenhouse *et al.* (80). DD by courtesy of B H Schofield, D F McDonald and S E Kopits, Dept. of Orthopaedic Surgery, Johns Hopkins University School of Medicine.]

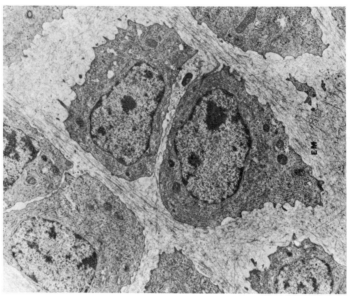

Fig. 9.9. Ultrastructural appearance of nanomelic chick cartilage. [From Pennypacker and Goetinck (1976) *Dev Biol* **50**: 35–47, with permission.]

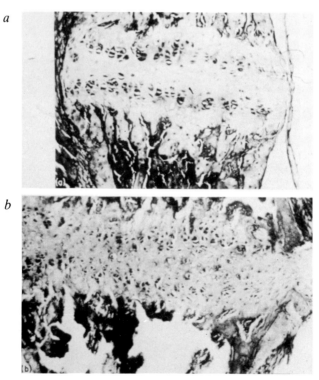

Fig. 9 10. Epiphyseal plates from normal (*a*) and *cn* (*b*) mice. [From Miller and Flynn-Miller (83), with permission.]

tion of dead cells, especially towards the centre of cartilaginous masses (90). Dead cells are not so commonly found elsewhere (muscle, liver, thymus). Less matrix than normal is present and cartilage columns are irregular. Electron microscopy showed only the increased number of dead and dying cells: the matrix appeared normal. Shepard supposed that the dead cells were those furthest away from a blood supply; perhaps they were unable to metabolize effectively at low oxygen concentrations. Shepard and Bass (91) used organ culture to study the uptake of radioactive precursors into *ac* cartilage. ^{3}H and ^{35}S showed normal uptake, but the amount of ^{14}C incorporated from glucose and galactose was almost doubled. Glucose acts as a source for both acid mucopolysaccharides and collagen, but relatively anaerobic cartilage also relies heavily on glycolysis for its respiratory needs. Bargman *et al.* (92) surmised that the defect in *ac* might be in oxidative energy metabolism. Using liver mitochondria as a substrate they demonstrated defective phosphorylation at site III (the cytochrome oxidase region).

The *ac* rabbit thus serves as a second example of a non-specific biochemical defect present in all cells in the body but manifesting as a chondrodystrophy, i.e., showing up only in the rather marginal conditions pertaining in cartilage. Mackler *et al.* (93, 94) have suggested that human achondroplasia also has a defect in oxidative phosphorylation, but other authors suggest that it is a matrix defect (69, 95).

Physical Defects in the Matrix

The strength of cartilage matrix in hereditary disorders such as chondrodystrophies seems to be unknown, but in degenerative joint diseases compositional variation occurs, and is usually detrimental. For instance, water content increases in experimentally induced osteoarthritis in dogs (96) and proteoglycan content may decrease with degeneration (97). This production of mechanically weak, less stiff, more permeable cartilage is also to be expected in chondrodystrophies, especially when a decrease in proteoglycans occurs or their core protein is absent.

In one sense the best model of this kind of defect is chondrodystrophy (68), where Seegmiller gives the cause of death in cyanosed homozygotes as suffocation due to the reduced structural strength of abnormal cartilage matrix, which in turn leads to failure of the trachea to maintain its patency. Freshly dissected cartilage is also described as 'floppy'. The histological and ultrastructural appearance of *cho* cartilage is characteristic and abnormal, with poor column formation and large areas of cartilage (mainly in the proliferation zone) devoid of chondrocytes. The matrix is heterogeneous, vesicular, stains poorly with toluidine blue, alcian blue and PAS. Ultrastructurally collagen fibres are wide (200 nm) and cross banded (*Fig.* 9.11). Why is the cartilage so mechanically unsound? Seegmiller *et al.* suggested that column formation fails to occur because of reduced acid mucopolysaccharides in the matrix, which renders it weak and unable to align daughter cells after mitosis. Unfortunately, later work does not support this hypothesis. Stephens and Seegmiller (98) and Seegmiller *et al.* (99) have examined *cho* matrix in detail and have found no abnormal biochemical parameters, save for a tendency to lose glycosaminoglycans rather more rapidly than normal by leaching. This is a common finding in chondrodystrophic mutants.

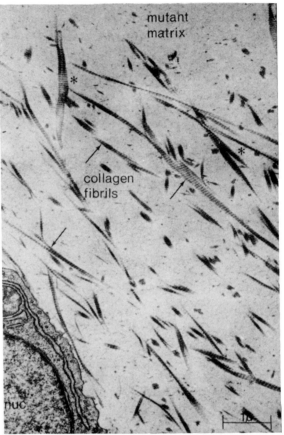

Fig. 9.11. Ultrastructural appearance of cartilage from the *cho* mouse. [From Seegmiller *et al.* (68), with permission.]

cho is thus a rather frustrating mutant. The strength of the cartilage is certainly reduced, the histological and ultrastructural appearance is distinctive, but the biochemistry appears to be normal. Is the defect in the banded collagen? Probably not, since this often occurs in normal cartilage in other species.

Other Mutations

The conditions described above are some of the best worked out models of chondrodystrophy. Many others exist, which may be ascribed to one or other of these groups as further details become available. Thus, lethal chondrodystrophy in the turkey (100) has under-sulphation of glycosaminoglycans. More detailed studies show that there are fewer sulphated glycosaminoglycans than normal per proteoglycan molecule, although the core protein which binds them together is present and of normal length. Disproportionate micromelia in the mouse

(*Dmm*; 101) has chondrocytes longitudinally compressed and set in a poorly staining cystic matrix. *Dmm* cartilage, like that of *cho*, leaks labelled glycosaminoglycans rapidly. Collagen synthesis is also subnormal and Type II collagen is confined to a pericellular location.

The cartilage anomaly mouse (*can*; 102, 103) has a defect in protein synthesis from the 17th day of gestation to the 3rd day of postnatal life, compensated by a later increase in both protein and mucopolysaccharide synthesis. We await fuller explanations of all these conditions.

OVERVIEW

Taken altogether, the study of normal and abnormal epiphyseal plates presents us with food for thought. The epiphysis of a long bone is a device concerned primarily with rapid longitudinal growth. Sissons (45) suggested a rate of 7·5 new cells per column per day in the upper tibial growth plate of the 4 week old rat, and Kember (47) found 5 new cells per day in his 'standard' column of 25 cells. Transverse expansion is thought to be one fifth to one tenth of this figure (18).

Is the presence of cell columns merely a reflection of this rapid growth? In areas where growth is less rapid (e.g. the slower-growing end of the rabbit metatarsal; 28) columnar organization is not seen: instead cartilaginous cells are organized as cell nests. This seems to be identical to the embryonic condition described by Streeter (21). Dodds (27) described the situation in the distal end of the phalanx of the human infant. Here, before the development of an epiphysis, cell nests occur, growth is a little slower and not so polarized, and the bone produced has rather irregular trabeculae. Is the regular organization of cartilage columns the result of speeding up the division rate in cell nests? Groups such as birds manage to grow perfectly good long bones without the benefit of cell columns; I have not been able to find any data on the relative rates of growth of the long bones in birds and mammals. If columns are a specialization aimed towards rapid elongation, then bird long bones should elongate less quickly than those of mammals. In birds, as in the infant digit, bone is not so regularly structured as that seen in the mammalian epiphysis and rests of calcified cartilage are often seen, removed by later remodelling. Cell columns thus provide well structured bone quickly.

Although the formation of a column is not necessarily merely the result of a high rate of cell division, the converse may be true: a high rate of cell division may be necessary to maintain the regular arrangement of the columns. Transplantation experiments showing the formation of columns in cartilage placed in an epiphysis only work in the long term. Lacroix (28) demonstrated the formation of columns commencing 8 days after grafting and complete after 4 months. This is a long time scale in a standard column of 25 cells which adds 5 new cells per day.

If a reduction in growth rate leads to a disruption in cartilage columns, then we have a model for chondrodystrophy. The reduced growth rate could be due to either decreased mitosis or a decrease in hypertrophic cell height. What factors are capable of causing the decreased rate of growth? We have several clues to this. Mitotic upsets such as that seen in stumpy (*stm*) seem to be primary. However, other factors could limit the rate of mitosis. In the achondroplastic rabbit we see an extreme example: a metabolic defect which first lowers mitotic rate then actually kills the cells. It seems likely that other generalized metabolic defects manifesting themselves in cartilage, such as the APS-kinase/ATP-kinase defect in the brachymorphic mouse, work in a similar way, by depressing metabolic rate and hence mitosis and/or growth.

Specific defects in cartilage matrix probably affect cartilage in a similar manner. We have seen (36) how the physical structure of the matrix is determined by the arrangement of its biochemical components, and how diffusion through cartilage may be aided by this structuring. Loss of balance between matrix components can lead to a defective structure, e.g. the web of pericellular collagen fibres seen in *smc*, *cmd* and diastrophic dysplasia (71, 80, 82). This must surely affect the metabolic processes, which normally have to cope with only the mucopolysaccharide-rich pericellular matrix. In other conditions we know only part of the story: the biophysical defect in *cho* cartilage is plain to see, but its biochemical basis eludes us.

Other defects are even more elusive. The hypertrophic cell height in *cn* is reduced. Can this be all that is wrong? Extensive biochemical, histochemical and ultrastructural studies (summarized in 2) have failed to find anything further. The story in *can* (102, 103) is obviously complex but no clear first cause was ever established. The epiphyseal cartilage still holds many secrets.

CONCLUSIONS

The epiphysis is a specialization aimed at separation of growth of the articular surface from that of the shaft of the bone. Epiphyseal columns allow well structured bone to be produced quickly. Any factor which reduces the rate of production of cells within the cartilage column will decrease the efficiency of the system by reducing growth rate and/or the regularity of the bone produced. The use of mutant genes which lead to reduced growth rate allow us to identify some of these factors, which include defects in mitosis, generalized metabolic defects manifested specifically in cartilage, specific metabolic defects leading to defective matrix and biophysical defects which disrupt matrix properties.

PRACTICAL SIGNIFICANCE

Cartilage columns within the mammalian epiphysis are a specialization allowing rapid growth. Any defect slowing this growth will lead to disruption of columns. A large number of potential defects with this effect have been discussed. Cartilage seems to be vulnerable to these conditions because of its avascular structure and unique metabolic processes.

REFERENCES

1. Romer A S (1942) Cartilage, an embryonic adaptation. *Am Nat* **76**: 394–404.
2. Johnson D R (1986) *The Genetics of the Skeleton*. Oxford: Oxford University Press.
3. Thorogood P V (1983) Morphogenesis of cartilage. *In*: *Cartilage, Vol 2, Development, Differentiation, and Growth* (B K Hall, ed), pp. 223–54. New York: Academic Press.

4. Grüneberg H (1963) *The Pathology of Development*. Oxford: Blackwell.
5. Hale L J (1956) Mitotic activity during early skeletal differentiation of the scleral bones in the chick. *Q J Microsc Sci* **97**: 333–53.
6. Jacobson W and Fell H B (1941) The developmental mechanisms and potencies of undifferentiated mesenchyme of the mandible. *Q J Microsc Sci* **82**: 563–86.
7. Janners M Y and Searles R L (1970) Changes in the rate of cellular proliferation during the differentiation of cartilage and muscle in the mesenchyme of the embryonic chick wing. *Dev Biol* **23**: 136–65.
8. Thorogood P V (1972) *Patterns of Chondrogenesis and Myogenesis in the Limb Buds of Normal and Talpid Chick Embryos*. PhD Thesis, Aberystwyth, University College of Wales.
9. Searls R L (1973) Newer knowledge of chondrogenesis. *Clin Orthop* **96**: 327–44.
10. Abbot J and Holtzer H (1966) The loss of phenotypic traits by differentiated cells. III. The reversible behaviour of chondrocytes in primary cultures. *J Cell Biol* **28**: 473–8.
11. Flickinger R A (1974) Muscle and cartilage differentiation in small and large explants from the chick embryo limb bud. *Dev Biol* **41**: 202–8.
12. Thorogood P V and Hinchliffe J R (1975) An analysis of the condensation process during chondrogenesis in the embryonic chick hind limb. *J Embryol Exp Morphol* **33**: 581–606.
13. Ede D A, Flint O P, Wilby O K and Colquhoun P (1977) The development of precartilage condensations in limb bud mesenchyme of normal and mutant embryos *in vitro* and *in vivo*. In: *Vertebrate Limb and Somite Morphogenesis* (D A Ede, J R Hinchliffe and M Balls, eds), pp. 161–79. London: Cambridge University Press.
14. Newman S (1977) Lineage and pattern in the developing wing bud. In: *Vertebrate Limb and Somite Morphogenesis* (D A Ede, J R Hinchliffe and M Balls, eds), pp. 181–97. London: Cambridge University Press.
15. Aniken A W (1929) Das morphogene Feld der knorpelbildung. *Wilhelm Roux' Arch Entwicklungsmech Org* **114**: 549–78.
16. Ede D A (1976) Cell interactions in vertebrate limb development. In: *The Cell Surface in Animal Embryogenesis and Development* (G Poste and G L Nicholson, eds), pp. 495–543. Amsterdam: Elsevier.
17. Hall B K (1978) *Development and Cellular Skeletal Biology*. New York: Academic Press.
18. Stockwell R A (1979) *Biology of Cartilage Cells*. London: Cambridge University Press.
19. Messier B and Leblond C P (1960) Cell proliferation and migration as revealed by radioautography after injection of thymidine H^3 into male rats and mice. *Am J Anat* **106**: 1075–7.
20. Fitzgerald M J T and Shtieh M M (1977) Interstitial versus appositional growth in developing non-articular cartilage. *J Anat* **124**: 503–4.
21. Streeter G L (1949) Developmental horizons in human embryos. *Contrib Embryol Carnegie Inst* **34**: 165–96.
22. Hicks M J (1982) *Analysis of the Differential Growth of Chondrogenic Elements in the Embryo Chick Limb*. Ph D Thesis, Aberystwyth, University College of Wales.
23. Haines R W (1935) Epiphyseal growth in the branchial skeleton of fishes. *Q J Microsc Sci* **77**: 77–97.
24. Haines R W (1937) The primitive form of epiphysis in the long bones of tetrapods. *J Anat* **72**: 323–43.
25. Heidsieck E (1928) Bau der Skelette bei der Reptilien. *Morph Jahrb* **59**: 343–92.
26. Lubosch W (1924) Bildung des Markknochens beim Huhnchen. *Morph Jahrb* **53**: 49–93.
27. Dodds G S (1930) Row formation and other types of arrangement of cartilage cells in endochondral ossification. *Anat Rec* **46**: 385–99.
28. Lacroix P (1949) *L'organisation des Os*. Liège: Editions Desoer.
29. Tonna E A (1961) The cellular component of the skeletal system studied autoradiographically with tritiated thymidine during growth and ageing. *J Biophys Biochem Cytol* **9**: 813–24.
30. Rigal W M (1962) The use of tritiated thymidine in studies of chondrogenesis. In: *Radioisotopes in Bone* (F C McLean and A M Budy, eds), pp. 197–225. Oxford: Blackwell.
31. Shimomura Y, Wezeman F H and Ray R D (1973) The growth cartilage plate of the rat and rib: cellular proliferation. *Clin Orthop* **90**: 246–54.
32. Shapiro F, Holtrop M E and Glimcher M J (1977) Organisation and cellular biology of the perichondral ossification groove of Ranvier. A morphological study in rabbits. *J Bone Joint Surg [Am]* **59**: 703–23.
33. Buckwalter J A, Mower D, Schafer J, Ungar R, Ginsberg B and Moore K (1985) Growth plate chondrocyte profiles and their orientation. *J Bone Joint Surg [Am]* **67**: 942–55.

34. Saltykov S A (1958) Stereometric Metallography. Moscow: Metallugizdat.
35. Moss-Salentijn L, Moss M L, Shinozuka M and Skalak R (1987) Morphological analysis and computer-aided, three-dimensional reconstruction of chondrocytic columns in rabbit growth plates. *J Anat.* **151**: 157–67.
36. Eggli P S, Herrman V, Hunziker E B and Schenk R K (1985) Matrix components in the growth plate of the promixal tibia of rats. *Anat Rec* **211**: 246–57.
37. Engfeldt B and Hjertquist S O (1968) Studies on the epiphyseal growth zone. *Virchow's Arch [Cell Pathol]* **1**: 222–9.
38. Speer D P (1982) Collagenous architecture of the growth plate and perichondral ossification groove. *J Bone Joint Surg [Am]* **64**: 399–407.
39. Wuthier R E, Majeska R J and Collins G M (1977) Biosynthesis of matrix vessels in epiphyseal cartilage. *Calcif Tissue Res* **23**: 135–9.
40. Schenk R K, Hunziker E B and Herrmann W (1982) Structural properties of cells related to tissue mineralization. *In: Biological Mineralization and Demineralization.* (G H Nancollas, ed), pp. 143–60. Berlin: Springer Verlag.
41. Pita J C and Howell D S (1978) Microbiochemical studies of cartilage. *In: The Joints and Synovial Fluid. Vol. I* (L Sokoloff, ed), pp. 273–330. New York: Academic Press.
42. Lufti A M (1970) Study of cell multiplication in the cartilaginous upper end of the tibia of the domestic fowl by tritiated thymidine autoradiography. *Acta Anat [Basel]* **76**: 454–63.
43. Folkman J and Moscona A (1978) Role of cell shape in growth control. *Nature (London)* **273**: 345–9.
44. Folkman J and Tucker R W (1980) Cell configuration, substratum and growth control. *In: The Cell Surface, Moderator of Developmental Processes.* (S Subtenly and N K Wessels, eds), pp. 259–75. New York: Academic Press.
45. Sissons H A (1956) Experimental study of the effect of local irradiation on bone growth. *In: Progress in Radiology* (J S Michel, B E Holmes and C L Smith, eds), pp. 436–48. Edinburgh: Oliver & Boyd.
46. Haines R W (1933) Cartilage canals. *J Anat* **68**: 45–64.
47. Kember N F (1960) Cell division in endochondral ossification. *J Bone Joint Surg [Br]* **42**: 824–39.
48. Gardner E, Gray D and O'Rahilly R (1963) *Anatomy.* Philadelphia: Saunders.
49. Serafini-Fracassini A and Smith J W (1974) *The Structure and Biochemistry of Cartilage.* Edinburgh: Churchill-Livingstone.
50. Hall-Craggs E C B (1969) Influence of the epiphyses on regulation of bone growth. *Nature (London)* **221**: 1245.
51. Hall-Craggs E C B and Laurence C A (1969) The effect of epiphyseal cartilage stapling on growth in length of the rabbit tibia and femur. *J Bone Joint Surg [Br]* **51**: 359–65.
52. Johnson D R (1974) The *in vivo* behaviour of achondroplastic cartilage from the cartilage anomaly (*can/can*) mouse. *J Embryol Exp Morphol* **31**: 313–8.
53. Krompecher S (1937) *Die Knochenbildung.* Jena: Fischer.
54. Westerborn O (1961) The effect of papain on epiphyseal cartilage. A morphological and biochemical study. *Acta Chir Scand [Suppl]* **270**: 1–84.
55. Hulth A (1959) Experimental retardation of endochondral growth by papain. *Acta Orthop Scand* **28**: 1–21.
56. Rönning O V (1971) Alterations in craniofacial morphogenesis induced by parenterally administered papain. An experimental study in the rat. *Proc Finn Dent Soc* **67**: (Suppl III): 1–94.
57. Johnson D R (1978) The effect of a single injection of papain on growth of the limb bones of the mouse. *Growth* **42**: 27–30.
58. Wirth C R, Augello F A, Mow V C and Roth V (1980) Variation of tensile properties of human patellar cartilage with age and histological indices. *Trans Ann Meet Orthop Res Soc* **5**: 38.
59. Mankin H J and Lippiello L (1971) Biochemical and metabolic abnormalities in articular cartilage from osteoarthritic human hips. *J Bone Joint Surg [Am]* **53**: 523–37.
60. Armstrong C G and Mow V C (1980) Friction lubrication and wear of synovial joints. *In: Scientific Foundations of Orthopaedics and Traumatology* (R Owen, J Goodfellow and P Bullough, eds), pp. 223–32. London: Heinemann Medical.
61. Kempson G E, Muir H, Polard C and Tuke M (1973) The tensile properties of the cartilage of human femoral condyles related to the content of collagen and glycosaminoglycans. *Biochim Biophys Acta* **297**: 456–72.

62. Salter R B and Field P (1960) The effects of continuous compression on living articular cartilage. An experimental investigation. *J Bone Joint Surg [Am]* **42**: 31–49.
63. Trias A (1961) Effect of persistent pressure on the articular cartilage. *J Bone Joint Surg [Br]* **43**: 376–86.
64. Evans E B, Eggers G W N, Butler J K and Blumel J (1960) Experimental immobilization and remobilization of rat knee joints. *J Bone Joint Surg [Am]* **42**: 737–58.
65. Lane P W and Dickie M M (1968) Three recessive mutations producing disproportionate dwarfing in mice. *J Hered* **58**: 300–8.
66. Bingel S A, Sande R D and Newbrey J (1983) Dwarfism in the Alaskan malamute: ultrastructural features of the growth plate chondrocyte. *Calcif Tissue Int* **35**: 216–24.
67. Silberberg R and Lesker P (1975) Skeletal growth and development of achondroplastic mice. *Growth* **39**: 17–33.
68. Seegmiller R, Fraser F C and Sheldon H (1971) A new chondrodystrophic mutant in mice. Electron microscopy of normal and abnormal chondrogenesis. *J Cell Biol* **48**: 580–93.
69. Ponseti I V (1970) Skeletal growth in achondroplasia. *J Bone Joint Surg [Am]* **52**: 701–16.
70. Smeets T and Van Buul-Offers S (1983) A morphological study of the development of the tibial proximal epiphysis and growth plate of normal and dwarfed Snell mice. *Growth* **47**: 145–59.
71. Johnson D R (1984) The ultrastructure of mandibular condylar and rib cartilage from mice carrying the spondylo-metaphyseal chondrodysplasia gene. *J Anat* **138**: 463–70.
72. Thurston M N, Johnson D R, Kember N F and Moore W J (1983) Cell kinetics of growth cartilage in stumpy: a new chondrodystrophic mutant in the mouse. *J Anat* **136**: 407–15.
73. Johnson D R (1977) Ultrastructural observations on stumpy (*stm*) a new chondrodystrophic mutant in the mouse. *J Embryol Exp Morphol* **39**: 279–84.
74. Thurston M N, Johnson D R and Kember N F (1985) Cell kinetics of growth cartilage of achondroplastic (*cn*) mice. *J Anat* **140**: 425–34.
75. Thurston M N, Johnson D R and Kember N F (1985) Cell kinetics of growth cartilage in spondylo-metaphyseal chondrodysplasia (*smc*) mice. *J Anat* **140**: 435–45.
76. Landaur W (1965) Nanomelia, a lethal mutation of the fowl. *J Hered* **56**: 131–8.
77. Mathews M B (1967) Chondroitin sulphate and collagen in inherited skeletal defects of chickens. *Nature (London)* **213**: 1255–6.
78. Fraser R A and Goetinck P F (1971) Reduced synthesis of chondroitin sulfate by cartilage from the mutant nanomelia. *Biochem Biophys Res Comm* **43**: 494–503.
79. Argraves W S, McKeown-Longo P J and Goetinck P F (1981) Absence of proteoglycan core protein in the cartilage mutant nanomelia. *FEBS Lett* **132**: 265–8.
80. Rittenhouse E, Dunn L C, Cookingham J, Calo C, Spiegelman M, Dooher G B and Bennett D (1978) Cartilage matrix deficiency (*cmd*), a new autosomal recessive lethal mutation in the mouse. *J Embryol Exp Morphol* **43**: 71–84.
81. Kimata K, Barrach H J, Brown K S and Pennypacker J P (1981) Absence of proteoglycan core protein in cartilage from *cmd/cmd* (cartilage matrix deficiency) mouse. *J Biol Chem* **256**: 6961–8.
82. Walker B A, Scott C I, Hall J G, Murdoch J L and McKusick V A (1972) Diastrophic dwarfism. *Medicine (Baltimore)* **51**: 41–59.
83. Miller W A and Flynn-Miller K L (1976) Achondroplastic, brachymorphic and stubby chondrodystrophies in mouse. *J Comp Pathol* **86**: 349–64.
84. Orkin R W, Pratt R M and Martin G M (1976) Undersulphated chondroitin sulphate in cartilage matrix of brachymorphic mice. *Dev Biol* **50**: 82–94.
85. Sugahara K and Schwartz N B (1979) Defect in 3' phosphoadenosine 5' phosphosulphate formation in brachymorphic mice. *Proc Natl Acad Sci USA* **76**: 6615–81.
86. Schwartz N B, Belch J, Henry J, Hupert J and Sugahara K (1982) Enzyme defect in PAPS synthesis of brachymorphic mice. *Fed Proc* **41**: 852.
87. Brown W H and Pearce L (1945) Hereditary achondroplasia in the rabbit. I. Physical appearance and general features. *J Exp Med* **82**: 241–61.
88. Pearce L and Brown W H (1945) Hereditary achondroplasia in the rabbit. II. Pathological aspects. *J Exp Med* **82**: 261–80.
89. Pearce L and Brown W H (1945) Hereditary achondroplasia in the rabbit. III. Genetic aspects: general conclusions. *J Exp Med* **82**: 281–95.
90. Shepard T H, Fry L R and Moffett B C (1969) Microscopic studies of achondroplastic rabbit cartilage. *Teratology* **2**: 13–22.
91. Shepard T H and Bass G L (1971) Organ culture studies of achondroplastic rabbit cartilage:

92. Bargman G J, Mackler B and Shepard T H (1972) Studies of oxidative energy deficiency. I. Achondroplasia in the rabbit. *Arch Biochem Biophys* **150**: 137–46.
93. Mackler B, Haynes B, Inamadar A R, Pedeyana L R, Hall J G and Cohen M M Jr (1973) Oxidative energy deficiency. II. Human achondroplasia. *Arch Biochem Biophys* **159**: 885–8.
94. Mackler B, Grace R, Davis K A, Shepard T H and Hall J G (1986) Studies of human achondroplasia: oxidative metabolism in tissue culture cells. *Teratology* **33**: 9–13.
95. Maynard J A, Ippolito E G, Ponseti I V and Mickelson M R (1981) Histochemistry and ultrastructure of the growth plate in achondroplasia. *J Bone Joint Surg [Am]* **63**: 969–79.
96. McDevitt C A and Muir H (1976) Biochemical changes in the cartilage of the knee in experimental and natural osteoarthritis in the dog. *J Bone Joint Surg [Br]* **58**: 94–101.
97. Mankin H J and Lippiello L (1970) Biochemical and metabolic abnormalities in articular cartilage from osteo-arthritic human hips. *J Bone Joint Surg [Am]* **52**: 424–33.
98. Stephens T D and Seegmiller R E (1976) Normal production of cartilage glycosaminoglycan in mice homozygous for the chondrodysplasia gene. *Teratology* **133**: 317–26.
99. Seegmiller R E, Myers R A , Dorfman A and Horowitz A L (1981) Structural and associative properties of cartilage matrix constituents in mice with hereditary chondrodysplasia (*cho*). *Connect Tissue Res* **9**: 69–77.
100. Goetinck P F (1983) Mutations affecting limb cartilage. *In: Cartilage, Vol. 3. Biomedical Aspects* (B K Hall, ed), pp. 165–89. New York: Academic Press.
101. Brown K S, Cranley R E, Greene R, Kleinman H K and Pennypacker J P (1981) Disproportionate micromelia (*Dmm*), an incomplete dominant mouse dwarfism with abnormal cartilage matrix. *J Embryol Exp Morphol* **62**: 165–82.
102. Johnson D R and Wise J M (1971) Cartilage anomaly (*can*) a new mutant gene in the mouse. *J Embryol Exp Morphol* **25**: 21–31.
103. Johnson D R and Hunt D M (1974) Biochemical observations on the cartilage of achondroplastic (*can*) mice. *J Embryol Exp Morphol* **31**: 319–28.
104. Hinchliffe J R and Johnson D R (1983) Growth of Cartilage. *In: Cartilage, Vol. 2. Development, Differentiation, and Growth* (B K Hall, ed), pp. 255–95. New York: Academic Press.

Chapter 10

Adaptation and Remodelling of Articular Cartilage and Bone Tissue

I. V. Knets

CONTENTS

INTRODUCTION
ARTICULAR CARTILAGE
CANCELLOUS BONE
COMPACT BONE

CONCLUSIONS
PRACTICAL SIGNIFICANCE
REFERENCES

INTRODUCTION

The mechanical behaviour of the biological tissue of synovial joints – the articular cartilage, cancellous and compact bone – depends significantly upon the conditions of its loading and changes with age. Moreover, the mechanical behaviour has to be analysed in a complex way taking into account that the tissue and the interstital fluid in cartilage form a united system. This chapter is a survey of investigations devoted to the determination of adaptational peculiarities of the structure and mechanical behaviour of articular cartilage and bone, and to the analyses of remodelling under the influence of different factors, especially those of mechanical loads.

ARTICULAR CARTILAGE

The articular cartilage of synovial joints has a specific 4-layered structure which ensures its unique mechanical and metabolic behaviour. Cartilage is a composite material with collagen fibres as reinforcement, cartilage cells (chondrocytes) and proteoglycans as a matrix. The 'pores' in cartilage which occupy about 60–80% of the entire volume are filled with interstitial fluid in the unloaded state.

The upper, so-called superficial, layer of cartilage is composed mainly of thin collagen fibres (with a diameter of about 35 nm) oriented along the outer contact surface of the joint. Its thickness is about 10% of the cartilage thickness. The load-bearing ability of the whole cartilage depends largely upon the integrity of this layer, which fulfils the function of a biomechanical protecting membrane. The metabolic activity of the chondrocytes in this layer is probably insignificant.

The middle layer is composed of randomly oriented collagen fibres (with a diameter of about 60 nm) and small chondrocytes embedded in the proteoglycan matrix. In the third or deep layer there are the same components, but collagen fibres (with a diameter of about 80 nm) are oriented mainly perpendicularily to the joint's surface and the chondrocytes, which are larger in size, form columns oriented in the same direction. In these 2 layers chondrocytes are metabolically active and play a significant role in the natural remodelling of articular cartilage. The cartilage cells are covered with a net of collagen fibres and form indpendent structural elements. As the collagen fibres in cartilage are stronger than collagen fibres of many other biological tissues such as blood vessels and bone, these reinforced chondrocytes partly fulfil the function of dampening dynamic excitations in the cartilage.

It is known that mechanical stresses and strains stimulate the process of cartilage remodelling by increasing the activity of chondrocytes in their synthesis of proteins, both of collagen and of proteoglycans. However, excessive compressive strains in cartilage can cause serious disturbances in the activity of chondrocytes. For example, strain of 25% causes the death of chondrocytes in the superficial layer, but strain of 50% results in the total death of the chondrocyte population over the whole thickness of the cartilage (1).

The fourth and deepest layer of cartilage is the calcified cartilage. It fulfils two functions: joining together the cartilage and the subchondral bone, and providing growth and remodelling of underlying bone tissue. Large collagen fibres become interlaced in this layer and join the cartilage to the bone. In the calcified layer, which has a thickness of about 10% of the whole thickness of the cartilage, there is a basophilic sheet called 'tidemark' which separates the uncalcified cartilage from the calcified layer. The thickness of the calcified layer decreases with age, but the number of tidemarks increases, particularly over the age of 60 (2). The remodelling and growth of the underlying bone tissue is ensured by the penetration of blood capillaries from subchondral bone into the calcified layer, which stimulates further cartilage calcification. However, the intensity of this process decreases with age.

Investigations of the mechanical behaviour of articular cartilage has been carried out by many scientists, but the values for the mechanical properties determined by them differ rather significantly. This may be explained by the fact that articular cartilage is extremely complicated from the standpoint of material mechanics – it may be considered as a multilayered, heterogeneous, anisotropic, physically non-linear, viscoelastic, 2-phase and porous solid. For example, the stiffness value of articular cartilage in compression depends on the structure of the loading plates. This is because of the fact that normal articular cartilage is saturated by interstitial fluid and its behaviour during compression will depend upon fluid loss. If the cartilage is compressed between two non-porous plates by a pressure of 0·6 MPa, the displacement after 2 min will be 4 times less than the value that could be reached by compressing it between porous plates (3). In the latter case, the large deformation is due to the penetration of interstitial fluid into the pores of the loading plates. It must be noted that after loading the cartilage with fluid squeezed out will return to its initial undeformed state only if the cartilage is placed in a fluid bath.

All this leads to different values for the elastic characteristics of cartilage determined under different test conditions. So, the value of the modulus of elasticity varies from 2 to 15 MPa (in some publications there are even values up to 160 MPa), the value of the shear modulus from 1 to 4 MPa and the value of

Poisson's ratio from 0·4 to 0·49. However, these are the average values of elastic characteristics only. Because of the lack of uniformity of *in vivo* loading conditions, the cartilage in fact has topographical differences in stiffness. In femur, the stiffest cartilage is located in a band which extends from the superior surface of the head around to the anterior and posterior aspects, while the softest cartilage is situated near the fovea (4). There is also a non-uniform distribution of the stiffness over different layers of cartilage. The highest modulus of elasticity in tension is in the superficial layer along the direction of collagen fibres (5). With an increase in the distance from the cartilage surface, i.e. in the middle and deep layers, the stiffness decreases. It becomes almost independent of the direction of loading in the deep layer of cartilage.

There is a complex reaction of collagen fibres, matrix and interstitial fluid in articular cartilage subjected to loading. Collagen fibres restrict the proteoglycans' ability to saturate with water and therefore prevent their swelling. Under a compressing load acting on the joint surface, the water of proteoglycans is squeezed out from the regions of high pressure. Since a net of collagen fibres resists such a process, high tensile stresses may appear in these fibres. Therefore, it is important to investigate not only the stiffness but also the strength of cartilage. It has been determined (6) that the tensile strengths of the cartilage of human femoral condyles along and across the direction of collagen fibres in the superficial layer are 26 and 10 MPa respectively, but the ultimate strains are 25% and 39%. In the deep layer the values of ultimate stresses decrease (17 and 7·5 MPa, respectively), but values of strains increase (85% and 120%).

The experimental investigation of the stress–strain state of cartilage and underlying bone is a very complicated technical problem. Therefore, different mathematical models have been developed to numerically analyse the different peculiarities of the mechanical behaviour of articular cartilage. There is an interesting analysis of the stress–strain state of articular cartilage under loading (7).

It was assumed that an axisymmetric compressive load acting on the cartilage has a parabolic distribution over the circular area (diameter = 2a). Two different cases with respect to the elastic properties of material were analysed. In the first case, the articular cartilage was assumed to be isotropic ($E = 12$ MPa), with the modulus of elasticity of the subchondral bone much higher, 300 MPa. In the second case, the superficial layer of articular cartilage was taken as transversely isotropic (the modulus of elasticity along the surface 30 MPa, that perpendicular to the surface 12 MPa). It was shown that when the ratio of loaded area radius (a) to the thickness of cartilage (d) = 5 (i.e. a:d = 5), only radial compressive stresses will appear in the superficial layer of articular cartilage. At the same time, the radial strain may change its sign. If in the centre of the loaded area there is maximum tensile strain, then with the increase of distance from the centre the strain will decrease and will become compressive, reaching its maximum near the periphery of the loaded area.

If the ratio a:d = 1, i.e. the load is applied over a small area of the cartilage surface, then the radial stress in the centre of the loaded area will be compressive again, but it will decrease rapidly and will become tensile, with the maximum occurring at the border of the loaded area. The radial strain below the load will be tensile with non-uniform distribution. Behind the loaded area, it decreases gradually and becomes compressive. The general conclusions of this investigation are that the soft cartilage lying on the much stiffer bone foundation provides no harmful tensile stresses to the superficial layer of cartilage under normal physiological loading and strain concentration in the cartilage. In cyclic loading, which takes place during normal human motion, tensile and compressive stresses appear in cartilage. These stresses could be the more obvious cause of degenerative cartilage changes with age rather than local fracture sites caused by the appearance of large tensile stresses.

Some investigations (5, 8, 9) show that the articular cartilage has a low tendency for cellular and matrix repair. Local cartilage destruction does not regenerate quickly and therefore must be considered a serious injury which may cause degeneration of the whole joint. The reason for the initiation of cartilage destruction may be long-term loading or forced immobilization (10).

The investigation of the viscoelastic behaviour of cartilage has a significant practical meaning. It has been determined that the character of the stress–strain curves of the superficial layer in tension depends upon the strain rate $\dot{\varepsilon}$ (11). In the initial stage of deformation the increase of $\dot{\varepsilon}$ causes the increase of stiffness, but, in the region of high strains (40–60%), the modulus of elasticity stays practically constant. However, an increase of $\dot{\varepsilon}$ leads to an increase in the stress level over the whole region of deformation at fixed strain values.

The consideration of cartilage as a 2-phase, permeable material allows us to analyse the processes of strain creep and stress relaxation in more detail (12–16). It was determined that cartilage treatment with trypsin, which decreases the content of proteoglycans, causes a significant increase in both strain creep and stress relaxation (17). Treatment with leucocytic elastase acting on the collagen structure of cartilage causes a decrease in strength characteristics. Thus, placing articular cartilage from the human femoral head in elastase of a given concentration during a 72 h period leads to a 37% decrease of ultimate tensile stress and a 22% decrease in stiffness at the stress level of 1 MPa (18). Increasing the concentration of the NaCl solution in which the specimens of articular cartilage were immersed caused anisotropic and heterogeneous decreases of their dimensions (19). The largest change took place in the transverse direction, i.e. over the thickness of the cartilage, while the smallest change took place along the orientation of collagen fibres in the superficial layer. The relationship between the concentration of NaCl solution and the decrease of cartilage dimensions along the direction of collagen fibres is linear and its intensity decreases with the increase of the distance from the cartilage surface.

This shows that the articular cartilage has a geometric non-uniformity and both a heterogeneity and an anisotropy of mechanical properties. These are the main factors affecting the adaptation of cartilage to physiological loads and providing it with a high working efficiency at load transfer and keeping the coefficient of friction between joint surfaces low (0·005–0·012). However, such an adaptation may be disturbed not only by overloading but also by normal ageing. Cartilage becomes less heterogeneous and anisotropic with age, and more fluid permeable, decreasing its working ability.

Since the structural components of articular cartilage have different metabolic activities, they become subjected to a different number of loading cycles during their lifetime. Therefore, it is important to investigate the behaviour of cartilage under long-term cyclic loading at different ages. The cyclic loading of articular cartilage *in vivo* has shown (20) that there can be some fibrillation of cartilage and loss of proteoglycans. The loading of cartilage specimens from the human femoral head at age 20–81 has revealed that the increase of applied cyclic stress magnitude leads to the decrease of the number of cycles to fatigue failure (21). This process increases with age. Mathematical analysis of the experimental results allows us to determine the relationship between the number of cycles to failure and age and cyclic stress magnitude. It shows that fatigue characteristics of cartilage decrease with age in such a manner that fatigue failure may already occur at age 50–60. So, articular cartilage at age 70 loaded by a cyclic tensile stress of 2 MPa will have a fatigue failure after 35×10^6 cycles. If we consider that the human cartilage during a year undergoes 1 million loading cycles on the average, then the fatigue fracture of the cartilage of this individual may occur after 35 years. But the risk of fatigue failure becomes more evident if the cartilage is subjected to a higher cyclic stress level. For instance, the articular cartilage of a person at age 50 loaded by a cyclic stress of 5 MPa will have a fatigue failure after only 10×10^6 cycles, i.e. after 10 years. However, it should be mentioned that these results are obtained on the basis of experiments *in vitro*. Certainly, the living tissue may be protected from fatigue by metabolic turnover which will increase resistance to fatigue failure.

CANCELLOUS BONE

The cancellous bone tissue of the epiphysis of long bones functions as a shock absorber of different dynamic loads acting on the joint and to transfer the load to the compact bone tissue. However, the structure of this tissue and the peculiarities of its remodelling under load has attracted the attention not only of biomechanicists and medical doctors, but also architects and engineers. The unique construction of this tissue allows us to view different possibilities for creating optimum forms of man-made structures.

During the development of cancellous bone tissue, primary and secondary structures can be distinguished. The primary cancellous bone is formed during remodelling of cartilage whose cells are replaced by connective tissue rich in blood vessels. These vessels penetrate the cartilage and form calcified plates which strengthen the tissue mechanically. The secondary cancellous bone has a spatial structure whose frame is formed from the calcified columns and/or plates. These columns and plates, also called trabeculae, are formed from thin lamellae joined together in the transverse direction by collagen fibres. In the trabeculae there are no Haversian canals, yet there is a large number of small canaliculi (in 1 mm^3 of cancellous bone there are about 1 million canaliculi). The spaces between trabeculae are filled with blood, yellow and red marrow, nerves, blood vessels, cells and intercellular fluid.

The investigation of bone remodelling began from the study of cancellous bone tissue. The well known Wolff's law, which was postulated more than 100 years ago, states that when the loads on a bone are changed the functional remodelling reorientates the trabeculae so that they align with the new trajectories of principal stresses. The experimental verification of this law and its mathematical description was carried out by many researchers. From the most interesting survey papers of recent years, the publications of Pugh *et al.* (22), Hayes and Snyder (23), Regirer and Stein (24) and Cowin (25) must be noted.

The mechanical properties of cancellous bone tissue depend upon its structure and density (26). The increase in density is connected with the accumulation of bone tissue in the structural elements, changing it from the column system to a system of interconnecting plates. Such a process of remodelling is stimulated by the action of external loads. The column system of low density cancellous bone is located in those regions of bone which are subjected to the smaller loads. Conversely, the system of plates having a higher density is located in regions where the largest loads are acting.

The stress–strain curve of cancellous bone in compression is typical for porous materials and depends significantly upon its density (27). An increase in density leads to an increase in both the stiffness and the strength of the tissue. In asymmetric loading the cancellous bone acquires an asymmetric structure too (28). The stress–strain curves in compression and tension differ significantly. The modulus of elasticity in compression varies widely depending upon different factors: type of bone, location and orientation of the specimen in bone, age, etc., but it is always less than the modulus of elasticity in tension.

The results of the investigation of cancellous bone strength are contradictory. Some publications (29–31) show that strength in tension and compression is practically one and the same. However, Kaplan *et al.* (32) have demonstrated that specimens of bovine cancellous bone tissue from the proximal humerus cut out perpendicularly to the long axis of bone have higher strengths in compression ($12 \cdot 4 \pm 3 \cdot 2$ MPa) than in tension ($7 \cdot 6 \pm 2 \cdot 2$ MPa).

The distribution of elastic and strength characteristics of cancellous bone tissue over the volume of bone is non-uniform, and the character of anisotropy of these properties (33) also changes. The survey of some investigations devoted to the determination of this lack of uniformity is presented in (34). Investigation of Brinnel's hardness of the cancellous bone tissue of the femoral head has shown that directly below the cartilage, bone hardness is 8–9 MPa, at a depth of 3–5 mm from the surface it decreases to 2–4 MPa, but in the centre of the head it reaches its maximum, 10–11 MPa (35).

The reaction of this tissue to cyclic loading is also non-uniform. The investigation of the deformation of the femoral head under cyclic compressive loading in the range of frequencies 1–100 Hz has revealed that tissue in the upper part of the head, which is subjected to large loads during a lifetime, is much stiffer than in the lower hemisphere (36). The long-term exposure of knee joints to cyclic loading *in vivo* has shown that subchondral bone starts to increase in stiffness after 3–5 days of loading (20, 37). Such a phenomenon, not understandable at first, is explained by the accumulation of microfractures in the trabeculae causing an intensive process of remodelling and trabecular healing. However, after more prolonged loading (3 weeks) when the distinct degeneration of articular cartilage is seen, the stiffness of subchondral bone decreases to its initial value.

The stress–strain state in the femoral head has been investigated by mathematical modelling using the finite elements method (38–42). For example, it has been determined that the presence of necrosis zones in cancellous bone causes redistribution of stresses in the femoral head (40). The bone tissue next to the necrosis site starts to work more intensively. It is assumed that the possible fracture of subchondral bone may take place because of large compressive hoop stresses arising during such remodelling. The distribution of pressure along the acetabulum caused by contact with the femoral head depends on the configuration of subchondral bone and the thickness of articular cartilage (43).

There is a significant influence of age on the adaptation and remodelling of cancellous bone caused by load. It has been determined that if, for a young man, an increase of physical activity causes an increase in both the stiffness and strength of the bone, then for an old man it may cause, conversely, a decrease in these characteristics (44). If we compare the bone tissue of young and old individuals we can see that both the stiffness and the strength decrease with age. In senility, with the attendant decrease of metabolic activity, it is especially dangerous to become subjected to long-term, high stress, cyclic loading because overloaded and partly fractured trabeculae are unable to remodel.

COMPACT BONE

Compact bone tissue is the main load-bearing component of long tubular bones. It represents a specific form of connective tissue with calcified intercellular substance. This tissue is a self-regulating system which reacts to changes in the stress–strain state, nutrition and biochemical content.

The main structural components of bone tissue are lamellae formed by collagen fibres of a particular orientation and interconnected by a proteoglycan matrix. The bone lamellae may form two structures, lamellae and osteons. In the lamellar structure the lamellae with different orientations of collagen fibres are tightly adjoined together and envelop the tubular bone circularly. In the osteon structure the thin cylindrical lamellae (with thickness of about 5–7 μm) form layered cylinders with diameters of about $0\cdot2$ mm, called osteons. In the centre of each osteon there is an Haversian canal through which the nutrition of bone tissue is ensured. The bone cells are located between lamellae and they are responsible for bone remodelling.

The mechanical properties of the tissue of different bones have been investigated by many researchers. The main results of those investigations are presented in several surveys (34, 45–48).

The distribution of different characteristics of mechanical properties over the volume of bones is non-uniform. This non-uniformity is one of the principal factors accounting for bone's ability to become adapted to external mechanical load and to ensure optimum working conditions. Thus, this lack of uniformity, together with the anisotropy of bone tissue, allows the increased blood supply, e.g. in the tibia under cyclic loading arising during normal walking (34, 49, 50). The distribution of ultimate shear stress τ_1^* and ultimate shear strain γ_{12}^* determined by torsion of specimens cut out along the longitudinal axis of the tibia from 6 zones of its cross-section (3 corner zones and 3 intercorner zones) is also specific (34). The highest value of τ_1^* is seen in the bone tissue in the medial and posterior intercorner zones. As the tibia has an almost triangular form in cross-section, during torsion of the whole bone with respect to its longitudinal axis, maximal shear stresses will arise precisely in the intercorner zones. However, the possibility of overloading these zones is compensated for not only by an increase of material strength in these zones, but also by much smaller shear modulus than in the corner zones. This leads to the smoothing of the bone strain state which indicates a good bone adaptation ability to mechanical loads.

The change of structure and mechanical properties of the bone tissue with age is also specific; there is an increase in the degree of calcification of osteons, a decrease of osteon dimensions but an increase in their number, a penetration of osteons into the region of lamellar bone, an increase of the cross-sectional area of Haversian canals located near the medullary cavity, a filling of old Haversian canals by inorganic substances, an increase in the size of bone crystals, a decrease of ultimate stress and strain and a decrease of bone stiffness. There is not only a change in their magnitude, but also in the anisotropy of elastic and strength properties, and the heterogeneity of structure and mechanical properties over zones of bone cross-section.

An interesting example is the character of the change with age of shear modulus G_{12} responsible for torsion stiffness with respect to the longitudinal axis over zones of human tibia cross-section (34). If the largest value of G_{12} in age group IV (19–44 years) is in the posterior-medial corner zone and in age group V (45–59 years) it does not change its location, then in age groups VI (60–74 years) and VII (75–89 years) it consecutively transfers clockwise to the posterior lateral and anterior corner zones. At the same time, the minimum value of G_{12} over the cross-section is located in the intercorner zone next to the zone where G_{12} is maximal. Thus, in age group IV, for example, minimum G_{12} is in the medial intercorner zone, in age group V it transfers to the posterior zone, but in age groups VI and VII it stays in the lateral zone. Both the average value over the cross-section and the maximum value of G_{12} decrease with age. At the same time, the heterogeneity of G_{12} over the cross-section decreases and, subsequently, decreases the ability of old bones to carry the load effectively.

Such a specific character in the change of G_{12} may be explained by a more intensive remodelling of bone tissue in corner zones. If, at a young age, the bone is able to remodel, then with ageing its activity decreases, the bone becomes more porous and unable to repair itself. This causes a marked decrease of G_{12} in the more loaded corner zone compared with other zones, thus leading to the transfer of maximum G_{12} from one corner zone to the other.

The increase of age also causes some decrease of the bone's ability to carry dynamic loads (51). It has been shown that impact energy absorption of human bone tissue at the age range of 3–90 years decreases almost 3 times. This behaviour is explained by the increased calcification and porosity of bone tissue.

The complex investigation of the viscoelastic properties of compact bone at different strain rates in cyclic loading and during creep testing has shown that the specific peculiarity of this material is a significant increase of ultimate specific energy of deformation in the range of strain rates corresponding to the normal physiological conditions of functioning (52). The magnitude of strain in these experiments depends primarily on the age of the samples, location of specimens in the bone, moisture of bone tissue and moisture conditions of testing. Thus, for example, the non-uniformity of creep properties over zones of tibia cross-section practically disappear after age 50. This result once again indicates that there is a decrease of rheological adaptation of bone to the loads with age. The change of bone moisture significantly affects its character of fracture (53–55).

The questions of growth, resorption and reinforcement in bone remodelling have been investigated both theoretically and experimentally. The more significant contribution to the theoretical analysis of surface and internal remodelling is given by Cowin and his co-authors (48, 58–64). A detailed review of the investigations of these questions is also given by Regirer and Stein (24).

The main cause for the reaction of biological tissue to the changes of loading conditions is considered to be piezoelectricity and alterations of calcium ion content. One of the first models connecting remodelling of bone tissue with piezoelectricity was proposed by Gjelsvik (56, 57) and was based on four assumptions:

1. The signal for surface remodelling is the piezoelectric polarization vector normal to the surface.
2. The material symmetry direction of new bone deposited follows the direction of the bone on which it is growing.
3. A new surface bone is deposited so that no residual stresses result.
4. The material symmetry directions try to keep aligned with the time average of the principal stress directions in the bone.

Fatigue microfractures are also considered as one of the stimulators of compact bone remodelling (65–69). Their development in bone is restricted to some degree by the lamellar structure of osteons stopping the fracture at the interfaces between the lamellae. The appearance of a fatigue microfracture in the osteon causes a change in its stress state and stimulates the forming of a new, secondary osteon in the fracture's pathway. If such a remodelling, i.e. healing of the microfracture, takes place before the fracture reaches its critical length, then the fatigue fracture of material is delayed and the bone has become even more dense, more load resistant.

The experimental accumulation of a sufficient amount of microfractures to start bone remodelling at a relatively small number of loading cycles indicates that even normal physical activity during a few days will accumulate a sufficient number of microfractures, so that their healing becomes significant for retaining the mechanical unity of the bone (69). The formed bone resorption sites are associated with microfractures 44 times more often than expected by chance alone.

However, it is necessary to mention that some believe that other factors of loading history could cause bone remodelling. Such factors could be the maximum value of applied strain, the amplitude of cyclic strain, the amplitude of only those strains which cause microfractures, the strain rate, the average value of load applied during the day, etc.

During the loading of bone tissue by specific loads, it is important to take into account the influence of age peculiarities on the process of remodelling (70, 71). For example, in experiments with animals kept under conditions of hypokinesis and hypodynamia it was found that, for older animals, hypodynamia causes a decrease in femoral external diameter at the almost constant diameter of the medullary cavity. For young animals, both hypokinesis and hypodynamia cause an increase in the diameter of medullary cavity at the constant external diameter of femur.

CONCLUSIONS

The disturbance of the equilibrium of articular cartilage and bone tissue can be provoked in two ways. First, the stress–strain state in the articular cartilage may change because of alterations in the loading conditions of the joint. If such alterations have a long-term character, then there will be a gradual change both in the structure and the mechanical properties not only of articular cartilage, but also of underlying structural components of the system - the cancellous and compact bones. Second, changes in structural and mechanical properties may be caused by alterations in the biochemical composition of articular cartilage. This alteration will change the cartilage's stress–strain state with all its ensuing consequences. Certainly in such a system the opposite reaction may exist too, i.e. changes in bone tissue lead to alterations both in the stress–strain state and the mechanical properties of articular cartilage.

All these changes are connected with the ability of biological tissue to adapt to mechanical loading and to undergo remodelling. If adaptation of the tissue to loading is already determined by its initial geometric shape and dimensions, by a lack of non-uniformity in the distribution of mechanical properties over different regions of the bone or cartilage, and by the anisotropy and physical nonlinearity of continuum, then remodelling takes place during the individual's lifetime under the influence of different factors, including mechanical ones. Such remodelling may be both surface remodelling, when the geometric shape and dimensions of bone or cartilage change, or internal remodelling, when the mechanical properties of the material undergo some changes.

PRACTICAL SIGNIFICANCE

The investigation of the process of adaptation of articular cartilage and bone to physiological mechanical loads and their remodelling due to changes in loading conditions has practical significance. It consists of the following:

1. The relationship between structure and mechanical behaviour of biological tissue is determined. It allows us to understand the mechanical principles of normal functioning and to evaluate the degree of injury caused by possible deviations from the normal conditions.
2. The possibility of determining optimum conditions of mechanical loading of biological tissue which gives the best improvement of long-term working ability.
3. The character of the changes with age in the functional adaptation of biological tissue to mechanical loading is analysed and the peculiarities of remodelling under long-term constant or cyclic loading are determined.
4. Criteria for new artificial materials used for replacement of damaged biological tissue which cause minimum stress concentration at the interfaces between natural and artifical materials are determined from the point of view of biomechanics.
5. New mathematical models of solids with more complex properties are developed, e.g. a model for a solid with internal degrees of freedom and finite deformation which allows one to investigate the mechanical behaviour in close relation with different physical and chemical processes proceeding in the material.

REFERENCES

1. Finley J B and Repo R U (1976) Controlled impact testing of living articular cartilage. *Proceedings of 4th New England Bioengineering Conference, New Haven*, pp. 69–71.

2. Lane L B and Bullough P G (1980) Age-related changes in the thickness of the calcified zone and the number of tidemarks in adult human articular cartilage. *J Bone Joint Surg [Br]* **62**: 372–5.
3. McCutchen C W (1962) The frictional properties of animal joints. *Wear* **5**: 1–17.
4. Kempson G E, Spivey C J, Swanson S A V and Freeman M A R (1971) Patterns of cartilage stiffness on normal and degenerate human femoral heads. *J Biomech* **4**: 597–610.
5. Woo S L-Y, Akeson W H and Jemmott G F (1976) Measurements of nonhomogeneous directional mechanical properties of articular cartilage in tension. *J Biomech* **9**: 785–91.
6. Kempson G E, Muir H, Pollard C and Tuke M (1973) The tensile properties of the cartilage of human femoral condyles related to the content of collagen and glycosaminoglycans. *Biochem Biophys Acta* **297**: 456–72.
7. Askew M J and Mow V C (1978) The biomechanical function of the collagen fibril ultrastructure of articular cartilage. *J Biomech Eng* **100**: 105–15.
8. Mankin H J (1974) The reaction of articular cartilage to injury and osteoarthritis. *N Engl J Med* **291**: 1285–92.
9. Frankel V H and Nordin M (1980) *Basic Biomechanics of the Skeletal System*. Philadelphia: Lea & Febiger.
10. Salter R B and Field P (1960) The effect of continuous compression on living articular cartilage. *J Bone Joint Surg [Am]* **42**: 31–49.
11. Li J T, Armstrong C G and Mow V C (1983) The effect of strain rate on mechanical properties of articular cartilage in tension. *In: 1983 Biomechanics Symposium*, pp. 117–20. New York: ASME United Engineering Center.
12. Mow V C and Lai W M (1979) Selected unresolved problems in synovial joint biomechanics *In: 1979 Biomechanics Symposium*, pp. 19–52. New York: ASME United Engineering Center.
13. Mow V C and Lai W M (1979) Mechanics of animal joints. *Ann Rev Fluid Mech* **11**: 247–88.
14. Mow V C, Kuei S C, Lai W M and Armstrong C G (1980) Biphasic creep and stress relaxation of articular cartilage in compression: theory and experiments. *J Biomech Eng* **102**: 73–84.
15. Armstrong C G, Lai W M and Mow V C (1981) Unconfined compression of articular cartilage. *In: 1981 Biomechanics Symposium*, pp. 133–6. New York: ASME United Engineering Center.
16. Simon B R, Coats R S and Woo S L-Y (1984) Relaxation and creep quasilinear viscoelastic models for normal articular cartilage. *J Biomech Eng* **106**: 159–64.
17. Stahurski T M, Armstrong C G and Mow V C (1981) Variation of the intrinsic aggregate modulus and permeability of articular cartilage with trypsin digestion. *In: 1981 Biomechanics Symposium*, pp. 137–40. New York: ASME United Engineering Center.
18. Kempson G E (1981) The effects of leucocytic elastase on the tensile properties of adult human articular cartilage. *In: 1981 Biomechanics Symposium*, pp. 141–4. New York: ASME United Engineering Center.
19. Myers E R, Lai W M and Mow V C (1984) A continuum theory and an experiment for the ion-induced swelling behaviour of articular cartilage. *J Biomech Eng* **106**: 151–8.
20. Radin E L, Parker H G, Pugh J W, Steinberg R S, Paul I L and Rose R M (1973) Response of joints to impact loading. III: Relationship between trabecular microfractures and cartilage degeneration. *J Biomech* **6**: 51–7.
21. Weightman B (1976) Tensile fatigue of human cartilage. *J Biomech* **9**: 193–200.
22. Pugh J W, Rose R M and Radin E L (1973) A possible mechanism of Wolff's law: trabecular microfracture. *Arch Int Physiol Biochem* **81**: 27–40.
23. Hayes W C and Snyder B (1981) Toward a quantitative formulation of Wolff's law in trabecular bone. *In: Mechanical Properties of Bone*, pp. 43–68. New York: ASME United Engineering Center.
24. Regirer S A and Stein A A (1985) Application of continuum mechanics methods to problems of living tissue growth and development. *In: Modern Problems of Biomechanics, Vol 2. Mechanics of Biological Tissue*. Riga: Zinatne (in Russian).
25. Cowin S C (1986) Wolff's law of trabecular architecture at remodelling equilibrium. *J Biomech Eng* **108**: 83–8.
26. Pugh J W, Rose R M and Radin E L (1973) Elastic and viscoelastic properties of trabecular bone. Dependence on structure. *J Biomech* **6**: 657–70.
27. Hayes W C and Carter D R (1976) Post-yield behaviour of subchondral trabecular bone. *J Biomed Res Symp* **7**: 537–44.
28. Gibson L J (1985) The mechanical behaviour of cancellous bone. *J Biomech* **18**: 317–28.
29. Carter D R, Schwab G H and Spengler D M (1980) Tensile fracture of trabecular bone. *Acta Orthop Scand* **51**: 733–41.
30. Bensusan J S, Davy D T, Heiple K G and Verdin P J (1983) Tensile, compressive and torsional testing of cancellous bone. *Trans Orthop Res Soc* **8**: 132.

31. Neil J L, Demas T C, Stone J L and Hayes W C (1983) Tensile and compression properties of vertebral trabecular bone. *Trans Orthop Res Soc* **8**: 344.
32. Kaplan S J, Hayes W C and Stone J L (1985) Tensile strength of bovine trabecular bone. *J Biomech* **18**: 723–7.
33. Saha S, Pal S and Rao V (1981) Anisotropic nature of the ultrasonic characteristics of cancellous bone. In: *1981 Biomechanics Symposium*, pp. 279–82. New York: ASME United Engineering Center.
34. Knets I V, Pfafrod G O and Saulgozis J Z (1980) *Deformation and fracture of hard biological tissue*. Riga: Zinatne (in Russian).
35. Shargorodski V S and Kresnij D I (1983) The mechanical properties of femoral head and the peculiarities of its loading depending upon the changes of the form of femur proximal end. *Proceedings of 3rd USSR Conference on the Problems of Biomechanics*, Vol 1, pp. 196–7. Riga (in Russian).
36. Miganaga Y, Tateishi T and Shirasaki Y (1976) The viscoelastic properties and strength of healthy and pathological cancellous bones. *Proceedings of 19th Japanese Congress on Materials Research: Non-metallic Materials*, pp. 238–43. Kyoto University.
37. Simon S R, Radin E L, Paul I L and Rose R M (1972) The response of joints to impact loading. II. *In vivo* behaviour of subchondral bone. *J Biomech* **5**: 267–72.
38. Villiappan S, Svensson N L and Wood R D (1977) Three-dimensional stress analysis of the human femur. *Comput Biol Med* **7**: 253–64.
39. Brown T D and Ferguson A B Jr (1978) The development of a computation stress analysis of the femoral head – mapping tensile, compressive and shear stress for the varus and valgus position. *J Bone Joint Surg [Am]* **60**: 619–29.
40. Brown T D, Way M E and Ferguson A B Jr (1980) Stress transmission anomalies in femoral heads altered by aseptic necrosis. *J Biomech* **13**: 687–99.
41. Rohlmann A, Bergmann G and Koelbel R (1982) The relevance of stress computation in the femur with and without endoprostheses. In: *Finite Elements in Biomechanics*, pp. 361–77. New York: Wiley.
42. Brown T D, Mutschler T A and Ferguson A B Jr (1982) A non-linear finite element analysis of some early collapse processes in femoral head osteonecrosis. *J Biomech* **15**: 105–15.
43. Rushfeldt P D, Mann R W and Harris W H (1981) Improved techniques for measuring *in vitro* the geometry and pressure distribution in the human acetabulum. II. Instrumented endoprosthesis measurement of articular surface pressure distribution. *J Biomech* **14**: 315–23.
44. Podrushnjak E P (1972) *Age changes in the human joints*. Kiev: Naukova dumka (in Russian).
45. Yamada H (1970) *Strength of Biological Materials*. Baltimore: Williams and Wilkins.
46. Evans F G (1973) *Mechanical Properties of Bone*. Springfield: Charles C Thomas.
47. Fung Y C (1981) *Biomechanics. Mechanical Properties of Living Tissue*. New York-Heidelberg-Berlin: Springer-Verlag.
48. Cowin S C (1983) The mechanical and stress adaptive properties of bone. *Ann Biomed Eng* **11**: 263–95.
49. Yanson H, Knets I and Saulgozis Y (1974) Physiological significance of changes in bone volume associated with deformation. *Polymer Mechanics* **10**: 594–601 (Translation from Russian by Consultants Bureau, New York).
50. Yanson H (1975) *Biomechanics of the Human Leg*. Riga: Zinatne (in Russian).
51. Currey J D (1979) Changes in the impact energy absorption of bone with age. *J Biomech* **12**: 459–69.
52. Melnis A E and Knets I V (1985) Viscoelastic properties of compact bone tissue. In: *Modern Problems of Biomechanics, Vol. 2. Mechanics of Biological Tissue*, pp. 38–69. Riga: Zinatne (in Russian).
53. Piekarski K (1970) Fracture of bone. *J Appl Physics* **41**: 215–23.
54. Hermann G and Liebowitz H (1972) Mechanics of bone fracture. In: *Fracture, Vol 7, Fracture of Nonmetals and Composites* (H Liebowitz, ed), pp. 771–840. New York and London: Academic Press.
55. Knets I V and Melnis A E (1982) Peculiarities of the fracture of dry and wet compact bone tissue. In: *Fracture of Composite Materials* (G C Sih and V P Tamuzs, eds), pp. 451–63. The Hague, Boston and London: Martinus Nijhoff.
56. Gjelsvik A (1973) Bone remodelling and piezoelectricity. I. *J Biomech* **6**: 69–77.
57. Gjelsvik A (1973) Bone remodelling and piezoelectricity. II. *J Biomech* **6**: 187–93.
58. Cowin S C and Hegedus D H (1976) Bone remodelling. I: Theory of adaptive elasticity. *J Elasticity* **6**: 313–26.

59. Hegedus D H and Cowin S C (1976) Bone remodelling. II. Small strain adaptive elasticity. *J Elasticity* **6**: 337–52.
60. Cowin S C and Nachlinger R R (1978) Bone remodelling. III. Uniqueness and stability in adaptive elasticity theory. *J Elasticity* **8**: 285–95.
61. Firoozbakhsh K and Cowin S C (1980) Devolution of inhomogeneities in bone structure; predictions of adaptive elasticity theory. *J Biomech Eng* **102**: 287–93.
62. Cowin S C and Firoozbakhsh K (1981) Bone remodelling of diaphyseal surfaces under constant load: theoretical predictions. *J Biomech* **14**: 471–84.
63. Meade J B, Cowin S C, Klawitter J J, Van Buskirk W C and Skinner H B (1984) Bone remodelling due to continuously applied loads. *Calcif Tissue Int* **36**: 25–30.
64. Cowin S C, Hart R T, Balser J R and Kohn D H (1985) Functional adaptation in long bones: establishing *in vivo* values for surface remodelling rate coefficients. *J Biomech* **18**: 665–84.
65. Carter D R, Hayes W C and Schurman D J (1976) Fatigue life of compact bone. II. Effect of microstructure and density. *J Biomech* **9**: 211–8.
66. Carter D R and Hayes W C (1977) Compact bone fatigue damage. I. Residual strength and stiffness. *J Biomech* **10**: 325–38.
67. Carter D R, Caler W E, Spengler D M and Frenkel V H (1981) Fatigue behaviour of adult cortical bone: the influence of mean strain and strain range. *Acta Orthop Scand* **52**: 481–90.
68. Martin R B and Burr D B (1982) A hypothetical mechanism for the stimulation of osteonal remodelling by fatigue damage. *J Biomech* **15**: 137–9.
69. Burr D B, Martin R B, Schaffler M B and Radin E L (1985) Bone remodelling in response to *in vivo* fatigue microdamage. *J Biomech* **18**: 189–200.
70. Dobelis M A and Saulgozis J (1982) Effect of the functional adaptation on non-uniformity in the mechanical properties of the tibia. *Mechanics of Composite Materials* **18**: 229–34 (Translation from Russian by Consultants Bureau, New York).
71. Dobelis M and Saulgozis J (1985) The role of structural components in deformation and load-carrying capacity of compact bone tissue. *In*: *Modern Problems of Biomechanics, Vol 2. Mechanics of Biological Tissue*, pp. 70–102. Riga: Zinatne (in Russian).

Chapter 11

Influence of Load Bearing on the Fluid Transport and Mechanical Properties of Articular Cartilage

V. C. Mow, M. H. Holmes and W. M. Lai

CONTENTS

INTRODUCTION

Articular cartilage probably experiences the highest compressive stresses and the most severe mechanical shocks of any connective tissue in the body (1–7). Yet, in spite of its low capacity for repair, articular cartilage can endure these high levels of mechanical stress and strain for many decades (8, 9). It has been axiomatically accepted that this is due to the superb friction and lubrication qualities of diarthrodial joints, which are in turn due to the intrinsic mechanical properties of articular cartilage and synovial fluid (10–13). However, the mechanisms responsible for these superb lubrication qualities have never been fully elucidated (11–15). One of the reasons for this is that, until very recently, little was known about how articular cartilage behaves under the high and rapidly fluctuating loads, especially in the knee and hip, that exist under physiological conditions in most diarthrodial joints (16–19). For example, only recently has it been shown that articular cartilage, under infinitesimal strain and slow strain rates, can dissipate energy (20) and that an energy dissipation

264

mechanism in compression is due, to a large degree, to interstitial fluid flow through the tissue. There are other dissipation mechanisms due, for example, to the viscoelasticity of the solid phase. Thus, understanding the details of how such an energy dissipation mechanism works may be important for the understanding of how articular cartilage might function under physiological loading conditions.

Recent *in vivo* and *in vitro* experimental findings have documented that repetitive impulse loading and single episodes of indirect blunt trauma, at impact levels below fracture stength of the bone, can cause morphological alterations (21), biomechanical changes (22, 23) and biological reactions in articular cartilage *in vivo* (24). These changes will no doubt alter the continued normal biomechanical functioning of the articular cartilage in the diarthrodial joint under high physiological loading conditions. Presumably the friction and lubrication efficacies of the joint will also be affected by these impact-induced changes. Thus it is important to have a theory capable of describing the deformational behaviour of articular cartilage at high loads and loading rates (25, 26).

Throughout the years, various theories have been proposed to describe the deformational behaviour of articular cartilage. These theories have evolved from the simple, single-phase, linear elasticity theory such as that used by Hirsch (1944), Sokoloff (1966), Linn (1968), Kempson and co-workers (1971), and Hayes and co-workers (1972) (27–31), to single-phase viscoelastic theories such as those used by Hayes and Mockros (1971), Coletti and co-workers (1972), and Parsons and Black (1977, 1979) (32–35), to biphasic poroelastic theories such as those used by McCutchen (1962), Zarek and Edwards (1965), Maroudas (1975), Torzilli and Mow (1976), Mansour and Mow (1976), and Mow and co-workers (1980) (36–41). The most significant advance in cartilage biomechanics in recent years, however, has been the development of the *finite deformation biphasic theory*, improving on the commonly used linear KLM infinitesimal biphasic theory (41), to describe the deformational behaviour of articular cartilage at high loads and loading rates (25, 26). This new theory incorporates both *nonlinear permeability effects* and *finite deformation effects* into a single comprehensive theory. The object of the present theoretical investigation is to utilize the new finite deformation biphasic theory to develop some basic concepts on how normal articular cartilage might behave under high loads and rapid loading rates. Subsequently, we may learn how damaged articular cartilage might behave under similar loading conditions. Specifically, in the present investigation, we wish to determine theoretically how the energy dissipation mechanism in articular cartilage depends on load bearing and loading rates, the latter measured by the frequency of cyclic excitation.

BIPHASIC NATURE OF CARTILAGE

The Composition of the Soft, Porous, Solid Matrix

To appreciate why this finite deformation biphasic theory is needed and to understand some of the implications of this new theory, it is necessary to present a brief review of the currently accepted concepts regarding cartilage composition and structure. Recent biochemical investigations of the composition of the tissue (42), of the structure of the extracellular matrix (43–45), and of the molecular structure of the component parts of the extracellular matrix, collagen (46) and proteoglycans (47–49), and recent biomechanical and physicochemical studies have led to the concept that the organic matrix of articular cartilage is a porous, fibre-reinforced, solid material, swollen with water (38, 50–52). Water and inorganic salts comprise about 70–80% of the total tissue mass (50, 53–55). The intrinsic mechanical properties of collagen (56–60) and proteoglycans (49, 61, 62), and the low volumetric ratio of the solid matrix volume to the fluid volume, ~20%, render this matrix very soft in compression. Indeed, the intrinsic equilibrium modulus of cartilage in compression has been measured to be only about 1·0 MPa at small compressive strains (34, 35, 50, 51, 63). Thus large deformations can and will *readily* occur *in situ* (64) when the tissue is loaded in compression at physiological levels (1–4) and rates of loading (65, 66).

Fluid Transport through the Soft, Porous, Solid Matrix

Many investigators have focused on the transport of the interstitial water, as well as ions, through the porous matrix by diffusion (38, 50, 67), by consolidation (36, 38, 63, 68) and by application of hydrostatic pressure gradients (36, 38, 40, 50, 68, 69). The results from some of these investigations have provided a simple method to estimate an equivalent 'pore size' for this highly hydrated, fibre-reinforced matrix. Using Poiseuille's law for the steady flow of viscous fluids through straight tubes with circular cross-sections, it has been estimated that the average pore size of undeformed cartilage is approximately 6.0 nm (36, 38, 51). However, if the ratio of the solid volume to the fluid volume increases, as can occur during compression, then the size of the 'pores' within the matrix will decrease. This decrease can be estimated by using the same procedure, i.e., measuring the permeability of the tissue as a function of increasing compression, and subsequently determining the equivalent 'pore size'. Following this procedure, Mow and co-workers (51) estimated that the equivalent 'pore size' of the porous fibre-reinforced solid matrix reduces from ~6.0 nm to ~3.0 nm, assuming a constant tortuosity factor. Thus, even though the tissue is highly hydrated, approximately 75% water, its pores are of molecular size. This indicates that the macromolecules comprising the solid matrix, collagen, proteoglycans and other glycoproteins, are *highly dispersed* into the interstitial fluid. A schematic representation of this view of the tissue is shown in *Fig. 11.1*. One consequence of this design is that the biphasic fluid/solid interaction occurring within the tissue must necessarily play a fundamental role in determining the deformational behaviour of articular cartilage under loads.

Non-linear Permeability Effects

Experimentally, Mansour and Mow (40) and Lai and Mow (69) determined that the permeability of cartilage does decrease with increasing compression. This is confirmed in an indirect measurement of this phenomenon by Maroudas (38), where the permeability of cartilage correlated inversely with the tissue

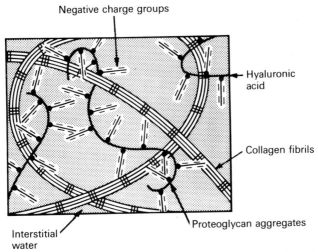

Fig. 11.1. Schematic representation of the biphasic nature of articular cartilage depicting the fibre-reinforced proteoglycan–collagen solid matrix, its molecule pores, and interstitial water. [From Mow *et al.* 1986 (26), with permission.]

hydration. Thus a *non-linear coupling effect* takes place where the deformation field within the tissue strongly affects one of the fundamental material properties of the tissue, i.e. its permeability. This has profound biomechanical consequences in terms of the mechanical response of articular cartilage under various loading conditions (65, 66). The non-linear coupling effect appears to be particularly important for cartilage function since, as stated above, the solid matrix of the tissue is extremely soft; thus large compressions are expected to occur in localized regions of the tissue under physiological loading conditions. Conversely, the large deformations within the tissue will regulate the manner and the rate of fluid transport through the tissue. For example, rapid rates of loading imposed by a porous, free-draining loading platen will cause rapid fluid efflux at the loading surface (41, 66). By virtue of the large frictional drag force exerted by the fluid onto the porous-solid matrix, large compressive strains will occur near the surface of the tissue (65, 66). Hence, any theory used to account for the deformational behaviour of cartilage at physiological loading levels must account for these large deformations occurring in the solid matrix. Consequently, theories describing the deformational behaviour of articular cartilage and other soft hydrated connective tissue must, by necessity, be highly complex; the motion and deformational behaviour of the tissues must be described by a generally valid *finite deformation non-linearly permeable biphasic theory*. Such a theory has been recently developed by Mow and co-workers (26) and Kwan and co-workers (25).

THEORETICAL FOUNDATION OF THE FINITE DEFORMATION BIPHASIC THEORY

In the following section we shall present a brief outline of the development of our finite deformation biphasic theory used to describe articular cartilage. Based upon our permeability and compressive equilibrium stress–strain measurements for human and bovine articular cartilage, the results of this theory will be used in the present investigation to describe how articular cartilage dissipates energy under various loading conditions.

Continuity Equations

One of the fundamental assumptions made in our biphasic theory for articular cartilage is that it is a *mixture* of 2 intrinsically incompressible materials: the interstitial water and the porous fibre-reinforced solid matrix are each by themselves incompressible. The continuity equation for such a mixture of an intrinsically incompressible solid and an intrinsically incompressible fluid was first derived in 1980 by Mow and co-workers (41) and is given by the expression:

$$\text{div} \left[(1 + \alpha)^{-1} (v^f + \alpha v^s) \right] = 0 \qquad (Eqn.\ 11.1)$$

where v^s, v^f are the velocities of the fluid and solid phases of the mixture respectively, and α represents the solid content ($= V^s/V^f$) within the mixture. Here, V^s and V^f are the volumes of the solid and fluid phases within the mixture, respectively. We note that the quantity $1/(1 + \alpha)$ in *Eqn.* 11.1 represents the porosity $\beta (= V^f/V^T)$ of the porous solid matrix; here V^T represents the total volume of the mixture given by $(V^s + V^f)$. For mixtures which are initially homogeneous, the initial solid content, $\alpha_0 = V_0^s/V_0^f$, is a constant. Under finite deformation conditions, Mow and co-workers (26) have shown that the solid content α of such a mixture is related to the matrix deformation by the equation:

$$\alpha = \frac{\alpha_0}{(1 + \alpha_0) \sqrt{\det \mathbf{B}} - \alpha_0}. \qquad (Eqn.\ 11.2)$$

Here, $\mathbf{B}$ denotes the left Cauchy–Green deformation tensor of the solid matrix. In any finite deformation problem involving such a biphasic mixture, these 2 equations must be solved along with the equations of motion governing the biphasic mixture. To accomplish this, it is necessary to specify the constitutive equations for the stress and diffusive drag. In the following section, we shall illustrate how we choose the appropriate constitutive equation governing the stress-strain behaviour of the porous, fibre-reinforced, solid matrix.

A Constitutive Equation for Soft Hydrated Materials

Articular cartilage is an example of a soft hydrated connective tissue whose predominant biomechanical role in the body is to resist compressive stresses. Under small compressive strains, the assumption of material isotropy seems to work very well (41, 65, 66). For finite deformation compression problems, the isotropy assumption also seems to be a reasonable one to make (25, 26). With this, the Helmholtz free-energy density functions A^s and A^f of the solid and fluid phases are functions only of the three scalar invariants of the left Cauchy–Green deformation tensor J_1, J_2, and J_3. In this case, the constitutive equations governing the solid and fluid phases are given by:

$$\sigma^s = -\alpha p\mathbf{I} + \rho^s(A^s - A)\mathbf{I} + 2\rho\left\{\left[J_2\frac{\partial A}{\partial J_2} + J_3\frac{\partial A}{\partial J_3}\right]\mathbf{I} + \frac{\partial A}{\partial J_1}\mathbf{B} - J_3\frac{\partial A}{\partial J_2}\mathbf{B}^{-1}\right\}$$
(Eqn. 11.3a)

$$\sigma^f = -p\mathbf{I} - \rho^s(A^s - A)\mathbf{I}. \qquad (Eqn.\ 11.3b)$$

Here $A = (\rho^s A^s + \rho^f A^f)/\rho$ is the Helmholtz free-energy of the mixture, ρ^s and ρ^f are the apparent densities of the solid and fluid phases, respectively, ρ is the total density of the mixture ($\rho^s + \rho^f$), and p is the interactive fluid pressure arising from the incompressible condition.

For biphasic mixtures, physical coupling between the solid and fluid phases gives rise to internal forces. These forces appear in the momentum equations as equal but opposite body forces acting on each phase. Under the previously stated assumptions, the equation governing these body forces is given by:

$$-\pi^s = \pi^f = -\alpha\rho\,\mathrm{grad}(\ln\rho^s) + \mathrm{grad}\,[\rho^s(A^s - A)] + K(\mathbf{v}^s - \mathbf{v}^f) \quad (Eqn.\ 11.4)$$

The first 2 terms are related to the effect of the gradient of chemical potential due to the deformation of the mixture. The last term represents the diffusive drag between the 2 phases as they move relative to each other. It is expected *a priori* that the diffusive drag coefficient K will depend on the strain in the solid matrix, since it was shown by Lai and Mow (69) that under slow flow conditions, K is inversely related to the permeability, k, of the tissue.

Equations of Motion

Each phase of the biphasic material must satisfy Cauchy's equation of motion given by:

$$\rho^{f,\,s}\mathbf{a}^{f,\,s} = \mathrm{div}\,\sigma^{f,\,s} + \rho^{f,\,s}\mathbf{b}^{f,\,s} + \pi^{f,\,s}. \qquad (Eqn.\ 11.5)$$

Here $\mathbf{b}^{s,\,f}$ are the body forces per unit mass, and $\mathbf{a}^{s,\,f}$ are the accelerations of the fluid and solid phases, respectively. Under quasi-static conditions, neglecting the body forces $\mathbf{b}^{s,\,f}$, these equations of motion become:

$$\mathrm{div}\,\sigma^{f,\,s} + \pi^{f,\,s} = 0. \qquad (Eqn.\ 11.6)$$

Inserting the constitutive relations defined by *Eqns.* 11.3–11.4 into *Eqn.* 11.6, the equations of motion may be expressed in terms of the Helmholtz free-energy function A for the mixture and the left Cauchy–Green deformation tensor **B** and its scalar invariants. Furthermore, the equation of motion for the solid and the fluid phases may be combined to yield the following equation of motion for the entire mixture:

$$\mathrm{div}\ 2\rho\left\{\left[J_2\frac{\partial A}{\partial J_2} + J_3\frac{\partial A}{\partial J_3}\right]\mathbf{I} + \frac{\partial A}{\partial J_1}\mathbf{B} - J_3\frac{\partial A}{\partial J_2}\mathbf{B}^{-1}\right\} - (1 + \alpha)K(\mathbf{v}^s - \mathbf{v}^f) = 0.$$
(Eqn. 11.7)

This is the general equation governing a non-linearly permeable biphasic material under finite deformation conditions. It may be used to describe any such material.

To use this equation to describe a *specific* material, a Helmholtz free-energy function must be chosen for that material. This is accomplished by judiciously choosing a function which satisfies certain constitutive restrictions, such as the tension-extension conditions, and by curve-fitting the relevant experimental data on the finite deformation behaviour of the *specific* material of interest. In the next Section, we outline the procedure we have used to choose the appropriate Helmholtz free-energy function for articular cartilage to describe the finite deformation effects. In addition, for a specific material, the strain-dependent permeability function must also be determined experimentally. For articular cartilage, these measurements were made by Mansour and Mow in 1976 (40) and by Lai and Mow in 1980 (69).

For uniaxial experimental conditions, *Eqn.* 11.7 (along with the continuity equation, *Eqn.* 11.1, and the kinematic condition on α, *Eqn.* 11.2) has been solved numerically to determine the non-linear creep and stress–relaxation behaviour of articular cartilage. For the infinitesimal strain theory, the results of the biphasic theory incorporating the non-linear strain-dependent permeability function have been proven to be remarkably accurate (65, 66). In this investigation, we wish to extend these results using our finite deformation biphasic theory to assess the implication of the ability of articular cartilage to dissipate or absorb energy at high loads and loading rates.

NON-LINEAR STEADY-STATE BEHAVIOUR OF ARTICULAR CARTILAGE

The deformational response of articular cartilage depends on 2 different types of nonlinear material behaviour: (1) non-linear strain-dependent permeability effect at all strain levels (40, 65, 66) and (2) non-linear equilibrium compressive behaviour when the strain is large (25, 26, 40). We hope to show in this investigation how these 2 non-linear effects act to influence the biphasic energy dissipation mechanism in the tissue at physiological loading levels and loading rates.

Non-linear Strain-dependent Permeability Effects

The first effect has been shown to dominate the compressive creep behaviour of cartilage (25). This is because the retardation force required for the observed creep behaviour is generated from the frictional drag force of interstitial fluid flow. The macroscopic measure of the diffusive resistance of the fluid flow through the porous-permeable solid matrix is the permeability coefficent (k). This coefficient is related to the diffusive drag coefficient K by the relation (69):

$$k = \frac{1}{(1 + \alpha_0)^2 K}. \qquad (Eqn.\ 11.8)$$

For articular cartilage, the permeability coefficient k has been shown to vary with strain, and this variation can be described by the following simple equation:

$$k = k_0 \exp[M(\sqrt{\det \mathbf{B}} - 1)] \qquad (Eqn.\ 11.9a)$$

or, in the case of small strain (69):

$$k = k_0 \exp(M \cdot \Delta). \qquad (Eqn.\ 11.9b)$$

Here Δ represents the dilatation within the solid matrix, and k_0 and M are intrinsic material parameters defining the intrinsic permeability function. Thus, with increasing compression, the permeability of the tissue decreases exponentially. For normal articular cartilage, the average value of k_0 is in the order of 10^{-15} m^4/N·s and the value of M is in the order of 10, based upon the infinitesimal strain theory (69). Although k_0 and M remain to be measured under finite deformation conditions, this result shows that significant reduction in tissue permeability can occur even under infinitesimal strain conditions.

The small permeability values mean that the frictional drag force of interstitial fluid flow is extremely high during deformation. The effects of these large drag forces on the compressive creep, stress–relaxation and dynamic oscillatory behaviour of cartilage have been studied (20, 51, 63, 65, 66). These experiments were all performed on precisely prepared circular osteochondral plugs under confined compression conditions. The confined compression configuration was used experimentally because the theoretical solution of the 1-dimensional problem may be readily solved analytically, as in the case of the linear problem (41, 64), and numerically or asymptotically as in the case of the non-linear problems (65, 66). The influence of this non-linear strain-dependent permeability effect on the stress–relaxation behaviour of cartilage, under infinitesimal strain and uniaxial confined compression conditions, has been derived asymptotically (66) where the asymptotic mathematical expressions were curve-fitted to a set of experimental results with remarkable accuracy.

Non-linear Finite Deformation Effects

Most of the information on the non-linear stress–strain behaviour of tendons, ligaments, and articular cartilage comes from tensile studies (56–60, 70). Some studies on the non-linear equilibrium compressive stress–strain behaviour also exist. Eisenfeld and co-workers in 1978 (71) and Mow and co-workers in 1980 (41) reported that the compressive equilibrium stress–strain behaviour of articular cartilage seems to be linear only up to 20% strain in confined compression. Thus, for finite strain conditions, an appropriate form of the Helmholtz free-energy function must be chosen such that the resulting stress–strain law, i.e., Eqn. 11.3a, can be used to describe the non-linear equilibrium compressive stress–strain behaviour of articular cartilage. The choice of the Helmholtz free-energy function $A(J_1, J_2, J_3)$ is restricted by various inequalities pertaining to material behaviour such as the pressure–compression condition, the tension–extension condition, and the invertibility of force–stretch condition proposed by such investigators as Baker and Ericksen (72), Truesdell and Toupin (73) and others. In addition, we impose the condition that the finite deformation stress–strain biphasic law will reduce to the linear KLM biphasic equations under infinitesimal strain conditions. Kwan (1985) showed that the Helmholtz free-energy function given by:

$$\rho_0 A = \frac{1}{8} J_3^{-1} [(3\lambda_s + 2\mu_s)J_1 + (\lambda_s + 2\mu_s)J_1^2 - (9\lambda_s + 10\mu_s)J_2]$$

$$(Eqn.\ 11.10)$$

satisfies all these criteria (25). Here ρ_0 is the initial total density of the tissue. Since this Helmholtz free-energy function yields a stress–strain law for the solid matrix which reduces to the linearly elastic stress–strain law, the coefficients (λ_s, μ_s) may be referred to as the Lamé constants of the solid matrix.

Under uniaxial confined-compression conditions, the kinematics of deformation may be written as:

$$\lambda_1 = \lambda_2 = 1, \qquad 0 < \lambda_3 \leqslant 1, \qquad (Eqn.\ 11.11a)$$

$$J = \lambda_3^2 + 2, \qquad J_2 = 2\lambda_3^2 + 1, \qquad J_3 = \lambda_3^2 \quad (Eqn.\ 11.11b)$$

where x_3 is the direction of compression along the axis of the osteochondral cylindrical specimen. The values of λ_i are the stretches along the x_i direction. At equilibrium, the pressure (p) = 0 and the stretches λ_i are constant. Inserting *Eqns.* 11.11a and b into *Eqn.* 11.10 and inserting the resulting form of the Helmholtz free-energy function into *Eqn.* 11.3, we obtain the finite deformation equilibrium stress–strain relation for the solid matrix in uniaxial compression:

$$\sigma_{zz}^s = (\lambda_s + 2\mu_s)\frac{[1 + d_1(\lambda_3 - 1)]}{4\lambda_3}\left(\lambda_3^2 - \frac{1}{\lambda_3^2}\right) \qquad (Eqn.\ 11.12)$$

where $d_1 = d_0(1 + \alpha_0)/(d_0 + \alpha_0)$, d_0 is the ratio of the true initial density of the solid matrix to the true initial density of the fluid, and $H_A = \lambda_s + 2\mu_s$ is the aggregate modulus of the solid matrix. The simplicity of *Eqn.* 11.12 makes it very easy to use for curve-fitting the experimental finite deformation equilibrium compressive stress–strain results for articular cartilage. We have performed a number of such compression tests with large strains on normal bovine and human articular cartilage. The experimental results and the theoretical curve-fits are shown in *Fig.* 11.2 along with the average aggregate modulus for the bovine and human specimens. The chosen Helmholtz free-energy function does yield a stress–strain law which can be used to describe the finite deformation behaviour of articular cartilage.

NON-LINEAR KINETIC BEHAVIOUR OF ARTICULAR CARTILAGE

Finite Deformation Compressive Creep Behaviour

Creep deformation of materials is a time-dependent process. Thus, the quasi-static equation of motion of the biphasic mixture, *Eqn.* 11.7, must be used. The Helmholtz free-energy function of the tissue for the uniaxial motion may be obtained by inserting *Eqns.* 11.11a and b into *Eqn.* 11.10. By inserting the resulting free-energy function into our equation of motion, *Eqn.* 11.7, and utilizing the continuity condition, *Eqn.* 11.1, we obtain the equation of motion for the tissue given by:

$$\frac{\lambda_s + 2\mu_s}{4}\frac{\partial}{\partial z}\left\{[1 + d_1(\lambda_3 - 1)]\left[\lambda_3 - \frac{1}{\lambda_3^3}\right]\right\} - (1 + \alpha)^2 K v_z^s = 0 \quad (Eqn.\ 11.13)$$

For finite deformation problems, it is more convenient to use the Lagrangian, or material, coordinates to formulate the problem by introducing a set of material coordinates (X_1, X_2, X_3) such that the motion is defined by:

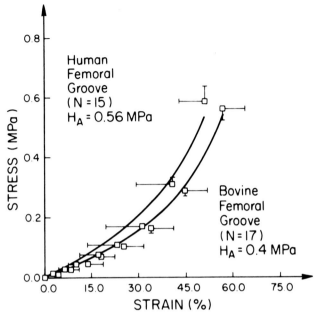

Fig. 11.2. Finite deformation equilibrium stress–strain data in compression for normal human and bovine articular cartilage. The solid lines are the curve-fitted theoretical results from *Eqn.* 11.12. The average aggregate moduli corresponding to the finite deformation theory are 0·56 MPa and 0·4 MPa, for normal human and bovine tissues, respectively.

$$x_1 = X_1, \; x_2 = X_2, \; x_3 = X_3 + u(X_3, t) \qquad (Eqn. \; 11.14a)$$

$$\lambda_1 = 1, \; \lambda_2 = 1, \; \lambda_3 = 1 + \frac{\partial u}{\partial X_3} \qquad (Eqn. \; 11.14b)$$

where $u(X_3, t)$ is the displacement component of the solid matrix in the X_3 direction. From now on, for convenience of notation, we will use Z to denote X_3. In these material coordinates, the equation of motion, *Eqn.* 11.13, becomes:

$$\frac{\lambda_s + 2\mu_s}{4} \left[1 + \frac{\partial u}{\partial Z}\right]^{-1} \frac{\partial}{\partial Z} \left\{ \left[1 + d_1\frac{\partial u}{\partial Z}\right] \frac{\left[1 + \frac{\partial u}{\partial Z}\right]^4 - 1}{\left[1 + \frac{\partial u}{\partial Z}\right]^3} \right\} = (1 + \alpha)^2 K \frac{\partial u}{\partial t}.$$

$$(Eqn. \; 11.15a)$$

Making use of the kinematic relation *Eqn.* 11.2, the relationship between the diffusive drag coefficient and permeability *Eqn.* 11.8, and the strain-dependent permeability relationship *Eqn.* 11.9, we arrive at the final governing equation for the tissue in finite deformation confined compression:

$$\frac{\lambda_s + 2\mu_s}{4} \frac{\left[1 + (1 + \alpha_0)\frac{\partial u}{\partial Z}\right]^2}{\left[1 + \frac{\partial u}{\partial Z}\right]^3} e^{M(\partial u/\partial Z)} \frac{\partial}{\partial Z} \left\{ \left[1 + d_1\frac{\partial u}{\partial Z}\right] \frac{\left[1 + \frac{\partial u}{\partial Z}\right]^4 - 1}{\left[1 + \frac{\partial u}{\partial Z}\right]^3} \right\} = \frac{1}{k_0} \frac{\partial u}{\partial t}.$$

$$(Eqn. \; 11.15b)$$

This non-linear diffusion equation describes the time-dependent behaviour of the solid matrix during uniaxial compression. In the case of creep, the boundary conditions are given by:

$$\sigma_{zz}^s(0, t) = \frac{\lambda_s + 2\mu_s}{4}\left\{1 + d_1\frac{\partial u}{\partial Z}\right\}\frac{\left\{1 + \dfrac{\partial u}{\partial Z}\right\}^4 - 1}{\left\{1 + \dfrac{\partial u}{\partial Z}\right\}^3} = -F_0, \ t > 0$$

(Eqn. 11.16a)

$$p = 0 \qquad\qquad (Eqn.\ 11.16b)$$

$$u(h, t) = 0 \qquad\qquad (Eqn.\ 11.16c)$$

where h denotes the initial thickness of the tissue. The initial condition of the problem is given by:

$$u(Z, 0) = 0. \qquad\qquad (Eqn.\ 11.16d)$$

This non-linear differential equation has been solved numerically using a finite difference scheme. The results shown in Fig. 11.3 are for the case when M = 0; the dimensionless creep responses [u(0, t)/h] are plotted against the dimensionless time $\tau = H_A k_0 t/h^2$ with loading factor $\sigma_0^* = F_0/H_A$ used as the parameter of the problem. Lightly loaded specimens correspond to $\sigma_0^* < 0.2$, while heavily loaded specimens correspond to $\sigma_0^* > 0.4$. For small loads, $\sigma_0^* = 0.1$, the linear infinitesimal (α_0 and k are constant) theory is very accurate. For $\sigma_0^* = 0.4$ or

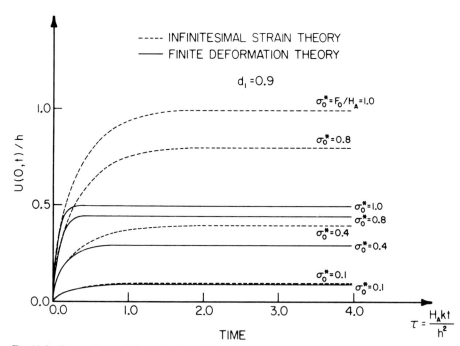

Fig. 11.3. Comparison of theoretical confined compression creep predictions from infinitesimal strain and finite deformation theories. The parameters used in these calculations are: $d_1 = 0.9$, M = 0, $\alpha_0 = 0.2$, and k_0 = constant; σ_0^* is the parameter of this computer simulation.

above, the results of the infinitesimal theory differ significantly from the predictions of the finite deformation theory. For $\sigma_0^* = 1{\cdot}0$, the infinitesimal theory predicts an equilibrium compressive strain of 100%, which is an obvious impossibility, while the finite deformation theory predicts a strain less than 50%. Finally, the finite deformation theory predicts a higher rate of creep at high loads than at low loads, thus the tissue reaches equilibrium much faster than at low loads. *Fig.* 11.4 shows the effect of strain-dependent permeability on the rate of creep. For this case of high load, $\sigma_0^* = 1{\cdot}0$, we see that with larger M, i.e. a more rapid shutdown of the permeability with compression, the creep response of the tissue is much slower. Thus the frictional drag of interstitial fluid flow has a predominant effect on the rate of creep of articular cartilage in uniaxial problems.

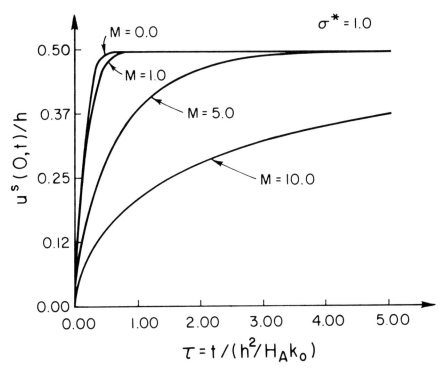

Fig. 11.4. Comparison of theoretical confined compression creep predictions for the finite deformation biphasic theory where the intrinsic strain-dependent permeability coefficient M (*Eqn.* 11.9) is used as the parameter of the problem. The other parameters required for this calculation are: $d_1 = 0{\cdot}9$, $\alpha_0 = 0{\cdot}2$, and k_0 and h are constants; $\sigma_0^* = 1.0$. The results clearly show that the shut-down of the permeability of the tissue causes greater creep retardation effects.

Biphasic Hysteresis Effect

One of the best ways to observe the dissipation of energy in a material is to perform precisely controlled oscillatory experiments where hysteresis loops may be observed. The area enclosed within the hysteresis loop is the energy dissipated per unit volume by the material during a cycle of excitation. *Fig.* 11.5 shows a schematic representation of the uniaxial biphasic confined compression experiment where 2 different types of cyclical motion are imposed. The sawtooth deformation pattern is traditionally used to obtain the hysteresis loop. For articular cartilage equilibrated and bathed in de-ionized water, under the uniaxial condition, a 10^{-3} Hz sawtooth excitation, 2% peak-to-peak strain, and 10% d.c. offset compressive strain were imposed by a rigid free-draining porous loading platen, *Fig.* 11.6. The typical experimental hysteresis loop for articular cartilage is shown in this figure. The solid curve is the prediction of the biphasic KLM theory where the exponential strain-dependent permeability function, *Eqn.* 11.9, has been used along with the linear infinitesimal stress–strain relationship for the porous-permeable solid matrix, and the appropriate boundary conditions have been imposed (20, 26). The solution was obtained by a finite difference numerical integration procedure. This result shows the accuracy of the linear KLM biphasic theory where the non-linear strain-dependent permeability has been incorporated into the equation (26). To perform this series of experiments in a manner consistent with the theory, care must be exercised to not generate large deformations in the solid matrix by either excessive loading or high loading rates. We have also studied the influence of interstitial ion concentration on this energy dissipation mechanism (74).

Cyclically Loaded Confined Compression Experiment

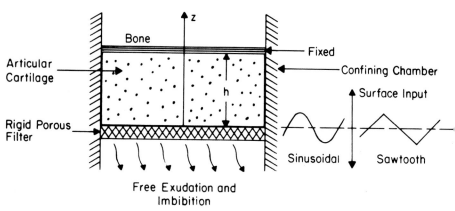

Fig. 11.5. Schematic representation of a confined compression test where the surface displacement inputs are the sawtooth function and the sinusoidal function. The rigid porous free-draining loading platen is interfaced against the articular surface. The cartilage–bone junction is assumed to be impervious.

Influence of Loading Rate on Cartilage Hysteresis

The above theoretical and experimental study was performed in such a manner as to ensure that the solid matrix experiences infinitesimal strains only. However, at physiological loads and loading rates, finite deformations readily occur (1–4, 64). In order to assess the effects of finite deformation on this biphasic energy dissipation mechanism, we solved *Eqn.* 11.15b for the finite

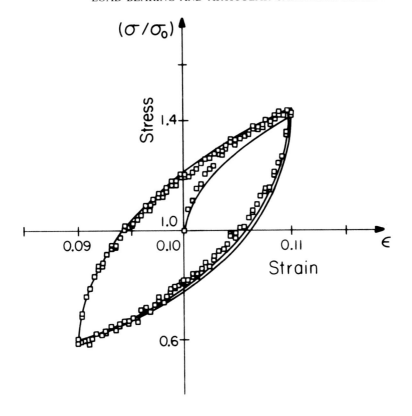

HYSTERESIS LOOP

Fig. 11.6. Comparison of experimental data (□) and theoretical prediction (——) of the biphasic theory when the material is subject to the sawtooth surface displacement shown in *Fig.* 11.5. The conditions of the experiment are: tissue is equilibrated in de-ionized water; compressed at 10% d.c. offset; 2% peak-to-peak strain; 10^{-3} Hz. The slow compression rate ensures that the strain field in the solid matrix will remain small. [From Mow *et al.* 1986 (26), with permission.]

deformation of articular cartilage under the uniaxial condition using the same finite difference scheme. In the present case, however, we impose a sinusoidal excitation, *Fig.* 11.5, onto the articular surface via the rigid, porous, free-draining loading platen. *Figs.* 11.7a and b show the theoretical predictions of the influence of frequency, 5×10^{-4}, 5×10^{-3}, 10^{-1} and $1 \cdot 0$ Hz, on the hysteresis loop under a 10% d.c. offset compressive strain and a 2% peak-to-peak strain. We note thatx the normalization constant σ_0 in *Figs.* 11.7a and b are compressive; for example, for the human and bovine specimens, corresponding to *Fig.* 11.2 and 10% d.c. offset compressive strain, they are $\sigma_0 = -0 \cdot 056$ MPa and $\sigma_0 = -0 \cdot 04$ MPa, respectively. The time parameter in these figures is the non-dimensional time given by $tk_0 H_A/h^2$. The other physical parameters of articular cartilage used were the initial solid content $\alpha_0 = 0 \cdot 2$, the intrinsic permeability coefficients $k_0 = 2 \cdot 5 \times 10^{-15}$ m^4/N·s, M = $2 \cdot 0$, h = $2 \cdot 0$ mm, and $d_1 = 0 \cdot 9$.

The salient features of this numerical simulation for these oscillatory tests are:
1. The results are highly dependent on the frequency of excitation, i.e., rate of loading.
2. There is a phase lag between the peak stress (σ_p) and peak strain (ε_p).
3. Tensile stress occurs at the surface of the tissue during the cycle going from T_1 to T_2 (*Fig.* 11.7b).
4. Steady-state excitation is reached within 2 cycles of excitation.

The first observation is understandable since the spread of interstitial fluid flow depends directly on the rate of compression and, at these higher rates, higher compressive strain also occurs. Thus, because of the strain-dependent permeability effect, the interstitial fluid must flow through a tissue of lower permeability, hence resulting in greater energy dissipation. *Fig.* 11.8 is a log–log plot of the area enclosed within the hysteresis loops versus the frequency of excitation corresponding to calculations such as those depicted in *Figs.* 11.7a and b. Thus, the energy dissipation is a power function of the frequency of excitation. Note that the scale of the ordinate in *Fig.* 11.7b is almost 25 times that of *Fig.* 11.7a. We have found that very high compressive strains are

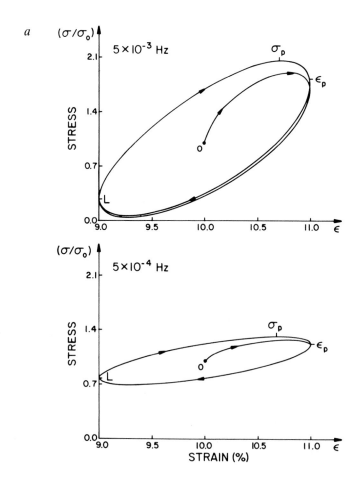

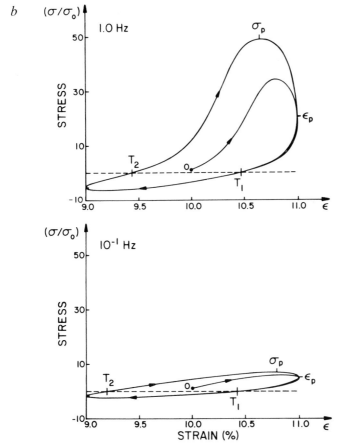

Fig. 11.7. *a*, Influence of frequency on the energy dissipation capacity of articular cartilage (*see* text for detailed discussion). Conditions for these calculations are: frequencies of excitation are 5×10^{-4}, 5×10^{-3}; 10% d.c. offset compressive strain; 2% peak-to-peak strain imposed by a sinusoidal input function; $\alpha_0 = 0.2$; $k_0 = 2.5 \times 10^{-15}$ m^4/N·s; M = 2.0; h = 2.0 mm, and $d_1 = 0.9$. *b*, Influence of frequency on the energy dissipation capacity of articular cartilage (*see* text for detailed discussion). Conditions for these calculations are: frequencies of excitation are 10^{-1} and 1.0 Hz; 10% d.c. offset compressive strain; 2% peak-to-peak strain imposed by a sinusoidal input function; $\alpha_0 = 0.2$; $k_0 = 2.5 \times 10^{-15}$ m^4/N·s; M = 2.0; h = 2.0 mm, and $d_1 = 0.9$.

occurring at the surface of the tissue when the rates of loading are beyond 5×10^{-1} Hz. In this simulation, we see that the non-linear coupling effect between fluid flow and solid matrix deformation causes more dissipation to occur within the material as the rate of loading increases.

The phase lag between σ_p and ε_p is due to the competition between the effects of interstitial fluid flow and the deformation effects in the solid matrix. The flow of the interstitial fluid (velocity) is dependent on the speed of compression, while solid matrix deformation (displacement) is dependent on the magnitude of the surface-to-surface displacement. In the sinusoidally imposed displacement function, as the surface-to-surface strain approaches ε_p, the velocity of the surface, which is proportional to $\cos(\omega t)$, is decreasing. These results imply that the effect of the decrease of the fluid velocity on the surface stress is greater than the increase of the surface-to-surface compressive strain. Related to this is the fact that the biphasic stress–relaxation effect occurring within the tissue is evolving more rapidly than the build-up of the stress as $\varepsilon \rightarrow \varepsilon_p$ in the downstroke of the cycle.

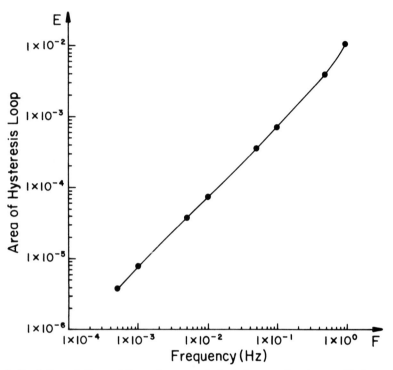

Fig. 11.8. Prediction of the variation of energy dissipated per unit volume with frequency of sinusoidal excitation by the non-linear finite deformation biphasic theory. The area within the hysteresis loop was obtained by numerically integrating the results shown in *Fig. 11.7.*

At 10^{-1} Hz, tensile stress (σ/σ_0) occurs at the surface during the cycle going from T_1 to T_2 even though the surface-to-surface strain is compressive. This is because at the higher frequencies, the rigid, free-draining, porous loading platen is moving faster than the natural rate at which the cartilage surface can recover. In order for the surface to follow the platen, a tensile stress must be imposed. Recovery of the compressed tissue is retarded by the rate at which fluid imbibition can occur at the surface. This indicates that interpretation of experimental results using theories unable to account for these non-linear effects, to explain compressive sinusoidal excitation behaviour of the tissue at frequencies greater than 10^{-2} Hz, may lead to serious erroneous conclusions. *Fig. 11.7b* also shows that dramatic asymmetric load-deformation pattern; for

$|\varepsilon| < |\varepsilon_p|$ during the upstroke at 1·0 Hz the surface stress drops precipitously and for $|\varepsilon| > L$ during the downstroke the stress does not increase precipitously. We believe this is due to the modulation of permeability via the strain-dependent permeability function and the formation of boundary layers of high compressive strains near the surface (66). This manifests as a strain-hardening effect with increasing strain rate. Finally, *Figs.* 11.7*a* and *b* show that the tissue reaches an equilibrium within 1 cycle of excitation. This is to be expected because the frictional drag of interstitial fluid causes the tissue to be a highly dissipative material.

Fig. 11.9 illustrates the dependency of the energy dissipation of articular cartilage on the compressive strain. Here the tissue is loaded under the same uniaxial motion condition; a 10^{-2} Hz sinusoidal excitation and 2% peak-to-peak strain is used. The d.c. offset compressive strain is imposed by a rigid, free-draining, porous loading platen and is used as the parameter in this computer simulation of the experiment with values of 10%, 20%, and 30%. The area enclosed within the hysteresis loop increases with compressive strain. At 10% d.c. offset compressive strain, tensile stress occurs for $T_2 < |\varepsilon| < T_1$ during the upstroke, but not for d.c. offset compressive strains of 20% and 30%. At these higher levels, there is sufficient strain energy stored within the porous solid matrix to cause a rapid fluid imbibition and recovery of the tissue such that no tensile stress needs to be applied to force the surface to follow the prescribed sinusoidal displacement. This simulation once again illustrates that as compressive strain increases, the drop in the permeability causes the tissue to be more dissipative, at least at 10^{-2} Hz.

CONCLUSIONS

The constitutive models used to describe the stress–strain behaviour of articular cartilage and other hydrated tissues have evolved from linear Hooke's law under infinitesimal strain conditions to linear viscoelastic laws (Kelvin model, other simple collection of spring and dashpot elements, and integral equation representation using Boltzmann's superposition principle) to poroelastic laws such as the linear KLM biphasic model. Each constitutive law is, by the very nature of Newtonian mechanics, an approximation of the real material. Each has a restricted range of applicability and utility. In this chapter, we have presented a formulation of a biphasic material for use under finite deformation conditions. This biphasic material is a mixture of an intrinsically incompressible solid and an intrinsically incompressible fluid. A specific choice of the Helmholtz free-energy function is made to model the equilibrium stress–strain behaviour of articular cartilage under finite deformation conditions, and a specific choice of strain-dependent permeability function is made to model the steady permeation behaviour of the tissue. The resultant theory is a non-linear finite deformation biphasic theory for articular cartilage. This methodology can be used to develop theories for other hydrated tissues of the body as well. The present finite deformation biphasic theory can now be used to describe the deformational behaviour of articular cartilage under high loads and high loading rates such as those found under physiological conditions.

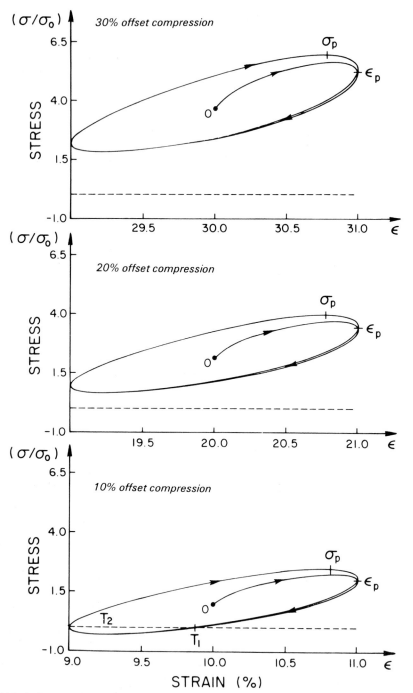

Fig. 11.9. Influence of compression on the energy dissipation capacity of articular cartilage (*see* text for detailed discussion). Conditions for these calculations are: d.c. offset compressive strains are 10%, 20%, and 30%; 2% peak-to-peak strain imposed by a sinusoidal input function at 10^{-2} Hz; $\alpha_0 = 0.2$; $k_0 = 2.5 \times 10^{-15}$ m^4/N·s; M = 2.0; h = 2.0 mm; and $d_1 = 0.9$.

PRACTICAL SIGNIFICANCE

Based upon the theory presented, articular cartilage can, under high and rapidly fluctuating physiological loads, dissipate energy due to interstitial fluid flow through the tissue. The deformations within cartilage regulate the manner and the rate of fluid transport. Energy dissipation by cartilage increases with increasing compressive strain and strain rate. Thus, load bearing in normal, working joints does influence the fluid transport and mechanical behaviour of cartilage. This non-linear mechanical behaviour is an essential mechanism behind the superb friction and lubrication qualities, which make possible the continued normal biomechanical functioning of the articular cartilage in the diarthrodial joint under high physiological loading conditions.

ACKNOWLEDGEMENTS

This research was supported by the National Institute of Arthritis, Diabetes and Digestive and Kidney Diseases grants AM19094 and AM26440, and National Science Foundation grant MSM8518501. Any opinions, findings, and conclusions or recommendations expressed in this publication are those of the authors and do not necessarily represent the views of the NSF.

REFERENCES

1. Ahmed A M and Burke D L (1983) *In vitro* measurement of static pressure distribution in synovial joints. Part. I: Tibial surface of the knee. *J Biomech Eng* **105**: 216–25.
2. Ahmed A M and Burke D L (1983) *In vitro* measurement of static pressure distribution in synovial joints. Part II: Retropatellar surface. *J Biomech Eng* **105**: 226–36.
3. Brown T D and Shaw D T (1983) *In vitro* stress distribution in the natural human hip. *J Biomech* **16**: 373–84.
4. Brown T D and Shaw D T (1984) *In vitro* contact stress distribution on the femoral condyles. *J Orthop Res* **2**: 190–99.
5. Radin E L, Paul I L and Lowy M (1970) A comparison of the dynamic force transmitting properties of subchondral bone and articular cartilage. *J Bone Joint Surg [Am]* **52**: 444–56.
6. Radin E L, Parker H G, Pugh J W, Steinberg R S, Paul I L and Rose R M (1973) Response of joints to impact loading. III. Relationship between trabecular microfractures and cartilage degeneration. *J Biomech* **6**: 51–8.
7. Radin E L (1980) Mechanical factors in the etiology of osteoarthrosis. In: *Epidemiology of Osteoarthrosis* (J G Peyron, ed), pp. 136–9. (Proceedings of Symposium, Paris).
8. Mankin H J and Brandt K D (1984) Biochemistry and metabolism of cartilage in osteoarthritis. In: *Osteoarthritis. Diagnosis and Management*. (R W Moskowitz, D S Howell, V M Goldberg and H J Mankin, eds), pp. 43–79. Philadelphia: Saunders.
9. Howell D S (1984) Etiopathogenesis of osteoarthritis, In: *Osteoarthritis. Diagnosis and Management*. (R W Moskowitz, D S Howell, V M Goldberg and H J Mankin, eds), pp. 129–46. Philadelphia: Saunders.
10. Swann D A and Radin E L (1972) The molecular basis of articular lubrication: I. Purification and properties of a lubricating fraction from bovine synovial fluid. *J Biol Chem* **247**: 8069–73.
11. Armstrong C G and Mow V C (1980) Friction, lubrication and wear of articular cartilage. In: *Scientific Foundation of Orthopaedic Traumatology* (R Owens, J W Goodfellow and P G Bullough, eds), pp. 223–32. London: Heinemann Medical.
12. Mow V C and Mak A F (1986) Lubrication of diarthrodial joints. In: *Bioengineering Handbook* (R Skalak and S Chien, eds), Chap. 5. New York: McGraw Hill.
13. Dowson D, Unsworth A, Cooke A F and Gvozdanovic D (1981) Lubrication of joints. In: *An Introduction to the Biomechanics of Joints and Joint Replacement* (D Dowson and V Wright, eds), pp. 120–45. London: Mechanical Engineering Publications.
14. Radin E L and Paul I L (1972) A consolidated concept of joint lubrication. *J Bone Joint Surg [Am]* **54**: 607–16.

15. Lipshitz H and Glimcher M J (1979) *In vitro* studies of wear of articular cartilage. II. Characteristics of the wear of articular cartilage when worn against stainless steel plates having characterized surfaces. *Wear* **52m**: 297–339.
16. Andriacchi T P, Andersson G B J, Fermier R W and Stern D (1980) A study of lower-limb mechanics during stair-climbing. *J Bone Joint Surg [Am]* **62**: 749–57.
17. Chao E Y, Laughman R K, Schneider E and Stauffer R N (1983) Normative data of knee joint motion and ground reaction forces in adult level walking. *J Biomech* **16**: 219–33.
18. Seireg A and Arvikar R J (1975) The prediction of muscular load bearing and joint forces in the lower extremities during walking. *J Biomech* **8**: 89–102.
19. Paul J P (1976) Force actions transmitted by joints in the human body. *Proc R Soc Lond (Biol)* **192**: 163–72.
20. Holmes M H, Hou J S and Mow V C (1984) Dissipation in articular cartilage under oscillatory compression. *In: 1984 Advances in Bioengineering*, (R L Spilker, ed), pp. 71–2. Translated by ASME.
21. Radin E L, Martin R B, Burr D B, Caterson B, Boyd R D and Goodwin C (1984) Effects of mechanical loading on the tissues of the rabbit knee. *J Orthop Res* **2**: 221–34.
22. Repo R U and Finlay J B (1977) Survival of articular cartilage after controlled impact. *J Bone Joint Surg [Am]* **59**: 1068–76.
23. Armstrong C G, Mow V C and Wirth C R (1985) Biomechanics of impact-induced microdamage to articular cartilage. A possible genesis for chondromalacia patella. *In: AAOS Symposium on Sports Medicine: The Knee*. (G Finerman, ed), pp. 70–84. St. Louis: Mosby.
24. Donohue J M, Buss D, Oegema T R Jr and Thompson R C (1983) The effect of indirect blunt trauma on adult canine articular cartilage. *J Bone Joint Surg [Am]* **65**: 948–57.
25. Kwan M K, Lai W M and Mow V C (1985) Finite deformation biphasic analysis of the confined compression behaviors of articular cartilage. *In: 1985 Advances in Bioengineering* (N Langrana, ed), pp. 3–5. Translated by ASME.
26. Mow V C, Kwan M K, Lai W M and Holmes M H (1986) A finite deformation theory for non-linearly permeable soft hydrated biological tissues. *In: Frontiers in Biomechanics* (G Schmid-Schonbein, S L-Y Woo and B Zweifach, eds), pp. 153–79. New York: Springer-Verlag.
27. Hirsch C (1944) The pathogenesis of chondromalacia of the patella. *Acta Chir Scand [Suppl]* **83**: 1–106.
28. Sokoloff L (1966) Elasticity of aging cartilage. *Fed Proc* **25**: 1089–95.
29. Linn F C (1967) Lubrication of animal joints. I. The arthrotripsometer. *J Bone Joint Surg [Am]* **49**: 1079–98.
30. Kempson G E, Spivey C J, Swanson S A V and Freeman M A R (1971) Patterns of cartilage stiffness on normal and degenerate femoral heads. *J Biomech* **4**: 597–609.
31. Hayes W C, Keer L M, Herrmann G and Mockros L F (1972) A mathematical analysis for indentation tests of articular cartilage. *J Biomech* **5**: 541–51.
32. Hayes W C and Mockros L F (1971) Viscoelastic properties of human articular cartilage. *J Appl Physiol* **31**: 562–8.
33. Coletti J M, Akeson W H and Woo S L-Y (1972) A comparison of the physical behavior of normal articular cartilage and the arthroplasty surface. *J Bone Joint Surg [Am]* **54**: 147–60.
34. Parsons J R and Black J (1977) The viscoelastic shear behavior of normal rabbit articular cartilage. *J Biomech* **10**: 21–9.
35. Parsons J R and Black J (1979) Mechanical behavior of articular cartilage: quantitative changes with alteration of ionic environment. *J Biomech* **12**: 765–73.
36. McCutchen C W (1962) The frictional properties of animal joints. *Wear* **5**: 1–17.
37. Zarek J M and Edwards J (1965) Dynamic consideration of the human skeletal system. *In Biomechanics and Related Bio-Engineering Topics* (R M Kenedi, ed), pp. 187–203. New York Pergamon.
38. Maroudas A (1975) Biophysical chemistry of cartilaginous tissues with special reference to solute and fluid transport. *Biorheology* **12**: 233–48.
39. Torzilli P A and Mow V C (1976) On the fundamental fluid transport mechanisms through normal and pathological articular cartilage during function. I. *J Biomech* **9**: 541–52.
40. Mansour J M and Mow V C (1976) The permeability of articular cartilage under compressive strain and at high pressure. *J Bone Joint Surg [Am]* **58**: 509–16.
41. Mow V C, Kuei S C, Lai W M and Armstrong C G (1980) Biphasic creep and stress relaxation of articular cartilage. *J Biomech Eng* **102**: 73–84.
42. Muir H (1983) Proteoglycans as organisers of the extracellular matrix. *Biochem Soc Trans* **11** 613–22.

43. Broom N D (1982) Abnormal softening in articular cartilage; its relationship to the collagen framework. *Arthritis Rheum* **27**: 1209–16.
44. Broom N D and Marra D L (1985) New structural concepts of articular cartilage demonstrated with a physical model. *Connect Tissue Res* **14**: 1–8.
45. Hascall V C and Hascall G K (1981) Proteoglycans. *In: Cell Biology of the Extracellular Matrix* (E D Hay, ed), pp. 39–63. New York: Plenum.
46. Eyre D R (1980) Collagen: molecular diversity in the body's protein scaffold. *Science* **207**: 1315–22.
47. Hardingham T E (1981) Proteoglycans: their structure, interactions and molecular organization in cartilage. *Biochem Soc Trans* **9**: 489–97.
48. Buckwalter J A and Rosenberg L C (1982) Electron microscopic studies of cartilage proteoglycans. Direct evidence for the variable length of the chondroitin sulfate rich region of proteoglycan subunit core protein. *J Biol Chem* **257**: 9830–9.
49. Mow V C, Mak A F, Lai W M, Rosenberg L C and Tang L-H (1984) Viscoelastic properties of proteoglycan subunits and aggregates in varying solution concentrations. *J Biomech* **17**: 325–38.
50. Maroudas A (1979) Physicochemical properties of articular cartilage. *In: Adult Articular Cartilage*, 2nd Ed (M A R Freeman, ed), pp. 215–90. Kent: Pitman Medical.
51. Mow V C, Holmes M H and Lai W M (1984) Fluid transport and mechanical properties of articular cartilage: a review. *J Biomech* **17**: 377–94.
52. Eisenberg S R and Grodzinsky A J (1985) Swelling of articular cartilage and other connective tissues: electromechanochemical forces. *J Orthop Res* **3**: 148–59.
53. Torzilli P A, Dethmers D A, Rose D E and Schryver H F (1983) Movement of interstitial water through loaded articular cartilage. *J Biomech* **16**: 169–70.
54. Myers E R, Lai W M and Mow V C (1984) A continuum theory and experimental verification of the ion-induced swelling behavior of articular cartilage. *J Biomech Eng* **106**: 165–73.
55. Myers E R, Armstrong C G and Mow V C (1984) Swelling pressure and collagen tension. *In: Connective Tissue Matrix* (D W L Hukins, ed), pp. 160–86. London: MacMillan.
56. Woo S L-Y, Akeson W H and Jemmott G F (1976) Measurement of non-homogenous, directional mechanical properties of articular cartilage in tension. *J Biomech* **9**: 785–91.
57. Woo S L-Y, Simon B R, Kuei S C and Akeson W H (1980) Quasi-linear viscoelastic properties of normal articular cartilage. *J Biomech Eng* **102**: 85–90.
58. Fung Y C (1972) Stress-strain-history relations of soft tissues in simple elongation. *In: Biomechanics, its Foundations and Objectives* (Y C Fung, N Peone and M Anliker, eds), pp. 181–208. Englewood Cliff: Prentice-Hall.
59. Viidik A V and Gottrup F (1986) Mechanics of healing soft tissue. *In: Frontiers in Biomechanics* (G Schmid-Schonbein, S L-Y Woo and B Zweufach, eds), pp. 263–79. New York: Springer-Verlag.
60. Roth V and Mow V C (1980) The intrinsic tensile behavior of the matrix of bovine articular cartilage and its variation with age. *J Bone Joint Surg [Am]* **62**: 1102–17.
61. Hardingham T E and Muir H (1974) Hyaluronic acid in cartilage and proteoglycan aggregation. *Biochem J* **139**: 565–81.
62. Hardingham T E, Muir H, Kwan M K, Lai W M and Mow V C (1987) Viscoelastic properties of proteoglycan solutions with varying proportions present as aggregates. *J Orthop Res* **5**: 36–46.
63. Armstrong C G and Mow V C (1982) Variations in the intrinsic mechanical properties of human articular cartilage with age, degeneration and water content. *J Bone Joint Surg [Am]* **64**: 88–94.
64. Armstrong C G, Bahrani A S and Gardner D L (1979) *In vitro* measurement of articular cartilage deformations in the intact human hip joint under load. *J Bone Joint Surg [Am]* **61**: 744–55.
65. Lai W M, Mow V C and Roth V (1981) Effects of a non-linear strain-dependent permeability and rate of compression on the stress behavior of articular cartilage. *J Biomech Eng* **103**: 61–66.
66. Holmes M H, Lai W M and Mow V C (1985) Singular perturbation analysis of the non-linear flow-dependent, compressive stress–relaxation behavior of articular cartilage. *J Biomech Eng* **107**: 206–18.
67. Torzilli P A, Adams T C and Mis R J (1986) Transient solute diffusion in articular cartilage. *J Biomech* In press.
68. Edwards J (1967) Physical characteristics of articular cartilage. *Proc Inst Mech Eng* **181**: 3J: 16–24.
69. Lai W M and Mow V C (1980) Drag-induced compression of articular cartilage during a permeation experiment. *Biorheology* **17**: 111–23.

70. Kempson G E, Muir H, Pollard C and Tuke M (1972) The tensile properties of the cartilage of human femoral condyles related to the content of collagen and glysaminoglycans. *Biochim Biophys Acta* **297**: 456–72.
71. Eisenfeld J, Mow V C and Lipshitz H (1978) Analysis of stress relaxation in articular cartilage during compression. *J Math Biosci* **39**: 97–111.
72. Baker M and Ericksen J L (1954) Inequalities restricting the form of the stress deformation relations for isotropic elastic solids and Reiner-Rivlin fluids. *J Wash Academic Sci* **44**: 33–35.
73. Truesdell C and Toupin R (1963) Static grounds for inequalities in finite strain of elastic materials. *Arch Rat Mech Anal* **12**: 1–33.
74. Hou J-S, Holmes M H and Mow V C (1986) Variation of the energy dissipation and permeability of cartilage with salt concentration. *Trans Orthop Res Soc* **11**: 454.

Chapter 12

Response of Tendons and Ligaments to Joint Loading and Movements

S. L-Y. Woo and W. H. Akeson

CONTENTS

INTRODUCTION

Biology

On gross examination, tendons and ligaments belong to a family of dense, regular connective tissues with closely packed, parallel collagenous bundles having a shiny white appearance (1). Under microscopic examination, these tissues contain a meshwork of interlacing fibres, flattened cells and ground substance. The fibre bundles are regularly arranged and oriented in the direction of functional need. Polarized light and special stains are used to differentiate and isolate the fibrous elements and similarly distinguish ground substance and fibroblasts in the interfibrillar spaces (*Fig. 12.1a*). Ultrastructural methods are used to define detailed hierarchies of arrangement down to microfibril size in tendons (2) with presumably similar arrangements in ligaments.

The insertions of ligaments and tendons to bone progress from fibril through fibrocartilage (usually less than 0·6 mm) to mineralized fibrocartilage (less than 0·4 mm) and finally to bone (3, 4) (*Fig. 12.1b*). Zones of fibrocartilage and calcified fibrocartilage are separated by a narrow line of unknown

287

significance. Two types of collagen fibre insertions into bone are seen. The first and more common crosses the mineralization front and the second, less common, inserts directly into bone relative to the periosteum (*Fig.* 12.1*c*)(3–5). Stress and joint motion are important in maintaining the functional integrity of these insertion sites (6, 7).

Tendons and ligaments consist of functional complexes of interdependent aggregations of collagen, elastin, glycoproteins, protein polysaccharides, glyco-lipids, water, and cells. The nature of the constituents is complex, and our understanding of their interaction continues to evolve. Roughly 70–80% of normal tendon or ligament is composed of collagen by dry weight. The collagen is mainly Type I, also found in skin and bone, but is thought to remain relatively inert metabolically with a half-life of 300–500 days (8) (a turnover rate even slower than that of bone collagen). Certain components of the collagen molecule, however, may turn over faster than others (9) and may therefore be of greater functional importance in adaptations to environmental, traumatic, or pathological processes.

Collagen obtains its structural stability from its unique molecular coil configuration and the quarter-staggered packing of tropocollagen units (4). It also has the ability to form covalent intramolecular (aldol) and intermolecular (Schiff base) cross-links (10–12), which are the key to the tensile strength characteristics and resistance to chemical or enzymatic breakdown.

On a dry weight basis, the ground substance constituents of tendons or ligaments comprise less than a few % of the total tissue. Water, however, comprises 60–80% of the total wet weight, and a significant part of that water is associated with the ground substance. The water and proteoglycans (PGs) probably provide lubrication and spacing crucial to the gliding function at intercept points in periarticular connective tissues where fibres cross in the tissue matrix. (The water and PGs also confer viscoelastic properties to tendons and ligaments. The movement of water in the system is inhibited by its entrapment between the large, highly charged molecules of proteoglycans.)

PGs are relatively uniform chemically in tendons and ligaments. The PG sub-unit consists of a core protein with protein-linked glycosaminoglycan (GAG) side chains. Except for hyaluronic acid, the GAGs are covalently linked to proteins to create aggregate molecules of massive molecular weight. They are highly negatively charged and possess a large number of hydroxyl groups, which attract water through hydrogen bonding and contribute important features to the collagen fibre–ground substance interaction.

Tensile Properties

Many important contributions concerning the biomechanical behaviour of ligaments and tendons have been published during recent decades. These tissues exhibit complex rheological characteristics, as portrayed by their non-linear elastic as well as time- and history-dependent viscoelastic properties (13, 14). Further, irregular shapes and geometry as well as the complex anatomical construction of ligaments and tendons contribute to the difficulties in testing for their biomechanical properties (15). Periarticular ligaments are attached to bone on either side of a joint and insertions are often broad-based, so that accurate

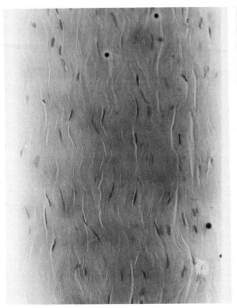

a

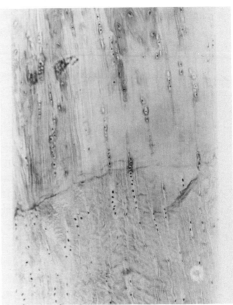

b

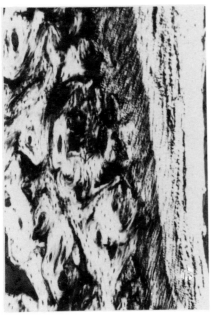

c

Fig. 12.1. *a*, Normal rabbit medial collateral ligament. *Note* longitudinal orientation of matrix seen
under low power magnification. (Haematoxylin-
eosin stain, × 140). *b*, Femoral insertion of normal rabbit medial collateral ligament. There is a
progression from bone (*top*) to mineralized fibrocartilage and fibrocartilage to normal ligament
(*bottom*). *Note* a narrow line separating fibrocartilage and mineralized fibrocartilage passing obliquely through this specimen (× 35). *c*, Polarizing
light photomicrograph of low power section of
normal rabbit medial collateral ligament tibial
insertion, showing some fibrils confluent with the
periosteum while others course directly and insert
into bone (× 35).

measurement of ligament length is impossible. Mounting of the isolated ligaments into clamps for testing often results in slippage at the clamp–specimen interface and damage to the underlying tissue which leads to premature failure. Thus, most testing has been conducted utilizing bone-ligament-bone preparations, since the loading conditions can be made to more closely approximate *in situ* conditions. However, a distinct difficulty has been the inability to separate the biomechanical properties of the ligament substance from those properties contributed by its insertion sites. Therefore, special devices such as the buckle transducer (16) and magnetic field displacement transducer (17) have been designed to measure the ligament load and strain during tensile loading. These systems, however, depend on direct contact with the ligament and therefore artifacts may be imposed upon ligament properties.

In our laboratory, we have used a non-contact video technique to measure the surface strains of the ligament substance when testing a bone-ligament-bone preparation (14) (*Fig. 12.2*). In this system, a television camera is used to transmit a picture of the ligament specimen to a video monitor, where an electronic dimensional analyser projects 2 windows. These windows can then be placed over any 2 stained lines (gauge length) placed on the ligament. The horizontal scan time of the gauge length is converted to an output voltage which increases proportionately as the gauge length increases under tensile loading. Therefore, the ligament strain can be automatically determined and recorded. The frequency response of the video dimensional analyser (VDA) system is as high as 120 Hz and errors in linearity and accuracy are less than 0·5% (14).

Significant time- and history-dependent viscoelastic properties of ligaments include creep (increasing deformation with time under constant load) and stress

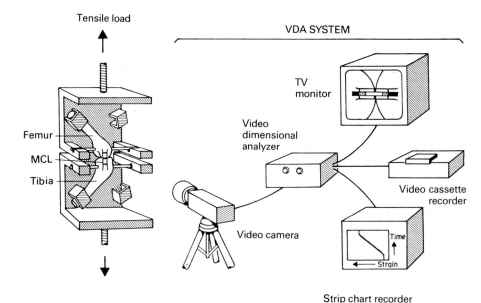

Fig. 12.2. The experimental apparatus designed to measure the tensile characteristics of the femur–MCL–tibia (FMT) complex as well as the ligament substance. For detailed principles of the VDA system, *see* references (14, 73).

relaxation (decreasing stress with time under constant deformation). Through a combination of these non-linear viscoelastic properties, the originally described quasi-static stress–strain relationship for tendons and ligaments at various strain rates has been predicted mathematically and shown to conform to experimental data (18).

Viscoelastic properties not only play a role in the case of single-cycle loading and unloading, but also during multiple-cycle loading, such as during walking or exercise. If applied strains and strain rates are constant (14, 18), transient softening of tissue substance with slight decreases in peak loads occurs as cycling proceeds. Similarly, deformation increases slightly during early cycles to a constant load showing creep effects on the tendon and ligament. These changes have been noted clinically with temporary softening and increases of test excursion (laxity) in exercised joints. After a short recovery period there is a return to normal joint stiffness and apparent length. The ultimate strength of muscle-tendon-bone and ligament-bone complexes may also be decreased during such repeated cycling and may thus predispose such joints to failure during ongoing exercise (19).

Relationships of Structure and Function

Tendons and ligaments are well-suited to the physiological functions they perform. Recruitment of collagen fibres from their resting crimp state can provide stable joint motion in anatomically determined positions of bony congruence. Neural feedback mechanisms protect static stabilizers by adding dynamic control and prevent displacement that would exceed their mechanical limits. Multiple tendons and ligaments serve a single joint, providing a mechanism for the maintenance of static and dynamic protection through wide ranges of movement.

The parallel fibre arrangement of tendons and ligaments allows for early tensile resistance once the crimp pattern is straightened. Their viscoelastic nature is similarly adapted to resisting sudden loads. The chemical structure and intermolecular cross-linking of the collagen, its interaction with the ground substance, and the water-binding capacity of the proteoglycans and collagen are all mechanically significant characteristics. Collectively they serve to maintain fibre orientation and distance in an organized meshwork for optimal load distribution and response. As fast loading rates cause increases in ultimate failure loads, joints are maximally protected during rapid movements. At slow loading rates and at lower loads, tendons and ligaments are extensible and have minimal mechanical impediment to normal ranges of motion.

Tendon and ligament insertions to bone are functionally adapted to force dissipation by passing through fibrocartilage to bone, and are less susceptible to disruption in the transition area than the extremes on either side (bone or peri-insertional ligament substance). Loading rates and failure modes will be discussed in a later section. As with all physiological systems, there are functional adaptations to age, temperature and sex. The mechanism of adaptation may well involve changes in content and organization of ligament substance secondary to any number of extraligamentous parameters (e.g. growth, sex, hormones, or activity).

RECENT FINDINGS ON THE BIOMECHANICAL PROPERTIES
OF NORMAL TENDONS AND LIGAMENTS

In the following section we will discuss some of our recent studies in tendon and ligament research as it pertains to the biomechanical properties. The readers may refer to our previous work for background information concerning the detailed methodology used to measure these biomechanical properties of ligaments and tendons (14, 15).

Effects of Maturity

The effects of age (maturation) on tendons, ligaments and their insertions have been demonstrated. Many authors, using rat tail tendons, have shown age-dependent increases in collagen fibril size, ultimate load and tensile strength from puberty to adulthood (20–22); afterwards, no changes were observed until senescence, where decreases in these properties may result (23). There exists limited information on changes in ligament properties as a function of age, however.

Four age groups of male New Zealand white rabbits were studied. Group I animals were aged 1.5 months (open epiphysis by radiological examination); Group II, 4–5 months (open epiphysis); Group III, 6–7 months; and Group IV, 12–15 months. All animals in Groups III and IV had closed epiphyses. The methods of procedures used have been described previously (14, 15). The structural properties of the femur-MCL-tibia (FMT) complex were represented by area of hysteresis, load-deformation curves, ultimate load and energy absorbed. The mechanical properties of the ligament were expressed by stress–strain curves.

The structural properties of the FMT complex increased dramatically from 1 to 6 months of age, at which time the magnitude of differences between groups diminished. The mechanical properties of the ligament substance demonstrated relatively early maturation, in that by 4–5 months of age, the stress–strain curves in the functional range, were similar to those of the adults (*Fig.* 12.3). However, the structural properties of the FMT complex did not reflect plateau values until closure of the epiphyses, at about 7 months. It was also noted by histological examination that the insertion site of the MCL on the tibial side is affected by its proximity to the growth plate, where osteoclastic activity in this region weakens the subperiosteal attachment, and part of the ligament insertion is at the area of the metaphysis. These findings are supported by the failure modes, as the rabbits with open epiphyses all failed by tibial avulsion. At maturity (closed epiphyses) only 12% failed by tibial avulsion.

Thus, it seems that the age of the animals has a significant effect on the relative strength of the various components in the FMT complex. For young animals, the ligament tissues (stress–strain) reflect adult properties prior to epiphyseal closure (*Fig.* 12.4). However, the insertion sites are directly affected by growth plate activity and remain structurally inferior until epiphyseal closure. Much interest has been generated on the changes in soft tissue with senescence and additional studies must be performed.

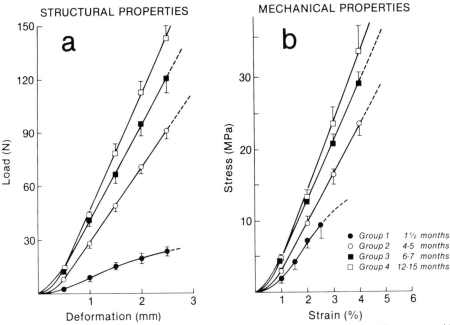

Fig. 12.3. *a*, The structural properties of the FMT complex for 4 age groups. There are rapid changes in the stiffness characteristics between the 2 younger groups, with smaller changes between the older groups. *b*, The mechanical properties of the MCL substance for 4 age groups. *Note* that the age-related changes were much less, as compared to those for the structural properties (*a*).

Temperature-dependent Properties

An important consideration when testing tendons and ligaments is the influence of the environmental temperature on their biomechanical behaviour. Most tests have been performed with the specimens in air at room temperature. Some immerse the specimen in a bath, such as an isotonic solution, where pH and temperature can be closely controlled. Rigby *et al.* suggested that no changes occur in the mechanical properties of ligaments between 0 and 37 °C (24). Apter reported that collagen has a negative temperature–elastic modulus relationship from 0 to 70 °C (25). Hunter and Williams found an inverse relationship between joint stiffness and temperature (26). We have also revealed a similar temperature dependence for articular cartilage (27).

The adult canine FMT complex was studied. The specimen was clamped and submerged into a 0·9% saline bath in a specially designed tank (approximately 8 l in volume) equipped with a heating and cooling system. The temperature was monitored and controlled by a thermostat (accuracy within 0·5 °C). Because of the length of time required to complete each test, the study was performed in 2 parts.

Study 1: Temperatures ranged from 22 to 37 °C (*Table* 12.1). Each specimen was sequentially tested at 22, 22, 27, 32, 37 and 22 °C. After applying a 2 N

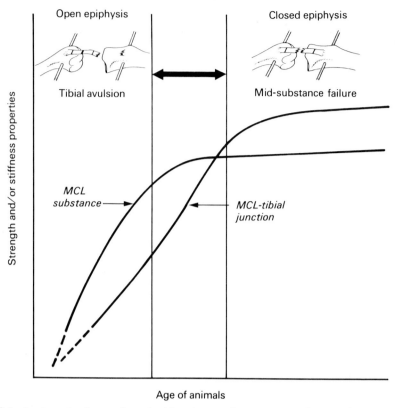

Fig. 12.4. A schematic diagram hypothesizing the asynchronous rates of maturation between the FMT complex and the MCL substance.

preload, the specimen was cycled between 0–2 mm extension (approximately 3% ligament strain) for 10 cycles at an extension rate of 2 cm/min. The specimen was then unloaded for 1 h at 22 °C and the same cyclic test was performed. A minimum of 1 h was required to allow recovery of the initial, untested condition due to the viscoelastic nature of the ligaments. Thereafter, the specimen was unloaded for 1 h between each cyclic test at 27, 32 and 37 °C. For the final test at 22 °C, a 2 h recovery period was allowed.

Study 2: Temperatures ranged from 2 to 22 °C (*Table* 12.1). Each specimen was sequentially tested at 22, 22, 2, 6, 14 and 22 °C. An identical testing procedure (as in *Study 1*) was used for each temperature except that the recovery period between tests ranged from 1.5 to 2.5 h. Note that the repeated cyclic tests at 22 °C for the beginning and end of each study were to check the repeatability and reliability of our experimental technique.

Loads and areas of hysteresis for each cycle at each temperature were recorded and normalized with respect to the first cycle load at 22 °C. The results demonstrate that the ligament reflects increasing stiffness in terms of cyclic loading as the temperature declines, and can be expressed by a simple linear

Table 12.1 Canine MCL cyclic testing. Algorithm demonstrating the testing protocol to study the effects of temperature on the biomechanical properties of canine MCL. Repeated test at 22 °C at the beginning and end are for checking the repeatability of the testing procedure as well as results.

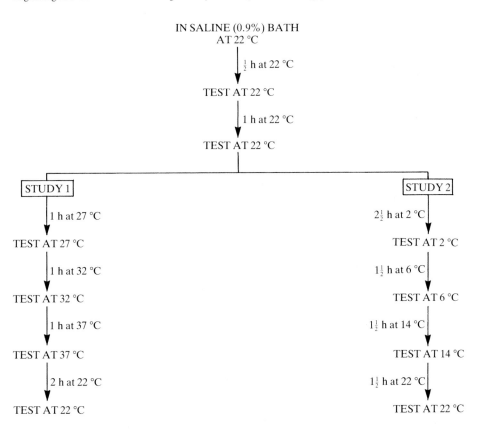

relationship (*Fig.* 12.5). For cyclic stress, the relaxation behaviour levelled out to lower values as the testing temperature was increased. The area of hysteresis reflected a similar temperature dependency. It is important to note that between temperature changes, the ligament requires between 1 and $2\frac{1}{2}$ h for it to return to its untested, resting characteristics. This may be of particular importance in explaining why our findings differ from those obtained by others. It also demonstrates how critical the use of a standardized procedure is to obtain dependable data and that temperature must be reported and controlled, as it can have profound effects on soft tissue behaviour.

Effects of Storage by Freezing

Biomechanical testing of ligaments and tendons has evolved into very complex methodologies. This often requires a considerable period of time for each

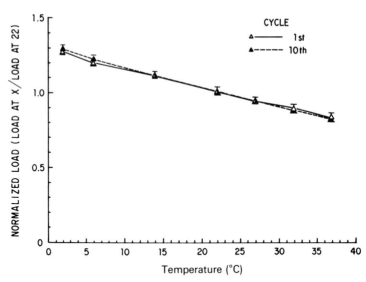

Fig. 12.5. Least square best fit curve of the normalized load (with respect to the load at 22 °C) *vs.* temperature, demonstrating a linear relationship (1st cycle: $y = -0.012X + 1.283$, $r = -0.999$; 10th cycle: $y = -0.013X + 1.304$, $r = -0.999$).

individual test, and therefore storage by freezing of the specimens becomes a necessity. Consequently, the effects of frozen storage on the mechanical properties of these tissues must be addressed. Furthermore, the results obtained will aid the current clinical interest of using frozen cadaver tendons and ligaments as allografts for transplantation.

Several biomechanical studies comparing the properties of fresh soft tissues with those following storage have been conducted, but with conflicting results (28-31). Most recently, several authors examined the effect of freezing storage for 4 weeks (at -15 °C) on monkey anterior cruciate ligaments (ACLs), and found no changes in the structural properties of bone-ligament-bone specimens (23, 32), while others reported a slight increase in stiffness (33).

In our laboratory, a study was designed to evaluate possible changes in the mechanical properties of the rabbit medial collateral ligament substance and/or of the structural properties of the FMT complex following 3 months of limb storage at -20 °C (34). Fresh contralateral limbs were dissected immediately at sacrifice and tested as controls.

There were no significant differences between fresh and frozen samples in most of the parameters measured (*Table* 12.2) except for the area of hysteresis, where the frozen samples demonstrated significant decreases during the first few cycles of loading and unloading when compared to fresh, contralateral controls. These differences diminished and became insignificant with further cycling. Thus, the area of hysteresis may be a sensitive indicator of minor changes in the properties of bone-ligament complex secondary to storage by freezing. It is conjectured that these changes may result from some insult to cellular integrity or associated ground substance (30) or from changes in ligament fluid dynamics (35).

Table 12.2 Structural properties of B-L-B complex (animals with closed epiphysis). Comparison of the biomechanical properties of fresh and frozen ligaments. P_{max} is the ultimate load in Newtons. Def_{max} is the deformation at failure. A_{max} is the ultimate energy absorbed.

	Fresh (n = 5)		Stored 45 days (n = 5)
Area of Hysteresis			
1st cycle (N·mm)	5·86 ± 1·60	$P < 0·05^*$	2·20 ± 0·54
10th cycle (N·mm)	1·36 ± 0·50	$P > 0·10$	0·58 ± 0·30
Structural Properties (at failure)			
P_{max} (N)	368·4 ± 15·0	$P > 0·05$	316·2 ± 22·3
Def_{max}(mm)	6·6 ± 0·6	$P > 0·50$	6·6 ± 0·5
A_{max} (N·mm)	1330·0 ± 200·0	$P > 0·50$	1170·0 ± 200·0

* paired t-test, statistically significant

Freezing did not appear to affect the ligament insertion sites, as the modes of failure were not altered between the experimentals and the controls. However, it is crucial to reiterate the care taken in preparing the tissue sample prior to freezing and in protecting the sample from dehydration. The ligaments were stored with muscle and other tissues left in place rather than in the completely dissected state. Each sample was then double-wrapped in saline-soaked gauze and sealed in airtight plastic bags. Thawing was carried out at refrigerator temperatures (4 °C) overnight and specimens were tested soon after thawing.

FAILURE MODES OF TISSUE-BONE COMPLEX

The functional support provided by a tendon is the muscle-tendon-bone complex and by a ligament is the bone-ligament-bone unit. Clinically, failure in adult tissue-bone complexes is more common by substance tear rather than by avulsion, yet many investigators using cadavers and experimental animals have commented on the difficulty of producing substance injuries, and have traditionally stated that the bone is the weakest component of the system (36–39). Identifiable factors for such discrepancies include species and ligament type, axis of loading, activity levels, strain rate and age. Investigations by our laboratory have been concerned with several of these factors.

Axis of Force Application

The structural properties of the bone-ligament complex have been shown to change when the load is applied along the longitudinal axis of the ligament or along the longitudinal axis of the tibia (40). In the case of the rabbit femur-ACL-tibia complex (FATC), if the load was directed along the ACL axis, angle of knee flexion had no significant effect on the ultimate load values and most failures were by bony avulsion. However, when directing forces along the longitudinal axis of the tibia, progressively lower strengths of the FATC were found as knee flexion increased, and failures occurred primarily by progressive fibre failure of the ACL at the insertion site. Thus, it appears that when the load was applied along the ligament axis, the ligament fibrils were oriented so that an even distribution of forces occurred and maximum strength resulted. Force application along the tibial axis resulted in uneven loading along the ligament, and the fibrils resisting most of the load failed in a progressive fashion. Similar results have also been observed for porcine and human ACL specimens in our laboratory.

Effects of Animal Activity

Findings in our laboratory and others (4, 41) have demonstrated that immobilization of a joint for several weeks leads to a precipitous decline in ligament–bone junction strength, particularly for those ligaments that insert via the periosteum and do not pass through well defined zones of fibrocartilage (e.g. the tibial insertion of the MCL). Most failures occur by bony avulsion and histological observation identifies the compromised bone–ligament junction as subperiosteal resorption.

Effects of Strain Rates

Considerable attention has been given to the effects of the rate of stretch on the failure mode of a bone–ligament–bone complex. Some investigators feel that the reason others have been unsuccessful in obtaining ligament substance failure is primarily due to employing slower strain rates (5, 20, 42).

In our laboratory, however, we have shown that the effects of maturation on ligament insertion strength can be even more significant than strain rate. For example, using a moderate strain rate (0·3/sec), we have found that for animals with open epiphyses, all failures occurred by tibial avulsion, whereas for those older animals (12–15 months) with closed epiphyses there was no failure by tibial avulsion (43).

The effect of strain rate on the MCL mid-substance material properties, as well as its effects on mode of failure of the FMT complex, have been investigated by selecting 2 groups of New Zealand white rabbits, 1 group with open epiphysis ($3\frac{1}{2}$ months old) and the other with closed epiphysis ($8\frac{1}{2}$ months old). The FMT complex was subjected to uniaxial tensile tests at 5 different extension rates (0·008–113 mm/sec). The corresponding strain rates of the ligament substance were 0·011–155%/s and 0·001–222%/s for Groups I and II, respectively. In the case of high strain rates, a high speed video recording system was used to tape the test history at 2000 frames/s (normal videotaping speed is 60 frames/s).

In Group I, the structural properties of the FMT complex were found to be dependent on the extension rates (*Fig.* 12.6a). The ultimate load and energy absorbed increased 2·5 and 3·0 times, respectively. For Group II, the ultimate load and energy absorbed also increased with increasing extension rates, but to a lesser degree (*Fig.* 12.6a). Significant differences were obtained only between the slowest and fastest strain rate tests (a range of 4 decades). The mechanical properties of the MCL substance in the pre-failure range paralleled the results on the structural properties (*Fig.* 12.6b). The tensile strength of the MCL increased significantly with strain rate, but by only 60% from the lowest to the highest strain rates. Failure modes, on the other hand, were independent of strain rate. All failures in animals with open epiphyses occurred by tibial avulsion, whereas all failures in animals with closed epiphyses occurred by ligament disruption. These results were confirmed by photomicrographs. We therefore concluded that the age of the animals was the most influential factor determining failure mode (*Fig.* 12.4).

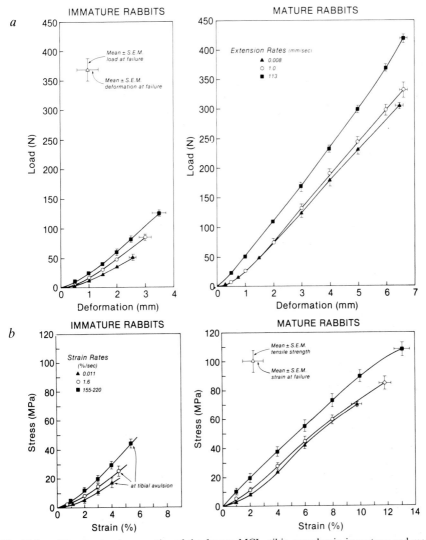

Fig. 12.6. *a*, The structural properties of the femur–MCL–tibia complex in immature and mature rabbits as a function of extension rates. *b*, The mechanical properties of the MCL substance in immature and mature rabbits as a function of strain rates.

FUNCTIONAL ADAPTATION – STRESS AND MOTION EFFECTS ON TISSUE HOMEOSTASIS

Similar to Wolff's law for bone (44), a generalized statement on the adaptation of applied stress and motion for tendons and ligaments can also be made. Roux (45) recognized this 'law of functional adaptation' by stating that 'an organ will adapt itself structurally to an alteration, quantitative or qualitative, of function'. Therefore, it is not surprising that ligaments are morphologically, biomechanically, and biochemically sensitive to both stress enhancement and stress deprivation.

Stress and Motion Deprivation (Immobilization)

The effects of stress deprivation on synovial joints are profound. Intra-articular changes include pannus formation to the point of obliterating the joint space. If the process is allowed to continue for months, cartilage necrosis is seen in contact areas (46) and erosion and ulceration occur in non-contact areas (47). Gross inspection of ligaments and tendons reveals them to be less glistening and more woody in appearance. Intercellular collagen fibre bundles may be decreased in thickness and number secondary to immobilization (i.e., atrophy of collagen) (48).

Increased joint stiffness after immobilization has been well known clinically. Quantitatively it has been demonstrated in experimental animals by using an arthrograph (49). After 9 weeks of immobilization, the amount of torque initially required to extend the rabbit knee and the area of hysteresis (measuring the energy requirements) were significantly increased (50). Increases in knee joint stiffness have been attributed to the adhesions, pannus, and decreased lubrication, but probably also include restricted extensibility of loose periarticular collagen weave by fixed contact at strategic sites (49, 51). Newly produced collagen fibrils are hypothesized to form these interfibrillar contacts and would be expected to restrict normal fibre sliding and motion in extensible structures such as capsule of the shoulder or posterior aspect of the knee.

In a recent study, rabbit knees were immobilized and remobilized for varying periods, viz. Group I, 9 weeks of immobilization; Group II, 12 weeks of immobilization; Group III, 9 weeks of immobilization followed by 9 weeks of remobilization; and Group IV, 12 weeks of immobilization followed by 9 weeks of remobilization. Significant changes in the structural properties of the FMT complex following immobilization were found (52). For Group I, the ultimate loads and energy-absorbing capabilities of the experimental complexes were only 29% and 16%, respectively, of the contralateral controls ($P < 0.01$). Group II had still further reduction. Ligament substance is also affected by immobility. Rather than becoming relatively more stiff in tension, however, as may be postulated from increased joint stiffness (contracture), ligaments become less stiff. Stress–strain curves revealed a significant softening of the ligament substance after immobilization (*Fig.* 12.7).

Following remobilization, the mechanical properties of MCL substance rapidly returned to normal control values after 9 weeks (*Fig.* 12.8), but the structural properties of the FMT complex remained inferior to controls. Mode of failure for Groups III and IV reflect this continued disruption at the bony

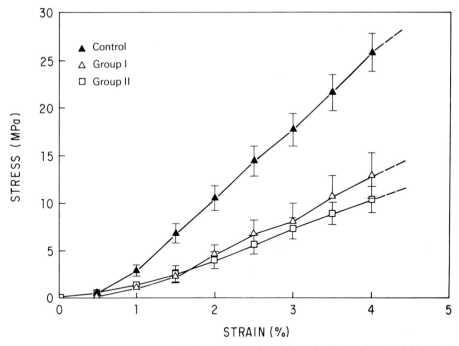

Fig. 12.7. Mechanical properties of MCL from normal and 9 week (Group I) and 12 (Group II) week immobilized MCL.

insertion sites. These findings are supported by histological results obtained. At 9 weeks of immobilization, the disruption of the ligament–tibia junction was complete and the ligament was secured by only its superficial periosteal attachment. This was reflected by large decreases in ultimate load. As such, an additional three weeks of immobilization (Group II) resulted in little further decline of the ultimate load. For the recovery groups (Groups III and IV), the structural strength of the FMT complex continued to lag behind their respective controls. These findings are supported by others and by the histology which demonstrated incomplete reorganization at the resorption sites (4, 41).

The mechanical properties of the ligament substance were presented in the pre-failure region. Contrary to most research which has been concerned with loads at failure, and as such have left the changes in the functional properties following stress-deprivation unnoticed, this study demonstrated significant deterioration in the tensile properties of the MCL following immobilization, but rapid recovery following remobilization. Such complete recovery of the MCL tissue has important implications not previously revealed. It should be mentioned that these results were for the medial collateral ligament and may not be generalized to other ligaments. For example, the ACL is positioned in a 'hostile' synovial fluid environment, thus immobilization may be of greater detriment to the ACL's physiological balance, while remobilization may not be as effective in restoring homeostatic conditions.

The collagen turnover study (53) further explains the changes seen in the mechanical properties of the ligament tissue. Gamble *et al.* (54) demonstrated

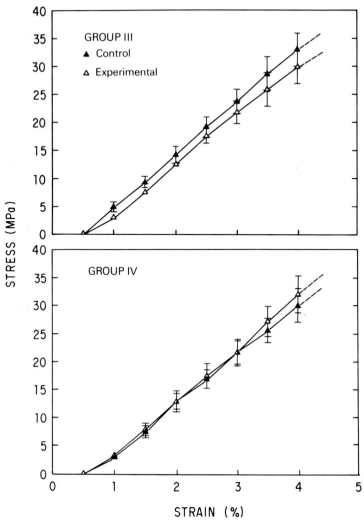

Fig. 12.8. Mechanical properties of normal and experimental MCLs. For the experimentals, the rabbit knees were subjected to 9 weeks of immobilization with 9 weeks remobilization (Group III), and 12 weeks of immobilization with 9 weeks remobilization (Group IV).

the enzymatic adaptation of the MCL fibroblasts to a state of catabolism following knee immobilization which may affect collagen and other matrix materials. The lysosomal enzymes degrade GAGs, and earlier studies in our laboratory (51) have shown a 20% reduction in GAGs from MCLs of immobilized rabbit limbs. Thus, the significant changes in the mechanical properties of the ligament substance may be due to the drastic reduction in GAGs (55). During remobilization, we have observed recovery of overall collagen mass in the MCL, and also presumably the fibre orientation and hence the mechanical properties (53), whereas the incomplete recovery of the FMT complex implies an asynchronous recovery rate of the tibial insertion site, especially the subperiosteal area.

Stress and Motion Enhancement (Exercise)

The effect of exercise on tendons and ligaments has only recently been investigated but with confusing and contradictory results. Reasons for discrepancies may include the use of various animal models, inadequate intergroup matching of important variables, different experimental procedures, and inconsistent definition of controls and exercised animals. There is a suggestion of decreased water content with a more dull appearance and a slight loss of fibre waviness immediately after exercise (19). An increase in cross-sectional area and weight have been reported after certain long-term exercise programmes (56). Microscopically, this increase in mass has been suggested as secondary to fibre bundle hypertrophy (with increased collagen matrix between cell bodies) as opposed to cellular hyperplasia (48, 56).

As noted above, ligament insertions are particularly sensitive to stress and motion, especially those which are in concert with the periosteum (4, 41). Many of these changes are probably influenced by specific ligaments or types, but one may suggest that a spectrum exists for tissue response to activity levels, i.e. each ligament or tendon has a unique threshold level of activity required to maintain normal homeostatic conditions.

Tipton *et al.* demonstrated definitive improvement of strength of the bone-ligament-bone complex of dogs by keeping the animals in open pens (56). The separation force of these complexes in various models generally have been higher following exercise (39, 48, 56, 57). Such results were obtained for medial collateral (58, 59), lateral collateral (60), and anterior cruciate knee preparations (5, 6).

In our laboratory, the effects of exercise on the biomechanical properties of swine digital tendons were studied (61, 62). Swine were randomly divided into 2 groups: one was trained for 3 months (short term) and the other for 12 months (long term). The running speeds were 6–8 km/h and the average distance run by each animal was 40 km/week. Non-exercised, age-matched swine were used as controls. It was found that short-term (3 months) exercise had little or no effect on the digital extensor and flexor tendon properties. However, the long-term exercise group had positive changes. The tensile strength of the extensor tendons was 22% higher, partially due to increase in the tendon mass.

For the flexor tendons, the mechanical properties of the tendon substance exhibited no statistical changes, even after 12 months of training. However, the ultimate load of the exercised flexor-tendon complexes increased 19%, secondary to changes at the bony insertion sites. Tipton *et al.* also noted that FMT complexes of caged, exercised dogs had higher strength/body weight ratios than those from caged, control, non-exercised dogs (48).

Summary of Findings

From these findings we can construct hypothetical curves to describe the homeostatic responses for connective tissues such as tendons and ligaments (*Fig.* 12.9). The relationship between the levels and durations of stress and motion, and the resulting changes in tissue properties and tissue mass, could be represented by a series of highly non-linear curves. With stress and motion deprivation (immobilization) a rapid reduction in tissue properties and mass may occur. For example, a short period of immobilization of the rabbit knee resulted in a significant alteration of the mechanical properties of the MCL substance, as well as the structural properties of the FMT complex. On the contrary, with exercise training, the resulting changes may not be as pronounced. For example, with 3 months of exercise training, the tendon had little change in mechanical properties and mass. Only with long-term (12 months) training were the positive responses on the mechanical properties (and mass) seen.

In terms of recovery following immobilization, one should separately consider the individual constituents of the tissue-bone complex. The mechanical integrity of the uninjured, immobilized ligament returns to normal in the functional range quite rapidly following remobilization. However, the recovery of the ligament-bone junction is slow and asynchronous with the ligament substance. It will take many months before the ligamentous insertion sites can complete the remodelling and return to normal.

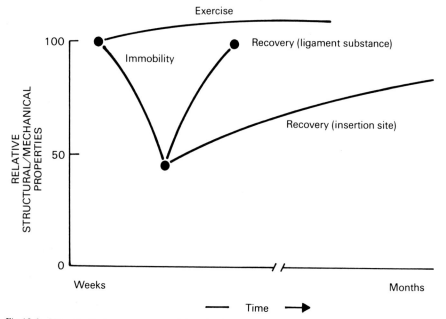

*Fig.*12.9. Hypothetical curves summarizing the homeostatic response of the structural/mechanical properties of tendons and ligaments subjected to different levels of physical activity (the Woo–Akeson–Amiel–UCSD hypothesis).

HEALING AND TREATMENT

The treatment of damaged ligaments and tendons is a difficult and challenging orthopaedic problem. The approach in determining the most adequate treatment protocols has yet to be determined. Accurate descriptions of other types of soft tissue healing have provided a springboard for current interests in tendon and ligament healing (63). Those interests include *(1)* non-repaired *vs.* repaired and *(2)* motion and activity level effects on the healing of tendons and ligaments.

Flexor Tendon Repair

A concept has prevailed that the gliding surface between the flexor tendon and fibrous digital sheath is not maintained after tendon injury and repair. Three factors contributing to the formation of adhesions – tendon suture, digital sheath injury and immobilization – have been considered essential, if unavoidable, components of the injury and repair process.

Mason and Allen's pioneer work of 1941 influenced the clinical and research communities (64). They concluded that the early stages following repair were characterized by a profound drop in strength (lowest values at 4–5 days), and that after 19 days, the strength of the repair increased directly with the stresses applied to it. These findings encouraged clinicians to immobilize tendons for 3 weeks and concentrate on the remodelling stages for stimulating increased tendon strength and gliding.

The paradox of the 'one-wound' healing precipitated by immobilization, however, is that the remodelling process involves a conflict between the needs for strength at the repair site and the needs for flexibility of the ingrowing tissue. In our laboratory, the flexor tendons of the second and fourth toes of adult mongrel dogs were lacerated and repaired by a technique described by Kessler and Missim (65). Animals were divided into 3 groups to determine the effects of mobilization on repair site strength, gliding, and scar remodelling (66), i.e. Group I was treated with continuous immobilization, Group II with delayed mobilization and Group III with immediate controlled mobilization. At sacrifice, the toes of forepaws were disarticulated at the metacarpophalangeal joints. For each repaired tendon a contralateral control tendon was prepared and tested for comparison.

The excursion (gliding) function of the tendon through the sheath was evaluated by means of an apparatus designed to measure the angular rotation of the distal interphalangeal joint when a small load of 1·5 N was applied. The mechanical properties of the repairs and controls were measured by determining the load and deformation of the 'tendon–bone composite' (61). The ultimate load, maximum percentage elongation and linear slope were determined.

The continuous immobilization group (Group I) did not exhibit significant increases in strength of the repaired tendons until 12 weeks of immobilization (*Fig.* 12.10). The delayed, passive mobilized tendons (in Group II) showed increased strength at each time interval beyond 3 weeks when compared to the immobilized tendons. Those for the immediate mobilization tendons (in Group III) showed significantly higher values for ultimate load at each time interval than either Group I or Group II tendons. A similar trend was also observed in the stiffness values of the tendons.

Gliding function, represented by the angular rotation data, was also greatest in the early mobilization group (*Fig.* 12.10) at both 6 and 12 weeks. For Group I (immobilized tendon), the angular rotation 6 weeks after repair was only $21 \pm 5\%$ of the intact controls. At 12 weeks, the rotation was further reduced to $19 \pm 2\%$. The Group II (delayed mobilization) tendons had better gliding than the Group I tendons, with angular rotation at 6 and 12 weeks, nearly 3 times that of the immobilized tendons. The angular rotation of the Group III (immediate mobilization) tendons at 6 weeks was $79 \pm 16\%$ and at 12 weeks was equal (100%) to that of the controls.

Further investigation by microangiography demonstrated that the mobilized groups had vessels oriented longitudinally and were more normal in density. DNA content at the repair site and in the digital sheath was significantly greater in the mobilized groups. Furthermore, scanning electron microscopy showed that the repaired site of the early mobilized tendons and sheath had a smooth surface and were free of adhesions. Light microscopy also showed that the mobilized tendons had a smooth covering over the repair site by cells from the epitenon at 10 days. This smooth, glistening surface remained unchanged and free of adhesions through 42 days. At the ultrastructural level, cells between the tendon ends were active in protein synthesis and collagen production at 21 and 42 days.

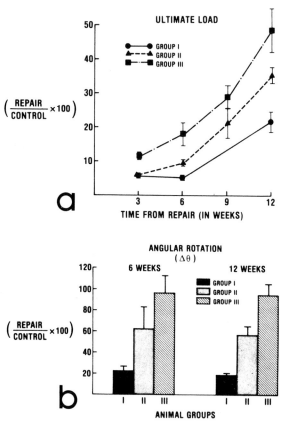

Fig. 12.10. Comparison of normalized (*a*) ultimate load (strength) and (*b*) angular rotation ($\Delta\theta$) excursion of repaired tendon from immobilization (Group I), delayed mobilization (Group II) and early mobilization (Group III) treatment groups.

These studies demonstrated that controlled passive mobilization exerted tensile forces and motion on the repair site that appeared to accelerate strength of the repaired tendon. Of equal importance were the tendon excursion properties. The decreased range of motion with prolonged immobilization was due to scar formation between the repaired tendon and surrounding sheath.

Medial Collateral Ligament Healing

The first histological description of the states of ligament healing in an animal model appeared in the work of Miltner (37) and subsequently a series of specific and multidisciplinary studies has been published.

Non-repaired ligaments

In complete disruptions, free ligament ends usually recoil with the tortuous appearance of the relaxed ligament bodies and are connected only by the forming haematoma (67). Vascular granulation tissue begins in the first few days and proliferates through haemorrhagic tissues to fill potential spaces in the area. Inflammation and granulation predominate for 2–3 weeks as progressive fibrosis occurs. At about 1 month, resorption of joint fluid and oedema reveals a considerable extent of underlying scar formation and maturation begins. Contraction and remodelling of this scar in the animal model is sufficiently advanced at 6 weeks for some to note 'complete healing' (68). However, months or years may be required to even approach normality. Eighteen months after injury, the bridging scar of the rabbit MCL has become relatively hypocellular, is still slightly disorganized, and has a different staining quality than normal (68).

Reports of tensile tests of healing ligaments suggest that the return to normal strength and elastic stiffness in ligaments is slow (69). The rate of return of the ligament's structural and mechanical properties is probably dependent on stress, however, and may therefore be controlled to some extent by physical means (57, 70, 71).

Repaired ligaments

With repair, there may be certain qualitative and quantitative alterations in the processes just described. Clayton and Weir (55, 70) noted diminution of separation in ligament ends and therefore a significant decrease in scar formation with repair. O'Donoghue et al. (50), using a similar model, noted more orderly healing in the early stages as a result of repair. Repaired ligaments appeared 'more taut' and had increased collagenization with shorter stages of inflammation and proliferation (50).

There is evidence of an early advantage in strength properties of repaired ligaments over those that are not repaired (50, 55). This advantage, however, may not be sustained. Sutured and unsutured ligaments had nearly equal length when measured at rest and failure strength when both had been subjected to exercise (70) but the non-repaired may be more distensible when stressed because of the scar.

Current studies

In our laboratory, we have studied complete surgical injuries to the mid-substance of the right rabbit MCLs (experimentals) and exposures only of their contralateral, left MCLs (sham controls) (69). There was no repair or immobilization and all animals had unrestricted cage activity until sacrifice in groups at 10 days, 3 weeks, 6 weeks, 14 weeks and 40 weeks after injury.

Additional age-, sex- and activity-matched animals (normal controls) were used at each of these time intervals to provide a baseline of all parameters.

Histological evaluation revealed that healing of the disrupted, non-repaired ligament is similar to the classic descriptions as detailed earlier. Biochemical results correlated well with the histological findings (69). Water content was significantly elevated at the injury site but returned to normal after 6 weeks. GAG content was elevated early and continued to be so even at 40 weeks. Collagen content dropped significantly after injury, and then steadily recovered, but never reached control values. The healing MCLs also contained significant amounts of Type III collagen.

The mechanical and structural properties of the healing MCL were persistently inferior to the sham controls even at 40 weeks post-injury. The MCL was larger, weaker and less stiff in tension than normals. Cyclic and stress–relaxation properties of the healed MCL, however, did show more complete recovery, indicating that the properties of the MCL may be more normal in the functional low loading range.

In a second model, adult mongrel dogs were separated into 3 groups. In Group 1, the early mobilization group, the MCL of the left knee was transected at the joint line and not repaired. The animals were each allowed 6, 12 and 48 weeks of cage and farm activities, and sacrificed. In Group 2, the short-term immobilization group, the MCL was repaired after transection. The knee joint was immobilized for 3 weeks and then remobilized for either 3 or 9 weeks with cage activity. In Group 3, the longer-term immobilization group, the MCL was transected and repaired as before. Immobilization was extended to 6 weeks and additional animals were each remobilized with cage and farm activities for 6 and 42 weeks. The right knee of all animals were sham operated, leaving the MCL intact.

At sacrifice, each knee was then attached to a device specially designed to measure varus–valgus (V–V) laxity at 90 °C flexion (72). A cyclic torque of ± 0.6 Nm was applied to the joint and the angular deformation (θ) was recorded. The $\Delta\theta$ value between ± 0.6 Nm was defined as the V– V joint laxity. After laxity testing, all soft tissue except the MCL was removed and the FMT complex was then subjected to tensile tests to failure following Woo *et al.* (72, 73).

At 6 weeks postoperatively, all experimental knees had significantly higher V–V laxities (*Fig.* 12.11). At 12 and 48 weeks, the experimental knees from Group 1, the early mobilization group, achieved the best results, as their values were similar to those of the controls, while Group 3, the longer-term immobilization group, continued to exhibit higher V–V laxity (174% of the controls at 48 weeks). An identical trend was observed for the structural properties of the FMT complex and the mechanical properties (stress–strain curves) of the healing MCL (*Fig.* 12.12). In Group 1, the ultimate load of the FMT complex recovered to the level of the control by 12 weeks (98%) and remained so up to 48 weeks (105%). However, the tensile strength of healing MCL was only 66% and 46% of the controls for Groups 1 and 3, respectively, at 48 weeks.

Both short- and long-term results obtained indicate that surgical repair with subsequent immobilization did not enhance the strength of healing MCL nor reduce the V–V laxity. These findings confirmed the clinical practice that

KNEE
VARUS-VALGUS LAXITY

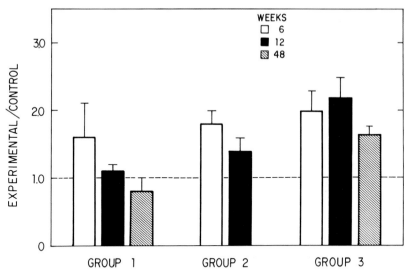

Fig. 12.11. The normalized varus–valgus laxity for experimental canine knees as a function of time (6, 12, and 48 weeks) post-operatively. Group 1 is the early mobilization group (without repair). Group 2 is the short-term immobilization group (with repair) and Group 3 is the longer-term immobilization group (with repair).

primary surgical repair may not be necessary for isolated tears of the MCLs in patients (74). These findings further demonstrate that the recovery of the mechanical properties of the healing MCL is slower than that of the structural properties of the FMT complex. Also, the animal species used (dog, rabbit) and postoperative activities (size of cage and farm) may have significant effects on the end points of the remodelling process for the healing MCL.

It is important to note that healing is dependent on ligament type. For example, the ACL is not known to heal unless approximated with sutures, and even then, healing is often incomplete, leading some surgeons to challenge the use of primary repair of the cruciates (74, 75). This has led to much recent interest on autograft, allograft, and xenograft, as well as synthetic replacement of the torn ACL. The important question is whether there is a mechanical difference between repaired or non-repaired ligaments which heal. More studies in this area are encouraged, as well as studies on the mediators of stress effects such as blood supply and hormones. Hopefully, additional research will result in a complete understanding of its function and nutritional source, so that the dismal sequelae associated with ACL injuries will be of only historic interest.

CONCLUSIONS

Much of our current understanding of the biomechanical properties of ligaments and tendons has come from the development and application of new

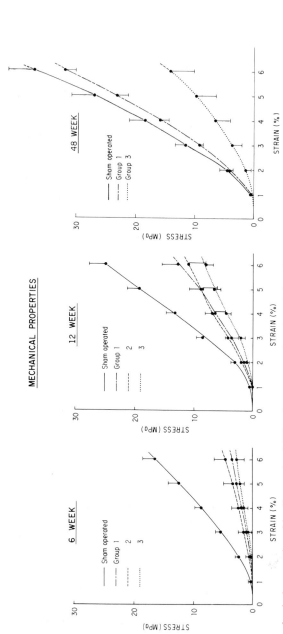

Fig. 12.12. Mechanical properties of healing canine MCL substance as a function of time (6, 12 and 48 weeks) post-operatively. *Refer to Fig.* 12.11 for group description.

technologies such as accurate determination of stress and strain of the ligament mid-substance. These technical breakthroughs have afforded us the ability to examine old ideas more thoroughly and accurately. Even more important is the stimulation that these examinations have provided for exploring new ideas and possibilities. Through utilization of normal and high speed video recording, together with the video dimensional analyser system and other bioengineering advances, we have presented new insights into the knowledge of the biomechanics of ligaments and tendons. We have shown that the tensile behaviour of ligaments (and probably all soft tissue) is based upon an inverse relationship between ligament stiffness and temperature. This study reinforces the need for a standardized testing procedure, since any change in environmental temperature may influence the results.

Other studies in this chapter include the identification of the differences between the ligament substance and its insertion sites under various conditions. The investigations concerning the strain-rate sensitivity of ligaments have reinforced the concept that tensile properties of the ligaments, like most other soft tissues, are not as sensitive to rates of stretch, but are more dependent on the animal's age. Through 4 decades of strain-rates, the MCL from animals with open epiphyses all failed by tibial avulsion, but those that had reached skeletal maturity failed by tearing of the MCL substance. Also, the differences in mechanical properties of the MCL between the younger and older groups were not nearly as large as those for structural properties of the FMT complex, and the asynchronous rate of maturation in the FMT complex has been demonstrated, i.e. the ligament substance matures earlier than the ligament–bone junction.

Our results concerning the homeostatic adaptation of ligaments and tendons to varying activity levels have revealed that each component of the bone–ligament–bone complex has unique time-dependent responses to stress. Ligament properties can completely recover following short-term remobilization, but recovery of the FMT complex structural properties is incomplete, due to persistent weakness at the insertion sites. The response of tendons and ligaments to exercise seems to be type specific. The mechanical properties of the flexor tendons underwent no significant changes following prolonged exercise when compared to non-exercised controls. However, the extensor tendons demonstrated significant increases, as well as tendon hypertrophy. Animal studies conducted by Tipton *et al.* have demonstrated an increase in junction strength of bone–ligament–bone preparations following exercise (48). They also reported that the strength of repaired ligaments is increased with training and decreased following immobilization.

Studies concerning tendon and ligament healing continue to generate much enthusiasm. We have been able to isolate the mechanical properties of the healing site as it undergoes continual reorganization. From a clinical standpoint, an important observation has been that for an isolated MCL tear, primary surgical repair seems to offer no lasting benefit in terms of varus–valgus laxity and of mechanical properties at the healing site. On the other hand, prolonged immobilization proves to be detrimental to the healing process, as well as to the overall bone–ligament–bone strength. Since many of these functional adaptations of ligament and tendon healing are type-specific, activity level-specific, and animal-specific, continued investigations are necessary to understand the unique responses of all ligaments (ACL, PCL, spinal ligaments, etc.) and tendons (Patellar, Achilles, etc.). Additional developments in biomedical engineering and technology will be required to expand our fundamental understanding of ligament and tendon function.

CLINICAL SIGNIFICANCE

Ligament and tendon disorders may be more important to clinical practice than is commonly appreciated. They are involved in congenital disorders, e.g. congenital dysplasia of the hip, Ehlers–Danlos syndrome, talipes equinovarus, arthrogryposis and a number of acquired conditions. They can be affected either primarily or secondarily in many of these conditions, including the connective tissue disorders (rheumatoid arthritis, ankylosing spondylitis, gout, Marfan's syndrome, and ochronosis), degenerative joint diseases (osteoarthritis, haemophiliac arthritis), infection (septic joints or bursae), neoplasms (bony or soft tissue), neurological conditions (Charcot's joint), toxins (lathyrism), and trauma.

Trauma is the best recognized cause of tendon and ligament pathology. Although the significance of catastrophic tendon and ligament failures at the hand, knee, ankle, or shoulder are well known, so-called sprains (probably the majority of injuries) are often diagnosed and treated with relative ease. Perhaps the most common entities in orthopaedic practice are injuries of the back and neck, and these often involve tendon and ligament injuries.

Commonly used clinical modalities including immobilization, traction, and physiotherapy clearly have a positive and negative influence on ligaments and tendons. Preoperative correction of joint deformity often relies on ligament softening and stretching by using combinations of these techniques.

The understanding of normal tendon and ligament physiology is an important prerequisite for the study of their healing processes. Correlations of morphology, biochemistry and biomechanics of normal ligaments provide an appreciation of their complexity and functional abilities. Normal tendons and ligaments are not inert structures. Although limited by metabolic activity and blood supply, they are nevertheless able to respond to joint loading and movement.

Commonly used orthopaedic modalities, such as rest and exercise, have dramatic effects on tendon and ligament properties. These effects should be considered in treatment planning that will affect the joint function. Recovery of strength in injured tendons and ligaments is exceedingly slow as a result of their physiological processes, and they must be treated accordingly.

The biological story of tendons and ligaments is far from complete. Only through a better understanding of the processes of their physiology (morphology, biochemistry and biomechanics) will mechanisms of injuries and healing be understood, and treatment of all conditions be optimized.

ACKNOWLEDGEMENTS

The authors gratefully acknowledge the financial support of the RR&D of the Veterans Administration, NIH Grants GM 24900 and AM14918, and the Malcolm and Dorothy Coutts Institute for Joint Reconstruction and Research.

We would also like to recognize the important contributions and technical assistance of students, residents and fellows of the Orthopaedic Bioengineering laboratory, La Jolla, CA, during the course of this work.

REFERENCES

1. Bloom W and Fawcett D W (1975) *A Textbook of Histology.* Philadelphia: Saunders.
2. Baer E (1978) The multicomposite structure of tendon collagen: relationships between ultrastructure and mechanical properties. *Proceedings of Third International Congress of Biorheology* La Jolla, California, p.43
3. Cooper R R and Misol S (1970) Tendon and ligament insertion. *J Bone Joint Surg [Am]* 52: 1–20
4. Laros G S, Tipton C M and Cooper R R (1971) Influence of physical activity on ligament insertions in the knees of dogs. *J Bone Joint Surg [Am]* 53: 275–86.
5. Noyes F R, DeLucas J L and Torvik P J (1974) Biomechanics of anterior cruciate ligament failure: an analysis of strain rate sensitivity and mechanisms of failure in primates. *J Bone Joint Surg [Am]* 56: 236–53.
6. Noyes F R, Torvik P J, Hyde W B and DeLucas J L (1974) Biomechanics of ligament failure. II. An analysis of immobilization, exercise and reconditioning effects in primates. *J Bone Joint Surg [Am]* 56: 1406–18.
7. Tipton C M, Matthes R D and Martin R R (1978) Influence of age and sex on the strength of bone-ligament junctions in knee joints of rats. *J Bone Joint Surg [Am]* 60: 230–4.
8. Neuberger A and Slack H G B (1953) The metabolism of collagen from liver, bones, skin and tendon in the normal rat. *Biochem J* 53: 47–52.
9. Grant M E and Prockop D J (1972) The biosynthesis of collagen. *N Engl J Med* 286: 194–9.
10. Bailey A J (1968) *Comprehensive Biochemistry.* Amsterdam: Elsevier.
11. Mechanic G L (1974) An automated scintillation counting system with high efficiency for continuous analysis: cross-links of [^{3}H]NaBH$_4$ reduced collagen. *Anal Biochem* 61: 349–54.
12. Tanzer M L (1973) Cross-linking of collagen. *Science* 180: 561–6.
13. Fung Y C B (1973) Biorheology of soft tissues. *Biorheology* 10: 139–55.
14. Woo S L-Y, Gomez M A, Woo Y K and Akeson W H (1982) Mechanical properties of tendons and ligaments. I. Quasi-static and nonlinear viscoelastic properties. *Biorheology* 19: 385–96.
15. Woo S L-Y, Gomez M A and Akeson W H (1985) Mechnical behaviours of soft tissues: measurements, modifications, injuries and treatment. *In: Biomechanics of Trauma.* (A M Nahum and J Melvin, eds), pp. 109–33. Norwalk: Appleton Century Crofts.
16. Lewis J L and Bhybut G T (1981) *In vivo* forces in the collateral ligaments of canine knees. *Trans Orthop Res Soc* 6: 4.
17. Arms S W, Pope M H, Boyle J B, Davignon P J and Johnson R J (1982) Knee medial collateral ligament strain. *Trans Orthop Res Soc* 7: 47.
18. Woo S L-Y, Gomez M A and Akeson W H (1981) The time and history dependent viscoelastic properties of medial collateral ligaments. *J Biomech Eng* 103: 293–8.
19. Tipton C M, Schild R J and Tomanek R J (1967) Influence of physical activity on the strength of knee ligaments in rats. *Am J Physiol* 212: 783–7.
20. Haut R C (1983) Age-dependent influence of strain rate on the tensile failure of rat-tail tendon. *J Biomech Eng* 105: 296–9.
21. Morein G, Goldgefter L, Kobyliansky E, Goldschmidt-Nathan M and Nathan H (1978) Change in mechanical properties of rat tail tendon during postnatal ontogenesis. *Anat Embryol (Berl)* 154: 121–4.
22. Nathan H, Goldgefter L, Kobyliansky E, Goldschmitt-Nathan M and Morein G (1978) Energy absorbing capacity of rat tail tendon at various ages. *J Anat* 127: 589–93
23. Noyes F R and Grood E S (1976) The strength of the anterior cruciate ligament in humans and rhesus monkeys. *J Bone Joint Surg [Am]* 58: 1074–82.
24. Rigby B, Hirai N, Spikes J and Eyring H (1958) The mechanical properties of rat tail tendon. *J Gen Physiol* 43: 265–83.
25. Apter J (1972) Influence of composition on thermal properties of tissues. *In: Biomechanics: Its Foundations and Objectives* (Y C Fung, N Perrone and M Anliker, eds), pp. 217–35. Englewood Cliffs: Prentice-Hall.

26. Hunter J and Williams M G (1951) A study of the effect of cold on joint temperature and mobility. *Can J Med Sci* **29:** 255–62.
27. Kuei S, Woo S L-Y, Gomez M A and Akeson W H (1979) The viscoelastic, thermoelastic, and time dependent properties of the knee ligaments. *Trans Orthop Res Soc* **4:** 25.
28. Wertheim M G (1847) Memoirs sur l'elasticite et la cohesion des principaux tissus du corps humain. *Ann Chim (Phys)* **21:** 385–414.
29. Smith J W (1954) The elastic properties of the anterior cruciate ligament of the rabbit. *J Anat* **88:** 369–80.
30. Viidik A, Sanquist L and Magi M (1965) Influence of post-mortem storage on tensile strength characteristics and histology of rabbit ligaments. *Acta Orthop Scand [Suppl]* **79:** 1–38.
31. Matthews L S and Ellis D (1968) Viscoelastic properties of cat tendon: effects of time after death and preservation by freezing. *J Biomech* **1:** 65–71.
32. Barad S, Cabaud H E and Rodrigo J J (1982) Effects of storage at −80 °C as compared to 4 °C on the strength of rhesus monkey anterior cruciate ligaments. *Trans Orthop Res Soc* **7:** 378.
33. Dorlot J M, Ait ba Sidi M, Gremblay G M and Drouin G (1980) Load-elongation behavior of the canine anterior cruciate ligament. *J Biomech Eng* **102:** 190–3.
34. Woo S L-Y, Orlando C A, Camp J F and Akeson W H (1986) Effects of post-mortem storage by freezing on ligament tensile behavior. *J Biomech* **19:** 399–404.
35. Stouffer D C and Butler D L (1984) An analysis of crimp unfolding, fluid expulsion and fiber failure in collagen fiber bundles. *In: 1984 Advances in Bioengineering,* (R L Spilker, ed), pp. 46–47. Translated by ASME.
36. Horwitz M T (1939) Injuries of the ligaments of the knee joint. An experimental study. *Arch Surg* **38:** 946–54.
37. Miltner L J, Hu C H and Fang H C (1937) Experimental joint sprain. Pathologic study. *Arch Surg* **35:** 234–40.
38. Viidik A (1966) Biomechanics and functional adaptation of tendons and joint ligaments. *In: Studies on the Anatomy and Function of Bone and Joints* (Evans F G, ed). pp.17–39. Berlin: Springer.
39. Zuckerman J and Stull G A (1969) Effects of exercise on knee ligament separation force in rats. *J Appl Physiol* **26:** 716–9.
40. Roux R D, Hollis J M, Gomez M A, Inoue M, Kleiner J B, Akeson W H and Woo S L-Y (1986) Tensile testing of the anterior cruciate ligament (ACL): a new methodology. *Trans Orthop Res Soc* **11:** 237.
41. Noyes F R (1977) Functional properties of knee ligaments and alterations induced by immobilization. A correlative biomechanical and histological study in primates. *Clin Orthop* **123:** 210–42.
42. Crowninshield R D and Pope M H (1976) The strength and failure characteristics of rat medial collateral ligaments. *J Trauma* **16:** 99–105.
43. Woo S L-Y, Orlando C A, Frank C B, Gomez M A and Akeson W H (1986) Tensile properties of medial collateral ligament as a function of age. *J Orthop Res* **4:** 133–41.
44. Wolff J (1892) *Das Gesetz der Transformation der Knochen.* Berlin: Hirschwald.
45. Roux W (1905) Uber die Selbstregulation der Lebewesen. *Arch Entwicklungsmech Org* **13:** 610–50.
46. Salter R B and Field P (1960) The effects of continuous compression on living articular cartilage: an experimental investigation. *J Bone Joint Surg [Am]* **42:** 31–49.
47. Evans E B, Eggers G W N, Butler J K and Blumel J (1960) Experimental immobilization and remobilization of rat knee joints. *J Bone Joint Surg [Am]* **42:** 737–58.
48. Tipton C M, James S L, Mergner W and Tcheng T K (1970) Influence of exercise on strength of medial collateral knee ligaments of dogs. *Am J Physiol* **218:** 894–902.
49. Woo S L-Y, Akeson W H, Amiel D, Convery F R and Matthews J V (1975) The connective tissue response to immobility: a correlative study of the biomechanical and biochemical measurements of the normal and immobilized rabbit knee. *Arthritis Rheum* **18:** 257–64.
50. O'Donoghue D H, Rockwood C and Zarecnyj B (1961) Repair of knee ligaments in dogs. I. The lateral collateral ligament. *J Bone Joint Surg [Am]* **43:** 1167–78.
51. Akeson W H, Amiel D and Woo S L-Y (1980) Immobility effects on synovial joints: the pathomechanics of joint contracture. *Biorheology* **17:** 95–110.
52. Woo S L-Y, Gomez M A, Woo Y-K and Akeson W H (1982) Mechanical properties of tendons and ligaments. II. The relationships of immobilization and exercise on tissue remodelling. *Biorheology* **19:** 397–408.
53. Amiel D, Akeson W H, Harwood F L and Frank C B (1983) Stress deprivation effect on metabolic turnover of the medial collateral ligament collagen. *Clin Orthop* **172:** 265–70.

54. Gamble J G, Edward C and Max S (1984) Enzymatic adaptation of ligaments during immobilization. *Am J Sports Med* **12:** 221–8.

55. Clayton M L and Weir G J (1959) Experimental investigations of ligamentous healing. *Am J Surg* **98:** 373–8.

56. Tipton C M, Matthes R D, Maynard J A and Carey R A (1975) The influence of physical activity on ligaments and tendons. *Med Sci Sports Exerc* **7:** 165–75.

57. Cabaud H E (1980) Exercise effects on the strength of the rat anterior cruciate ligaments. *Am J Sports Med* **8:** 79–86.

58. Tipton C M, Matthews R D and Sandage D S (1974) *In situ* measurement of junction strength and ligament elongation in rats. *J Appl Physiol* **37:** 758–61.

59. Woo S L-Y, Kuei S C, Gomez M A, Winters J M, Amiel D and Akeson W H (1979) Effect of immobilization and exercise on the strength characteristics of bone-medial collateral ligament-bone complex. *Amer Soc Mech Eng Biomech Symp* **32:** 67–70.

60. Zuckerman J and Stull G A (1973) Ligamentous separation force in rats as influenced by training, detraining and cage restriction. *Med Sci Sports Exerc* **5:** 44–9.

61. Woo S L-Y, Gomez M A, Amiel D, Ritter M A, Gelberman R H and Akeson W H (1981) The effect of exercise on the biomechanical and biochemical properties of swine digital flexor tendons. *J Biomech Eng* **103:** 51–56.

62. Woo S L-Y, Ritter M A, Amiel D, Sanders T M, Gomez M A, Garfin S R and Akeson W H (1980) The biomechanical and biochemical properties of swine tendons. Long term effects of exercise on the digital extensors. *Connect Tissue Res* **7:** 177–83.

63. Brofkis J G (1972) *The Scientific Fundamentals of Surgery*, pp. 186–209. New York: Appleton Century Crofts.

64. Mason M L and Allen H S (1941) The rate of healing of tendons. An experimental study of tensile strength. *Ann Surg* **113:** 424–59.

65. Kessler I and Missim F (1969) Primary repair without immobilization of flexor tendon division within the digital sheath. *Acta Orthop Scand* **40:** 587–601.

66. Gelberman R H, Vande Berg J, Lundborg G N and Akeson W H (1983) Flexor tendon healing and restoration of the gliding surface. *J Bone Joint Surg [Am]* **65:** 70–80.

67. Jack E A (1950) Experimental rupture of the medial collateral ligament of the knee. *J Bone Joint Surg [Br]* **32:** 396–402.

68. Frank C B, Schachar N and Dittrich D (1983) The natural history of healing in the repaired medial collateral ligament: a morphological assessment in rabbits. *J Orthop Res* **1:** 179–88.

69. Frank C B, Woo S L-Y, Amiel D, Gomez M A, Harwood K F L and Akeson W H (1983) Medial collateral ligament healing. A multidisciplinary assessment in rabbits. *Am J Sports Med* **11:** 379–89.

70. Clayton M L, Miles J S and Abdulla M (1968) Experimental investigations of ligamentous healing. *Clin Orthop* **61:** 146–153.

71. Vailas A C, Tipton C M, Matthew R D and Gant M (1981) Physical activity and its influence on the repair process of medial collateral ligaments. *Connect Tissue Res* **9:** 25–31.

72. Woo S L-Y, Gomez M A, Inoue M and Akeson W H (1987) The development of new experimental procedures to evaluate the mechanical properties of healing medial collateral ligament (MCL). *J Orthop Res* (In press.)

73. Woo S L-Y, Gomez M A, Seguchi Y, Endo C and Akeson W H (1983) Measurement of mechanical properties of ligament substance from a bone-ligament-bone preparation. *J Orthop Res* **1:** 22–9.

74. Indelicato P A (1983) Non-operative treatment of complete tears of the medial collateral ligament of the knee. *J Bone Joint Surg [Am]* **65:** 323–9.

75. O'Donoghue D H, Frank C R and Jeter G L (1971) Repair and reconstruction of the anterior cruciate ligament in dogs: factors influencing long term results. *J Bone Joint Surg [Am]* **53:** 710–8.

Chapter 13

The Epidemiology of Degenerative Joint Disease: Occupational and Ergonomic Aspects

J. S. Lawrence

CONTENTS

INTRODUCTION

Degenerative joint disease may be considered under two main headings, depending on whether it affects the diarthrodial or the amphiarthrodial joints. As it affects diarthrodial joints it is termed osteoarthrosis or osteoarthritis, depending on whether it is in an inflammatory phase or not. The most frequent amphiarthrodial joints to be affected are those which involve the intervertebral discs. Collins in 1949 (1) recommended that this be called disc degeneration and that a diagnosis of osteoarthritis of the spine be restricted to apophyseal joint affection, though no doubt some would include the uncovertebral joints. I seldom use the term osteoarthritis because, as an epidemiologist looking at population samples, I seldom see individuals during a painful inflammatory episode, but I recognize that clinicians seldom see patients except during a painful episode and thus prefer to use this term. 'Spondylosis' is a popular term, but I prefer to avoid it since it does not differentiate between osteoarthrosis of the apophyseal joints and disc degeneration, although admittedly the two often occur together.

In a population sample lumbar disc degeneration occurs chiefly in males, whereas arthrosis of the lumbar apophyseal joints occurs with about the same frequency in both sexes. Moreover, disc degeneration occurs with roughly the same frequency in persons with and without Heberden's nodes (2).

316

DISC DEGENERATION

This is probably the type of degenerative joint disease which is most affected by occupation. It was first recognized by Wenzel in 1824 (3). Extensive studies by Schmorl of Dresden (4), begun in 1925 on routine autopsy material, revealed the great frequency of degenerative changes in the intervertebral discs and their relationship to disc prolapse (5). Little attention, however, was paid to degenerative changes not associated with prolapse, although it was realized that in many instances of sciatic and brachial pain no protrusion was found at operation. Instability associated with disc degeneration in the lumbar spine was noted by Knutson in 1944 (6). In 1945 Kay (7) emphasized the importance of degenerative disc disorders in attacks of low back and sciatic pain, and Friberg (8) stressed the greater importance of disc degeneration than of disc prolapse as a cause of disability and indicated the triad – disc narrowing, osteophytes around the vertebral margins and sclerosis of vertebral plates by which it can be recognized on X-ray. An early feature is atrophy of the vertebral lip. This is due to chronic bulging of the annulus in an interior or lateral direction, which lifts the periosteum away from the adjacent vertebral body. This precedes osteophyte formation and, when osteophytes subsequently develop, it results in the osteophyte sprouting from the vertebral body away from the vertebral lip. In this respect osteophytes differ from the syndesmo-osteophytes of spondylitis and the osteophytes of early ankylosing hyperostosis (Forestier's disease).

In *Fig.* 13.1, Grade 1 is a very early stage of disc degeneration. There is only slight atrophy of the anterior or lateral vertebral lip above and below the third lumbar disc. The disc at this stage is beginning to lose water and probably to protrude forward slightly as a result of loss of turgor. In Grade 2 there is definite osteophyte formation and the anterior wear is more marked. The disc is becoming narrower and the third lumbar vertebra (L3) is beginning to sublux posteriorly. This is the standard Grade 2 of the Atlas of Standard Radiographs of Arthritis (9). In Grade 3 the L3 disc has lost so much water that it has shrunk to a third of its original thickness and there is marked protrusion forward. There is a secondary arthrosis in the corresponding apophyseal joint. In Grade 4 disc degeneration the disc has shrunk to a quarter of its original thickness. The narrowing of the disc space is most marked anteriorly and there is a definite posterior slip of vertebrae L2 and L3. There is marked sclerosis of the vertebral plates. The presence of intranuclear gas is an occasional feature (10) but is not shown here.

In the dorsal spine (*Fig.* 13.2) anterior wear is a less striking feature and may be absent even in quite severe disc degeneration. In the cervical spine (*Fig.* 13.3) it may be altogether lacking, reflecting no doubt the type of stress involved, weight bearing in the lumber spine and sudden whiplash and rotary movement in the cervical spine.

Observer differences as to grading inevitably arise when reading X-rays. In *Table* 13.1 a series of 171 lumbar spine X-rays were read by 4 observers before the above gradings were introduced for disc degeneration. Two were rheumatologists, 1 a radiologist and 1 an orthopaedic surgeon. They had no agreement as to the dividing line between 'slight' disc degeneration and 'none' (11), the surgeon (observer 4) finding more with none, actually 42%, and one of the rheumatologists (observer 1) fewer, 32% ($P \simeq 0 \cdot 05$). Severe disc degeneration was noted most by a rheumatologist (observer 2) and least by the radiologist

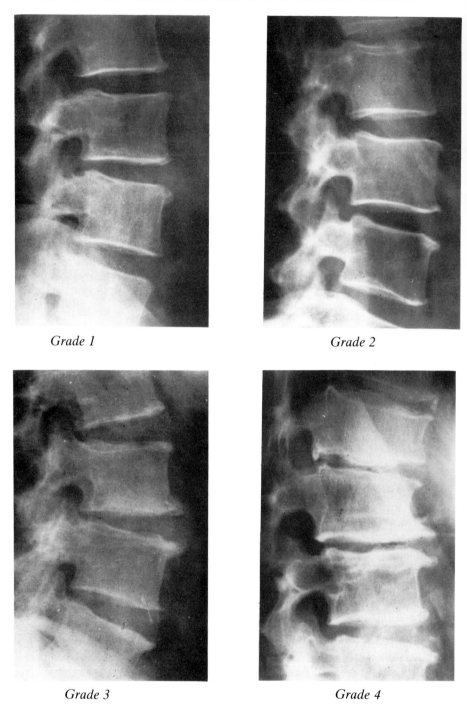

Grade 1

Grade 2

Grade 3

Grade 4

Fig. 13.1. Standard gradings for lumbar disc degeneration.

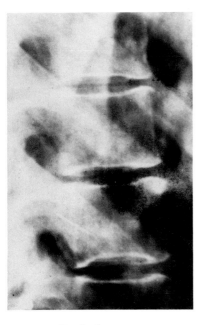

Grade 1

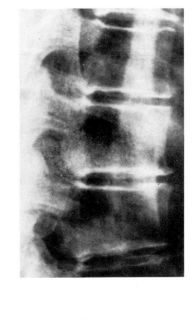

Grade 2

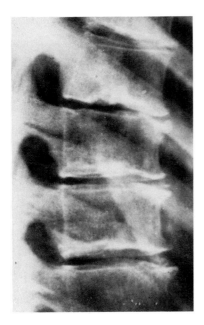

Grade 3

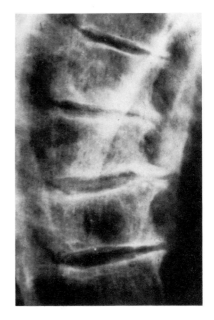

Grade 4

Fig. 13.2. Standard gradings for dorsal disc degeneration.

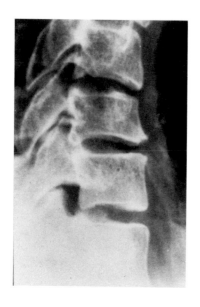

Grade 1

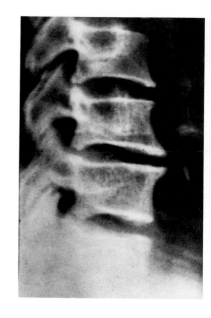

Grade 2

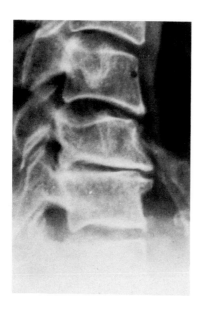

Grade 3

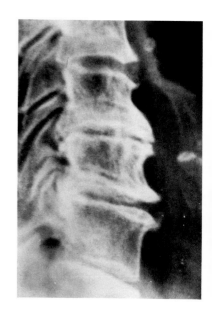

Grade 4

Fig. 13.3. Standard gradings for cervical disc degeneration.

Table 13.1 Observer error in X-ray diagnosis of lumbar disc degeneration (severity)

Category and Observer	Grading			Total
	None	Slight	Severe	
Miners				
Observer 1	7	41	36	
2	10	29	45	
3	9	50	25	84
4	18	30	36	
Manual workers				
Observer 1	19	18	8	
2	25	9	11	
3	20	16	9	45
4	21	12	12	
Office workers				
Observer 1	28	11	3	
2	29	10	3	
3	30	12	0	42
4	33	6	3	
Observer 1	32%*		27%	
2	37%		35%**	
3	34%		19%**	
4	42%*		30%	

*$P \simeq 0.05$ **$P \simeq 0.001$

(observer 3) ($P \simeq 0.001$). All observers agreed as to the main conclusions of the survey, namely a higher prevalence and greater severity of disc changes in miners than in light manual and office workers ($P \simeq 0.001$). Similarly there were differences of opinion as to the number of discs affected, but general agreement that multiple disc involvement is a feature of the miner's spine. Intra-observer differences are similar. When 186 X-rays were read together and independently by 2 observers, comparison of their readings indicated a maximum error of ± 11%, 12% higher and 10% lower (12). Later readings in 1967–1972 by one of these observers (*Fig.* 13.4) gave a higher grading in 10% and a lower grading in 21%. There was a difference of 2 grades in 8% and 3 grades in 0.3%. Thus it is apparent that the observer's ideas may change and that, with time and experience (or perhaps with increasing age), he may become more conservative in his views. It is therefore important, when comparing 2 populations seen at different times, to mix their X-rays and if possible to read them 'blind'.

Prevalence

In 4253 post-mortem examinations Schmorl (4) found that 80% of males and 60% of females had spondylosis, mainly disc degeneration, by age 50. By age 70 this had risen to 95%. Even by age 30, 10% had degenerative changes in one or more discs.

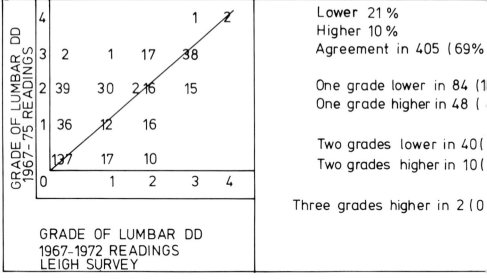

Fig. 13.4. Reproducibility of lumbar disc degeneration gradings.

Radiological evidence of disc degeneration, at least in the cervical spine, has a somewhat lower prevalence. In population samples in the UK the cervical spine was affected in 55% of males and 51% of females by age 50, and in 87% of males and 74% of females by age 70. Some 23% of males and 13% of females had Grade 1–4 disc degeneration in at least 4 discs. At age 30, 10% of males and 3% of females had X-ray changes (*Table* 13.2) (*Fig.* 13.5).

The prevalence of lumbar disc degeneration, as determined radiologically, is known in random population samples only from age 35 (*Table* 13.3), by which age 36% of males and 25% of females already have definite evidence of lumbar disc degeneration. By age 50, 58% of males and 39% of females are affected and by age 70 84% of males and 68% of females. Some 41% of males and 19% of females have 4 or more discs affected by age 70. Thus at all ages the preponderance in males is greater in the lumbar than in the cervical spine.

In the dorsal spine the position is reversed. By age 50 some 59% of males and 83% of females have degenerative changes in their dorsal discs, but from age 65 95% of males and 92% of females (*Table* 13.4).

The 5-year incidence of cervical disc degeneration in a longitudinal study in Oberhörlen in Hessen was 16% in males and 11% in females. In both sexes the incidence was maximal around age 50, when it was 33% in men and 24% in women, but in men there was a second peak at age 65 and over (*Table* 13.5).

Looking at the discs individually, the disc most commonly affected is the 8th dorsal in males and the 7th dorsal in females (*Fig.* 13.6). This may seem surprising, but it should be pointed out that dorsal disc degeneration is seldom associated with symptoms, probably because the dorsal spine is supported by the rib cage. In the cervical spine the disc most commonly affected is C5 and in the lumbar spine L3.

As regards neurological complications, a fundamental difference exists between disc degeneration in the cervical and lumbar spine (13). In the lumbar

Table 13.2 Radiological evidence of disc degeneration in cervical spine in Leigh, Wensleydale, Watford, and Rhondda, by sex and age group

Enlarged Sample

Age Group (yrs)	Males								Females							
	Total X-rayed	Grade of Disc Degeneration					No. with grade 1–4 in four or more discs		Total X-rayed	Grade of Disc Degeneration					No. with grade 1–4 in four or more discs
		0	1	2	3	4				0	1	2	3	4	
15–24	220	208	9	3	—	—	—		205	197	7	1	—	—	—
–34	220	185	15	19	1	—	—		220	192	18	8	2	—	—
–44	377	237	32	82	26	—	2		246	177	18	37	14	—	—
–54	450	161	42	149	93	5	7		265	102	26	72	63	2	7
–64	350	80	33	101	121	15	36		379	87	36	155	95	6	26
65+	186	10	13	48	96	19	42		257	42	26	85	95	9	33
Total	1803	881	144	402	337	39	87		1572	797	131	358	269	17	66

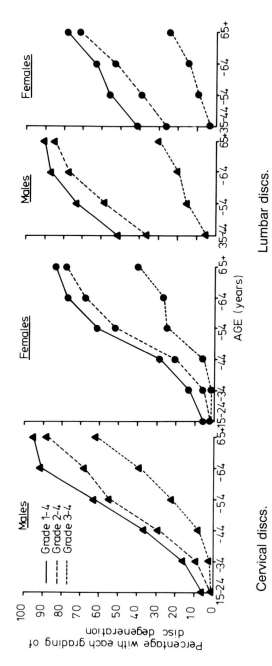

Fig. 13.5. Grades of disc degeneration (cervical and lumbar) by age and sex.

Table 13.3 Radiological evidence of disc degeneration in lumbar spine in Leigh, Wensleydale, and Watford

Enlarged Sample

Age Group (yrs)	Males							Females						
	Total X-rayed	Grade of Disc Degeneration					No. with grade 1–4 in four or more discs	Total X-rayed	Grade of Disc Degeneration					No. with grade 1–4 in four or more discs
		0	1	2	3	4			0	1	2	3	4	
35–44	185	90	29	56	9	1	3	211	125	33	47	5	1	4
–54	236	64	33	103	35	1	34	236	104	39	72	19	2	10
–64	154	20	14	89	25	6	56	182	66	19	72	20	5	17
65+	138	12	9	65	44	8	56	180	40	13	84	34	9	35
Total	713	186	85	313	113	16	149	809	335	104	275	78	17	66

Table 13.4 Dorsal disc degeneration (DD) in population samples

Age Group (yrs)	Males						Females					
	Total X-rayed	Grade of DD				% 2–4	Total X-rayed	Grade of DD				% 2–4
		1	2	3	4			1	2	3	4	
15–24	53	9	11	2		22	20	1	4			20
–34	100	11	32	2		34	44	7	21	2		52
–44	74	5	39	3		57	53	3	39	3		79
–54	71	6	33	9		59	66	3	46	9		83
–64	69	7	37	20		83	22	1	14	5		86
65+	66	2	42	20	1	95	36	2	12	16	5	92
	438						241					
15+	Unweighted mean 58						Unweighted mean 69					

Table 13.5 5-year incidence of disc degeneration in the cervical spine

Age	Total	New cases		1963–68 %
		2–4	3–4	2–4
Males				
15–24	40	0	0	0
25–34	43	0	1	0
35–44	28	8	2	29
45–54	15	5	0	33
55–64	27	1	5	4
65+	20	6	2	30
			Unweighted mean	16
Females				
15–24	30	0	0	0
25–34	32	1	0	3
35–44	47	7	4	15
45–54	42	10	2	24
55–64	37	6	3	16
65+	32	2	8	6
			Unweighted mean	11

spine neural compression is usually caused by a large fragment of displaced nuclear material, which either causes a localized protrusion beneath the annulus or herniates through an annular tear into the spinal canal following a spinal strain or injury. In the neck it is annular bulging and the consequent osteophytes which compress the cord and roots, a slowly progressive process. Osteophytes on the uncovertebral joints also cause root pressure (14) and also root sleeve fibrosis (15).

Disc prolapse occurs at an earlier age than disc degeneration. In a series of 500 cases requiring surgery (16), 4% were aged 11–20, 35% were 21–30, 38% 31–40, 18% 41–50 and 5% 51–60. It would appear that in the terminal fibrotic stage of disc degeneration nuclear extrusion cannot occur.

A history or signs of cervical nerve root pressure was found in 0·2% of 1953 adults aged 15 and over with Grade 0–1 disc degeneration in 3 English population samples, which I examined in 1954–62. The proportion with neuronal involvement rose to 1·7% in those with Grade 3–4 disc degeneration ($P < 0.001$).

A history suggestive of pressure on the lumbar nerve roots, usually sciatica, with or without weakness or paresthesiae or objective sensory loss and with absent knee or ankle jerk or muscle wasting, was noted in 4% of the 710 patients with Grade 0–1 lumbar disc degeneration, in 6% of those with minimal disease and in 10% with moderate or severe disease (*Table* 13.6). Thus those with Grade 3–4 disc degeneration are more likely to have nerve root pressure, but this is only a small proportion of those with local or referred pain in the segmental distribution of the degenerate disc, which comprises 61% of those with Grade 3–4 lumbar disc degeneration (17).

In some of the respondents with nerve root pressure in the lumbar or cervical canal, stenosis may have played a part. Lumbar canal stenosis depends on a combination of a basically narrow spinal canal, which may be inherited, with

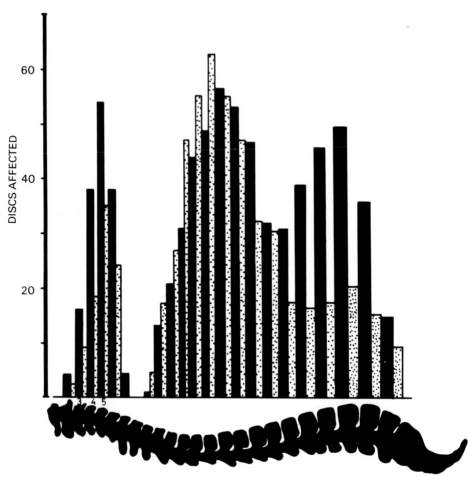

Fig. 13.6. Prevalence of Grade 2–4 degenerative change in individual discs in random samples of 100 males and 100 females aged 35 and over. Males: black. Females: stippled.

Table 13.6 Cervical nerve root pressure in relation to grade of disc degeneration in three English and one Welsh population

| | Grade of disc degeneration | | | | | |
| | Cervical | | | Lumbar | | |
	0–1	2	3–4	0–1	2	3–4
Total X-rayed	1953	760	662	710	528	224
Nerve root pressure	6	3	11	29	29	22
	0.15%	0.39%	1.7%	4%	6%	10%
	***		***	***		***
Local or referred pain	40%	44%	60%	48%	54%	61%
	**		**	***		***

$**P < 0.01$ $***P \simeq 0.001$

superimposed degenerative changes from middle age onwards (18). It gives rise characteristically to the symptom 'neurogenic claudication' (19). After walking a certain distance the patient develops a tingling in the legs, beginning in the feet and spreading up the legs. When the patient stops the symptoms often take up to 20 min to subside (13) and he may have to lie down or crouch down bending forward (20).

The narrowing of the lateral recesses may be due either to a bulging degenerate disc, osteoarthrosis of the facet joints, or disc space narrowing so that the vertebrae move closer together.

Lumbar canal stenosis affects an older group of patients than disc prolapse, though it may begin as early as the 30s. Men outnumber women by about 3:1. Radiographs reveal dense, hypertrophied facet joints. The pedicles are short, the intervertebral foramina flattened and the interlaminar gap narrow. Axial tomography reveals that the canal is trefoil shaped and the distance between the base of the spinous process and the back of the centrum of the corresponding vertebral body is usually less than 15 mm (21).

Ultrasound has been used by Porter (22) to detect spinal canal stenosis, using echoes from bony surfaces. A transducer is placed just lateral to the spinous process of a lumbar vertebra 15° to the sagittal plane and at the level of the laminar window. The measurements of the spinal canal at this level are remarkably repeatable, the intra- and inter-observer error being at most 0·5 mm and sometimes as low as 0·2 mm. The spinal canal diameter decreases with age, approximately 1·5 mm in 4 decades. However, a patient with a canal measuring 1·3–1·5 cm with disabling symptoms that have not settled on conservative treatment probably has a large herniated disc. So far as I know ultrasound has not been used for epidemiological studies.

Computed tomography can demonstrate the shape of the canal and bony encroachment (23) and the whole body scanner will permit canal measurement. This method also does not appear to have been used for occupational surveys.

Occupational Factors

Miners. Gantenberg in 1929 (24) and 1930 (25) first noted that miners were prone to degenerative changes in their discs, having more disc involvement than factory workers or artisans. There followed a radiological survey by Fischer in 1930 (26), probably the first of its kind. Fischer found that 79% of miners had rheumatic complaints and 34% had lost work because of them. X-ray changes, mostly in the spine, were present in 51%; more than in any other occupation. In a survey of 84 coalminers undertaken at the Bedford Colliery in Lancashire by the University of Manchester, moderate or severe lumbar disc degeneration (Grade 3–4) was noted in 43% of miners compared with 7% of office staff (*Table* 13.7). All 5 lumbar discs were affected in 14% of miners but in none of the office staff. The lower dorsal discs were also involved to an excessive extent in miners, 50% of whom had radiological evidence of disc degeneration in this region compared with 18% of light manual workers and 7% of office staff aged 40–50 (11).

A feature of the lumbar spines in miners is the frequent finding of wedging of the lumbar and lower dorsal vertebral bodies. This was present in 8 out of 24 miners and was lacking in a group of 31 non-mining controls ($P < 0.005$).

Table 13.7 Lumbar disc degeneration

Occupation	Total Workers	Severity (Grading)						No. of Discs Affected				
		None		Slight		Severe		1	2	3	4	5
Miners	84	7	8%	41	49%	36	43%	16	21	19	9	12
Manual workers	45	19	42%	18	40%	8	18%	8	7	9	1	1
Office workers	42	28	67%	11	26%	3	7%	8	1	2	3	0

Cervical disc degeneration was marginally increased in miners in West Virginia surveyed by Lockshin and his colleagues (27), but not in miners in the UK.

Lumbar disc involvement in miners is related mainly to the duration of heavy lifting (12). This applies regardless of age. A worker aged 40–50 who has undertaken heavy lifting for more than 30 years is more likely to have lumbar disc degeneration than a worker of the same age who has engaged in heavy lifting for less than 25 years. In association with these disc changes there is increased incapacity due to back pain in relation to the duration of heavy lifting. It is thus clear that the effect of heavy lifting is gradual and does not depend on a single injury or a sudden acute strain but on repeated minor stresses.

Work in cold damp conditions is also associated with low back pain and resulting incapacity, but not with more radiological evidence of disc degeneration.

The position which a miner adopts at work depends on the seam height. If this is greater than 5 ft 6 in (1.7 m) he can stand with a straight back, if 4 ft 5 in (1.35 m) he stands and bends. If the seam height is below 4 ft 5 in (1.35 m) he kneels but has a straight back. If it is less than 3 ft 6 in (1.1 m) he kneels and bends. Disc degeneration is most frequent and most severe in miners working at a roof height less than 3 ft 6 in (1.1 m), but loss of work due to back pain is greatest at a roof height of 4 ft to 4 ft 5 in (12).

Four groups of miners have been examined by the Miners' Welfare Commission in the UK (*Fig.* 13.7). Three were face workers and 1 was a group of workers in underground roadways. Of the face workers 1 group worked in a wet low seam, 1 in a dry high seam and 1 in a dry low seam. The greatest prevalence of severe disc degeneration (58%) was found in the workers in the wet, low seam and the lowest (36%) in the roadway workers. Face workers in the low wet seam had the greatest loss of work and those in the dry low seam the least.

Dockworkers also have a high prevalence of lumbar disc degeneration, almost as great as in miners, but it is not quite so severe and affects fewer discs, although more than in light manual workers. Although 12% of miners show the highest grade of radiological change (Grade 4), only 2% of dockers fall into this category. 36% of miners show involvement of 4 or more discs, but only 18% of dockers ($P < 0.01$). The dockers on the other hand are considerably worse off

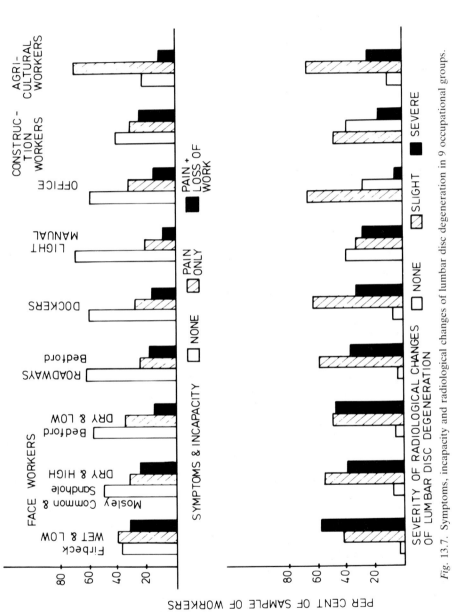

Fig. 13.7. Symptoms, incapacity and radiological changes of lumbar disc degeneration in 9 occupational groups.

than light manual workers. As in miners the worst affected disc is the third lumbar.

Construction workers have more than twice as much Grade 3–4 lumbar disc degeneration as controls, but have less disc degeneration than miners or dockers, indeed 43% aged 35–64 have no X-ray changes and only 15% show severe disease (*Fig.* 13.7). They fall somewhere between the light manual and office workers. They are closer to light manual workers than any other group, but lose more work from musculoskeletal pain.

Agricultural workers. Some 90% of agricultural workers have degenerative changes in the lumbar discs, significantly more than in construction or light manual workers but similar to that in miners and dockers. It is not however so severe as in these 2 groups. A remarkable feature is the high prevalence of musculoskeletal pain together with a low absence from work; only 10% of agricultural workers had lost work from back, hip or sciatic pain, less than in office workers.

Foundry workers. This is another occupation involving heavy lifting. These men have a high prevalence of lumbar disc degeneration but it is less severe than in miners (28). Only 23% of foundry workers aged 40–50 surveyed by the Arthritis & Rheumatism Council had Grade 3–4 changes, compared with 50% of miners working at the coal face. Despite a higher prevalence of lumbar disc degeneration in foundry workers there were fewer symptoms and there was less incapacity from pain in the D12–L2, L3–4 and L5–S2 segmental distribution.

Foundry workers are exposed to considerable radiation during the pouring of molten metal. The radiant heat incident on the body of the lightly clothed workman varies between 0·05 and 0·30 W/cm^2, with a mean value of 0·12 W/cm^2. In comparison a patient undergoing 'radiant heat' therapy can be exposed to 0·16–0·37 W/cm^2. Relief of pain occurs in some 80% of rheumatic sufferers during such therapeutic exposure. It seems reasonable to suppose that, in foundry workers, incapacity for work is reduced in the same way.

Other occupations which are associated with disc changes are *railway stokers* (29), *bus* and *tramway drivers* and *conductors*. Radiological changes of disc degeneration have been found in 80% of railway stokers, sometimes with crushing of vertebral bodies, but showing no relationship to symptoms. In bus and tramway drivers X-ray changes of spondylosis and scoliosis in the dorsal and lumbar spine rose from 28% to 59% with increasing age from 20 to 60 (30).

Relationship of Lumbar Disc Degeneration to Low Back and Leg Pain

Low back and leg pain is significantly related to lumbar disc degeneration in males from the age of 35–54 but is not so associated in the older age groups (17). In females the association is less definite.

In cervical disc degeneration there is a relationship between X-ray changes and neck, shoulder and brachial pain in both sexes. The onset of symptoms is mainly between ages 25 and 44 years in both sexes.

Using the responsibility index (*Fig.* 13.8) it is possible to gain an indication of the responsibility of various diseases for back pain (*Table* 13.8). Disc degeneration stands out, being responsible in 12% of cases in population

Responsibility index. The proportion of those with a given sympton in which a given disease is responsible for the symtoms

$$\text{Responsibility index} = \left(\frac{a}{a+b} - \frac{c}{c+d} \right) \times 100$$

a = the number with disease + symptoms
b = the number with symptoms without the disease
c = the number with the disease without the symptoms
d = the number with neither the disease nor the symptoms.

Fig. 13.8. Responsibility index.

Table 13.8 Responsibility index for low back and sciatic pain in population samples in the UK (Leigh, Wensleydale and Watford: age 35+)

Disease	With $D12$-S_2 Pain	Without $D12$-S_2 Pain	Responsibility Index
Total X-rayed	877	825	
Lumbar disc degeneration (Grade 2–4)	59%	47%	12%***
Lumbar osteoarthrosis (Grade 2–4)	22%	17%	5%**
Osteoarthrosis, sacroiliac joints (Grade 2–4)	8%	6%	2%NS
Sacroiliitis (Grade 2–4)	2·6%	1·4%	1·2%
Lumbar rheumatoid arthritis (Grade 2–4)	3·7%	0·5%	3%**
Lumbar ankylosing spondylitis (Grade 2–4)	0·8%	0%	0·8%NS
Lumbar disc prolapse (Grade 2–4) or root pressure from other causes	10%	Not Known	<10%
Total			35%

NS = Not significant   **$P \simeq 0\cdot01$ ***$P < 0\cdot001$

samples in the UK. Arthrosis of the apophyseal joints is responsible for 5% and of the sacroiliac joints for 2%.

Assuming that some disc prolapse is asymptomatic, the proportion of those with symptoms and signs of root pressure in whom disc prolapse is responsible for the symptoms must be less than 10%, possibly much less. The large numbers in which lumbar and sciatic pain is unexplained by known diseases indicates how much remains to be done to elucidate the causes of pain at these sites. Many of the as yet unexplained cases are quite trivial and may be due to slight ligamentous strain, possibly associated with minor subluxations such as our osteopathic colleagues treat with manifest, if sometimes transient, success. No doubt these will be elucidated by newer non-invasive techniques applied to population samples.

The responsibility of degenerative joint disease for neck–shoulder–brachial pain is shown in *Table* 13.9. At this site also, disc degeneration is the commonest known cause, being responsible for 14% of cases. Rheumatoid arthritis is responsible for 13%. These are mainly cases of shoulder pain. Generalized arthrosis is responsible for 9% and arthrosis in the apophyseal joints for only 4%. The remaining arthrosis is in the shoulders or possibly the uncovertebral joints. Less than 72% can be accounted for by known diseases.

Table 13.9 Responsibility of known diseases for neck-shoulder-brachial pain in population samples in the UK

	Neck-shoulder-brachial pain		
	With NSB pain	*Without NSB pain*	*Responsibility index*
Total	1,366	2,009	
Cervical DD (Grade 2–4)	50%	36%	14%***
Rheumatoid arthritis	30%	17%	13%***
Generalized OA (3+ joints Grade 2–4)	26%	17%	9%***
Cervical OA (Grade 2–4)	12%	8%	4%***
Ankylosing spondylitis	1·8%	0·05%	1·7%***
Chondrocalcinosis	0·26%	0·18%	0·08%NS
Psychoneurosis	8%	8%	0%
Local OA shoulder (clinical)	11%		<11%
Capsulitis	9%		<9%
Cervical disc prolapse	4%		<4%
Post-traumatic arthritis shoulder	4%		<4%
Bursitis	2%		<2%
Polymyalgia rheumatica	0·04%		<0·4%
Total	1,464	2,200	<72%

NS = Not significant

***$P < 0.001$

OSTEOARTHROSIS

Arthrosis may arise in any diarthrodial joint but is most common in the distal interphalangeal joints of the fingers, particularly the index finger (31). In young persons up to age 44 the first metatarsophalangeal joints are most often affected, but thereafter the distal interphalangeal joints take precedence (*Fig.* 13.9). Second in frequency are the knees in females and the lumbar spine in males. Females have more osteoarthrosis in the distal and proximal interphalangeal, metacarpophalangeal and carpometacarpal joints, knees and first metatarsophalangeal joints in European populations. These are the joints involved in the primary generalized form of osteoarthritis as described by Kellgren and Moore (32).

Arthrosis affecting one or more joints is almost universal in persons who survive beyond age 64. It is rare, about 10%, in the 15–24 age group, reaches a prevalence of 38% in males and 39% in females in the 40s and 86% in both sexes in the 60s.

Generalized or polyarthrosis may be defined as arthrosis in 3 or more joint groups (*Fig.* 13.10). It has much the same frequency in both sexes up to age 50 and then increases more rapidly in females, attaining a frequency of 38% in males and 51% in females in the 60s and 63% in males and 80% in females after age 64. If only those with 5 or more joint groups are considered, the prevalence at over 64 is 37% in males and 49% in females.

Usually arthrosis of the apophyseal joints is secondary to disc degeneration, but occasionally a primary involvement of these joints may occur as part of a generalized arthrosis (33).

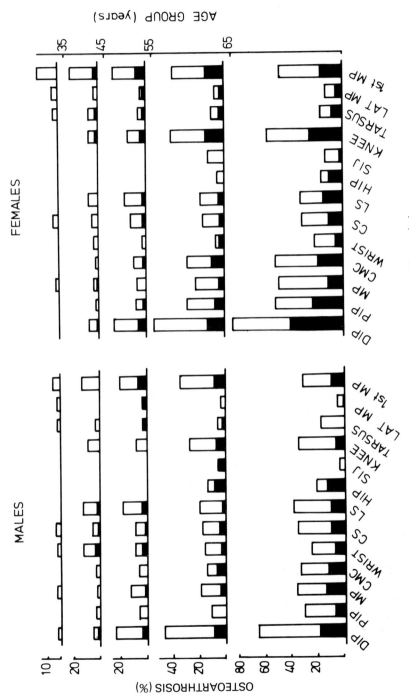

Fig. 13.9. Joint pattern of arthrosis in an English population.

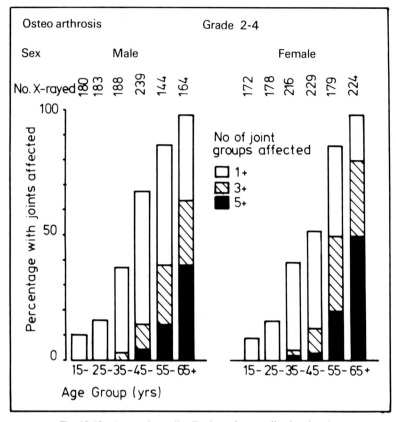

Fig. 13.10. Age and sex distribution of generalized arthrosis.

Generalized arthrosis may be divided into nodal and non-nodal forms, depending on whether or not it is associated with Heberden's nodes. The nodal form affects mainly the joints of the fingers and thumbs. The only occupation in which I have found an increased frequency of the nodal form is in textile workers. Genetic factors would seem to be much more important in this type of arthrosis, which is 4 times as common in female relatives as in controls (34) and is associated very significantly with the HLA A1 B8 haplotype in 31% of female relatives, compared with 9% of controls (35).

Traumatic arthrosis should always be suspected where a single joint is involved. In a proportion of individuals with arthrosis in a population sample there is either a history of previous trauma or radiological evidence of injury. The prevalence of traumatic arthrosis, as so defined, was 35% in males and 15% in females in a population sample aged 55–64 in the north of England (*Table* 13.10). In both sexes the knee was the joint most frequently affected, 12% of males and 9% of females having knee arthrosis which was considered to be the result of an injury; lumbar arthrosis was often found in those with such a history, usually in conjunction with disc degeneration.

Table 13.10 Traumatic arthrosis in an urban population aged 55–64

Traumatic arthrosis or disc degeneration (%)	Males		Females	
	Total X-rayed	Arthrosis(%)	Total X-rayed	Arthrosis(%)
Distal interphalangeal	173	2·3	206	0·5
Proximal interphalangeal	173	0·6	206	0·5
Metacarpophalangeal	173	1·7	206	0
Carpometacarpal	173	2·9	206	1·0
Wrist	172	1·2	205	0
Cervical spine	170	0	201	0
Lumbar spine	165	6·6	193	1·6
Hips	167	2·5	191	1·6
Sacroiliac	165	0	191	0
Knees	171	12·3	199	9·0
Tarsal	173	2·9	206	0·5
Lateral metatarsophalangeal	173	0·6	206	0·5
First metatarsophalangeal	173	1·7	206	1·0
Total	173	35***	207	15***
Disc degeneration				
Disc cervical	170	4·7	201	0
Disc lumbar	165	9·7	193	1·0

***$P \simeq 0·001$

Occupational Factors

Numerous surveys have been made of the relationship of arthrosis to occupational stress.

Agricultural workers have been reported to have a higher prevalence of hip arthrosis in French rheumatism clinics than in population surveys (29). This has been confirmed in Austria by Frank and Klemmayer (36). Pommier (37) observed primary osteoarthrosis in 33% of farmers and 19% of controls. It would seem likely that some degree of selection was involved since, in population samples submitted to routine hip X-rays, osteoarthrosis was present in only 12% of farmers and 11% of non-farmers (*Fig.* 13.11). No doubt farming includes many different activities and the strains involved differ greatly. In a survey in Wensleydale in the UK the farmers were mainly concerned with sheep-rearing and dairy farming and 25% of them had hip arthrosis, compared with 17% of non-farmers (*Fig.* 13.12). In a population in Azmoos in Switzerland 18% of farmers and 11% of non-farmers had hip arthrosis (*Fig.* 13.13). In Oberhörlen in West Germany the position was reversed. 6% of farmers and 13% of non-farmers had hip arthrosis (*Fig.* 13.14). These differences, however, are small and are not significant.

The most frequent sites of arthrosis in farmers as a whole are the knees and the distal interphalangeal joints of the fingers. The finger joints are affected in 30% of farmers and 22% of non-farmers ($P \simeq 0·01$). The difference is most

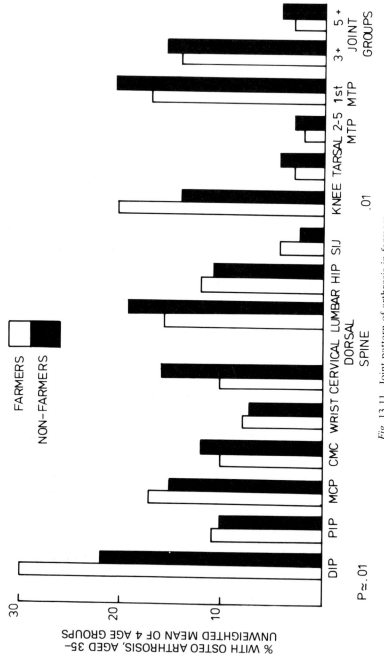

Fig. 13.11. Joint pattern of arthrosis in farmers.

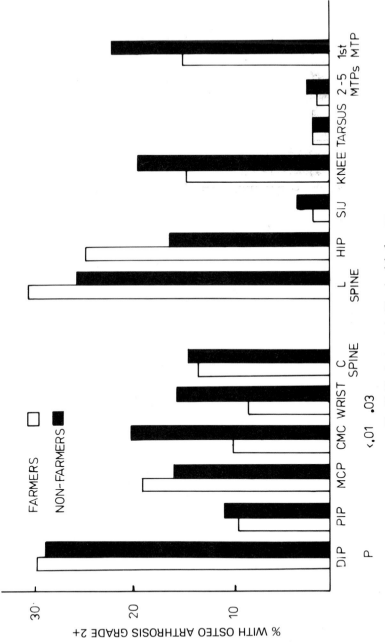

Fig. 13.12. Arthrosis in Wensleydale farmers.

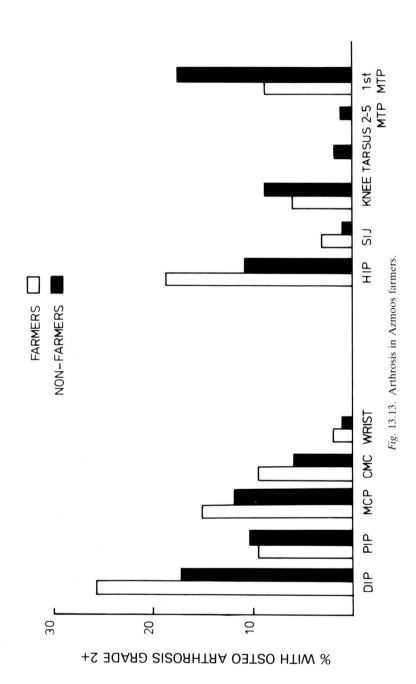

Fig. 13.13. Arthrosis in Azmoos farmers.

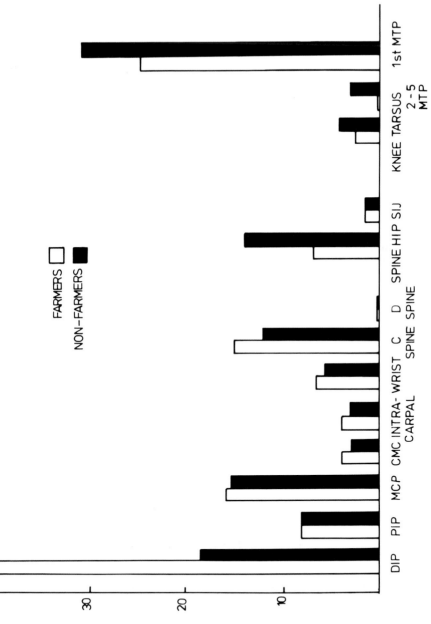

Fig. 13.14. Arthrosis in Oberhörlen farmers.

noticeable in the German and Swiss populations and is lacking in Jamaican farmers (*Fig.* 13.15). In this connection it is of interest that, of the 4 populations studied, the German and Swiss farmers were exposed to the lowest winter temperatures. Knee arthrosis was observed in 21% of farmers and 14% of non-farmers ($P \simeq 0.01$). This figure was largely influenced by the relatively high prevalence of arthrosis in this joint in the Jamaican farmers. This is not surprising in view of the large distances covered by farmers, mainly over rough ground.

Miners. Radiological evidence of arthrosis in miners has been encountered mainly in the knees which were affected (Grade 2–4) in 24% of a sample of 216 miners aged 41–50 (12). Those working in the underground roadways had the greatest frequency (36%). Of 170 light manual workers and office staff in the same age group, 11% had knee arthrosis ($P < 0.005$). Kneeling was not found to be a factor, and indeed knee pain and incapacity so arising were more frequent in miners who had worked predominantly in the higher seams of over 4 ft. Knee arthrosis was unaffected by either the duration of work in a kneeling position or the seam height. Only a few of the miners gave a history of injury to the knee, but surgery for meniscus tears is said to be common (38) and is a potent source of arthrosis. There is no relationship to distance walked underground. Locking of the joint often occurs first when the miner is walking on rough ground with a bent knee.

Schlomka and his colleagues (39) included the shoulders, knees, hands and hips in their examination of miners and found the highest prevalence of arthrosis in the shoulders. Some 52% of miners had involvement of this joint compared with 12% of porters. The hip was affected in 43% of miners and 28% of porters, the knee in 46% and 32% respectively. Spondylosis was more frequent in all areas of the spine in miners than in bank clerks, though rather less than in porters. It was related to the time spent in mining or other similar occupation.

Building workers have attracted considerable attention because of the heavy nature of their work and their exposure to unfavourable weather conditions. Tellefsen (40) recorded an annual loss of 420 days/100 bricklayers, which may be compared with a figure of 188 days for all occupations in males. Building workers do not, however, show any increase of arthrosis except in the first metatarsophalangeal joints, which are particularly liable to injury from being stubbed or having weights dropped on them (*Table* 13.11).

Foundry workers have significantly less arthrosis in the apophyseal joints of the lumbar spine and in the knees, hips and distal interphalangeal joints of the fingers than age-matched controls. In none of the joints is there significantly more arthrosis (28).

Textile workers. Radiological evidence of arthrosis in Lancashire cotton mills was found to be more common in males in whom spinning was the main occupation (41). In females the occupations were more evenly distributed between weavers, spinners and machine tenders, the last being the largest group and comprising mainly cardroom workers. The joints which were more affected in male cotton workers than in controls were all in the hands and included the distal ($P \simeq 0.02$) and proximal interphalangeal, and first carpometacarpal joints. There was no difference in the frequency and severity of these changes between the left and right hands. The difference between Grade 3 and Grade 4 arthrosis in the distal interphalangeal joints in male cotton workers and controls was

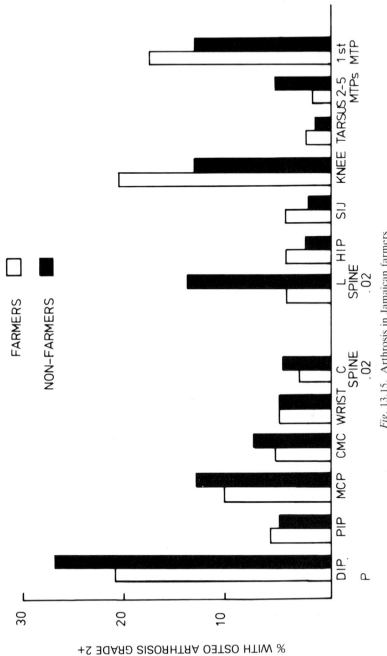

Fig. 13.15. Arthrosis in Jamaican farmers.

highly significant ($P \simeq 0.02$). In females the pattern of arthrosis was very similar in cotton workers and controls. The reason for this is far from clear. It would seem unlikely that the predominance of spinners in the males is responsible, since female spinners do not show a greater predominance than weavers. It is possible that genetic factors have a greater influence in females and result in a higher prevalence of arthrosis in female controls. An interesting feature is that sick absence of 3 months or more is less in male workers than in controls ($P \simeq 0.01$), due no doubt to the warm environment in the spinning room.

Table 13.11 Joint pattern of radiological osteoarthrosis in construction workers

Site of osteroarthrosis	Total X-rayed	Grade of osteoarthosis				Expected	
		1	2	3	4	2–4	3–4
DIP	248	16	21	3	1	36	10 NS
PIP	248	6	9	3	0	12	2
MCP	249	9	14	4	0	16	4
CMC	249	9	5	1	0	7	1
Wrists	249	3	10	2	0	8	2·5
C spine	234	12	13	1	0	10	2
Hips	131	7	4	2	1	10	5
Knee	56	7	11	1	2	11	2
Tarsal	248	2	4	1	0	10	0
Lat MTP	248	4	9	0	0	3	0
First MTP	248	24	62	7	1	48*	1

*$P \simeq 0.04$

Hadler (42) has since surveyed 3 groups of textile workers, curlers, winders and spinners assessed for range of motion, malalignment and radiological evidence of degenerative joint disease. There was more wrist arthrosis in those who did winding but not in those who did precision gripping. The latter had more arthrosis in the 2nd and 3rd metacarpophalangeal joints. It was possible to detect differences in the above parameters in relation to the type of work.

American *footballers* have more knee arthrosis, *soccer players* more knee, ankle and foot involvement and in *baseball pitchers'* shoulders and elbows are affected (43, 44, 45).

Fishermen. In a survey of rheumatism in North Sea fishermen by Behrend et al. (46), arthrosis was present in 1 or more joints in 65%. The controls, a sample of the local population, had an identical frequency but it was more generalized in the fishermen, 20% of whom had arthrosis in 3 or more joint groups, compared with 6% in controls ($P < 0.05$) (*Table* 13.12). The nodal form of generalized arthrosis, in which heredity plays such an important part, was not encountered. Heberden's nodes when they occurred were asymmetrical and of the traumatic type.

The fishermen had more arthrosis than the controls in all joints except the metatarsophalangeal (*Fig.* 13.16). In the hips the difference is negligible, but it is significant in the case of the distal interphalangeal joints of the fingers

EPIDEMIOLOGY OF DEGENERATIVE JOINT DISEASE 345

$(P \simeq 0.03)$. Disc degeneration was not increased in fishermen. A very significant relationship was noted between the grade of arthrosis by X-ray and the symptoms in the distal interphalangeal joints of the fingers, the carpometacarpal joints, spine, hips and first metatarsophalangeal joints.

Table 13.12 Osteoarthrosis in fishermen

Age	Total Examined	No. of Joints with Grade 2–4 Arthrosis							%		
		1	2	3	4	5	6	NX	1+	3+	5+
Fishermen											
35–44	47	17	2	3	1			6	48·9	8·5	0
–54	34	12	3	4	3	1		2	67·6	23	2·9
–64	34	9	0	4	4	1	1	6	56	29	5·9
35–64	115								58	20*	3
Controls											
35–44	18	8	1						50	0	0
–54	22	9	3	0	1				59	4·5	0
–64	20	10	4	2	0	1		2	85	15	5
35–64	60								65	6*	2

*$P < 0.05$ NX = Not X-rayed

In addition to arthrosis, fishermen in the North Sea have an increased prevalence of seronegative polyarthritis, but it is unlikely that that would explain the increased frequency of generalized arthrosis, since the joint pattern of their arthrosis is atypical of rheumatoid arthritis. Moreover, the polyarthritis was not associated with X-ray changes of arthrosis. It would seem more probable that the arthrosis in fishmen is due to repeated trauma and exposure to cold, as in farmers.

Some occupational influences are so obvious that they do not require a detailed statistical analysis. Holtzmann (47) ascribed arthrosis of the shoulder, elbow and hand to *vibrating tools*. This was associated occasionally with osteochondritis of the lunate (Kienböck's disease) and with pseudoarthrosis of the scaphoid. This has been confirmed by others and occupational differences in the pattern of these lesions have been noted in *boiler makers* and *steel girder and building workers*, who have arthrosis mainly in the elbow. *Stone drillers* show cystic changes in the region of the hand joints (48). 30% of *miners* using pneumatic drills have arthrosis in the elbow, compared with 16% of miners not using a pneumatic drill (12, 49). The use of a vibrating tool is sometimes associated with Raynaud's disease in the affected hand. The onset starts 6–40 months after starting the work and may persist after stopping.

Bus drivers have been reported by Nairn (50) to develop shoulder arthrosis on the same side as the gear lever.

Caisson workers. Arthrosis of the shoulders and hips and occasionally of the knees and ankles was reported as long ago as 1913 by Bassoe (51) and later by Kahlstrom et al. (52), Thomson and Young (53), Jaffres and Merer (54) and Gaultier et al. (55). The initial lesion is an osteonecrosis due to air embolism.

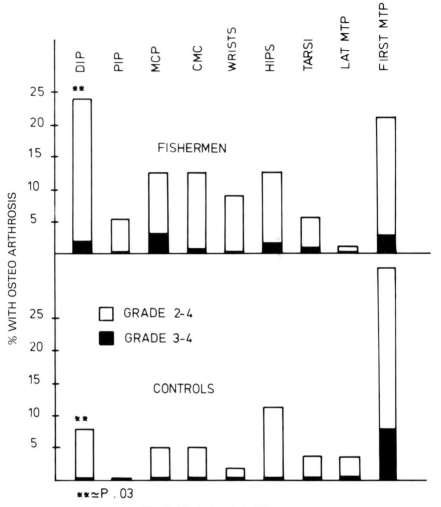

Fig. 13.16. Arthrosis in fishermen.

When the necrotic bone is situated in the epiphysis and borders on the joint, varying degrees of collapse of the weight-bearing portion occur, followed by invasion and replacement by new bone. Articular cartilage overlying the involved area breaks down and is replaced by fibrocartilage. This is followed after a year or two by degenerative changes in the joint. A feature of this type of arthrosis is the early onset, usually between the ages of 30 and 40 (56). In addition to degenerative joint disease the X-rays show irregularly branching stellate islands of sclerosis in the adjacent spongy bone.

Another form of arthrosis, involving the symphysis pubis in *footballers*, also occurs at a relatively early age (57).

Gout may be regarded as an occupational disease particularly amongst *executives* with large expense accounts. In a recent survey of *veterinary surgeons* I have found in them an increased prevalence of gout, probably dietetic. Gouty arthrosis is practically limited to the first metatarsophalangeal joints.

Surveys based on clinical data have been undertaken by Anderson and Duthie (58) in *dockyard workers*. Vague pains in the back were the most frequent complaint. This was noted in 23% of workers. Disc disease was diagnosed in 10% and osteoarthrosis in 7%. Some 50% had no symptoms. Nine per cent of workers had some degree of limitation and this was greater in outdoor than indoor workers ($P \simeq 0.01$).

In a *mining* population the same authors (59) discovered that 41% of miners had no symptoms, 14% had disc disease and 15% osteoarthrosis. 16% had undetermined back and neck pain. Face workers had more osteoarthrosis than non-face workers. Sickness absence due to disc disease was 27 weeks per 100 face workers, and 14 weeks in non-face workers. The figures for osteoarthrosis were 13 and 2 weeks respectively. Rheumatism was responsible for 15% of all sickness absence sustained by the whole group. Disc disease was the commonest cause of change of occupation.

Racial differences in the prevalence of arthrosis have been attributed to environmental stresses by some workers. Jurmain (60) in a survey of 798 skeletons belonging to four racial groups (black and white Americans, Pueblo Indians and Alaskan Eskimos) found a greater prevalence and severity of arthrosis in the shoulder, knee, elbow and hip in the Eskimos. He attributed this to the stresses associated with their lifestyle. The right side was usually more affected than the left. The Eskimos, moreover, had an earlier onset of arthrosis. Blacks were usually more affected than whites in the knee, shoulder and elbow.

In considering occupational influences it is important to remember that in some types of degenerative joint disease heredity plays a major role. The nodal form of generalized arthrosis is 4 times as common in first degree relatives of probands with nodal generalized osteoarthritis as in samples of the population, adjusted for age and sex (35). The heritability is 93% compared with 27% in the non-nodal form and there is an association with the A1 B8 haplotype.

THE PRODUCTION OF SPINAL PAIN

The mode of production of spinal pain in degenerative joint disease is uncertain. What evidence there is comes from the results of stimulating structures in the back during operations performed during local anaesthesia. Where the pain is due to root compression, retraction of the root reproduces the symptom and decompression of the root relieves it (61). Pressure on a normal disc seldom produces the pain, but pressure on an abnormal disc often does so and the pain may be referred to the hip or down the leg. A needle passed into the affected disc and injection of normal saline under pressure also reproduces the symptoms (62). Injection into the interfacetal joint similarly produces referred pain, but injection into the posterior ligaments produces only a local pain quite unlike the pain of which the patient complained. The most sensitive area is the posterior annulus.

THE EFFECT OF CLIMATE

Climate can be divided into macro- and micro-climate. In considering occupational factors we are concerned with microclimate, the climate within the factory or workplace. As we have already seen, foundry and textile workers spend their working lives mainly in a favourable climate, and although they have as much or more degenerative joint disease as the general population they have fewer symptoms and less incapacity due to rheumatic complaints (41).

Agricultural and construction workers are exposed to the outdoor macro-climate and, except when this is extreme and gives rise to frostbite, do not suffer any excess of degenerative joint disease. On the other hand, agricultural workers in the warm Caribbean climate have more disc degeneration but for Caribbean men, each grade of disc degeneration is associated with fewer symptoms and less incapacity than in agricultural workers in a temperate climate. Arthrosis is just as frequent in Jamaica as in England, but in all joints except the cervical spine Jamaicans with Grade 3–4 arthrosis have fewer symptoms than their counterparts in England.

TRENDS OF FUTURE SCIENTIFIC ENDEAVOURS

In future epidemiological studies the trend will be to use fewer X-rays and to substitute newer techniques in order to avoid radiation hazards. Personally I think the risk from diagnostic X-rays has been exaggerated. In a survey in Wensleydale in the UK, in which half the adult population had X-rays of the hands, feet, knees, hips, cervical and lumbar spine, the incidence of cancer 20 years later was lower in the half who were X-rayed. It is well recognized that X-rays in therapeutic doses carry a risk, but in small doses they may possibly be prophylactic. There is, so far as I know, no evidence that there is a straight-line relationship.

Of the newer methods of studying degenerative joint disease, magnetic resonance appears to hold out most promise. It has the advantage that it is non-invasive and avoids radiation risk. Clinical images clearly show the internal structure of the intervertebral disc and degenerate discs show a reduced level of hydration of the nucleus pulposus relative to the annulus, and make it possible to grade the degenerative changes in the disc (63). T2 values demonstrate age changes and T1 values can be used to differentiate degenerate from aged discs (64).

These newer techniques will make it possible to carry out more longitudinal studies, which at present are rather lacking. They would, no doubt, have been used in epidemiological studies in the past were it not for the matter of cost.

Computed tomography permits unique visualization of the spine and associated soft tissues in cross-section, and is particularly valuable in identifying and localizing spinal canal stenosis and apophyseal disease (65). So far as I know it has not been used in epidemiological studies.

I do not propose to discuss the results of invasive procedures such as discography, lumbosacral venography, myelography or radiculography, since these are unsuitable for epidemiological studies of healthy individuals.

CONCLUSIONS

Degenerative joint disease includes two main conditions, disc degeneration and osteoarthrosis. Many epidemiological studies of disc degeneration, in which radiological methods have been used, have demonstrated the relationship between occupational factors and disc degeneration. People occupied in hard labour such as miners were at higher risk. The same was true in the case of osteoarthrosis. In the future, new techniques like magnetic resonance will make it possible to carry out longitudinal studies on the development of degenerative joint disease in people with different occupations.

CLINICAL SIGNIFICANCE

This chapter emphasizes the importance of occupational factors in the aetiopathogenesis of degenerative joint disease. A correlation exists between the physical stress of work and the prevalence of disc degeneration and osteoarthrosis. New non-invasive techniques applied to human populations may help us to understand better the epidemiology, as well as the nature and course, of degenerative joint disease.

REFERENCES

1. Collins D H (1949) *The Pathology of Spinal and Articular Diseases.* London: Arnold.
2. Kellgren J H and Lawrence J S (1958) Osteo-arthrosis and disk degeneration in an urban population. *Ann Rheum Dis* **17**: 388–97.
3. Wenzel C (1827) *Über die Krankheiten am Rückgrate.* Bamberg: Wesche.
4. Schmorl G (1929) Zur pathologischen Anatomie der Wirbelsäule. *Klin Wochenschr* **8**: 1243–9.
5. Schmorl G and Junghanns H (1932) *Die gesunde und kranke Wirbelsäule in Röntgenbild und Klinik.* Stuttgart: Thieme.
6. Knutson F (1944) The instability associated with disc degeneration in the lumbar spine. *Acta Radiol* **25**: 593–609.
7. Kay J A (1945) Intervertebral disc lesions are the most common causes of low back pain with or without sciatica. *Ann Surg* **121**: 534–44.
8. Friberg S (1948) Anatomical studies on lumbar disc degeneration. *Acta Orthop Scand* **17**: 224–30.
9. Atlas of Standard Radiographs of Arthritis (1963) *In: The Epidemiology of Chronic Rheumatism,* Vol 2, (J H Kellgren, M R Jeffrey and J Ball, eds), pp. 22–3. Oxford: Blackwell.
10. Edeiken J and Pitt M J (1971) The radiological diagnosis of disc disease. Symposium on disease of the intervertebral disc. *Orthop Clin North Am* **2**: 405–17.
11. Kellgren J H and Lawrence J S (1952). Rheumatism in miners. II. X-ray study. *Br J Ind Med* **9**: 197–207.
12. Lawrence J S (1955) Rheumatism in coalminers. III. Occupational factors. *Br J Ind Med* **12**: 249–61.
13. Maurice-Williams R S (1981) *Spinal Degenerative Disease.* Bristol: Wright.
14. Cave A J E, Griffiths J D and Whiteley M M (1955) Osteoarthritis deformans of the Luselka joints. *Lancet* **1**: 176–9.
15. Frykholm R (1951) Lower cervical vertebrae and intervertebral discs. *Acta Chir Scand* **101**: 345–59.
16. O'Connell J E A (1951) Protrusions of lumbar intervertebral discs. *J Bone Joint Surg [Br]* **33**: 8–30.
17. Lawrence J S (1969) Disc degeneration. Its frequency and relationship to symptoms. *Ann Rheum Dis* **28**: 121–37.

18. Nelson M A (1973) Lumbar spinal stenosis. *J Bone Joint Surg [Br]* **55**: 39–59.
19. Wilson C B, Ehni G and Grollmus J (1971) Neurogenic intermittent claudication. *Clin Neurosurg* **18**: 62–85.
20. Kavanah G J, Svien H J, Holman C B and Johnson R M (1968) Pseudoclaudication produced by compression of the cauda equina. *J A M A* **206**: 2477–81.
21. Epstein J A, Epstein B S and Lavine L (1962) Nerve root compression associated with narrowing of the lumbar spinal canal. *J Neurol Neurosurg Psychiatry* **25**: 165–76.
22. Porter R W (1980) Measurement of the spinal canal by diagnostic ultrasound. In: *The Lumbar Spine and Back Pain, 2nd Ed* (M I V Jayson, ed), pp. 231–45. Tunbridge Wells: Pitman.
23. Sheldon J J, Sersland T and Leborgne J (1977) Computed tomography of the lower lumbar vertebral column. *Radiology* **124**: 113–8.
24. Gantenberg R (1929) Die Bedeutung deformierender Prozesse der Wirbelsäule unter besonderer Berücksichtigung. *Fortschr Röntgenstr* **39**: 650–6.
25. Gantenberg R (1930) Zur klinischen Bedeutung deformierender Prozesse der Wirbelsäule. *Fortschr Röntgenstr* **42**: 740–6.
26. Fischer A (1930) Über das Vorkommen und die soziale Bedeutung rheumatischer Erkrankungen bei der Industriebevölkerung. *Arch Gewerbepath Gewerbehyg* **1**: 703–30.
27. Lockshin M D, Higgins I T T, Higgins M W, Dodge H T and Canale N (1969) Rheumatism in mining communities in Marion County, W. Virginia. *Am J Epidemiol* **90**: 17–29.
28. Lawrence J S, Molyneux M K and Dingwall-Fordyce I (1966) Rheumatism in foundry workers. *Br J Ind Med* **23**: 42–52.
29. Louyot P and Savin R (1966) La coxarthrose chez l'agriculture. *Rev Rhum Mal Osteoartic* **33**: 625–32.
30. Barbaso E (1958) Sull'incidenza delle alterazioni della colonna vertebrale nel personale viaggiante di una azienda auto-tramviaria. *Med Lav* **49**: 630–4.
31. O'Brien W M, Clemett A R and Acheson R M (1968) Symptoms and pattern of osteoarthrosis in the hands. In: *Population Studies of Rheumatic Diseases: Proceedings of the Third International Symposium, New York, 1966 (Int Congr Ser No 148)* (P H Bennett and P H N Wood, eds). pp. 398–406. Amsterdam: Excerpta Medica Foundation.
32. Kellgren J H and Moore R (1952) Generalized osteo-arthritis and Heberden's nodes. *Br Med J* **1**: 181–7.
33. Jayson M I V (1978) Back pain, spondylosis and disc disorders. In: *Copeman's Textbook of the Rheumatic Diseases* (J T Scott, ed), pp. 960–85. Edinburgh: Churchill Livingstone.
34. Kellgren J H, Lawrence J S and Bier F (1963) Genetic factors in generalized osteo-arthrosis. *Ann Rheum Dis* **22**: 237–55.
35. Lawrence J S, Gellsthorpe K and Morrell G (1983) Heberden's nodes and HLA markers. *Rheumatol [Suppl]* **9**: 32–3.
36. Frank O and Klemmayer K (1968) Die Coxarthrose bei der Landbevölkerung. *Z Rheumatol* **27**: 371–9.
37. Pommier L (1977) *Contribution à l'étude de la coxarthrose chez l'agriculture.* Thèse Med Tours.
38. Sharrard W J (1965) Pressure effects on the knee in kneeling miners. *Ann R Coll Surg Engl* **36**: 309–24.
39. Schlomka G, Schroter G and Ochernal A (1955) Über die Bedeutung des beruflichen Belastung für die Entstehung der degenerativen Gelenkleiden. *Z Inn Med* **10**: 993–9.
40. Tellefsen A (1949) Uber die Rheumatismusmorbidität durch Krankenkassenmaterial beleuchtet. *Acta Med Scand [Suppl]* **233**: 1–63.
41. Lawrence J S (1961) Rheumatism in cotton operatives. *Br J Ind Med* **18**: 270–6.
42. Hadler N (1978) Hand structure and function in an industrial setting. *Arthritis Rheum* **21**: 210–20.
43. Rall K L, McElroy G L and Keats T E (1964) Study of long term effects of football injury to the knee. *Mo Med* **61**: 435–8.
44. Solonen K A (1966) The joints of the lower extremity of football players. *Ann Chir Gynaecol* **55**: 176–80.
45. Lee P, Rooney P J and Sturrock R D (1974) Aetiology and pathogenesis of OA. *Semin Arthritis Rheum* **3**: 189–218.
46. Behrend T, Zuric Z, Hach G and Lawrence J S (1987) Rheumatism in fishermen. (In preparation.)
47. Holtzmann F (1929) Erkrankungen durch Arbeit mit Pressluftwerkzeugen. *Umschau* **33**: 1002–3.

48. Bittersohl G (1960) Ergebnisse von Röntgenuntersuchungen an Knochen und Gelenken bei Pressluftwerkzeugarbeitern. *Arch Gewerbepath Gewerbehyg* **17**: 597–617.
49. Roche L, Maitrepierre J, Lejeune E, Marmet J (1961) Les atteintes du membre supérieur chez les ouvriers travaillant au marteau pneumatique. *Arch Mal Prof* **22**: 57–61.
50. Nairn S J G (1932) Rheumatism in the London busmen. *Br J Phys Med* **6**: 214–5.
51. Bassoe P (1913) The late manifestations of compressed-air disease. *Am J Med Sci* **145**: 526–42.
52. Kahlstrom S C, Burton C C and Phemister D B (1939) Aseptic necrosis of bone. I. Infarction of bones in caisson disease resulting in encapsulated and calcified areas in diaphyses and in arthritis deformans. *Surg Gynecol Obstet* **68**: 129–46.
53. Thomson J D and Young A B (1958) Aseptic necrosis of bone in caisson disease. *Br J Ind Med* **15**: 270–2.
54. Jaffres R and Mehrer P (1960) Pathogenic considerations on aseptic barotraumatic osteonecrosis of the hip and coxarthrosis. *Rev Rhum Mal Osteoartic* **27**: 467–74.
55. Gaultier M, Fournier E and Gervais P (1962) A propos de deux cas d'ostéo-arthrite baro-traumatique à révélation tardive. *Arch Mal Prof* **23**: 32–8.
56. Raymond V (1960) Arthroses baro-traumatiques. *Arch Mal Prof* **21**: 609–21.
57. Radochay L and Somogyi J (1957) Eigenartige Form der Osteoarthritis bei Fussballspieler. *Zbl Chir* **82**: 1322–6.
58. Anderson J D and Duthie J J R (1963) Rheumatic complaints in dockyard workers. *Ann Rheum Dis* **22**: 401–9.
59. Anderson J D, Duthie J J R and Moody B P (1962) Social and economic effects of rheumatic disease in a mining population. *Ann Rheum Dis* **21**: 342–52.
60. Jurmain R D (1977) Stress and the etiology of osteoarthritis. *Am J Phys Anthropol* **46**: 353–66.
61. Murphey F (1968) Sources and patterns of pain in disc disease. *Clin Neurosurg* **15**: 343–51.
62. Hirsch C (1948) An attempt to diagnose the level of a disc lesion clinically by disc puncture. *Acta Orthop Scand* **18**: 132–40.
63. Aspden R M, Hicken D S, Hukins D W L and Jenkins J P R (1986) Degenerative changes in lumbar intervertebral discs identified by magnetic resonance imaging. *Publ Univ Kuopio Med Orig Rep* **6**: Miniposter Bl.
64. Jenkins J P R, Hickey D S, Zhu X P, Machin M and Isherwood I (1985) MR imaging of the intervertebral disc: a quantitative study. *Br J Radiol* **58**: 705–9.
65. Isherwood I and Antoun N M (1980) CT scanning in the assessment of lumbar spine problems. *In: The Lumbar Spine and Back Pain, 2nd Ed* (M I V Jayson, ed), pp. 247–64. Tunbridge Wells: Pitman.

Chapter 14

Significance of Endogenous and Exogenous Mechanisms in the Development of Osteoarthritis

H. G. Fassbender

CONTENTS

INTRODUCTION

There are various aspects from which one can consider the pathogenesis of osteoarthritis. It is understandable that orthopaedic surgeons concentrate primarily on the exogenous aspects of this disease, for instance from the viewpoint of pre-arthritic alterations.

ANIMAL MODELS FOR STUDIES OF EXOGENOUS FACTORS

The association between already existing disturbances of the biomechanics and the subsequent development of osteoarthritis is quite clear. Numerous

352

animal models have been developed to clarify the exogenous pathomechanisms. Most of these animal models are based on an intervention into the joint mechanics. It appears that the impairment of the articular cartilage is less dependent on the quality of the intervention than on the degree of severity and its duration. It seems that experiments with totally different methods show similar results. Radin *et al.* (1) and Videman (2) applied repetitive impact loads to rabbit knees. The authors observed an increase in ^{99m}Tc labelling in the subchondral bone, followed by an increase in tetracycline labelling, bone formation, and a decrease in porosity, which has been associated with relative stiffening of bone.

Radin *et al.* consider subchondral osteosclerosis and the consequently reduced shock absorption to be of essential significance for the degradation of articular cartilage. He even regards bone fracture to be an efficient way of absorbing energy and protecting the joints.

Long-term immobilization of a joint causes degenerative articular changes similar to those seen in human osteoarthritis (3–14). Videman (2) showed, however, that repeated periods of immobilization also produce articular changes which correspond to those in human osteoarthritis. An immobilization period of 4 days had a cumulative effect in producing osteoarthritis, and an interval of 4 weeks between immobilization periods could not prevent this process. Videman argues that all situations which lead to the immobilization of a joint may cause osteoarthritis-like changes. Videman and co-workers (15) also discovered that, after an immobilization of only 4 days, the rabbit knee joint showed an increased uptake of ^{35}S-sulphate in ligaments and articular cartilage which progressed within 2–4 weeks also into the juxta-articular bone. The authors therefore concluded that the structural changes of the soft tissues around the osteoarthritic joint play a role in the pathogenesis of osteoarthritis.

Langenskjöld and co-workers (10) found the most severe osteoarthritic changes in rabbit joints after an immobilization period of 5–6 weeks. The articular cartilage was destroyed and osteophytes had developed. On the other hand, the investigations of Williams and Brandt (16) create the impression that exclusively exogenous factors are of significance in the development of osteoarthritis, since the hyaline cartilage in these experiments only plays a passive role. But these conceptions no longer correspond to the picture as described by modern ultrastructural and biochemical research, which considers the cartilaginous matrix to be a dynamic system which is continuously exposed to anabolic and catabolic factors.

The experiments of Stofft and Graf (17) with guinea-pigs demonstrate the significance of the well controlled functioning of intact chondrocytes for adjustment to mechanical overloading. Although the collagen fibres at the articular surface become partially unmasked, at the same time the chondrocytes increase their production of proteoglycans. After a rest period of 4 weeks, full recovery with complete re-masking of the collagenous framework takes place. These investigations therefore suggest that a continuous load may lead to superficial lesions of the hyaline cartilage, but that these lesions can be balanced by functioning chondrocytes. The increased stress on the joint may also lead to alterations in the subchondral bone (18).

THE CHONDROCYTE AND MECHANISMS IN THE DEVELOPMENT OF OSTEOARTHRITIS

The Chondrocyte and its Products

In the 6th embryonic week, the future cartilage cells begin to differentiate from the mesenchyme. The advanced differentiation is reflected in the complex ultrastructural equipment of the cartilage cell and its capacity to survive in nearly anaerobic conditions, a capacity not shared by other cells in the organism. This is achieved at the cost of its inability to regenerate after injury and its high sensitivity to toxic influences.

The chondrocyte is the only living element of the cartilage (*Fig. 14.1*). It lives 'walled-in' between its products, like a hermit. Its products, collagen and proteoglycans, have a quite different lifespan. Whereas the collagen fibre network is long-lived and stable, the proteoglycans are subject to constant turnover. The half-life of proteoglycans has been shown to be between 1 week and 200 days, depending on the joint and the measuring method.

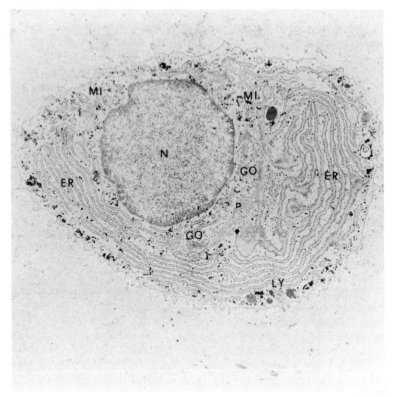

Fig. 14.1. Active chondrocyte of oval shape in the intermediate zone of rat articular cartilage. Nucleus (N) with smooth-walled membrane; strongly developed endoplasmic reticulum (ER); prominent Golgi apparatus (GO); a few small mitochondria (MI), and a few lysosomes (LY) (× 2880). (Electron micrograph: R. Raiss.)

The chondrocyte has a relatively low metabolic activity. Each individual chondrocyte, which lacks direct cell-to-cell interaction, receives its nutrients and eliminates its waste products by diffusion through the matrix, which consists of 2 types of macromolecules, collagen Type II and proteoglycan. Most of the proteoglycans of the articular cartilage exist as extremely large aggregate molecules, which are compressed into a 3-dimensional network of fine Type II collagen fibres (*Fig.* 14.2).

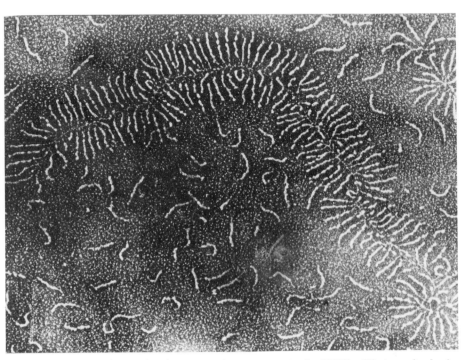

Fig. 14.2. Electron micrograph of a proteoglycan aggregate (× 28 000). (Photograph: J. A. Buckwalter.)

Each proteoglycan aggregate is assembled extracellularly and consists of many proteoglycan monomers bound non-covalently to a single strand of hyaluronic acid. This interaction is stabilized by link molecules. The proteoglycan monomer consists of a central core protein with covalently attached chondroitin sulphate and keratan sulphate chains.

The network of collagen fibres gives the tissue its tensile strength and shape and withstands the swelling pressure of the hydrophilic proteoglycans. The proteoglycan molecules have the ability to bind large amounts of water, which is most important for the elasticity of the articular cartilage. The water content amounts to 66–79%. In the normal cartilage matrix, the arrangement and complex interactions between these 2 macromolecules form a weight-bearing tissue with unique physical capacity to resist compressive forces (*Fig.* 14.3).

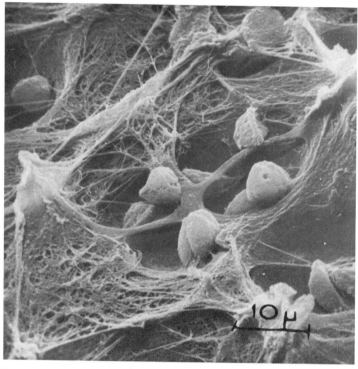

Fig. 14.3. Enzyme-induced (hyaluronidase) destruction of chondral intercellular substance in the mouse. The exposed collagen fibres of the chondral matrix are visible. In the centre there are several chondrocytes. (Scanning electron micrograph: I.-E. Richter.)

Threats to the Chondrocyte

The highly differentiated chondrocyte possesses an extremely complex ultra-structure and, compared with fibroblasts and other cells of mesenchymal origin, it is very sensitive to disturbing influences, although it is surrounded by its territorial matrix and thus has a degree of specific protection. Nevertheless, the integrity of the chondrocyte is exposed to various risks. A basic risk results from the chondrocyte's location in the avascular cartilage. The nutrition of the chondrocyte is only achieved by diffusion through the joint cavity. This process requires a long transit distance, which means that the essential supply of glucose must make its way from the synovial capillaries through the synovial fluid and the cartilage matrix until it finally reaches the chondrocyte. This long journey may be subject to disturbance in four places (*Fig.* 14.4). The consequence is deficient nutrition, with the further possibility of lesion and death of the chondrocyte. The final consequence is a regional proteoglycan deficit of the territorial matrix.

The synovium is the only surface of the organism which has no basement membrane and thus allows free passage of damaging substances into the synovial fluid. From there they may penetrate the matrix and are potentially hazardous to the chondrocyte. It is furthermore conceivable that substances which have proved to be 'antiproliferative' and 'cytostatic' in pharmacological experimentation will find a sensitive target in the highly differentiated ultrastructure of the chondrocyte.

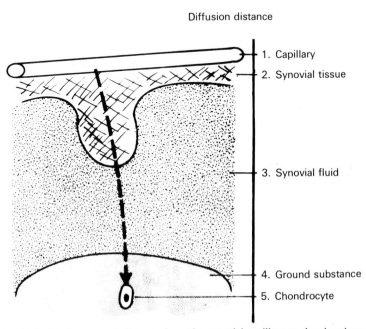

Diffusion distance

1. Capillary
2. Synovial tissue
3. Synovial fluid
4. Ground substance
5. Chondrocyte

Fig. 14.4. The long transit distance from the synovial capillary to the chondrocyte.

Ultrastructural Chondrocyte Test System (UCT)

In our institute, the effect of dexamethasone, non-steroidal anti-inflammatory substances, and chondroprotective substances on the ultrastructure of chondrocytes in the healthy rat articular cartilage has been determined morphometrically and evaluated statistically. Eleven different ultrastructural parameters have been included in the morphometric evaluation (standardized ultrastructural chondrocyte test system, UCT) (*Fig.* 14.5).

Effect of Antirheumatic Substances on the Chondrocyte

Our studies have shown that the most severe damage is caused by dexamethasone, followed by phenylbutazone and indomethacin (*Fig.* 14.6). In contrast to these results, the newer non-steroidal antirheumatic drugs cause only

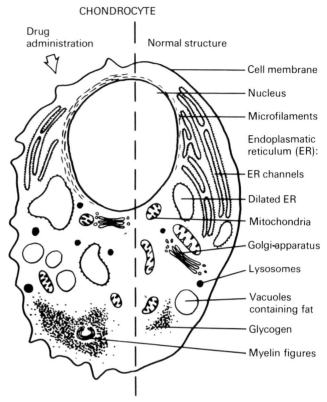

CHONDROCYTE

Drug
administration   Normal structure

Cell membrane

Nucleus

Microfilaments

Endoplasmatic
reticulum (ER):

ER channels

Dilated ER

Mitochondria

Golgi-apparatus

Lysosomes

Vacuoles
containing fat

Glycogen

Myelin figures

Fig. 14.5. Diagram of the organelles morphometrically evaluated in the ultrastructural chondrocyte test system (UCT). (R. Raiss.)

insignificant   degenerative   damage   in   the   chondrocytic   ultrastructure (19, 20, 21).

The question as to which other substances can also damage the chondrocytes remains to be clarified. It can only be answered for those substances which were tested in standardized experiments. Meanwhile, the suspicion must remain that in the course of their existence the chondrocytes are exposed to a series of toxic influences many of which are not yet known. However, we must also take into account the fact that once the chondrocyte is damaged, it has a considerable recuperative capacity. Another endogenous threat against the chondrocyte arises via a different mechanism. In addition to the structural elements of cartilage, proteoglycans and collagen, the chondrocyte also secretes degrading enzymes and protease inhibitors. It is undoubtedly important that these must be present in precisely regulated amounts to permit the slow turnover of proteoglycans and collagens, which is a characteristic of healthy adult cartilage (*Fig.* 14.7). It is thus conceivable that a disorder in the balance between anabolism and catabolism of cartilage matrix would be followed by destruction of the supporting joint cartilage.

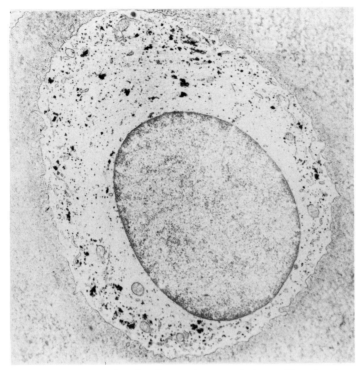

Fig. 14.6. Advanced damage to the chondrocyte in rat articular cartilage by dexamethasone: deposition of microfilaments displacing the organelles (× 8194). (Electron micrograph: R. Raiss.)

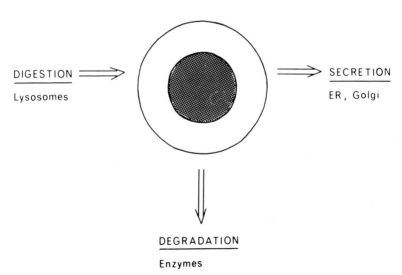

Fig. 14.7. Diagram illustrating turnover of proteoglycans and collagen in articular cartilage. ER, endoplasmic reticulum.

Effect of Chondroprotective Substances on the Chondrocyte

Using the same standardized ultrastructural chondrocyte test system (UCT) we have determined the influence of chondroprotective substances (glucosamine sulphate and glycosaminoglycan–peptide complex) on the ultrastructure of chondrocytes in the rat. We showed that these substances have no influence on any of the 11 ultrastructural parameters of the healthy untreated rat articular cartilage.

The effects of both chondroprotective substances on the ultrastructure of chondrocytes in impaired articular cartilage in the rat were tested by using our standardized morphometric method and gave the following results:

1. The extent of standardized damage (by dexamethasone) on cell size and nucleus size could not be influenced by chondroprotective substances.
2. Dexamethasone-induced reduction of the rough endoplasmic reticulum (RER) could be partly restored to normal by chondroprotective substances. The surface of the dilated RER-cisternae doubled in size, which accounts for an increased synthesis capacity of the chondrocyte.
3. Dexamethasone-induced reduction of the Golgi apparatus could be completely restored to normal by treatment with chondroprotective substances.
4. The number of mitochondria increased after treatment with dexamethasone, but this was also the case after simultaneous administration of chondroprotective substances. On the other hand, the dexamethasone-induced reduction of mitochondrial size was restored to normal by chondroprotective substances.
5. Lysosomes, lipid, and deposition of glycogen increased with dexamethasone treatment. The administration of chondroprotective substances seemed to restore these organelles largely to normal, except for the lipid inclusions.
6. With dexamethasone treatment the microfilaments of the cytoplasm increased from 16 to 70%. After treatment with chondroprotective substances this effect was reduced to 52%.
7. With dexamethasone treatment the cell mortality rate increased from 4·6 to 15·3%. After treatment with chondroprotective substances the cell mortality was reduced to 9%.

It thus appears that on the one hand chondroprotective substances are able to largely restore cell structure to normal after standardized damage of the chondrocytes by dexamethasone and, on the other hand, regressive changes of the organelles are reduced. Moreover, these substances show a protective influence on the vitality of the chondrocytes (22, 23).

Threats to the Chondrocyte from Chondrocytic Proteolytic Enzymes

In vitro studies by Aydelotte and Kuettner (24) provided evidence that it is precisely matrix degradation which, due to increased chondrocytic proteolytic activity, can play an essential role in the genesis of osteoarthritis. The fact that such matrix degradation can be triggered by external influences is confirmed by the administration of vitamin A in vivo and in vitro. The matrix rapidly becomes depleted of proteoglycans, and subsequently collagen is lost (Fig. 14.8).

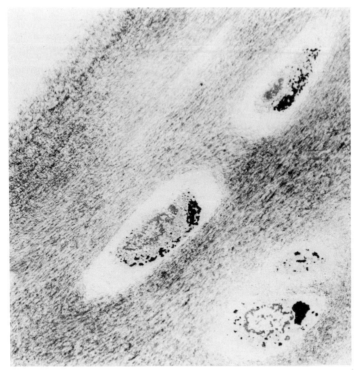

Fig. 14.8. Degradation of the chondrocytes' territorial matrix by chondrolytic enzymes in rat articular cartilage (× 2870). (Electron micrograph: M. Annefeld.)

A similar pattern of matrix degradation is observed when cartilage is co-cultured with synovial tissue or grown in synovium-conditioned medium. Catabolin, a small molecular weight protein isolated from the culture medium, acts as a 'messenger molecule' and stimulates degradation of matrix by living chondrocytes (25, 26).

ARTICULAR STRUCTURES AND THE DEVELOPMENT OF OSTEOARTHRITIS

Unmasking of the Collagen Fibres: First Step towards Mechanical Destruction

It thus becomes evident that there are two different mechanisms which jeopardize the integrity of the articular cartilage; firstly, secretory insufficiency of the chondrocytes, and secondly, matrix destruction by the degrading enzymes of the chondrocytes.

The particular importance to be attributed to the proteoglycans in masking the collagen fibre network makes it clear that, above all, a disturbed function or the destruction of chondrocytes will result in unmasking of the collagen fibres (*Fig.* 14.9). Denudation of the collagen fibre network, however, means that in consequence each movement will lead to traumatic lesions to the respective joint (*Figs.* 14.10, 14.11). A phase is then reached which progresses according to the mechanical laws of 'wear and tear': the joint surface becomes roughened and shows fissures and cartilage detachments up to complete abrasion of the cartilage substance (*Figs.* 14.12, 14.13).

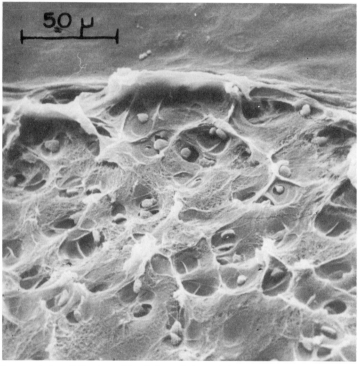

Fig. 14.9. Enzyme induced (hyaluronidase) degradation of the chondral intercellular substance in the mouse. In the upper part of the picture the surface of the cartilage is still intact, whereas in the lower part the collagen fibres and chondrocytes are already exposed (Scanning electron micrograph: I.-E. Richter.)

When the cartilage is damaged (being incapable of regeneration), the subchondral osseous tissue reacts to the changed strain with structural adaptation by new growth. Thus, the destruction of the cartilage is accompanied by osteosclerosis and osteophytosis (*Figs.* 14.14, 14.15). Similar secondary arthrotic transformation processes also occur after cartilage destruction in rheumatoid arthritis. However, the sclerotic bone, too, is subject to mechanical abrasion. Synovial fluid and detritus are pressed into the opened medullary spaces. Debris cysts are thus formed (*Figs.* 14.16, 14.17).

The process hitherto described is of purely morphological character, i.e. clinically it may be asymptomatic, as neither the cartilage nor the subchondral bone are provided with nerve endings. Pure, non-physiological strain on the capsule and ligaments, triggered by structural destruction, may cause distress.

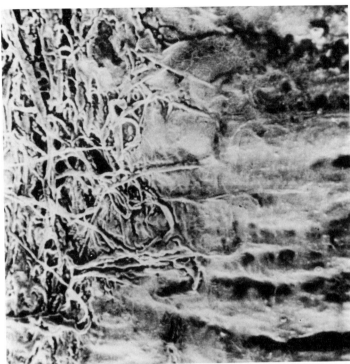

Fig. 14.10. Incipient osteoarthrosis: on the left side the collagen fibres are already exposed, whereas on the right side they are still embedded in the intercellular substance (Scanning electron micrograph: I.-E. Richter.)

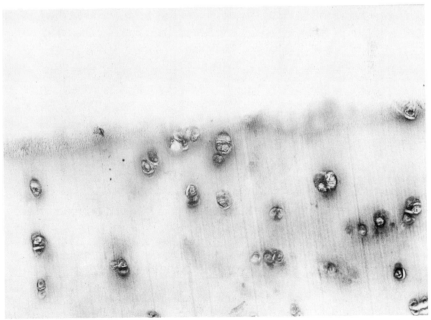

Fig. 14.11. Osteoarthrosis: superficial collagen fibres in the initial stage of exposure ($\times$ 140).

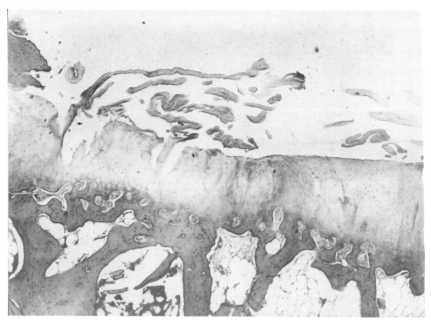

Fig. 14.12. Osteoarthrosis: deep fissures of articular cartilage, as well as detachment of cartilage fragments ($\times$ 21).

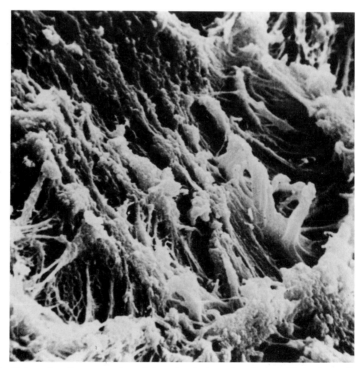

Fig. 14.13. Osteoarthrosis: exposed and largely destroyed collagen fibres from the chondral matrix. (Scanning electron micrograph: I.-E. Richter.)

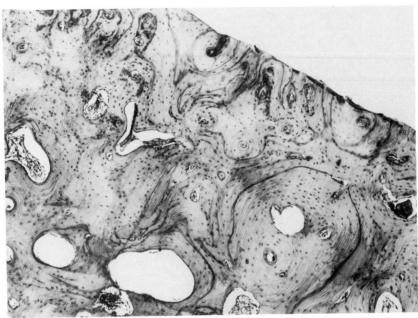

Fig. 14.14. Osteoarthrosis: eburnation of bone (× 55). *Note* the dense new osteons with smooth surface abrasion (right upper corner).

This also accounts for the unusually high number of morphologically (X-ray) proved, but clinically mute, arthrotic alterations in the epidemiological studies of Wagenhäuser (27).

Development of a Secondary Synovitis

All structural elements of the joint, collagen fibres, proteoglycans, chondrocytes (28), as well as calcium apatite crystals of the bone (29, 30), can trigger a synovitis by themselves or by their metabolites (*Fig.* 14.18). Considering the fact that during the entire process of cartilage detachment and abrasion the synovial tissue is flooded with detrital components, it is clear that the primarily degenerative process may be reinforced by a secondary synovitis.

Osteoarthrosis + Synovitis = Osteoarthritis

From this moment, the joint is painful and shows the symptoms of arthritis. The arthrotic person now becomes a rheumatic patient; the osteo*arthrosis* becomes osteo*arthritis*. In principle, secondary synovitis occurring in osteoarthritis shows no qualitative differences as compared with the primary synovitis encountered, for example, in rheumatoid arthritis. As in primary synovitis, all the various elements of the synovial tissue are involved; the pathomechanisms are exudation, proliferation, and infiltration (*Fig.* 14.19). Attention should also be drawn to one fundamental difference between secondary synovitis in

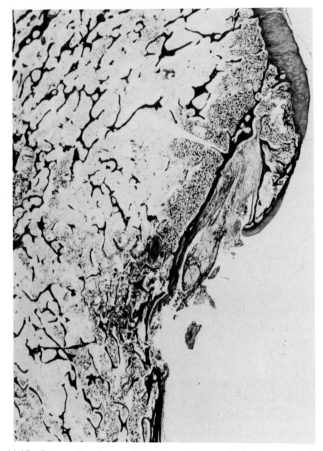

Fig. 14.15. Osteoarthrosis: marginal osteophyte; marked osteoporosis (× 21).

osteoarthritis and primary synovitis in rheumatoid arthritis (*Fig.* 14.20): the synovial tissue in osteoarthritis never attacks and destroys the articular cartilage in the way the tumour-like proliferation does in rheumatoid arthritis (*Figs.* 14.21, 14.22).

Hyalinization and Chondroid Metaplasia of the Synovial Membrane

As the osteoarthritic process progressively develops, the joint surfaces become increasingly deformed and incongruent, with the result that the synovial tissue is exposed to further mechanical damage. This mechanical force on the one hand, and the repeated inflammatory processes on the other, results in a marked fibrosis and hyalinization within the synovial tissue. It is of interest that in these hyalinized areas, which are avascular, the connective tissue cells

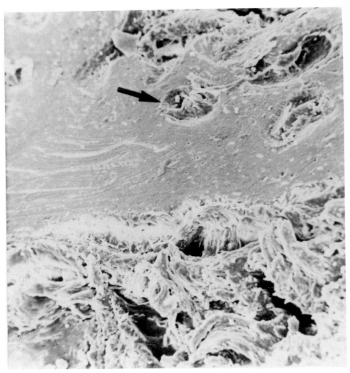

Fig. 14.16. Osteoarthrosis: exposed and abraded bone. *Note* the lamellar structure. In the centre (arrow) the medullary space lies open, and from it fibres are emerging. (Scanning electron micrograph: I.-E. Richter.)

have undergone a transformation into chondrocyte-like cells (*Fig.* 14.23). This shows that the chondrocyte itself is a form of mesenchymal cell specifically adapted to a life of hunger and existence under nearly anaerobic conditions.

Chondrocalcinosis within the Synovial Tissue

It is one consequence of chondroid metaplasia that the deposition of calcium pyrophosphate crystals, which normally only involves the cartilage, now also includes the chondroid transformed synovial tissue.

A Means of Repair

The opening of medullary spaces due to bone erosion, however, also shows a positive aspect, since collagen fibres and blood vessels can thus emerge into the superficial defect so that a scar pannus develops, which constitutes a certain superficial repair mechanism (*Fig.* 14.24). Although a new formation

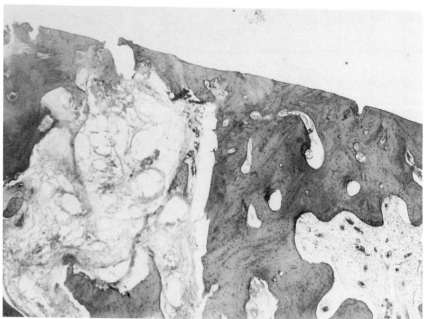

Fig. 14.17. Osteoarthrosis: destruction of the abraded subchondral bone and formation of a chondral debris cyst in the adjacent medullary space ($\times$ 55).

of hyaline cartilage is impossible, sometimes a functionally important repair is achieved by this scar pannus (*Fig.* 14.25).

CONCLUSIONS

Exogenous factors are able to break through the limit of tolerance of the healthy hyaline cartilage and thus damage its structure. Animal models, in this respect, are of significance as they allow us to study the effect of exogenous, mainly mechanical, factors in the articular cartilage. Human osteoarthritis, however, results from a combination of exogenous and endogenous components as long as there are no excessive mechanical factors involved. In the course of life the articular cartilage undergoes a reduction of quality which, on the one hand, results from the changing structure of the matrix molecules and, on the other hand, is due to deficient nutrition and toxic influences to the chondrocytes. The tolerance of the articular cartilage against load within physiological limits is determined by the balance between anabolic and catabolic processes in the cartilaginous matrix. Often osteoarthritis becomes clinically manifest only when a secondary synovitis supervenes. This synovitis is triggered by inflammation mediators, which develop from phagocytosed components of the detritus. In the course of the arthritic process degenerative changes, e.g. hyalinization, succeeded by a chondroid metaplasia, form the basis for the manifestation of a chondrocalcinosis.

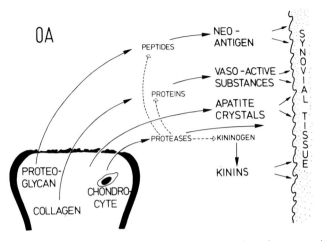

Fig. 14.18. Osteoarthrosis: provocation of a secondary synovitis by substances originating from disintegrated cartilage and bone.

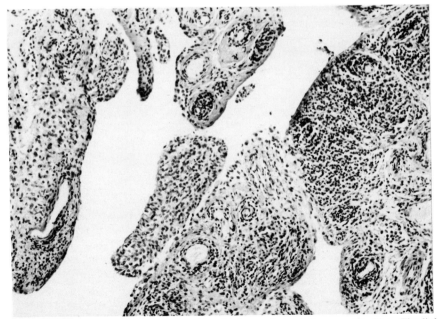

Fig. 14.19. Osteoarthritis: secondary synovitis with hyperplasia of the synovial villae. The lining cells are multi-layered and cuboid in shape. On the left slight proliferation of the local connective tissue cells; moderate lymphocyte and plasma cell infiltration on the right-hand side (× 55).

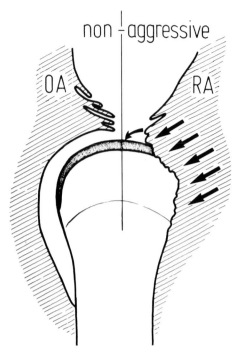

Fig. 14.20. Comparison between secondary synovitis in osteoarthrosis (OA) and primary synovitis in rheumatoid arthritis (RA). In contrast to the synovitis occurring in rheumatoid arthritis, secondary synovitis in osteoarthrosis is non-aggressive.

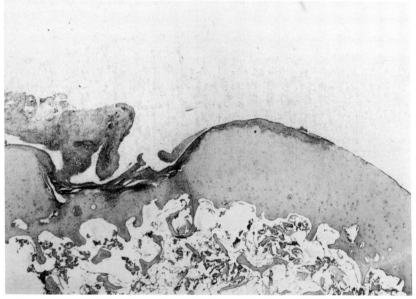

Fig. 14.21. Aggression of synovial cell masses encroaching onto the cartilage from the recessus in rheumatoid arthritis ($\times$ 21).

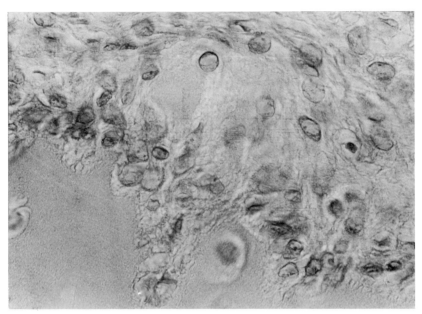

Fig. 14.22. Detail of *Fig.* 14.21 with cartilage remnants (× 140).

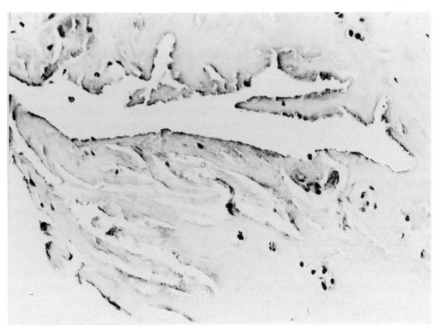

Fig. 14.23. Flattening and fraying of the hyalinized capsular tissue, together with chondroid metaplasia, in an advanced case of osteoarthrosis (× 21).

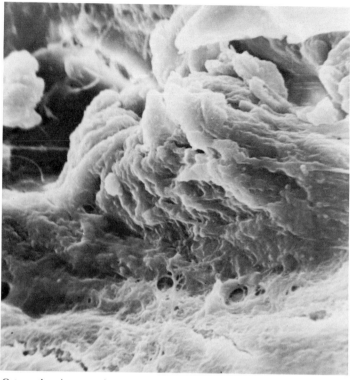

Fig. 14.24. Osteoarthrosis: vascular connective tissue emerging from a debris cyst in the medullary space and invading the joint cavity. (Scanning electron micrograph: I.-E. Richter.)

CLINICAL SIGNIFICANCE

In comparison with rheumatoid arthritis, osteoarthrosis seems not to be a true disease. Osteoarthrosis results from the disproportion between the articular load and the structural tolerance of the hyaline articular cartilage. Both vary in the course of life. While the exogenous components, e.g. body weight, quality of the stabilizing musculature, and defective position of the joints, basically may be corrected, the endogenous factors which disturb the balance between anabolism and catabolism evade therapeutic intervention. In this respect the chondroprotective substances may be useful. However, it is too early to come to any firm conclusion.

The transition from osteoarthrosis to osteoarthritis results from a supervening secondary synovitis. This synovitis can become a pathological factor itself and requires treatment. Together with the destruction of the articular cartilage it may lead to a mechanical grinding of the synovial membrane. The hyalinization of the tissue leads to destruction of the blood vessels and chondroid metaplasia may occur which in turn forms the basis for the development of chondrocalcinosis. It is of importance to reduce the exogenous risk factors to a minimum by living a reasonable life with sufficient physical exercise. Otherwise the limit of tolerance of the articular cartilage will be exceeded, since in any case its quality decreases with age.

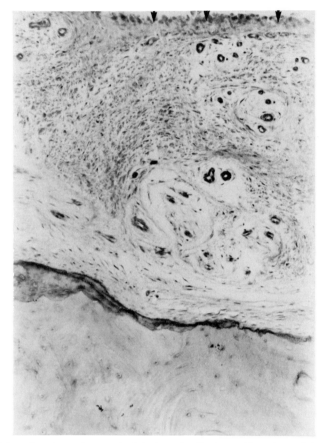

Fig. 14.25. Osteoarthrosis: replacement of destroyed articular cartilage by a plate of fibrous scar tissue. On the surface a layer of new synovial lining cells (arrows)($\times$ 55).

REFERENCES

1. Radin E L, Martin R B, Burr D B, Caterson B, Boyd R D and Goodwin C (1984) Effects of mechanical loading on the tissues of the rabbit knee. *J Orthop Res* **2**: 221–34.
2. Videman T (1982) Experimental osteoarthritis in the rabbit. *Acta Orthop Scand* **53**: 339–47.
3. Ely L W and Mensor M C (1933) Studies on the immobilization of normal joints. *Surg Gynecol Obstet* **57**: 212–5.
4. Evans E B, Eggers G W N, Butler J K and Blumel J (1960) Experimental immobilization and remobilization of the rat knee joints. *J Bone Joint Surg [Am]* **42**: 737–58.
5. Field P L and Hueston J T (1970) Articular cartilage loss in longstanding immobilization of interphalangeal joints. *Br J Plast Surg* **23**: 186–91.
6. Finsterbush A and Friedman B (1973) Early changes in immobilized rat knee joints: a light and electron microscopic study. *Clin Orthop* **92**: 305–19.
7. Finsterbush A and Friedman B (1975) Reversibility of joint changes produced by immobilization in rabbits. *Clin Orthop* **111**: 290–8.
8. Hall M C (1963) Cartilage changes after experimental immobilization of the knee joint of the young rat. *J Bone Joint Surg [Am]* **45**: 36–44.
9. Hall M C (1964) Articular changes in the knee of the adult rat after prolonged immobilization in extension. *Clin Orthop* **34**: 184–95.

10. Langenskjöld A, Michelsson J-E and Videman T (1979) Osteoarthritis of the knee in rabbits produced by immobilization: attempts to achieve a reproducible model for studies on pathogenesis and therapy. *Acta Orthop Scand* **50**: 1–14.
11. Salter R B and Field P (1960) The effect of continuous compression on living articular cartilage: an experimental investigation. *J Bone Joint Surg [Am]* **42**: 31–49.
12. Sood S C (1971) A study of the effects of experimental immobilization on rabbit articular cartilage. *J Anat* **108**: 497–507.
13. Thaxter T H, Mann R A and Anderson C E (1965) Degeneration of immobilized knee joints in rats: histological and autoradiographic study. *J Bone Joint Surg [Am]* **47**: 567–85.
14. Trias A (1961) Effects of persistent pressure on the articular cartilage: an experimental study. *J Bone Joint Surg [Br]* **43**: 376–86.
15. Videman T, Michelsson J-E, Rauhamäki R and Langenskjöld A (1976) Changes in ^{35}S-sulphate uptake in different tissues in the knee and hip regions of rabbits during immobilization, remobilization and the development of osteoarthritis. *Acta Orthop Scand* **47**: 290–8.
16. Williams J M and Brandt K D (1984) Exercise increases osteophyte formation and diminishes fibrillation following chemically induced articular cartilage injury. *J Anat* **4**: 599–611.
17. Stofft E and Graf J (1983) Rasterelektronenoptische Untersuchung des hyalinen Gelenkknorpels. *Acta Anat (Basel)* **116**: 114–25.
18. Radin E L, Ehrlich M M, Weiss C A and Parker H G (1976) Osteoarthrosis as a state of altered physiology. In: *Recent Advances in Rheumatology* (W W Buchanan and W C Dick, eds), pp. 1–18. Edinburgh, London, New York: Churchill Livingstone.
19. Annefeld M and Fassbender H G (1983) Ultrastrukturelle Untersuchungen zur Wirksamkeit antiarthrotischer Substanzen. *Z Rheumatol* **42**: 199–202.
20. Annefeld M, Raiss R and Cleres C (1984) Der Einfluss der Tiaprofensäure auf den Gelenkknorpel der Ratte im Vergleich zu Referenzsubstanzen – elektronenoptische und morphometrische Studie. *Arzneim Forsch* **34**: 1763–5.
21. Raiss R (1984) Einfluss eines NSAID (Lonazolac-Ca) auf den Gelenkknorpel der Ratte – Ultrastrukturelles Chondrozytentestsystem. *Therapiewoche* **34**: 3482–4.
22. Annefeld M and Raiss R (1984) Veränderungen in der Ultrastruktur des Chondrozyten unter dem Einfluss eines GAG-Peptid-Komplexes. *Akt Rheumatol* **9**: 99–104.
23. Raiss R (1985) Einfluss von D-Glucosaminsulfat auf experimentell geschädigten Gelenkknorpel. *Fortschr Med* **103**: 658–62.
24. Aydelotte M B and Kuettner K E (1984) A histochemical study of distributions of proteoglycans in cultures of adult bovine chondrocytes in agarose gel. *Transactions of the 30th Annual Meeting, Orthopaedic Research Society 1984;* **9**: 117.
25. Dingle J T, Horsefield P, Fell H B and Barrat M E (1975) Breakdown of proteoglycan and collagen induced in pig articular cartilage in organ culture. *Ann Rheum Dis* **34**: 303–11.
26. Dingle J T and Dingle T T (1980) The site of cartilage matrix degradation. *Biochem J* **190**: 431–8.
27. Wagenhäuser F J (1969) *Die Rheumamorbidität.* Bern, Stuttgart, Vienna: Huber.
28. Fassbender H G (1981) Pathomechanisms responsible for synovitis in osteoarthritis. XVth International Congress of Rheumatology, Paris. *Rev Rheum Mal Osteoartic* (Special Abstract) **1459**.
29. Schumacher H R and Kitridou R C (1972) Synovitis of recent onset. A clinicopathologic study during the first month of disease. *Arthritis Rheum* **15**: 465–85.
30. Dieppe P A, Huskisson E C, Crocker P and Willoughby D A (1976) Apatite deposition disease. A new arthropathy. *Lancet* **I**: 266–9.

Chapter 15

Physiology and Therapeutic Value of Passive Motion

W. H. Akeson, D. Amiel, and S. L-Y. Woo

CONTENTS

INTRODUCTION

The goal of this chapter will be to develop the rationale for application of passive motion to certain musculoskeletal disorders. The concept of the stress dependence of connective tissue is central to this rationale and will be described as the basis for the discussion to follow. For this purpose, effects of both stress deprivation and stress enhancement on joint physiology will be outlined and, finally, the existing knowledge of the efficacy of passive motion as a therapeutic modality will be summarized.

375

The understanding of the therapeutic value of passive motion is a relatively recent development. By contrast, rest has historically been accorded the key role in the management of a variety of disorders of the musculoskeletal system. In this history, the use of an infinite variety of braces, casts and assorted apparatus to impose the needed immobility on the spine or extremities has a long and colourful tradition. The treatment of fractures and dislocations and the correction of musculoskeletal deformities has provided the most obvious rationale for the use of enforced rest. Additional indications include bone and joint infections, arthritic deformity, and muscle imbalance secondary to neurological dysfunction. However, the basis for treatment decisions utilizing immobility as an essential adjunct has been largely empirical. Giants of early orthopaedic surgery figure prominently in this history.

Both stress deprivation and stress enhancement influence morphological and biomechanical characteristics of connective tissue. Data from experimental animals and from descriptive clinical studies on humans, which has accumulated over the past 2 decades, is sufficient to place stress deprivation effects on a secure foundation in qualitative terms (1, 2). Quantitative data on the process remains sketchy, but enough information has been accumulated to suggest a few generalizations which may be used to introduce the subject and provide guidelines for future research priorities. Unfortunately, data on exercise effects on connective tissue other than muscle and bone remain quite meagre. The available evidence infers that hypertrophy of tendon and possibly of ligament occurs in exercising animals (3). Recent studies on exercise effects in humans and animals clearly show that sustained exercise produces bone hypertrophy, a finding of importance with respect to the osteoporosis of an ageing population. The problem of recovery from stress deprivation has been shown to have a much greater time requirement than that which induced the effect, a matter of frustration to physicians who are required to use casts in the treatment of injuries or deformities, and a matter of even greater frustration to patients forced to undergo prolonged rehabilitation programmes to regain prior functional strength, mobility, and agility of the affected extremity (4). A brief resume of pertinent supporting data for these conclusions follows.

THE STRESS DEPENDENCE OF CONNECTIVE TISSUE

The interrelationship between skeletal form and function has long been accepted. The most explicit expression of the relationship was, of course, Wolff's Law, which states that bone adapts to the applied stresses. In more recent years, the expression has been found to apply equally importantly to the joint composite, including articular cartilage, ligament, tendon, capsule, and synovial membrane as well as to bone (4). This broader expansion of Wolff's Law is probably simply recognized with slight editorial license as Wolff's Law of connective tissue, although others, as is more often the rule in science, may have priority in recognition of the broader application of the more general interrelationship between form and function as applied to fibrous connective tissue and the joint composite (5).

ANATOMICAL PATHOLOGY OF STRESS DEPRIVATION OF SYNOVIAL JOINTS

It is instructive to review the protean manifestations of stress deprivation on synovial joints in order to put passive motion therapy into perspective. There are enough gross and microscopic observations on human anatomical pathology to feel confident that experimental animal and human changes are closely similar. The changes are conveniently divided into *(1)* periarticular and synovial tissue changes, and *(2)* articular cartilage and subchondral bone changes.

Periarticular and Synovial Tissue Changes

The consistent feature of the gross appearance of the periarticular and synovial tissues of immobilized joints is a fibro-fatty connective tissue proliferation within the joint space (6, 7). In knee immobilization models, this phenomenon is seen prominently in the inter-condylar notch, but is also observed in other joint recesses. The proliferative fibro-fatty connective tissue covers exposed intra-articular soft tissue structures such as the cruciate ligaments and the under-surface of the quadriceps tendon. It also blankets the non-articulating cartilage surfaces. With the passage of time, adhesions develop between the exposed tissue surfaces as the fibro-fatty connective tissue is transformed into more mature scar. The proliferation of this type of tissue is relatively the same in such diverse species as the rabbit, rat, dog and primate. Similar changes are also prominent in human posterior intervertebral joints and in human knee joints (7).

Articular Cartilage and Subchondral Bone Changes

The changes which occur secondary to immobility affecting articular cartilage can be separated into those in non-contact areas, and those in contact areas. The changes in non-contact areas are thought to be in part secondary to the fibro-fatty connective tissue proliferation described above. The ingrowth of connective tissue which fills the joint space soon covers the joint surfaces. In the rat model studied by Evans *et al.* (6), in which the progress was evaluated on a progressive time base, there was coverage of the articular surfaces by 30 days. The connective tissue became more dense and adherent during the subsequent month and remained relatively constant thereafter. The surface cartilage cells gradually became confluent with the overlying connective tissue. By 60 days the tangential layer of cartilage cells was lost in many of the animals. There was consistent evidence of thinning of the cartilage grossly, beginning peripherally where the adhesions first occured. Fibrillation of the cartilage was also seen and variable loss of staining of matrix was observed. Staining changes were also described by Baker *et al.* (8), in human spinal facet joints after anterior spine fusion. These changes included first a zone of loss of staining around the cells peripheral to the cellular lacunae. Ultimately, loss of definition of lacunae occurred, and the cartilage cells

became stellate with poorly defined margin. Such change in staining characteristics of cartilage matrix had been described much earlier by Reyher in
1874 (9). Baker *et al.* described similar changes and termed them 'Weichselbaum's space' (8, 10). Parker and Keefer observed this process in cartilage
beneath rheumatoid pannus and proposed that it represented a metaplastic
process of cartilage cells transformed into fibroblasts (11), a view which
Baker *et al.* endorsed.

In the contact areas, mild to severe changes of articular cartilage are
observed depending on the rigidity of immobilization, the position of
immobilization and, most important, the degree of compression. Typically,
the mild changes consist of loss of intensity of staining of the matrix. In areas
of greater compressive forces there are varying degrees of destruction, up to
and including full thickness ulceration of cartilage with cellular distortion and
necrosis, fibrillation of matrix, and erosion of matrix down to subchondral
bone (12, 13).

The major areas of alteration in the subchondral bone occur beneath
cartilage lesions in joints immobilized 60 days or longer. Hyperaemia in the
subjacent marrow spaces is noted with proliferation of vascular connective
tissue. In some areas this tissue penetrated the subchondral plate and
hindered the calcified layer of articular cartilage. Trabecular atrophy and
resorption in the areas subjacent to cartilage lesions are also seen. Subchondral cysts sometimes develop in this location in animals followed for longer
periods.

Not surprisingly, such profound alterations in gross and microscopic
architecture are associated with significant biomechanical and biochemical
changes.

EXPERIMENTAL STUDIES OF THE FIBROUS CONNECTIVE TISSUE RESPONSE TO STRESS ALTERATION

The changes in joint structure and function in immobilized limbs have been
the subject of considerable interest with respect to the underlying processes
involved, and with respect to the possibility of modifying the responses
through the use of drugs or hormones. In an experimental model designed to
evaluate the soft tissues' response to immobility in our laboratory, the hind
limbs of dogs (1) and rabbits (14) were immobilized using internal fixation
procedures for up to 12 weeks, and periarticular connective tissues were
examined.

Casts or internal fixation of the flexed knee with a threaded pin placed
through the tibia and femur well posterior to the knee joint give similar
results. The latter technique has generally been preferred to obviate pressure
sores from cast friction.

Biomechanical Changes in the Knee Composite

The knee contracture was assessed immediately after sacrifice, utilizing an
apparatus called an 'arthrograph' (15). The arthrograph is designed to

measure the joint stiffness in knees in terms of a torque–angular deformation (T–O) diagram. The knees of the experimental and control from each animal were mounted on the arthrograph and cycled at a frequency of 0·2 Hz. Two ranges of motion, 5 cycles each, were used in sequence: the first was 50–80°, and the second 45–95° of knee angles. Each cycle of flexion and extension was recorded on the X–Y recorder. Recording of the first cycle of the contracture knee was particularly important because subsequent cycles required substantially less energy. In addition, the amount of torque required to extend the knee from 50–65° from acute flexion during the first cycle was also significantly higher than that of subsequent cycles. The significant increases in torque and area of hysteresis were used as measures of increase in joint stiffness of severity of joint contracture. A progressive increase in the strength of contracture was observed on serial evaluations between 2 and 12 weeks. Detailed descriptions of the apparatus and technique are given in several earlier papers (14, 15). The arthrograph permits evaluation of the efficacy of therapeutic modalities such as drug or hormone injections on the process. Interestingly, hyaluronic acid has been shown to significantly inhibit contracture developed under stress deprivation conditions (16).

Biomechanical Changes in Ligaments

Following 9 weeks of immobilization, the linear slope, ultimate load, and energy absorbing capabilities of the rabbit medial collateral ligament (MCL)– bone complex during tension decrease to approximately one third of that of the contralateral non-immobilized control. The load–strain characteristics of the MCL substances become inferior. Further immobilization of up to 12 weeks causes additional degradation of the MCL substance (3). These data are obtained with the aid of the video dimensional analyser system, where the mechanical properties of ligament substance and structural properties of the bone–ligament complex can be simultaneously evaluated (17).

The failure mode is altered in this model, as well as reduction in the failure load and reduction in modulus of elasticity. The bone resorption at the ligament insertion site causes failure by avulsion at the insertion site, a problem noted by several investigators (18, 19, 20).

These mechanical alterations occur after a relatively brief stress deprivation period compared to common clinical treatment programmes for fractures and joint injuries. They have important implications to the rationale for selection of treatment options and, as we will see, equally dramatic implications for rehabilitation following recovery from the initial injuries.

Exercise Effects on Specialized Connective Tissue Structure

An animal model has been used to evaluate effects of exercise on bone, tendon and ligament in normals. In one study, miniature swine were exercised at intervals on a track over 1 year on a schedule which created cardiac hypertrophy (21) and increased cardiac output. At the end of 1 year, cortical bone showed improved structural properties of about one third, indicative of cortical hypertrophy. The material properties were unchanged, indicating that the changes observed were entirely due to bulk change rather than qualitative improvement. Similar changes were observed for digital extensor tendons. The cross-sectional areas 12 months after onset of the exercise period were increased 21% and the load to failure increased 62% (22). It is important to observe that, at 3 months after onset, differences in bone and extensor tendon were not significant, indicating that a long time and large effort are required for the improvement in structural properties to be seen. Furthermore, site and tissue specific factors are involved, since digital flexor tendons and ligaments were less responsive than bone and extensor tendon to the exercise programme.

Recovery from Stress Deprivation

Of interest here is that the recovery of the MCL substance following immobilization may be quite rapid. The load–strain curve of the MCL from the experimental knee of 9-week-immobilized animals recovered to the same level of that of the control after 12 weeks of cage activity. The recovery curve for the 12-week immobilized knees continued to be slightly inferior after a cage-activity recovery period of 12 weeks (23). The experimental knee ligaments continued to have inferior structural properties as compared to that of the control knees. The P_{max} and the A_{max} for the experimentals were approximately two-thirds that of the controls. The slower recovery of strength of the bone–ligament junction confirmed findings obtained by other investigators (18, 20, 24).

The surprising finding, however, is that following remobilization there was a rapid recovery of properties of the MCL substance in the functional range (up to 5% ligament strain), while the ultimate load and energy-absorbing capability of the MCL–bone complex were still considerably inferior (23). The tibial insertion sites continued to be the weakest link. These results added to the earlier conclusion made by Noyes *et al.* (24), where up to 1 year of reconditioning is required (following 8 weeks of immobilization) to regain the strength of anterior cruciate ligament (ACL)–bone complex. In this respect, our results on structural properties are similar to these authors. But additionally, our data indicate that the ligament substance will recover rapidly during remobilization and can function normally in the physiological range.

The implications for treatment are that prevention of stress deprivation effects are paramount to the success of rehabilitation efforts. This conclusion forms an important aspect of the scientific rationale of passive motion in the early phase of rehabilitation.

Biochemical Events Consequent to Stress Deprivation

The biochemical changes of periarticular connective tissue matrix are manifold. Space does not permit a detailed exposition of those changes. However, a summary will follow, along with key references to the literature on the subject. An important point, which has evolved from our laboratory, is that there are notable differences between biochemical matrix characteristics of ligaments and tendons and, furthermore, there are differences unfolding between various ligaments. The functional implications of these differences are not yet clear, and require further study.

Extracellular fluid volume changes

The water content of fibrous connective tissues is in the range of 65–70%. As the population of cells is relatively sparse in this tissue, the majority of this water is perforce in the extracellular space. On gross inspection, the dissected tissues from the immobilized limb appear less glistening and more 'woody' in texture. Chemical analysis shows a statistically significant decrease in water content of 4–6% as compared to the control side (25). It seems likely that this amount of water loss is functionally significant. Fluid movement, which plays such an important role in articular cartilage load bearing and lubrication, is probably equally important in performing the same role in fibrous connective tissue. It has recently been established that hyaluronic acid and its attached or entrapped water is the principal fibrous connective tissue lubricant (26).

It is presumed that the interstitial fluid in a densely fibrous 'connecting' anatomical structure serves as a spacer between individual collagen fibres or fibrils, permitting discrete movement of one fibre or fibril past the adjacent fibres. The importance of interstitial fluid to tissue rheology is obvious, as the concept of viscoelasticity of connective tissue rests upon the dual fluid and solid nature of these systems.

Glycosaminoglycan changes

The largest change found in the composition of the stress-deprived periarticular connective tissue is reduction in the concentration of glycosaminoglycans (GAG)(27). The decreases in chondroitin-4-sulphate and chondroitin-6-sulphate (30%) and hyaluronic acid (40%) are statistically significant, while the % change of dermatan sulphate thought to be associated with fibres is smaller. Decreased concentration of GAG and water would be expected to alter the plasticity and pliability of connective tissue matrices, and to reduce lubrication efficiency. Biochemical analyses of articular cartilage and meniscus from the experimental knees also show a reduction of 24% and 31% respectively of GAG content in these tissues (27).

Water content appeared to parallel the GAG ranges in concert with the known facts concerning the high water-binding capacity of GAG. The preferential loss of GAG is also consistent with known facts about their rapid turnover half-life (1·7–7·0 days)(28) as compared with collagen (half-life of 300–500 days)(29). Turnover studies utilizing tritium-labelled acetate show that the decrement in specific activity of hyaluronic acid with time after preliminary labelling is the same for control and immobilized limbs. The conclusion is therefore that there is no acceleration of degradation, but rather a reduction in the synthesis of hyaluronic acid in the immobilized extremities. The fibroblasts of the fibrous connective tissue matrix apparently respond to physical forces by a homeostatic feedback loop to maintain the proper balance of connective tissue constituents.

A gel-like structure created by the interaction between water and glycosaminoglycans is currently well accepted by physiologists working with interstitial fluid flow questions (30). Clearly, the gel structure is severely compromised in connective tissue deprived of mechanical stimulation. It is postulated that the GAG and water changes are permissive in so far as qualitative changes in collagen are concerned, as fibre–fibre distances must be reduced when water and GAG volumes are reduced.

It is presumed that the lubricating and volume separating effects provided by hyaluronic acid and water permit the independent gliding of microfibrils past one another, facilitating tissue adaptation to motion permitted by the particular connective tissue weave pattern. Loss of this volume-separating and lubricating property provides for fibril–fibril friction as well as the potential for adhesions or cross-linking between adjacent collagen fibrils. Any newly synthesized collagen is apt to be randomly dispersed and to create interference with the functional gliding between fibres necessary for normal mobility. This is particularly so, since in the stationary attitude maturation processes may encourage fibril growth in diameter by including these newly synthesized random fibrils within the fibre structural units. Such mismatch with respect to functional elongation needs and weave without regard to the usual physical force and motion is probably central to the pathomechanics of joint stiffness.

Collagen changes

The processes seen in the studies described above, which rely on the techniques of anatomical pathology, suggest that connective tissue proliferation or simple granulation tissue production is the basis of joint contractures. However, collagen turnover studies are difficult to reconcile with this concept at first examination. For example, the studies by Brooke and Slack (31) showed that collagen precursor uptake was actually reduced in denervated rat limbs compared to controls. However, the collagen synthesis did proceed, but at a reduced level. Peacock (32) used saline solubility of collagen to estimate the amount of new collagen synthesized and found no difference in immobilized and control joints except for the posterior capsular area where there was increased collagen solubility. However, as he used pin fixation with a placement proximal to the posterior capsule, the significance of finding total collagen mass changes became uncertain. Our laboratory was able to demonstrate reduction in total collagen of only 10% by total joint mass evaluation using the whole periarticular connective tissue unit (33). Studies of Klein (34) using long-term labelling techniques, which are more sensitive for this purpose, found small increases in collagen mass in denervated limbs.

We feel, however, that strategic placement of anomalous cross-links of newly synthesized collagen fibrils in the contracture process is of importance. These cross-links can act as bridges between existing functionally independent fibres with divergent tracking patterns. Using a simplified model, i.e. the Chinese finger trap mechanism, it can be seen that fixed contact at just a few nodal points defeats the functional gliding of the whole apparatus. Demonstration of such changes within the weave of the joint capsule is quite difficult because of right-to-left variability in microarchitecture and the small degree of change necessary to effect a mechanical impediment. However, it is easy to be convinced that such a process must play a role in the synovial joint contracture process. Disorganization which occurs in the cruciate ligament of a rabbit after 9 weeks of immobilization has been demonstrated in our previous work (35). The pattern of cellular alignment becomes distorted as well, almost certainly reflecting a more random matrix organization.

Collagen cross-link alterations

The studies of quantitative changes in the cross-linking of collagen from the immobilized rabbit knee periarticular connective tissue show significant increases in the sodium borohydride-reducible intermolecular cross-links (36). A typical radioactive elution profile from column 1 of a 3N p-toluene sulphonic acid hydrolysate of [^{3}H]NaBH$_4$ reduced periarticular connective tissue from control and immobilized joints, and the rechromatography on an extended basic column of the aldolhistidinedihydroxylysinonorleucine (DHLNL) peaks show a two-fold increase in DHLNL on the immobilized side. It was shown that dihydroxylysinonorleucine, hydroxylysinonorleucine (HLNL) and histidinohydroxymerodesmosine (HHMD) are the major cross-links which increase following immobilization. No change in hydroxylysine/lysine ratio between the immobilized and control periarticular connective tissue collagen was detected.

It can be speculated that the increased intra- and intermolecular collagen cross-links are important in the contracture process. How do such cross-links interact at a molecular level? To begin with, it is unlikely that a fibre-to-fibre distance is bridged by a lysine-lysine or lysine-hydroxylysine reaction. The distances are much too great and the forces too small to create the nodal fibre-to-fibre cross-link which is proposed to hamper joint motion. Rather, it is presumed that the nodal fibre-to-fibre cross-links are brought about by aggregation of new fibrils with preexisting fibres of the matrix. The process may proceed in the usual manner of aggregation of fibrils into fibres, then incorporating bridges of newly synthesized collagen fibril elements into pairs of existing fibres. Such structures become mechanically constraining at the time when the joint is freed from constraining devices.

Collagen type changes

Since the formation of reducible cross-links follows collagen synthesis (37) and since the presence and relative amounts of these cross-links may, in part, depend upon the type of collagen being synthesized (38), it is important to examine the type or types of periarticular connective tissue collagen synthesized during the period of immobilization. Examination of the densitometric scan of the SDS gel of the CNBr-cleaved peptides from control and immobilized tissue reveals no alteration in the type of collagen being synthesized during the period of immobilization (33). The peptides a_1 [III] CB characteristic of Type III collagen are absent in the CNBr-digest of the control and immobilized periarticular connective tissue collagen. Furthermore, these results are confirmed by amino acid analysis and SDS gel electrophoresis performed on intact a components separated by CM cellulose chromatography. These results provide additional supportive evidence that only Type I collagen is found in the dense fibrous structures of normal and contracture knees.

The significance of the changes in collagen type ratios and cross-linking patterns observed secondary to stress deprivation probably reflects the effects of increased collagen turnover. The altered mechanics, in turn, most probably result from the random orientation of newly synthesized fibrous matrix constituents. These new fibrils are disposed without regard to mechanical requirements because of the lack of input from the mechanical signals which are normally operative.

THE DEVELOPMENT OF CONCEPTS OF PASSIVE MOTION

The events described above indicate a disturbing and very harmful outcome of stress deprivation on synovial joints, which threatens the success of rehabilitation after treatment with casts or splints for trauma or other disorders requiring immobilization. It was not unexpected, therefore, in the past decade and a half, to observe the development of new concepts of treatment emphasizing early motion. The controversy about early motion had, in fact, erupted earlier still. The archetypal protagonists commonly identified as providing leadership for the 'motion-versus-rest' camps in the century past were Hugh Owen Thomas, called 'Hugh the Rester', and Championniere, whose philosophy of treatment was exemplified by his phrase 'in motion there is life'. The historical advocates of rest-versus-motion schools relied almost entirely on empirical observation and appeals to authority for the basis of therapeutic decisions. It remained for the clarification of effects of stress on synovial joints to properly prioritize the therapeutic decision on rehabilitation. Equally important in the evolution of modern rehabilitation philosophy were fundamental studies on the influence of stress and motion on repair of bone, tendon, ligament and cartilage. Furthermore, studies on stress and motion effects on disorders of the synovial joint composite have provided a foundation for musculoskeletal management decisions which are approaching a more logical construct. Technological advances have occurred which, hand-in-hand with these observations, have provided new avenues for treatment which could be coupled with the early motion philosophy of rehabilitation.

In fracture management, for example, it has been possible to achieve improved fracture stability with biomechanically sound internal fixation devices. These devices applied very early in the post-injury period have permitted not only early joint mobility, but mobilization of the total patient. The ability to accomplish patient mobilization after multiple trauma has resulted in a marked improvement in the survival rates in critically injured patients – a tribute to the modern trauma management system, and to the philosophy of early mobilization.

The philosophy of early mobilization has adapted passive motion in several forms: *(1)* occasional, *(2)* interrupted, and *(3)* continuous, with various combinations thereof, to the early post-injury or post-operative state where patient compliance with active motion programmes cannot reasonably be expected because of post-operative pain or weakness.

For successful application of passive motion to the post-injury state, the integrity of the repair – bone, ligament or tendon – must be maintained. Details of specific applications await further contributions from basic and clinical science. However, enough is known to make it possible to develop an understanding of some of the general principles of application which should find universal utility in musculoskeletal rehabilitation for the foreseeable future. What follows is a brief outline of the evidence of efficacy of passive motion in a variety of clinical applications and of the scientific basis of those applications.

SYNOVIAL JOINT SPACE CLEARANCE WITH CONTINUOUS PASSIVE MOTION (CPM)

Studies on clearance rates from synovial joints have demonstrated the value of passive motion in facilitating transport of intrasynovial contents. The clearest example of this application is the paper of O'Driscoll and colleagues (39) on the clearance of blood from the joint space. This data demonstrated convincingly that a haemarthrosis in a model system treated by CPM was more rapidly cleared than in contralateral mobilized joints. The clearance rate of indium-III-oxine-labelled erythrocytes was double that seen in the immobilized joints. After 1 week there was significantly less blood remaining in the joints treated with CPM.

This effect was seen directly in a paper by Skyhar et al. using $^{35}SO_4$ to study nutrition of anterior cruciate knee ligaments under conditions of CPM and rest (40). It was demonstrated that in CPM knees there was less $^{35}SO_4$ uptake than in a cage activity group. The effect of CPM on synovial fluid clearance was so large that the uptake of $^{35}SO_4$ in the CPM-treated knees was less than that in the immobilized knees, suggesting, at first, poor diffusion under conditions of CPM, but actually indicating that clearance of isotope occurred before diffusion into the ligament could occur.

These experiments demonstrate the importance of the convection effect of activity to the nutritional support of synovial joint components, especially articular cartilage and ligaments. Furthermore, the clinical application of CPM in the post-operative state is emphasized as a practical step in improved patient care post-operatively or post-trauma. The clearance of blood from the joint space is of undisputed advantage, knowing the harmful effects of chronic haemarthrosis in states such as haemophilia.

CONTINUOUS PASSIVE MOTION IN TREATMENT OF SEPTIC ARTHRITIS

The use of motion to favourably influence the outcome of septic arthritis has been demonstrated in papers by Salter et al. (41, 42) in a model system. The beneficial effect was most prominently seen in articular cartilage, where the damage of the septic process from proteolytic enzymes was reduced by the imposition of a passive motion programme. Presumably, clearance of the deleterious lysosomal enzymes which accumulate in joint fluid in septic arthritis was facilitated by motion-induced convection effects. The articular cartilages of joints treated by the activity protocols were presumably spared exposure to high levels of matrix-destructive enzymes by the acceleration of clearance of those products from the joint space by CPM.

PASSIVE MOTION EFFECTS ON REPAIR

Several repair models have been studied under the influence of one of the passive motion modalities. In several applications the quality of repair appears to be improved under motion conditions as compared to immobility. These applications require stability of the repair line in order for healing to proceed successfully. This is seen most clearly in flexor tendon repair, where failure of the suture line in the early postoperative state can result in tendon disruption. However, if the suture line is maintained, improved outcome has been observed in several respects (43). In certain circumstances intermittent passive motion has resulted in a successful outcome. In the case of ligament, cage activity has been shown to be superior to the immobilized condition (44). In still other circumstances, especially in cartilage healing, CPM was shown to provide a superior outcome (45). Generally speaking, the experimental models have indicated improved healing rates of bone, tendon, ligament and cartilage under motion conditions and also improved quality of repair. Indeed, in the flexor tendon case within the flexor tendon sheath, it has been shown that healing proceeds by different mechanisms under motion conditions (intrinsic healing) as compared to immobilization conditions (extrinsic healing – the one wound concept)(43). The available data is insufficient to describe optimum clinical protocols of frequency, intensity or duration of passive motion. We have spoken of the problem as analogous to the drug dose–response curve. In fact, the optimum values for passive motion may be found to vary in the spectrum of specific applications. Until that data is available, empirical rules will apply.

The examples below, however, will provide insights into the range of potential applications of passive motion to the problems of specialized connective tissue healing and the broad principles which underly these uses.

Continuous Passive Motion Influence on Cartilage Healing

The interaction between healing of the joint surfaces and motion had beginnings with the early concepts of cup arthroplasty. It was recognized that conversion of the new arthroplasty surface to fibrocartilage, following debridement of the degenerative hip and reaming to a concentric sphere of bleeding bone, required motion. Without motion the surface contained only fibrous tissue. In a few instances there was the opportunity to observe surfaces in patients who had not been able to move the hip for unrelated medical reasons. In these patients conversion of fibrous tissue to fibrocartilage was not observed. Mooney and Ferguson showed this effect in the rabbit metatarsophalangeal joint where immobilized segments did not develop fibrocartilage surfaces as well as mobilized joints (46). Hohl and Luck were able to demonstrate superior healing in drill hole defects in femoral cartilage of primates if motion occurred, as compared to immobilized knees (47). Convery and Akeson studied varying size drill hole defects in horse femoral condyles and observed that relatively small defects ($\frac{1}{8}$ inch diameter) healed readily on pasture-grazing activity, but larger defects ($\frac{1}{4}-\frac{7}{8}$ in) did not heal (48). The dimensional aspect of cartilage healing is important to recognize because, with or without motion regimens, large defects ($\frac{1}{4}$ in or larger) simply do not heal with hyaline cartilage. Nor do arthroplasty surfaces heal with hyaline cartilage. Large surface defects or craters cover a portion but usually not the entire surface and the composition of the surface replacement matrix is of fibrocartilage, not hyaline cartilage. This has been demonstrated convincingly by histological and biochemical methods. The biomechanical properties of the replacement tissue are inferior to hyaline cartilage, permitting approximately twice as much deformation on compression as compared to hyaline cartilage. These factors have obvious functional and clinical implications which must temper the interpretation of CPM effects on cartilage healing.

Salter and colleagues have been important contributors to the studies of facilitation of cartilage healing under the influence of CPM (45). They have shown convincingly that small defects of rabbit femoral articular cartilage of the order of magnitude of $\frac{1}{8}$ in diameter will heal with hyaline cartilage in a significant percentage of knees mobilized by CPM. This is an important observation which relates to several clinical circumstances in which small defects in hyaline cartilage of the joint surface occur. It is important to note that the facilitation of repair of primitive mesenchymal cells to hyaline cartilage occurs *only* in the very small defects, not in large defects or full surface defects.

Continuous Passive Motion Influence on Periosteal and Perichondrial Grafting

The fact that only very small cartilage defects heal with a satisfactory extracellular matrix of hyaline cartilage has led several investigators to search for improved techniques of treatment of such defects. Ohlsen (49) and Engkvist (50) studied rib perichondrial tissue as a potential source of primitive cells with chondrogenic potential for this purpose. The work was later confirmed by Coutts et al. (51). Because experimental studies indicated considerable promise, pilot clinical perichondrial arthroplasty studies for small joints of the hand were soon thereafter performed with some success (52). Poussa (53) showed similar chondrogenic potential of periostial grafts. O'Driscoll and Salter confirmed Poussa's work in a rabbit knee joint model (42). They were able to improve the result from 8% success in immobilized knees to 59% success in knees managed by CPM. Fixation of the periosteal or perichondrial membrane is crucial to the successful outcome of periosteal or perichondrial grafting. O'Driscoll et al. developed a method of stretching the periosteal membrane over a bone plug sized to fit the defect to be filled. This technique has worked effectively in the experimental application (42), but different methodology will be required for clinical application.

Continuous Passive Motion in Fracture Healing

The development of modern biomechanical devices and modern principles of application of those devices to fracture fixation permits the use of CPM early in the post-injury state. CPM is most effectively applied in intra-articular fractures where fracture lines through subchondral bone and articular cartilage are commonly observed. Following the observations of Salter *et al.* described above, it will frequently be the case that the width of the gap between fracture fragments is less than $\frac{1}{8}$ inch. If congruence of the joint is established and the cartilage fracture gaps are narrow, CPM should facilitate the cartilage healing process. Additional benefits should be anticipated in terms of facilitation of the rehabilitation programme by lessening stress deprivation effects and by providing stress enhancement to guide deposits of matrix components in an orderly and functionally useful alignment.

Intermittent Passive Motion Effects on Tendon Healing

The application of passive motion to flexor tendon healing in 'no man's land' in the flexor tendon sheath has been slow to evolve for two reasons: *(1)* concern about integrity of the suture line, and *(2)* concern about the mechanism of tendon healing requiring ingrowth of connective tissue from the flexor tendon sheath. The paradox of this process, termed the 'one wound concept' by Peacock (32), was that the very tissue ingrowth which caused healing also caused the tendon to be locked against the flexor sheath and limited the functional tendon excursion. Indeed the major failures are not with tendon healing, but with tendon adhesions which markedly reduce the range of motion of the tendon and affected joints. The fundamental studies of Gelberman *et al.* (43) reversed this thinking by demonstrating clearly that tendon healing could occur by an intrinsic mechanism of proliferation of epitenon and endotenon cells when the extrinsic mechanism was blocked by intermittent passive motion. The canine forepaw model was used for these flexor tendon studies. Not only did the tendon heal by the intrinsic route, but the healing occurred more rapidly and with greater mechanical strength while simultaneously preserving mobility of tendon and the joints of the affected finger.

It is important to note that the motion required for this effect is not of great duration. The mobilization schedule was only 5 min of careful manual passive motion conducted by a therapist twice a day. The remainder of the time the limb was immobilized in a fibreglass cast. This 'mini' passive motion schedule recognized the concerns for the potential of rupture of the suture line with a more aggressive range of motion protocol.

In this instance, motion therapy was able to convert the healing mode from extrinsic to intrinsic, while simultaneously providing improved healing strength and improved mobility, a string of therapeutic bonuses which are seldom so clearly identified from an alteration of treatment protocol.

Salter and colleagues have shown, in the patellar tendon laceration model, similar effects of improved healing associated with continuous passive motion. In this case, repair is necessarily an extrinsic and intrinsic mechanism due to the anatomical differences between patellar tendon and flexor tendon.

Intermittent Active Motion Effects in Ligament Healing

The discussion of ligament healing is confounded by the diversity of structures under the ligament classification with respect to anatomical and physiological idiosyncracies. For example, the anterior cruciate ligament of the knee will not heal, for reasons not precisely known, although the 'hostile' synovial environment in which the ACL resides is widely presumed to be an important or even decisive factor in that outcome. The ACL receives significant nutrition from synovial fluid and that nutritional source may not be adequate to support fibroblastic proliferation (although it will support a healing response in the case of flexor tendon). The enigma remains.

However, CPM is used by many clinicians in the postoperative period following replacement of the ACL by a grafting technique employing a tendon or synthetic substitute for the ligament. Interestingly, tendon and ligament are not identical biochemically (54). Distinctive differences between collagen cross-links and collagen types have been reported. Burks has cautioned that CPM can cause failure of the tendon graft if the graft is not isometric and is not firmly secured (55). However, if those conditions prevail, the graft is unlikely to survive in a rehabilitation setting. Tendon grafts actually become very weak mechanically at 3–6 weeks after insertion. The tendon cells undergo autolysis in this environment (56) and are replaced by cells from synovial sources. The matrix of the graft is gradually remodelled and assumes the matrix characteristics of ACL.

Unfortunately, none of the animal studies have shown recovery of mechanical strength of the graft substitute for ACL to the original tissue's mechanical and structural properties.

Better results can be reported for most other ligaments. In the medial collateral ligament of the knee, for example, an abundant surrounding soft tissue blood supply offers the opportunity for superior nutritional support of the needed fibroplasia. In this case, the recent work of Inoue et al. has provided strong evidence supporting the concept of early active motion of the knee (44). When compared to knees immobilized for the entire postoperative period, or knees immobilized for the first half of the postoperative period, the early activity group clearly showed superior mechanical and structural strength at the end of 12 weeks. Others have shown a favourable effect of CPM on reorganization of the fibrils of the scar into parallel arrays (57). It is to be emphasized that in these models the cruciate ligaments are intact, thus providing the stability necessary for early ambulation or CPM.

Continuous Passive Motion Effects in Total Knee Replacement

The total knee replacement procedures now frequently performed for degenerative or rheumatoid arthritis have provided a challenging problem for the application of CPM. Particular needs for improving range of motion postoperatively were felt in the rehabilitation of these patients. Slow recovery of flexion is commonly observed postoperatively, sometimes requiring forceful manipulation under anaesthesia.

A multi-institutional study of over 100 total knee replacement cases treated traditionally and compared to similar cases treated with CPM has provided data which clarifies the effectiveness of CPM in a clinical rehabilitation setting (58). The patients treated with CPM had a more rapid gain in knee motion and had a shorter hospital stay than patients treated traditionally. Data in this series showed a lower pain medication requirement than in the traditionally treated series. The theory commonly employed to explain the surprising tolerance of postoperative patients for passive motion is the 'gate' theory of Melzack and Wall (59). This theory postulates that non-painful afferent input into spinal cord ganglia can overwhelm pain fibre input, thereby blocking a part of the pain perception otherwise experienced. CPM provides considerable afferent input due to effects of motion on proprioceptive receptors. There is no universal acceptance of this effect in postoperative applications of CPM, but at least it seems clear that CPM does not increase pain medication requirements.

Finally, CPM in the postoperative patient does not inhibit wound healing. No wound disruptions were seen resulting from application of CPM and, furthermore, postoperative swelling and joint effusions were reduced. In total, the benefits of a relatively brief few days of application of CPM post operatively in this application appear to significantly outweigh questions of cost or of risk.

Continuous Passive Motion Effects on Prophylaxis Against Thrombophlebitis

The use of CPM in the variety of clinical applications described above has evoked interest in its use in prophylaxis against thrombophlebitis in the postoperative period of high risk (60). The physiological basis of the presumed effect is the pulsation in intramuscular pressure which occurs during passive motion (61). The passive pressure alteration almost certainly has the same functional effect as active muscle contraction in propelling venous blood back to the heart. Since venous stasis is presumed to be an important factor in venous thrombosis, the utilization of CPM, which would significantly reduce venous stasis, would be expected to have a salutory effect on reducing the rate of complications of postoperative thrombophlebitis and pulmonary embolism.

Preliminary results suggesting the validity of this line of reasoning have been presented by Lynch *et al.* (62). Several centres have ongoing studies on this problem and considerable information will be forthcoming in the near future to document the degree of effectiveness of CPM in this application.

CONTINUOUS PASSIVE MOTION AS A POTENTIAL MODALITY TO INFLUENCE CENTRAL NERVOUS SYSTEM ADAPTATION FOLLOWING BRAIN INJURY

Nickel (63) has proposed that CPM may be useful as a rehabilitation modality following stroke. There is an awakening interest in the concept of central nervous system plasticity and in the ability of the central nervous system to recover from injury by development of alternative neural pathways. The clinical question posed is whether passive motion might accelerate this process. The proposed mechanism would be increased afferent input from proprioceptive receptors in joints and muscles of the motion segment, which would modulate the central nervous system adaptive response. The local musculoskeletal benefits to be gained are obvious: reduced incidence of joint contractures at a relatively low cost in terms of equipment and therapy personnel. It is expected, for example, that much of the CPM application could be carried on in the home.

It is to be emphasized that this hypothesis is advanced on theoretical grounds and that data from carefully controlled studies are yet to be published.

CONCLUSIONS

This review describes the existing knowledge on the importance of stress and motion to synovial joint homeostasis. The deleterious effects of stress deprivation occur rapidly and are profound, influencing joint mechanics, biochemistry and physiology in fundamental ways. The recovery from this process is not symmetrical, requiring many months rather than weeks to re-establish near normal values. In fact, mechanical strength of composite ligament structures have not regained normal strength even after 12 months of resumption of activity.

Exercise at a level producing cardiac hypertrophy and increased cardiac output causes hypertrophy of specialized fibrous connective tissues such as tendons and ligaments. However, that effect occurs slowly at great effort: it requires 1 year to produce hypertrophy which is at nominal levels of significance.

The use of CPM to bypass some of the deleterious effects of stress deprivation and its application to repair of cartilage, tendon, ligament and fractures are described. Clinical use in the post-operative management of total joint replacement seems solidly in place and is widely applied to facilitate rehabilitation of the joint affected, to reduce swelling and joint effusion, possibly to reduce incidence of thrombophlebitis and to shorten the hospital stay.

Passive motion places in effect such fundamental cellular and tissue processes that we are probably observing only the infancy of its development. The next decade should see a dramatic increase in its application to problems in the field of synovial joint rehabilitation.

The manner in which cells interpret physical signals will be a likely field for fundamental science in parallel with, and in support of, the clinical efforts.

CLINICAL SIGNIFICANCE

The clinical utility of passive motion in synovial joint rehabilitation is on the threshold of a rapid expansion due to successes in the several uses described. Facilitation of repair processes by passive motion seems an almost universal observation for tendon, ligament, cartilage and bone. In recent years there has been a burgeoning of device development for application to the hand, large joints of the upper extremity, and large joints of the lower extremity. The utility of the passive motion concept to treatment of such widely divergent problems as septic arthritis, haemathrosis, total joint replacement and tendon repair indicates the breadth of application currently employed clinically. The future directions of passive motion utilization will almost certainly be expanded. Some of the potential applications discussed may be only the tip of the iceberg, due to the extremely fundamental nature of the cellular responses involved.

REFERENCES

1. Akeson W H (1961) An experimental study of joint stiffness. *J Bone Joint Surg [Am]* **43**: 1022–34.
2. Akeson W H, Amiel D and Woo S L-Y (1980) Immobility effects on synovial joints: the pathomechanics of joint contracture. *Biorheology* **17**: 95–110.
3. Woo S L-Y, Kuei S C, Gomez M A, Winters J M, Amiel D and Akeson W H (1979) Effect of immobilization and exercise on strength characteristics of bone–medial collateral ligament–bone complex. *Am Soc Mech Eng Symp* **32**: 67–70.
4. Akeson W H, Woo S L-Y, Amiel D and Frank C B (1984) The biology of ligaments. *In: Rehabilitation of the Injured Knee* (L Hunter and F Funk, eds), pp. 92–148. St. Louis: Mosby.
5. Frank C, Akeson W H, Woo SL-Y, Amiel D and Coutts R D (1984) Physiology and therapeutic value of passive joint motion. *Clin Orthop* **185**: 113–25.
6. Evans E B, Eggers G W N, Butler J K and Blumel J (1960) Experimental immobilization and remobilization of rat knee joints. *J Bone Joint Surg [Am]* **42**: 737–58.
7. Enneking W F and Horowitz M (1972) The intra-articular effects of immobilization on the human knee. *J Bone Joint Surg [Am]* **54**: 973–85.
8. Baker W C, Thomas T G and Kirkaldy-Willis W H (1969) Changes in the cartilage of the posterior invertebral joints after anterior fusion. *J Bone Joint Surg [Br]* **51**: 736–46.
9. Reyher C (1874) On the cartilages and synovial membranes of the joints. *J Anat Physiol* **8**: 261–73.
10. Weichselbaum A (1878) Die feineren Veränderungen des Gelenkknorpels bei fungoser Synovitis und Caries der Gelenkenden. *Virchow's Archiv* **73**: 461–75.
11. Parker F and Keefer C S (1935) Gross and histologic changes in the knee joint in rheumatoid arthritis. *Arch Path* **20**: 507–22.
12. Salter R B and Field P (1960) The effects of continuous compression on living articular cartilage. *J Bone Joint Surg [Am]* **42**: 31–49.
13. Thaxter T H, Mann R A and Anderson C E (1965) Degeneration of immobilized knee joints in rats. *J Bone Joint Surg [Am]* **47**: 567–85.
14. Akeson W H, Woo S L-Y, Amiel D, Coutts R D and Daniel D (1973) The connective tissue response to immobility: biochemical changes in periarticular connective tissue of the immobilized rabbit knee. *Clin Orthop* **93**: 356–62.
15. Woo S L-Y, Matthews J V, Akeson W H, Amiel D and Convery R (1975) Connective tissue response to immobility. Correlative study of biomechanical and biochemical measurements of normal and immobilized rabbit knees. *Arthritis Rheum* **18**: 257–64.
16. Amiel D, Frey C, Woo S L-Y, Harwood F and Akeson W H (1985) Value of hyaluronic acid in the prevention of contracture formation. *Clin Orthop* **196**: 22–7.
17. Woo S L-Y, Gomez M A, Seguchi Y, Endo C M and Akeson W H (1983) Measurement of mechanical properties of ligament substance from a bone–ligament–bone preparation. *J Orthop Res* **1**: 22–9.
18. Laros G S, Tipton C M and Cooper R R (1971) Influence of physical activity on ligament insertions in the knees of dogs. *J Bone Joint Surg [Am]* **53**: 275–86.
19. Cooper R R and Misel S (1970) Tendon and ligament insertion. *J Bone Joint Surg [Am]* **52**: 1–20.
20. Tipton C M, Matthes R D and Martin R R (1978) Influence of age and sex on the strength of bone–ligament junctions in knee joints of rats. *J Bone Joint Surg [Am]* **60**: 230–4.

21. Woo S L-Y, Kuei S C, Amiel D, Cobb N G, Hayes W C and Akeson W H (1980) The response of cortical long bone secondary to exercise training. *Trans Orthop Res Soc* **5**: 256.
22. Woo S L-Y, Ritter M A, Gomez M A, Kuei S C and Akeson W H (1980) The biomechanical and structural properties of swine digital flexor tendons secondary to running exercise. *Orthop Trans* **4**: 165–6.
23. Woo S L-Y, Gomez M A, Amiel D, Newton P O, Orlando C A, Sites T and Akeson W H (1987) The biomechanical and biochemical changes of the MCL following immobilization and remobilization. *J Bone Joint Surg [Am]* (In press.)
24. Noyes F R, Torvik P J, Hyde W B and DeLucas J L (1974) Biomechanics of ligament failure. II. An analysis of immobilization, exercise and reconditioning effects in primates. *J Bone Joint Surg [Am]* **56**: 1406–18.
25. Akeson W H, Woo S L-Y, Amiel D, Coutts R D and Daniel D (1973) The connective tissue response to immobility: biochemical changes in periarticular connective tissue of the immobilized rabbit knee. *Clin Orthop* **93**: 356–62.
26. Swann D A, Radin E L and Nazimiec M (1974) Role of hyaluronic acid in joint lubrication. *Ann Rheum Dis* **33**: 318–26.
27. Akeson W H, Amiel D and LaViolette D (1967) The connective tissue response to immobility. A study of chondroitin 4 and 6 sulfate and dermatan sulfate changes in periarticular connective tissue of control and immobilized knees of dogs. *Clin Orthop* **51**: 183–97.
28. Schiller S, Matthews M D, Cifonelli J and Dorfman A (1956) The metabolism of mucopolysaccharides in animals. Further studies on skin utilizing ^{14}C glucose, ^{14}C acetate, and ^{35}S sodium sulfate. *J Biol Chem* **218**: 139–45.
29. Neuberger A and Slack H G B (1953) The metabolism of collagen from liver, bones, skin and tendon in the normal rat. *Biochem J* **53**: 47–52.
30. Guyton A C, Barber B J and Moffatt D S (1980) Theory of interstitial pressures. *In: Tissue Fluid Pressure and Composition* (A Hargens, ed), pp. 11–19. Baltimore: Williams & Wilkins.
31. Brooke J S and Slack H G B (1959) Metabolism of connective tissue in limb atrophy in the rabbit. *Ann Rheum Dis* **18**: 129–36.
32. Peacock E E (1963) Comparison of collagenous tissue surrounding normal and immobilized joints. *Surg Forum* **14**: 440–3.
33. Amiel D, Akeson W H, Harwood F L and Mechanic G L (1980) Effect on nine week immobilization on the types of collagen synthesized in periarticular connective tissue from rabbit knees. *Trans Orthop Res Soc* **5**: 14.
34. Klein L, Dawson M H and Heiple K G (1977) Turnover of collagen in the adult rat after denervation. *J Bone Joint Surg [Am]* **59**: 1065–7.
35. Akeson W H, Amiel D, Woo S L-Y and Harwood F L (1978) Mechanical imperatives for synovial joint homeostasis: the present potential for their therapeutic manipulation. *Proceedings 3rd International Congress Biorheology* **47**.
36. Akeson W H, Amiel D, Mechanic G L, Woo S L-Y and Harwood F L (1977) Collagen cross-linking alterations in joint contractures: changes in the reducible cross-links in periarticular connective tissue collagen after nine weeks of immobilization. *Connect Tissue Res* **5**: 15–9.
37. Bailey A J and Robins S P (1973) Development and maturation of the cross-links in the collagen fibers of skin. *Front Matrix Biol* **1**: 130–56.
38. Jackson D S and Mechanic G (1974) Cross-link patterns of collagens synthesized by cultures of 3T6 and 3T3 fibroblasts and by fibroblasts of various granulation tissues. *Biochim Biophys Acta* **336**: 228–33.
39. O'Driscoll S W, Kumar A and Salter R B (1983) The effect of continuous passive motion on the clearance of a hemarthrosis. *Clin Orthop* **176**: 305–11.
40. Skyhar M J, Danzig L A, Hargens A R and Akeson W H (1985) Nutrition of the anterior cruciate ligament. Effects of continuous passive motion. *Am J Sports Med* **13**: 415–18.
41. Salter R B, Bell R S and Keeley F (1981) The protective effect of continuous passive motion on living articular cartilage in acute septic arthritis: an experimental investigation in the rabbit. *Clin Orthop* **159**: 223–47.
42. O'Driscoll S W and Salter R B (1984) The induction of neochondrogenesis in free intra-articular periosteal autografts under the influence of continuous passive motion. *J Bone Joint Surg [Am]* **66**: 1248–57.
43. Gelberman R H, Woo S L-Y, Lothringer K, Akeson W H and Amiel D (1982) Effects of early intermittent passive mobilization on healing canine flexor tendons. *J Hand Surg* **7**: 170–5.

44. Inoue M, Gomez M, Hollis V, Roux R D, Lee E B, Burleson E M and Woo S L-Y (1986) Medial collateral ligament healing: repair *vs* nonrepair. *Trans Orthop Res Soc* **11**: 78.
45. Salter R B, Simmonds D F, Malcolm B W, Rumble E J and MacMichael D (1980) The biological effects of continuous passive motion on the healing of full-thickness defects in articular cartilage: an experimental investigation in the rabbit. *J Bone Joint Surg [Am]* **62**: 1232–51.
46. Mooney V and Ferguson A B Jr (1966) The influence of immobilization and motion on the formation of fibrocartilage in the repair granuloma after joint resection in the rabbit. *J Bone Joint Surg [Am]* **48**: 1145–55.
47. Hohl M and Luck J V (1956) Fractures of the tibial condyle. *J Bone Joint Surg [Am]* **38**: 1001–18.
48. Convery F R, Akeson W H and Keown G H (1972) The repair of large osteochondral defects. An experimental study in horses. *Clin Orthop* **82**: 253–62.
49. Ohlsen L (1978) Cartilage regeneration from perichondrium. Experimental and clinical applications. *Scand J Plast Reconstr Surg* **62**: 507–13.
50. Engkvist O (1979) Reconstruction of patellar articular cartilage with free autologous perichondrial grafts. An experimental study in dogs. *Scand J Plast Reconstr Surg* **13**: 361–9.
51. Coutts R D, Amiel D, Woo S L-Y, Woo Y K and Akeson W H (1983) Establishment of an appropriate model for the growth of perichondrium in a rabbit joint milieu. *Trans Orthop Res Soc* **8**: 196.
52. Engkvist O and Johansson S H (1980) Perichondrial arthroplasty. A clinical study in twenty-six patients. *Scand J Plast Reconstr Surg* **14**: 71–87.
53. Poussa M, Rubak J and Ritsilä V (1981) Differentiation of the osteochondrogenic cells of the periosteum in chondrotrophic environment. *Acta Orthop Scand* **52**: 235–9.
54. Amiel D, Frank C, Harwood F, Fronek J and Akeson W H (1984) Tendons and ligaments: a morphological and biochemical comparison. *J Orthop Res* **1**: 257–65.
55. Burks R, Daniel D and Losse G (1984) The effect of continuous passive motion on anterior cruciate ligament reconstruction stability. *Am J Sports Med* **12**: 323–7.
56. Amiel D, Kleiner J and Akeson W H (1987) The natural history of the anterior cruciate ligament autograft of patella tendon origin. *Am J Sports Med* **14**(6): 449–462.
57. Fronek J, Frank C, Amiel D, Woo S L-Y, Coutts R D and Akeson W H (1983) The effect of intermittent passive motion (IPM) on the healing of the medial collateral ligament. *Trans Orthop Res Soc* **8**: 31.
58. Coutts R D, Toth C and Kaita J (1984) The role of continuous passive motion in the rehabilitation of the total knee patient. *In: Total Knee Arthroplasty. A Comprehensive Approach* (D Hungerford, K A Krackow and R V Kenna, eds, pp. 126–32. Baltimore: Williams & Wilkins.
59. Melzack R and Wall P D (1970) Psychophysiology of pain. Evolution of pain theories. *Int Anesthesiol Clin* **8**: 3–34.
60. Fisher R L, Kloter K, Bzdyra B and Cooper J A (1985) Continuous passive motion (CPM) following total knee replacement. *Conn Med* **49**: 498–501.
61. Coutts R. Personal communication.
62. Lynch J A, Baker P L, Polly R E, McCoy M T, Sund K and Roudybush D (1984) Continuous passive motion: a prophylaxis for deep venous thrombosis following total knee replacement. Unpublished paper. Presented at the American Academy of Orthopedic Surgery, Annual Meeting, Atlanta, Ga, 1984.
63. Nickel V. Personal communication.

Chapter 16

Drugs and Physical Therapy in the Treatment of Rheumatoid Arthritis Patients

S. L. Silverman, T. M. Spiegel, J. S. Spiegel and H. E. Paulus

CONTENTS

INTRODUCTION

Rheumatoid arthritis (RA) is a systemic disease of unknown cause, characterized by chronic inflammation of connective tissue, especially the synovium of joints and tendons as well as other organs. Granulation tissue from the proliferating synovium penetrates the joint cavity as pannus, invading the cartilage and causing pain, swelling, joint destruction and deformity. Inflammation usually affects the small joints of the hands and feet in a symmetrical fashion. The disease affects more women than men, usually beginning at age 35–45. Approximately 3% of the US adult population have rheumatoid arthritis. The natural history is that of a chronic progressive disease with a relapsing and remitting course (1).

Although RA primarily affects the joints, it may have diverse systemic manifestations including lung disease, vasculitis, pericarditis, neuropathy, myopathy, and eye lesions, as well as rheumatoid nodules. Patients with RA develop pain and stiffness associated with inflammation and then destruction of their joints leading to loss of function and loss of both the quality and style of life. Fatigue may be so profound that it may cause more disability than the joint changes. There may be weakness, weight loss and fever.

Rheumatoid arthritis patients often experience a progressive deterioration in their functional ability, becoming unable to work and dependent upon others for performing self-care and daily living activities. RA patients with severe disease have increased mortality (2). An American study examining employment status of RA patients estimated that the probability of work disability is 44% for patients with no joint deformity and 72% for those with deformity (3). Other studies have shown that RA patients earn only 50% of the income predicted for them if they did not have arthritis (3). Direct medical costs for RA patients are 3 times the national USA average, and indirect costs due to lost income are 3 times the direct medical costs (4). An English survey found that 61% of employed rheumatoid arthritis patients had been absent from work for at least 3 weeks because of illness during a 1 year period (5).

Appropriate measures should be initiated early in the course of the disease to help patients attain the following therapeutic goals:

1. Relief of symptoms.
2. Prevention of joint destruction and deformity.
3. Maintenance of function.
4. Preservation of quality and style of life.

Available to both the physician and patient is a variety of treatment modalities. Medications are available which reduce the signs and symptoms of inflammation which the patient perceives as pain and stiffness. Some medications are available which may modify the disease course and slow the disease progression. Education, rest, physical therapy, occupational therapy, and orthopaedic surgery all play an important role.

Each patient with RA is uniquely different, and requires an individual treatment plan. This treatment plan must reflect such factors as course and severity, response to treatment, and patient's lifestyle. This treatment plan is not fixed for each patient but needs to be adjusted continuously, based on the patient's response to treatment, disease progression and changes in psychosocial environment.

DRUGS IN THE TREATMENT OF RHEUMATOID ARTHRITIS

The drugs used to treat rheumatoid arthritis (RA) are directed at various aspects of inflammation. It is tempting to think that if we can just eliminate the inflammation, we can eradicate rheumatoid arthritis. Unfortunately, inflammation is a normal protective response to the tissue injury seen in rheumatoid arthritis. For the purpose of rationalizing drug therapy for rheumatoid arthritis, we must consider the following sequence to occur. An unknown aetiological factor or prime cause exists which initiates the inflammation and then produces toxic mediators that indirectly injure tissue. Ordinarily, the inflammatory response leads to eradication of the prime cause and results in healing of the injured tissue with restoration of its function.

However, in the case of RA, the normal protective inflammatory response is unable to eliminate the basic cause of the inflammation. Thus, the normal inflammatory process is amplified by the products of injured tissue, resulting in continued inflammation, progressive tissue injury, the manifestations of disease, and ultimately loss of function.

In rheumatoid arthritis, the striking feature is the persistence of both acute and chronic inflammation. The acute inflammation is dominated by polymorphonuclear leucocytes. The chronic inflammation is dominated by monocytes. Lymphocyte-produced lymphokines activate macrophages which have many functions including phagocytosis, presenting antigen to lymphocytes and producing interleukin-1, which induces the acute phase response. These macrophages also release proteases. In addition, antibodies form immune complexes which activate phagocytic cells.

This formulation of the inflammatory disease in rheumatic arthritis suggests that control of both acute and chronic inflammation is necessary and also suggests several targets for our therapy. First, if one could eliminate the primary cause or aetiological factor, the inflammatory process would express itself normally and heal the injured tissue and the disease would cease. This, in fact, happens when one treats a bacterial arthritis with an effective antibiotic. Secondly, if one is unable to eliminate the prime cause, perhaps mediators of tissue injury could be eliminated or otherwise inactivated. In the case of rheumatoid arthritis, suppression of immune responses approaches this target in some cases. If one is unable to prevent tissue injury, then an attempt can be made to moderate the non-specific inflammatory response evoked by tissue injury. Since non-specific anti-inflammatory medicines do not prevent tissue injury, it is not surprising that joint damage and other tissue injury progress during therapy with these drugs. Moreover, if the drugs completely suppressed the non-specific inflammatory response, the patient would not be protected from environmental insults and infections.

With these principles in mind, the drugs that are used in the treatment of RA can be rationally considered (6,7). The aspirin preparations, the non-steroidal anti-inflammatory drugs, and small doses of corticosteroids non-specifically moderate the inflammatory response, generally regardless of its cause. These drugs to various extents relieve pain, swelling and other characteristics of inflammation but do not eliminate the inflammation completely, nor do they prevent ongoing tissue damage.

The so-called disease-modifying antirheumatic drugs (DMARDs), the immunosuppressive drugs, and the immunomodulating drugs probably act on the immunological mediators of tissue injury, without effectively removing the prime cause of the disease. Examples include gold, D-penicillamine, azathioprine, cyclophosphamide, methotrexate and levamisole for rheumatoid arthritis and for treatment of autoimmune diseases, and very high doses of corticosteroids. Most of the time, these drugs only moderate the disease process and some level of chronic inflammation persists, but sometimes the disease process appears to be completely suppressed in a drug-induced remission. However, the patient is not cured because when the drug is removed the disease recurs, usually with some delay in the onset of symptoms.

Non-steroidal Anti-inflammatory Drugs

An important part of this treatment plan is the appropriate use of medication (6,7). Initial therapy of rheumatoid arthritis should begin with the use of non-steroidal anti-inflammatory drugs (NSAIDs)(6). NSAIDs reduce but do not eliminate the signs and symptoms of inflammation. They have a rapid onset. They have no effect on the underlying disease course, nor do they protect against tissue or joint injury. NSAIDs inhibit synthesis of prostaglandins, prostacyclin and thromboxanes. In addition NSAIDs inhibit bradykinin release, granulocyte and monocyte migration and phagocytosis. NSAIDs are also analgesic and antipyretic.

The number of NSAIDs available continues to increase. There are currently 7 basic families of NSAIDs: salicylates, proprionic acids, indoles, fenamates, pyrroles, pyrazoles, and oxicams. Aspirin is the prototype. Salicylates and other NSAIDs are analgesic at lower doses and anti-inflammatory at higher doses. Thus it is important to administer a dose sufficient for anti-inflammatory effect. This dose will vary from patient to patient and doses should be titrated.

When administered at an optimal anti-inflammatory dose, all of the NSAIDs have approximately equal efficacy to aspirin. Nevertheless, therapeutic response varies from patient to patient. Poor response to one NSAID does not predict a similar response to another NSAID.

In rheumatoid arthritis either aspirin or one of the other NSAIDs is used to initiate therapy. If aspirin is used the dose is adjusted to achieve a serum salicylate level of 20–30 mg/dl. If salicylates are ineffective or toxic they are discontinued and one of the other NSAIDs is substituted. The dose of the NSAID is increased to the optimal tolerated level and continued for at least 2 weeks to determine efficacy. Therapeutic trials of different NSAIDs may continue until the patient has achieved adequate control of the signs and symptoms of inflammation with minimal side effects. If patients continue to have evidence of joint inflammation despite treatment with NSAIDs for a treatment period of 2–3 months, or if radiographic evidence of bone erosions develop, a disease-modifying antirheumatoid drug (DMARD) is added to the NSAID.

Adverse Effects of the NSAIDs

Although NSAIDs are generally safe and well tolerated, they are associated with a wide spectrum of clinical toxicities (6,7). The frequency of particular side effects varies with the compound; available data are not sufficient to recommend any one of these agents as safer than the others. The major toxicities occur in the gastrointestinal tract, central nervous system, haematopoietic system, special senses, kidney, skin and liver. Generally side-effects tend to be dose related.

Perhaps because of their effects on prostaglandin synthetase, NSAIDs as a group tend to cause gastric irritation and to exacerbate peptic ulcers. They make gastrointestinal bleeding worse both by increasing acid production in the stomach and by decreasing platelet adhesiveness. Suppression of prostaglandins increases acid production and decreases gastro-oesophageal sphincter tone, thus permitting acid regurgitation into the oesophagus. NSAIDs also have been reported to decrease the production of gastric mucus and to decrease the rate of cellular proliferation of the gastric mucosa. Further, indomethacin and sulindac have an extensive enterohepatic recirculation, which increases gastrointestinal exposure to these drugs and enhances their gastrointestinal toxicity.

The anticoagulant effects of NSAIDs are of 2 types. The drug may displace warfarin from plasma protein binding sites, thus increasing warfarin's anticoagulant effect. This is clinically significant only for phenylbutazone, and for salicylates in toxic concentrations. Secondly, NSAIDs decrease platelet adhesiveness by inhibiting a prostaglandin-initiated sequence that is necessary for platelet activation. Acetylation by aspirin irreversibly decreases platelet aggregation, and this effect persists until the acetylated platelets are replaced by newly produced platelets that have not been exposed to aspirin (10–12 days). For the other NSAIDs, the platelet effects are reversible and persist only so long as the drug is present.

Reversible hepatocellular toxicity, characterized by elevations of 1 or more liver function tests, has been observed in up to 5% of patients treated with aspirin and is also seen with other NSAIDs. Transaminase elevations revert to normal after discontinuation of the drug, and sometimes become normal even though the drug is continued. Rarely, NSAID-induced hepatic dysfunction may be more severe, causing elevation of bilirubin and/or prolongation of prothrombin times, in which case discontinuation of the drug is mandatory. In the case of benoxaprofen, failure to recognize early evidence of hepatic toxicity led to hepatorenal syndrome in some patients.

NSAIDs may decrease creatinine clearance and increase creatinine concentrations in patients predisposed by hypovolaemia or impaired renal function, probably by suppressing the vasodilatory function of renal prostaglandins. These creatinine elevations often revert to normal even with continued use of the drug, but NSAIDs should be used cautiously in patients with conditions that may impair renal function or in patients with decreased circulating blood volume, and in the elderly who are predisposed to these conditions.

Disease-modifying Antirheumatic Drugs

The disease-modifying antirheumatic drugs (DMARDS) are so named because it is thought that these drugs may modify the progression of the disease as measured by X-ray evidence such as joint erosions or joint destruction. These drugs may also alter the progression of disability in RA as measured by disability index scores. Common to all these drugs are certain features such as slow rate of onset of benefit (weeks to months) and increased toxicity requiring frequent laboratory monitoring and multiple physician visits (7).

Disability develops most rapidly during the first years of disease and then progression of disease is relatively slow (8). This suggests that effective disease-modifying therapy should be initiated as soon as possible during the initial period of rapid disease progression.

It is unclear if remittive drugs affect long-term radiographic outcome (9). There is considerable debate whether DMARDS affect X-ray progression of the disease. A recent population study by Fries (10) of 1043 RA patients shows that part of the problem may be the way in which these drugs are used. The number of years of treatment with remittive agents was generally less than 30% of the total number of years of illness. The duration of remittive drug therapy may have been too short. Most patients started remittive drug therapy late in their disease. The average duration of illness prior to the start of remittive therapy was 12·8 years.

Hydroxychloroquine, originally an antimalarial drug, is often the first DMARD used (7). Initial dosage is 200 mg twice daily with meals, reduced to 200 mg daily after 2–3 months. Hydroxychloroquine is usually well tolerated with low toxicity. The major toxicity is retinal damage with deposition of the drug in the pigment layer of the retina. However, the incidence of retinal toxicity appears low in patients taking no more than 400 mg per day. Patients should be examined for signs of retinal toxicity by an ophthalmologist every 3–6 months. Other side effects include rash, gastrointestinal symptoms and haemolytic anaemia.

Gold has been used in the treatment of RA for more than 50 years. Gold is available as either a parenteral or oral preparation (7). Two parenteral preparations, gold sodium thiomalate and aurothioglucose are available, both of which are 50% metallic gold. Gold sodium thiomalate is water soluble and therefore easier and less painful to inject than aurothioglucose, which is an oily suspension and is less rapidly absorbed. Nitritoid reactions (flushing, dizziness and syncope) are more common with gold sodium thiomalate. Parenteral gold is usually administered intramuscularly on a weekly basis with weekly blood counts and examination of the urine for albumin. If improvement occurs the interval between injections is gradually increased to a maximum of once monthly. Minor side effects occur in about 30–50% of patients. The most common reactions include pruritic skin rashes, proteinuria, stomatitis, and haemotological abnormalities. Although rare, thrombocytopenia, aplastic anaemia and pancytopenia may be fatal.

Oral gold, auranofin, is an incompletely absorbed lipid-soluble preparation of gold which is 30% gold by weight. It appears effective at a daily dose of 6 mg. As compared to parenteral gold, loose stools or diarrhoea is a common side-effect occurring in up to 49% of patients but is usually well tolerated. In summary, parenteral gold appears more effective than oral gold but is associated with more side-effects. It is unknown if the more serious haematological reactions will occur with less frequency with oral gold.

D-penicillamine is a structural analogue of cysteine and a metabolite of penicillin. Its mechanism of action in RA is unknown. D-penicillamine is similar to gold in terms of onset of action and toxicity. The starting dose is 250 mg daily which is increased slowly at 2–3 month intervals until total daily dosages of 750–1000 mg are attained. D-penicillamine is equally as effective as gold but is reserved for patients who cannot take gold therapy. Like gold therapy, D-penicillamine therapy requires careful monitoring of clinical and laboratory parameters. However, unlike gold, D-penicillamine is associated rarely with autoimmune syndromes such as myasthenia, polymyositis, systemic lupus, pemphigus and pemphigoid.

Three groups of immunosuppressive drugs have been used in patients with RA, methotrexate (a folic acid antagonist), the purine antagonist, azathioprine, and alkylating agents, cyclophosphamide and chlorambucil. These drugs should be reserved for RA patients with disease refractory to customary therapy including antimalarials, gold and penicillamine because of significant and sometimes lethal side-effects.

Methotrexate is being used increasingly in RA (7). It is currently prescribed more often than penicillamine for patients with RA. Methotrexate works more rapidly than most DMARDs with onset of improvement in pain, stiffness and joint swelling within 3–8 weeks. Methotrexate usually is given orally or intramuscularly in doses from 7·5 mg to 25·0 mg weekly. Reversible toxicity includes nausea, stomatitis, rash, drug fever, hepatocellular toxicity and bone marrow suppression. Toxicity is less if the drug is given once weekly rather than more frequently. Methotrexate-induced hepatic fibrosis, which may progress to cirrhosis, appears to be related to the cumulative total dose. Liver biopsy should be done after each 1500 mg increment in total dose, to detect this otherwise silent toxicity at an early stage.

The long hiatus lasting weeks to months between beginning DMARD therapy and the onset of effect poses a management problem. Available to the rheumatologist are a variety of modalities which may assist the RA patient. Intra-articular corticosteroids may be used to treat individual joints that are more symptomatic than other joints. Since infection may produce similar symptoms, joint fluid should be examined whenever corticosteroids are injected. Systemic corticosteroids are used, but once started on corticosteroids the patient with RA may be unable to withdraw. Chronic corticosteroids predispose patients to the risk of systemic or articular infection and osteoporosis as well as the many other known steroid complications such as diabetes. Low dose corticosteroids in the range of 5 mg daily have been suggested. Such doses appear *in vitro* to inhibit synthesis and release of proteases and collagenases without altering matrix component production. Low dose prednisolone is often clinically beneficial in patients who cannot tolerate adequate doses of non-steroidals, but there is no clinical evidence that it prevents progressive joint damage, and long-term therapy is associated with osteoporosis.

REST

Rest of inflamed joints is one of the basic principles of the management of acute and chronic arthritis (11). In experimental models of acute urate crystal-induced inflammation, joint motion enhanced the synovial inflammation. However, prolonged joint immobilization causes cartilage damage and loss of matrix glycosaminoglycans. Here is the dilemma of the rheumatic disease physician: encourage rest to decrease inflammation, yet simultaneously encourage activity to prevent functional loss.

Rest may be general, localized or modified. Systemic features of rheumatoid arthritis, such as fever, anaemia and malaise, benefit from general rest in bed. However, we lack the evidence that general bed rest favourably influences a long-term course of the disease. Local rest may be of benefit for specifically inflamed joints. Immobilization of rheumatoid arthritis joints for as long as 4 weeks reduces inflammation without significant loss of mobility, although strength is diminished (12,13).

In modified rest, activities are permitted but painful stress is avoided by *(1)* using splints and supports which achieve a form of partial rest; *(2)* educating the patient in joint protection – this teaches the patient how to decrease the stresses of activities of daily living on small joints; *(3)* increasing the amount of time in bed by 2–3 h through the day – by the patient learning to pace his activities, the efficacy of drug therapy can be increased; and *(4)* modified rest may serve as a form of posture training (14).

EXERCISE THERAPY

Exercise therapy for the patient with rheumatoid arthritis is designed to meet the needs of the individual patient. Both short- and long-term goals are established, including *(1)* maintaining or increasing range of motion; *(2)* maintaining or increasing strength; and *(3)* increasing endurance. The method of achieving these goals is modified by the activity of the disease. When there is acute inflammation in a given joint, the patient will benefit from passive exercises or exercises with gentle assistance. It is essential to put all joints through their range of motion at least once daily to maintain mobility. Stretching exercises prevent contractures; oedema and pain restrict joint motion and predispose to contractures. Immobilization may affect capsular structures without inflammation. Inflammation, however, increases the effect.

As the inflammation subsides, the patient can use active exercises and exercises against resistance. With restoration of active joints, motion is an additional goal. Exercises are best performed when stiffness is at its least and after preparation with heat, cold, analgesics or hydrotherapy.

In the presence of joint disease, muscle weakness is a common problem. Muscle weakness may be secondary to atrophy and/or reflex inhibition. Reflex inhibition is not voluntary but occurs by spinal reflex action from damaged joints. This has been shown in normal subjects receiving infusion of physiological saline in knee joints.

Rheumatoid arthritis patients as a group have lower than expected aerobic capacity in physical performance. In 1 study, their muscle strength was 60% below that of age-matched control subjects (15). Patients have been shown to tolerate both short- and long-term exercise regimens with considerable improvement in both functional and other outcome measures (15).

COMPREHENSIVE CARE

We believe that optimal use and coordination of currently available medical, physical and surgical management can reduce the disease activity, moderate the crippling deformities, and help patients maintain or improve their functional ability. We believe that poorly coordinated care fragmented among the various health professions does not optimally utilize existing knowledge or produce the best results for RA patients. Treatment does not just happen – it must be planned, and decision points must be set so that programmed changes can be instituted at agreed times. There must be a 'game plan' for each patient.

Successful care of the patient with rheumatoid arthritis requires more than a single physician. Most patients with RA early in their course will need evaluation by several physician specialists including a rheumatologist, orthopaedic surgeon and physiatrist. Physical therapists, occupational therapists, psychiatrists, and social workers play an important role. This multidisciplinary team of arthritis specialists first became available with the creation of inpatient and then outpatient rheumatic disease units.

PHYSICAL THERAPY

The physical therapist can help the physician and patient by evaluating *(1)* strength and range of motion of both upper and lower extremities; *(2)* transfer activities (including sit-to-stand, stand-to-sit etc.); *(3)* balance (both sitting and standing); *(4)* ambulation (on both level surface and stairs); *(5)* gait; and *(6)* endurance. The physical therapist will recommend an individualized daily range of motion and strengthening exercise programme for each patient. The therapist may also recommend orthopaedic shoes, walking or transfer aids, and various therapeutic modalities for pain relief including superficial heat and cold, ultrasound, hydrotherapy, transcutaneous nerve stimulation, and biofeedback.

OCCUPATIONAL THERAPY

The occupational therapist evaluates the need for assistance in performing certain daily living activities. This includes eating, dressing, personal hygiene, general hand activities, mobility, kitchen work, transportation, and endurance. Whenever possible the patient's performance of these tasks is observed, preferably in the home setting. The occupational therapist will also inquire about the patient's living situation, including type of access, vocational and recreational activities, use of assistive equipment, and sexual history. The therapist will also enquire about problems encountered at the patient's work place. Finally the occupational therapist will instruct the patient in principles of joint protection and energy conservation in performing daily activities. Joint protection teaches patients how to perform daily activities so as to minimize stress on involved joints. For many patients the therapist will provide adaptive equipment and joint splints.

PSYCHOSOCIAL INTERVENTIONS

Social workers, as well as other team members such as psychologists, psychiatrists and vocational counsellors, can help patients with RA to maximally utilize family, community and agency resources. Common psychological problems include loss of independence and self-esteem, uncertainty about the disease process, sexuality, fear of becoming crippled and dependent, concern about altered body image, feelings of frustration and depression associated with continuing disease (16).

EDUCATION

Effective management of RA requires regular medical care interspersed with long periods of self-management where the patient rather than the physician is the initiator of care. Patients with RA must be able to detect acutely worsening disease and side-effects which they must report to their physician. They must be able to adhere to a regular treatment regimen which often causes side effects. They must take medicines like DMARDs for which benefit may not occur for weeks or months. They must adhere to a regimen of frequent clinical and laboratory monitoring. It is therefore not surprising that studies of patient adherence to treatment regimens in RA put the non-compliance rate at roughly 50%. Education of the patient in terms of the disease, its natural history and treatment are imperative for a succesful treatment plan.

ORTHOPAEDIC SURGERY

Surgery may be prophylactic to prevent deformity. Extensor tenosynovitis of the dorsum of the hand unresponsive to medical therapy is an indication of surgical tenosynovectomy to prevent extensor tendon rupture.

Surgery is an important means of relieving pain and improving function. Individual joint synovectomy such as knee synovectomy is only temporarily effective and does not prevent recurrences. The evaluation of newer techniques for radioactive synovectomy by intra-articular injection of radioisotopes into single joints is not complete.

The development of the low friction hip arthroplasty by Charnley (17) using a metal femoral head with a polyethylene acetabular socket and poly(methylmethacrylate) bone cement is considered the most important reconstructive surgical advancement of the twentieth century and has revolutionized treatment for rheumatoid arthritis. Patients with longstanding painful hip joint destruction can benefit from pain relief, improved range of motion and increased walking distance. Considerable progress has been made in the development of total knee replacement. Total joint replacement is being developed for other joints including wrists, elbows, shoulders, ankles, and feet. A particular problem in the RA patient is maintenance of post-operative range of motion. In patients with painful feet, deformity can be ameliorated by surgical metatarsal head resection.

Hand surgery can release an entrapped median nerve in a carpal tunnel. Silicone implants can restore function and decrease deformity of metacarpophalangeal and to a lesser extent proximal interphalangeal joints. In some joints such as the wrist and thumb where loss of motion is not functionally significant, surgical fusion can provide dramatic relief of pain. When multiple joints are involved, generally distal joints assume first priority. When decision is made for surgery the whole patient must be considered. For example, if lower extremity surgery is contemplated, one must be certain that the upper extremities can bear the weight of a crutch. The patient's general medical condition and endurance must be assessed.

MULTIDISCIPLINARY RHEUMATIC DISEASE UNITS

Multidisciplinary rheumatic disease units provide comprehensive care, but in the changing health-care economic climate it is important to document their efficacy. Spiegel *et al.* have recently reviewed the literature on rheumatic disease units (18). They reviewed 15 studies, 11 of inpatients and 4 of outpatients, with a total of 1712 patients studied. In 12 studies, functional data was obtained at follow-up (19–28). In 10 of these 12 studies, function improved in approximately 41% of patients. Five of these studies had control groups. Of these 5, 3 did show differences between the patients receiving rheumatic disease unit care and controls. One of these 5 studies was performed by Spiegel *et al.* on our inpatient rheumatic disease unit at UCLA (28).

We have studied patients hospitalized in our inpatient unit in a 1-year prospective controlled trial. The results of this trial have been published elsewhere (28). In this study we enrolled 92 adults with classic or definite rheumatoid arthritis with disease duration greater than 1 year. All patients had some functional deterioration in the 3-month period prior to entry in the study. The experimental group was 49 RA patients admitted to the UCLA inpatient rheumatology rehabilitation unit. In the first 72 h after admission all patients were seen by a study physician and completed a functional and health status questionnaire. The control group consisted of 43 RA patients with deteriorating functional ability who were followed as outpatients by one of 14 rheumatologists at Cedars Sinai Medical Center. At the time of the study there was no outpatient or inpatient arthritis rehabilitation programme at Cedars Sinai. All patients were evaluated at study entry and at 6 weeks, 6 months, and 12 months after entry. Study measures included self-reported information as well as objective and clinical measures. All patients completed a self-administered functional and health status questionnaire based on scales from the Rand Corporation's Health Insurance Experiment and the Arthritis Impact Measurement Scales (AIMS). The programme for the experimental group consisted of hospitalization in our multidisciplinary rheumatology rehabilitation unit. Members of the UCLA team included rheumatologists, physical and occupational therapists, a nurse-educator and a social worker. The mean length of stay was 13 days, and the mean total hospital charges were $7000.

Our study patients are described in *Table 16.1*. The patients were predominantly white females with a mean age of 58. Most were unemployed (88%), half had RA greater than 10 years, and 25% were living alone. Experimental patients had significantly more joint deformity than controls. During the year following entry into the study, medical care varied between the 2 groups as shown in *Table 16.2*. Experimental patients underwent orthopaedic surgery more often. Changes in DMARD regimens occurred more often in the experimental group. Use of oral and injectable steroids was similar. Although numbers of outpatient visits were not significantly different between the 2 groups, more experimental patients were admitted for non-arthritis problems, while more control patients were admitted for arthritis problems. The same physician provided care throughout the study for almost all control patients; however, about half the experimental patients received care from their referring community physician.

Table 16.1. Rheumatoid arthritis (RA) patient characteristics at study entry

	Experimental (n = 49)	Control (n = 43)
Age, years (mean ± SD)	59 ± 12	57 ± 13
Women	80	83
White	76	71
College education ≥ 1 year	37	36
Income ≤ $15,000/year	57	69
Living with spouse	47	47
Living alone	24	23
Employed	12	12
Other medical problems		
Hypertension or heart disease	16	16
Obesity	27	35
Non-arthritis problems which may limit function	18	12
Duration of RA > 10 years	49	45
Mean joint deformity	1·8	1·4*
Medications		
Gold	12	37**
Penicillamine or other antirheumatic drug	16	30
Cytotoxic drug	2	5
Steroids	41	33
Narcotic analgesics	33	42

All values are expressed as percentages, except age and mean joint deformity, for which a score of 0 = none, 4 = severe.
* $P < 0.05$
**$P < 0.01$

Table 16.2. Patient characteristics during 12-month follow-up period

	Experimental (n = 49) (%)	Control (n = 43) (%)
Orthopaedic Surgery		
Lower extremity	22	12
Upper extremity	4	2
Neck	8	0
Medical hospitalization		
For arthritis problem	20	28
For non-arthritis problem	29	19
Changes in medication		
Gold		
Patients beginning	10	0**
Patients stopping	12	5
Penicilllamine or other antirheumatic drug		
Patients beginning	20	0**
Patients stopping	6	14
Cytotoxic drug		
Patients beginning	12	2**
Patients stopping	0	2
Steroids		
Patients beginning	19	14
Patients stopping	14	9
Same teaching centre-affiliated physician providing care throughout study	53	91**
Did not complete study	2	5

**$P < 0.01$

The outcome measures for both groups were examined over the 12 month period of the study, and compared between the 2 groups. Functional status scales included manual dexterity, household activities, activities of daily living, physical activity and mobility. Mental and social measures included depression, psychological well-being, anxiety and social activity. The experimental patients showed more deterioration in the 3 month period prior to study entry and were often worse on entering the study than the controls. As shown in *Fig.* 16.1, during the study the experimental patients showed greater improvement than the controls. At study termination the experimental patients were usually better than at study entry, while the controls had little if any change. This included all questionnaire measures for functional status, depression, psychological well-being and social activity, as well as all disease activity and performance measures. The sustained improvement noted in the experimental group was not simply explained as regression to the mean of a functionally more ill group. Both functionally ill and functionally less ill subgroups of both experimental and control patients showed the same changes over time. Covariate analysis of process measures of patient characteristics of the 2 groups did not explain these differences. *Table 16.3* shows the scores of the questionnaire outcome scales at study entry, and at 12 months with and without adjustment for covariate variables. At 12 months the experimental group scored significantly higher than the control group in manual dexterity, household activities, depression, psychological well-being and social activity. As shown in *Table 16.4*, there was also more significant improvement in the experimental group than the control group in measures of disease activity such as joint tenderness and sedimentation rate. Measures of objective performance such as grip strength and walking time were improved but were not statistically significant.

It is our belief that the major beneficial component of this programme is the coordination and optimization of therapy plans formulated by the multidisciplinary team. During the initial evaluations, each member of the therapy team has a particular area of expertise and sees the same patient differently, and thus will often obtain different information. When this information and differing perspectives are shared during the team conference, the result is a more comprehensive and realistic patient assessment. With this assessment standard treatment modalities can be optimized for each patient.

On the UCLA inpatient unit every team member independently evaluated each patient. The synthesis of these separate evaluations into a comprehensive management plan occurred in a formal weekly patient conference. Each professional discussed his evaluation. Then, based on each member's input, a comprehensive team list of problems and therapy plans was formulated. The group interaction of the patient conference produced significant changes in individual listing of patient problems and therapy plans by each team member. When compared before and after team conferences, the patient's problem lists changed an average of 15% per team member and therapy plans changed an average of 38% per team member (29). Future studies are needed to examine in closer detail the various components of the inpatient programme to see which components account for the greatest change. It will be important to see if benefits persist for longer than 1 year and if repeated hospitalization is needed to maintain the effect. With the advent in the United States in 1984 of prospective payment for Medicare patients, known

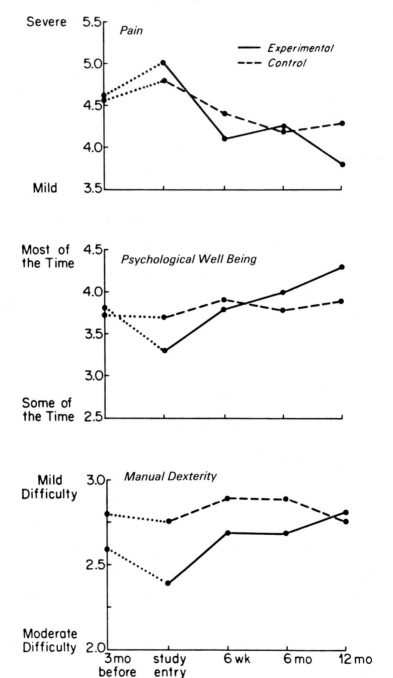

Fig. 16.1. Changes over time in specific outcome measures for experimental and control patients. [From Spiegel *et al.*, 1986 (128); with permission.]

Table 16.3. Questionnaire outcome measures for experimental and control patients at study entry and at 12 months

	Score at study entry		Unadjusted score at 12 months		Adjusted score at 12 months#	
	Exp.	Control	Exp.	Control	Exp.	Control
Functional status measure†						
Manual dexterity	2·3	2·8*	2·8	2·8	2·9	2·6**
Household activities	2·6	3·1*	2·9	3·1	3·1	2·9**
Activities of daily living	2·9	3·4*	3·3	3·5	3·4	3·3
Physical activity	1·8	2·2*	2·2	2·3	2·3	2·2
Mobility	1·5	1·9*	1·7	1·9	1·8	1·6
Mental and social health measure†						
Depression	4·1	4·6**	5·0	4·7	5·1	4·5*
Psychological well-being	3·2	3·7**	4·2	3·9	4·3	3·7*
Anxiety	3·8	3·8	4·0	3·9	4·0	3·9
Social activity	3·3	3·3	3·8	3·3	3·8	3·3*

Adjusted for entry value of the measure and modification during the 12-month follow-up period by treatment factors, including orthopaedic surgery and steroidal, antirheumatic, or cytotoxic drugs.
† Possible range for functional status measures = 1–4, except for mobility = 1–3; possible ranges for all mental and social health measures = 1–6. Higher score means better functional status, better mental and social health. Statistically significant differences between the 2 groups for entry and 12-month adjusted score are indicated.
** $P < 0.01$.
* $P < 0.05$.

Table 16.4 Disease activity, performance, and process measures for experimental and control patients at study entry and at 12 months

	Possible range	Score at study entry		Unadjusted score at 12 months		Adjusted score at 12 months#	
		Exp.	Control	Exp.	Control	Exp.	Control
Disease activity and performance measures†							
Joint tenderness	0–4	1·7	1·0**	0·8	0·9	0·6	1·0*
Joint swelling	0–4	1·1	0·8**	0·5	0·6	0·4	0·6
Sedimentation rate (mm/h)	3–99	55	47	39	47	37	49
Disease activity by physician	1–4	3·2	2·7**	1·9	2·2	1·9	2·2*
Disease activity by patient	1–4	3·7	3·3**	2·8	3·0	2·7	3·0
Pain by patient	1–6	5·0	4·7	3·8	4·3	3·7	4·4**
Morning stiffness by patient	1–6	4·5	4·0	3·5	3·7	3·4	3·8
Grip strength (mmHg)	30–183	62	82*	75	81	84	72
50-foot walktime (seconds)	9–76	40	18**	25	19	20	24
Questionnaire process measures†							
Compliance	1–4	3·3	3·1	3·8	3·0	3·8	3·1*
Knowledge of arthritis	1–4	2·9	3·1	3·4	3·2	3·4	3·1*
Use of equipment	0–16	4·1	2·7	5·4	4·0	5·2	4·3
Use of outpatient services	1–4	2·4	2·5	1·8	1·8	1·7	1·9

Adjusted for the entry value of the measure and modification during the 12 month follow-up period by treatment factors, including orthopaedic surgery and steroidal, antirheumatic, or cytotoxic drugs.
† Higher score means more of an item or concept. Statistically significant differences between the 2 groups for entry and 12-month adjusted score are indicated.
** $P < 0.01$.
* $P < 0.05$.

as DRG or diagnosis-related grouping system, we developed at UCLA in 1985 an outpatient rheumatology rehabilitation clinic. In team conferences in this clinic we have attempted to stress the importance of information obtained from home and workplace evaluation obtained by direct observation by therapists sent to the site. If this intervention proves beneficial and cost effective, we hope to develop it to the point where practising rheumatologists would be able to incorporate team conferences into the routine care of their patients. Studies are currently in progress.

In summary, coordinated multidisciplinary care can produce significant improvement in the medical, functional and psychological problems which RA patients experience as a result of their disease.

CONCLUSIONS

Multidisciplinary care can produce significant improvement in the medical, functional, and psychological problems which individual RA patients experience as a result of their disease. Therapy plans formulated by the members of the multidisciplinary team are coordinated and optimized by sharing of information and perspective. Central to the multidisciplinary team is the measurement of the functional outcomes rather than simply deformity or disease activity. Participating in this multidisciplinary team is the rheumatologist, who brings expertise in the medical management of RA. The medical management of RA begins with the NSAIDs and with onset of erosions or severe, systemic or unresponsive disease progresses to DMARDs. Patients with disease unresponsive to DMARDs may be advanced if needed to experimental drugs such as methotrexate. The orthopaedist brings expertise not only in repair and total joint replacement but in prophylactic surgery such as tenosynovectomy. The occupational therapist and physical therapist bring expertise in evaluating and treating disorders of mobility and problems with activities of daily living. The social worker and/or psychologist brings expertise in coping with chronic disease and its impact on the individual and family.

CLINICAL SIGNIFICANCE

This chapter emphasizes the importance of comprehensive care for rheumatoid arthritis patients. Coordinated application of currently available medical, physical and surgical treatments by multiple medical specialties can reduce the activity of disease, moderate the crippling deformities, and help patients maintain or improve their ability to function. Multidisciplinary rheumatic disease units have achieved promising results in the treatment of RA patients.

REFERENCES

1. Mikkelsen W M, Dodge H J, Duff IF and Kato HJ (1967) Estimate of the prevalence of rheumatic disease in the population of Tecumseh, Michigan, 1959–60. *J Chronic Dis* **20**: 351–69.

2. Pincus T, Callahan L F, Sale W G, Brooks A L, Payne L E and Vaughn W K (1984) Severe functional declines, work disability, and increased mortality in seventy-five rheumatoid arthritis patients studied over nine years. *Arthritis Rheum* **27**: 864–72.
3. Yelin E, Meenan R, Nevitt M and Epstein W (1980) Work disability in rheumatoid arthritis: effects of disease, social and work factors. *Ann Intern Med* **93**: 551–6.
4. Meenan R F, Yelin E H, Nevitt M and Epstein W V (1981) The impact of chronic disease: a sociomedical profile of rheumatoid arthritis. *Arthritis Rheum* **24**: 544–9.
5. Anderson J A D (1971) Rheumatism in industry: a review. *Br J Ind Med* **28**: 103–21.
6. Paulus H E and Furst D E (1985) Aspirin and other nonsteroidal anti-inflammatory drugs. *In: Arthritis and Allied Conditions, 10th Ed* (D J McCarty, ed), pp. 453–86. Philadelphia: Lea and Febiger.
7. Paulus H E (1983) Antirheumatic drug therapy agents. *In: Internal Medicine* (J H Stein, ed), pp. 1094–9. Boston: Little Brown.
8. Sherrer Y S, Bloch D A, Mitchess D M, Young D Y and Fries J F (1986) The development of disability in rheumatoid arthritis. *Arthritis Rheum* **29**: 494–500.
9. Iannuzzi L, Dawson N, Zein N and Kushner I (1983) Does drug therapy slow radiographic deterioration in rheumatoid arthritis? *N Engl J Med* **309**: 1023–8.
10. Fries J F, Spitz P W, Mitchess D M, Roth S H, Wolfe F and Bloch D A (1986) Impact of specific therapy upon rheumatoid arthritis. *Arthritis Rheum* **29**: 620–7.
11. Mills J A, Pinals R S, Ropes M W, Short C L and Sutcliffe J (1971) Value of bed rest in patients with rheumatoid arthritis. *N Engl J Med* **284**: 453–8.
12. Harris R and Copp E P (1962) Immobilization of the knee joint in rheumatoid arthritis. *Ann Rheum Dis* **21**: 353–8.
13. Partridge R E H and Duthie J J R (1963) Controlled trial of the effect of complete immobilization of the joints in rheumatoid arthritis. *Ann Rheum Dis* **22**: 91–9.
14. Swezey R L (1974) Essentials of physical management and rehabilitation in arthritis. *Sem Arthritis Rheum* **3**: 349–61.
15. Nordemar R, Bjorn E, Zachrisson L and Lundvist K (1981) Physical training in rheumatoid arthritis: a controlled long-term study. I. *Scand J Rheumatol* **10**: 17–23.
16. Rogers M P, Liang M H and Partridge A J (1982) Psychological care of adults with rheumatoid arthritis. *Ann Intern Med* **96**: 344–8.
17. Charnley J (1972) The long-term results of low friction arthroplasty of the hip performed as the primary intervention. *J Bone Joint Surg [Br]* **54**: 61–2.
18. Spiegel J S, Spiegel T M and Ward N B (1987) Are rehabilitation programs for rheumatoid arthritis patients effective? *Semin Arthritis Rheum* (In press.)
19. Barraclough D, Alderman W W and Popert A J (1975) Rehabilitation of non-walkers in rheumatoid arthritis. *Rheumatol Rehabil* **15**: 287–91.
20. Brattström M and Berglund K (1970) Ambulant rehabilitation of patients with chronic rheumatic disease. *Scand J Rehabil Med* **2**: 133–42.
21. Conaty J P and Nickel V L (1971) Functional incapacitation in rheumatoid arthritis: a rehabilitation challenge. *J Bone Joint Surg [Am]* **53**: 624–37.
22. Duthie J J R, Brown P E, Truelove L H, Baragar F D and Lawrie A J (1964) Course and prognosis in rheumatoid arthritis. A further report. *Ann Rheum Dis* **23**: 193–202.
23. Karten I, Lee M and McEwen C (1973) Rheumatoid arthritis: five-year study of rehabilitation. *Arch Phys Med Rehabil* **54**: 120–8.
24. Katz S, Vignos P J Jr, Moskowitz R W, Thompson H M and Svec K H (1968) Comprehensive outpatient care in rheumatoid arthritis. A controlled study. *JAMA* **206**: 1249–54.
25. Robinson H S (1969) How do rheumatic diseases relate to economic potential as influenced by the rehabilitation specialist. *Pa Med* **72**: 70–3.
26. Rosenthal A M. Five-year follow-up study of the patients admitted to the rehabilitation center of the hospital of the University of Pennsylvania. *Amer J Phys Med* **41**: 198–211.
27. Scott D L, Coulton B L, Chapman J H, *et al.* (1983) The long-term effects of treating rheumatoid arthritis. *J R Coll Physicians Lond* **17**: 79–85.
28. Spiegel J S, Spiegel T M, Ward N B, Paulus H E, Leake B and Kane R L (1986) Rehabilitation for rheumatoid arthritis patients: a controlled trial. *Arthritis Rheum* **29**: 628–37.
29. Spiegel J S and Spiegel T M (1984) An objective examination of multidisciplinary patient conferences. *J Med Educ* **59**: 436–8.

Chapter 17

Loading and Motion in Relation to Ageing and Degeneration of Joints: Implications for Prevention and Treatment of Osteoarthritis

L. Sokoloff

CONTENTS

INTRODUCTION

Although it is a fundamental premise of the orthopaedic approach that osteoarthritis is a mechanically-derived disorder – and the premise warrants proper weight – the concept has less rigorous documentation than one might expect. How else can one explain the wide divergences in the relative frequencies reported for primary and secondary varieties of hip osteoarthritis in the literature? The classic teachings of Pauwels (1), that excessive pressure causes degeneration of the joint surface, were formulated in static terms. An analysis of the relationship between stress and osteoarthritis ultimately has to take into account not only the amplitude of the stress but also its duration, frequency and rate of change. Obviously this sort of information is hard to come by, and we must also draw on occupational and athletic data.

The following remarks are intended to review the varieties of evidence on this score, delineate several factors in degenerative joint disease that current biomechanical theories cannot explain, and recognize some mechanical bounds within which methods for preventing or reversing osteoarthritis must operate.

412

LOADING OF JOINTS

Kinetics

Although this subject is nominally concerned with the motions, forces and pressures transmitted across joints, least is known about what is of greatest importance in the context of degenerative joint disease: the actual pressures (force/area) in localized contact points on the bearing surfaces. The forces arise from the effects of gravity and external loads on the joints as well as the tension in the muscles, tendons, capsule and ligaments. Methods for measuring these in different joints have been reviewed succinctly by Paul (2).

Bulk estimates of pressures are based on mean values of areas of contact between the apposed surfaces, determined with varying degrees of accuracy. The values measured indirectly in different joints in ordinary use fall within a narrow range: 2–4·3 megapascals (MPa), i.e. 300–850 lbf/in² (PSI). Average pressures gauged this way are actually way off the mark for individual areas within a given joint. More direct measurements are made with small strain gauge transducers placed at multiple points on the articular surface of cadaveric material mounted in rigs that simulate normal angular motion and applied forces. Rushfeldt and coworkers (3) found peak pressures of 6·8 MPa (1000 PSI) in the hip joint, but most values fell into the lower range indicated above. An instrumented hemiprosthesis in a living subject yielded higher values than those predicted *in vitro* (4). They varied from point to point in the acetabulum as the hip passed through its range of motion in various functions. Pressure rates were as high as 107 MPa (16 000 PSI) sec⁻¹ when rising out of a chair.

Contact Area

The contact area, for a given load, has several determinants.

Conformation. The geometry of the surfaces necessarily governs the degree of incongruence of the articulating members in different phases of the joint motion (5). Because area and volume of the contact regions are exponential functions, small differences in linear dimension have enormous effects on the pressures generated.

Compliance of the cartilage increases the contact area as joint surfaces are forced together. The deformation of the cartilage surface is time dependent, and it has been questioned whether sufficient time elapses during ordinary locomotion for a large change in contact area to occur. The elastic modulus is a function of the water and proteoglycan content of the matrix as well as the weave of its collagen. Topographic variations occur in each of these as well (6–8) and impart a distinct anisotropy to the cartilage. The surface of the cartilage ordinarily is not parallel to the bone. As a result a proportion of the internal strain in the cartilage is of shearing type rather than compressive, and the resulting deformations are larger (9).

Thickness of the cartilage also influences the deformation of the cartilage and thereby the contact area. Compliance is not uniform throughout the thickness of cartilage (7). There is often an inverse relationship between th thickness of apposed cartilage surfaces, the convex member being thicke centrally and the concave, peripherally (10). Thicker cartilages have a lowe cell density, more proteoglycan, more water (6) than thinner ones, feature conducive to greater compliance and load distribution (11). This is mechanism compensating for incongruences as joints move into differer positions (8). In the previously cited study of Rushfeldt *et al.* (3), the highl irregular pressure profile of the hip joint was found due primarily to th distribution of the thickness of the cartilage and to irregularities at th interface with the underlying calcified layers.

Subchondral Bone

This is much stiffer than cartilage but undergoes measurable deformatio when it supports load. According to Radin and Paul (12), there is so muc bony tissue relative to the amount of cartilage in the extremities that th deformation involved in the absorption of energy under impact loading take place in the former rather than in the latter. There is a general correlatio between the density of subchondral bone, compressive loading of the joir and the thickness of the cartilage. Bone density is greater on the convex tha on the concave mating surface in most joints, but even this is not uniforml true (13). Pugh (14) has marshalled evidence that the internal architecture c subchondral bone is important in affecting the overlying cartilage. A prefei red arrangement of trabeculae favours load transfer to cortical bone and als has secondary effects on the deformation of the cartilage. This view i predicated on the assumption that it is only the bony tissue within the bon that supports load. Whether the marrow contributes a hydraulic componer as well is a debated point (15). The observation that local stiffness gradient rather than stiffness *per se* are associated with foci of chondromalacia doe not establish whether they are the cause rather than the concomitant c consequence of the cartilage degeneration.

REMODELLING OF JOINTS

Definition

The concept of remodelling was originally derived from Wolff's law c functional adaptability of bone: every stress applied to bone engenders change in the internal or external architecture such as to minimize the strair Remodelling, the change in the architecture, involves a structural removal c tissue at one point and its deposition at another. L C Johnson first articulate the concept of osteoarthritis as an exaggerated process of remodelling of th articular ends of the bone. This has sometimes been interpreted as indicatin that the primary expression of Wolff's law in this instance takes place in th bone. However, remodelling may also be extrapolated to a more genera condition: the articular cartilage may also have its own functional adaptabilit n response to mechanical loading. The theory is less well developed than in the case of bone (16) and tools for handling it not well defined. One way or another, there is evidence that the shape of joints changes throughout life, even in the apparent absence of gross osteoarthritis (17). It is hypothesized that a presently undefined feedback mechanism governs the shape of the joints in relation to stress; and that the attending redistribution of load to a formerly unloaded cartilage may be instrumental in degeneration of the joint surface.

Histogenesis

The histogenetic processes in articular remodelling are akin to but more complex than the classic findings in bone. They involve three distinct compartments: *(1)* the cartilage proper; *(2)* the osteochondral junction; *(3)* the adjacent bone and capsular attachments. Furthermore there are differences related to the pace and degree of degeneration.

Cartilage substance is lost by several means: chondrolysis, atrophy, single cell death, fibrillation and detachment. Alterations of the osteochondral junction are of 2 sorts: *(1)* advancing endochondral calcification of the base of the cartilage, manifested by reduplication of the tidemark; and *(2)* focal vascular resorption and ossification of the calcified layer. These are consistent features of the osteochondral junction in adult life and strong *prima facie* evidence of an ongoing remodelling of this portion of the joint (18).

Proliferation of osteoarticular tissue adds substance to joints in the *capsular attachments* and *subchondral bone marrow*. Marginal osteophytosis is a variable age-related phenomenon in non-osteoarthritic joints and, indeed, often at insertions of tendons at a distance from joints. The contour of the joint is altered by variously adding bone, mixed types of cartilage, fibrous and synovial tissue.

The changes present a morphological spectrum in which ageing, degeneration and osteoarthritis merge imperceptibly. It is possible to reconstruct the sequences with limited confidence. The proliferative components are like those of callus formation and at times are clearly the consequence of microfractures in the articular cortex. In advanced osteoarthritic lesions, this cannot always be documented, but the mechanical contribution, whether abrupt in the form of a fracture or more slowly evolving as a trophic process, may be inferred from the similarity of the end product. New cartilage is laid down on the articular surface of the osteophytes. It also protrudes through gaps in the eburnated surface. Rapid progress is being made in unravelling the molecular events in the induction of these tissues (19, 20) but it goes beyond the scope of this review.

Gross Changes with Age

Increasing congruence has been described as a feature of ageing in several joints. In each instance it was achieved by a variable fibrillation or other loss of the cartilage surface. The loss was first seen in areas considered to bear the least compressive stress. From this arose the idea that disuse atrophy was the mechanism involved. In the femoral head, the infrafoveal portion was predilected (21); in the elbow joint, the rim of the radial head (22). There also is a disparity in the localization of age-related fibrillation vis-a-vis osteoarthritic erosion of the patella: the former occurring on the medial, and the latter on the lateral facet (23). In the ankle, flattening of the superior talar profile has been reported as a function of age (24). There was no simple relationship between the flattening and severity of osteoarthritis developing in the same structure.

These measures have not dealt with the contour of the subchondral and marginal bone or the ongoing changes in the osteochondral junction described above. X-ray films of the head of the femur reveal remodelling and osteophytosis of the fovea as a consistent concomitant of the local degenerative changes seen in the cartilage with ageing. Changes in the parachondral bone must enter into the thickness, material properties and shearing stress in the cartilage for reasons already discussed.

LESIONS OF AGEING AND DEGENERATION

The usual teaching about osteoarthritis is that it begins with superficial degeneration of articular cartilage; and that progressive denudation of the surface leads to structural disintegration of the joint. Minor degrees of cartilage damage are common and widespread in older people; severe or symptom-producing deformities, far less so. This has raised a basic question about the relationship of the mild to the severe lesions. It has been sometimes formulated as non-progressive vis-a-vis progressive alteration of articular cartilage (25) or as ageing changes vis-a-vis osteoarthritis. Occam' razor notwithstanding, some have challenged the idea that ageing changes are the precursors of osteoarthritis. Topographical differences between the abnormalities have already been noted: osteoarthritic erosion predominates in regions of high compressive loading; ageing changes predominate in low compressive loading.

One way in which a progressive relationship might be established is to follow a time curve of the distribution of articular degeneration in a cross-sectional population. Few quantitative anatomical data are available for such an analysis, but existing necropsy information indicates that the findings vary from joint to joint. There was a roughly linear correlation of the degree of joint degeneration with age in the knee (26). This was not the case in the hip, and some local aetiological factor must have overwhelmed any ageing contribution. The findings are consistent with the possibility that, within a given individual, a mechanical factor may operate exponentially while the ageing change *per se* progresses linearly.

ASSOCIATION OF LESIONS WITH LOADING PATTERNS

Primary and Secondary Coxarthrosis

No one questions that overloading is the mechanism by which hip dysplasia cause osteoarthritis. There is, however, a wide divergence of opinion as to whether there is a mechanical basis for the usual sorts of hip osteoarthritis encountered clinically. Stulberg and associates (27) attribute at least 85% of their cases to structural abnormalities, sometimes subtle, and speculate that the same may be true in other joints as well. Other investigators place the figures at a much lower level and recognize primary osteoarthritis as a valid and frequent entity (28, 29).

Genu valgum, Genu varum

The conventional principles of abnormal loading associated with these conditions as causes of osteoarthritis have been spelled out by Maquet (30). As in hip disease, it is difficult to be confident about the extent to which the altered angulation of the osteoarthritic knee, on which the mechanical analyses are based, is a primary or secondary abnormality.

Heberden's Nodes

A distinction has often been made between mechanically- and constitutionally-derived forms of osteoarthritis of the distal interphalangeal joints of the fingers. The constitutional concept rests largely on the symmetry of the lesions, association with generalized osteoarthritis, familial occurrence and assumption that the particular joints are exposed to low compressive stress.

The biomechanical explanation is based on habitual uses of the hands and the relative sizes of the contact areas in the finger joints. Emphasis has been placed on pinch *vs.* grasp actions in explaining the greater frequency of distal than proximal finger joint involvement and a higher prevalence in women than men (31). Hadler and coworkers (32) found that textile workers engaged in pinch operations for at least 20 years are more prone to develop distal interphalangeal joint involvement than are winders, whose actions and lesions occur primarily at the wrists. Further evidence for mechanical contributions to finger osteoarthritis was the association of the lesions with handedness (33), and the finding among 16 categories of top-notch athletes in Switzerland (34): judo was a single sport in which Heberden's nodes occurred with high frequency. An *in vitro* analysis of the contact areas of cadaver fingers by Moran *et al.* (35) led to the conclusion that the average compressive stress was indeed greater in the distal interphalangeal than in the more proximal hand joints in pinch loading; but higher in the metacarpophalangeal than the interphalangeal joints during grasp function. Parenthetically, the compressive stress levels were about one fourth of those already indicated in the large joints. The concordance of the epidemiological and the biomechanical data is impressive but not conclusive that loading is the sole or even dominant factor in the development of the finger lesions. They do not account for the association with generalized osteoarthritis. The handedness data, while supported by the findings of Hadler (32), were statistically significant but the magnitude of the differences was small: handedness accounted for only 10% of the osteoarthritis observed (33). Nor were the findings internally consistent with the mechanical loading theory: the left first metacarpophalangeal joint was more severely affected than the right, even in right-handed persons. There are also methodological difficulties in evaluating the data, e.g. the frequency and severity of the lesions in different hand joints did not necessarily coincide with each other (36).

Cartilage Defects of other than Mechanical Origin

Sometimes discontinuities and depressions develop in previously normal articular cartilages, for which there is no ready mechanical explanation. Fossae nudatae are normal developmental features of the trochlear notch of the ulna in many mammalian species (37, 38), and occasionally are seen in man (39). Polyarticular degeneration is so widespread a feature of generalized osteoarthritis (29) that peculiar loading or motion patterns are unlikely causes.

BIOMECHANICAL ANIMAL MODELS

Instability

These models depend on a greater or lesser degree of abnormal loading of joints with respect to magnitude, distribution, duration and character of the stress. The relevant literature has been reviewed recently by Adams and Billingham (40). The lesions recapitulate those of human osteoarthritis in proportion to the severity of the instability employed. They differ pathogenetically in the explosive onset of the insult, in contrast to that usually observed clinically. Abnormal loading is not the only mechanism involved in the destruction of cartilage in these models – synovial proliferation and vascular disturbance are also integral components of the reaction (41).

Immobilization and Disuse

There is some anatomical support (42) for an old view that disuse of joints leads to atrophy of articular cartilage. The effect of immobilization *per se* in this circumstance must be distinguished from 2 other mechanical phenomena often associated with it: diminished compressive loading or excessive compressive loading. It is a common experience at the autopsy table that, in patients with long standing post-hemiplegic flexion contractures of the knee, gross indentation of the cartilage occurs only at the immediate contact areas. This suggests that the thinning resulted from relatively high compressive stress rather than disuse. These problems have been examined experimentally in several laboratories and disclosed a surprising lability of cartilage. Non-strenuous exercise for a period of several weeks resulted in a measurable increase in the size of articular cartilage in the knees of young rabbits (43).

Immobilization of joints has led to alteration of the proteoglycans of the matrix: a reduced quantity, biosynthesis and aggregatability with hyaluronate over the course of 4–6 weeks (44, 45). Morphological damage to cartilage has also been interpreted as evidence that immobilization is a model for osteo-arthritis (46, 47). The changes were relatively mild and bring into perspective difficulties in defining what one means by osteoarthritis, and determining the relationship between non-progressive and progressive degenerative joint dis-ease.

When previously healthy dog knees have been allowed to move, but not bear weight following amputation of the foot, the quantity and quality of the proteoglycans synthesized by the cartilage decreased greatly over the course of 6 weeks (48). Thus a certain degree of load-bearing, as distinct from the motion itself, is required for the health of cartilage. This finding must be juxtaposed to other sorts of evidence. Salter and co-workers (49) found that passive motion facilitated cartilaginous repair of surgically-induced osteochon-dral defects in rabbits. Temporary immobilization favoured repair of cartilage damage in guinea pig knees following chemical damage from intra-articular instillation of iodoacetate (50). Separate effects of immobilization were seen on the damage to the cartilage and the formation of osteophytes.

Actions of pharmacological agents on the evolution of experimental osteo-arthritis may also involve mechanical as distinct from metabolic mediation. The non-steroidal anti-inflammatory agent benoxaprofen reduced osteophyte formation in the previously mentioned idoacetate-induced lesion (51). Was this achieved by suppressing discomfort, thus allowing more favourable locomotion and loading of the joints? Analogous considerations enter into the interesting findings of O'Connor (52) that sensory deprivation of the knee in dogs did not harm the joints, but when an additional exercise burden was superimposed, cartilage damage ensued. The observation has fuelled specula-tions about presently unidentified mechanoreceptor defects as aetiological mechanisms in primary osteoarthritis. These might cause subtle but major differences in locomotion and loading of joint surfaces over the long run.

BIOMECHANICS IN CLINICAL MANAGEMENT

Prevention

The following remarks are confined to 3 topics of current interest: obesity, running and menisscectomy. Many ergonomic and orthotic measures continue to be tested empirically.

The role of *obesity* as an aetiological factor in degenerative joint disease remains a controversial subject. The literature has been reviewed in part recently by Hartz et al. (53) who analysed a large cross-sectional population sample in the United States. They found significant association of osteoarth-ritis of the knee with relative body weight. The relationship between overweight and osteoarthritis of the hip was less secure and there was none with sacroiliac involvement. The investigators interpreted the data as indicat-ing that obesity was an aetiological factor, and that it accomplished this by mechanical rather than metabolic means. Furthermore, they suggested that the precise loading mechanism responsible for the damage varied from joint to joint – in some instances excessive load proper was the culprit, while in others altered kinetics of locomotion or posture were responsible. Smith and coworkers (54), using the same data base, concluded that obesity was the cause rather than the consequence of the joint disease. Obesity was no more frequent in osteoarthritic individuals who complained of pain than in those who did not; hence pain did not restrict physical activity and so lead to obesity.

This type of thinking is in accord with some reports (55), but is at variance with other clinical and experimental studies (56).

Current enthusiasm for the virtues of *physical exercise* must be juxtaposed to clear clinical evidence that athletic injuries may eventuate in degenerative joint disease. Even here, the evidence is incomplete as to the nature of the injury and the mechanism by which it leads to osteoarthitis. Wright (57), for example, has not found more osteoarthritis among parachute jumpers and certain other sportsmen than in a control population.

Recent American experience (58, 59) indicates no excess of knee osteoarthritis among inveterate joggers as compared with non-joggers. The findings are in accord with previous findings in Finnish long distance runners (60). Perhaps what these data tell us is that people with poor joints do not become champion racers, i.e. there may be a selection bias in evaluating the morbidity. Although protracted impact loading of joints may not be damaging – perhaps even be salubrious – for individuals with good musculoskeletal structure, it may be harmful for those not so endowed.

Meniscectomy in man, as in experimental animals, is a mechanical precursor of knee osteoarthritis. Even here, there is a biological component: this complication of meniscectomy occurs more frequently in patients who have Heberden's nodes than those who do not (61). Replacement of meniscectomy by arthroscopic repair of meniscus injuries offers promise of preventing this form of osteoarthritis.

Reversal of Osteoarthritis

Resurfacing of osteoarthritic joints by cartilage is not only permissible biologically but in at least a few instances has proven a reality when pressure on joints has been relieved surgically. Anatomical documentation for this is almost nonexistent. In 1965, Professor J. Thurner of Salzburg let me have sections of the hip joints obtained at necropsy of a patient operated on by Pauwels. One hip had been treated by a Voss procedure; the other, by a Pauwels osteotomy. Excellent restoration of function was established. When the patient died 5 years later, a thick cartilage covered the acetabulum and femoral head bilaterally. Much of the regenerated surface had a fibrocartilaginous character, but it was functionally adequate.

CONCLUSIONS

I have been asked not only to review the state of the art but to express personal views about future avenues of research. The requirements for this particular subject cannot be satisfied with any degree of confidence, given the unknowns and contradictions indicated above. If there is one plea, it is that we not be parochial in approaching the problems of osteoarthritis. The scientific method requires that one not only reduces a complex problem to its simple elements but also recognizes the interactions of its components. Here we include with the biological, the physical, temporal and spatial relationships.

Articular cartilage is intimately associated with subchondral bone. Together they act as a *system* that mediates and adapts to mechanical stress. It is difficult to isolate events in one compartment that do not affect the other. At the osteochondral junction, articular cartilage is subject to endochondral ossification, a process too often overlooked by workers in our field. All recent evidence indicates that cartilaginous tissue possesses an intrinsic capacity for repair, in terms of both chondrocytic proliferation and biosynthetic activity. Furthermore, new cartilage is formed from pluripotential skeletal mesenchyme at joint surfaces by mechanisms analogous to induction of fracture callus. It may be overly pedantic to remark that the term 'repair' has 2 rather different meanings; one, a restoration of structure and function to normal; the other, in the parlance of pathologists, a response in which cells divide and do what they are supposed to do – independent of a *restitutio ad integrum*.

Repair capability must operate within bounds of mechanical loading and time. If these limits are not met, the tissue repair processes not only fail to restore function but may generate mechanical disadvantages that procreate further damage at varying paces – some rapidly progressive, others not. In this sense, osteoarthitis is not so much an inability of articular surface to repair as it is an aberration of the repair.

Pharmacological methods designed to arrest enzymic destruction of cartilage or to stimulate its proliferation or biosynthetic activities (62, 63) could only be successful within a mechanically permissible range. In deformed joints, any putative reparative action – unless confined to areas of cartilage loss and without change in subchondral architecture – might only increase the abnormalities of the loading and intensify the pathological process. These considerations should enter into the interpretation of experimental animal models of osteoarthritis that are based on changes from a normal rather than deformed baseline.

Four categories of future study seem particularly interesting:
1. *Biological.* Elucidation of the mechanisms by which physical signals are transduced into cellular and molecular events in the differentiation of connective tissues is central to understanding and manipulating the remodelling process.
2. *Engineering.* It would be valuable, albeit difficult, to formulate a systems analysis to gauge the mechanical bounds on the modulation of cartilage biology in the pathogenesis of osteoarthritis. Some components of this have appeared in qualitative schemes by several authors (64).
3. *Clinical.* Detection of articular degeneration, while still in a reversible stage, would seem a prerequisite to rational restorative drug therapy. Measurements of breakdown products released into body fluids are one possible approach and remarkably sensitive tests for some of these are currently being reported.

4. *Epidemiological.* Two major forms of endemic osteoarthritis, Kashin-Beck and Mseleni diseases, are timely subjects for study (65). Although they have distinct differences from banal osteoarthritis, there also are important similarities. They are acquired disorders and so must tell us something special about the pathophysiology of osteoarticular structures in general. As such, epidemiological and experimental investigations may empirically open up new vistas in defining the biological and mechanical interactions of ordinary degenerative joint disease.

PRACTICAL SIGNIFICANCE

It is well known that joint overloading is the mechanism by which hip dysplasias give rise to coxarthrosis and genu valgum or varum osteoarthritis of the knee. Also, meniscectomy, which increases the load in the knee joint, presents a mechanical challenge to the health of the joint. On the other hand, when mechanical pressure on a joint has been relieved surgically, resurfacing of the osteoarthritic joint by cartilage has been shown to occur, at least in a few instances. However, it has been more difficult to demonstrate any relationship between increased joint loading and joint degeneration in other common conditions affecting human joints, e.g. in obesity or after physical exercise, which means that further studies concerning the effects of mechanical stress on articular cartilage are needed.

REFERENCES

1. Pauwels F (1980) *Biomechanics of the Locomotor Apparatus.* Berlin and New York: Springer-Verlag.
2. Paul J P (1980) Joint kinetics. *In: The Joints and Synovial Fluid,* Vol 2 (L Sokoloff, ed), pp. 139–76. New York: Academic Press.
3. Rushfeldt P D, Mann R W and Harris W H (1981) Improved techniques for measuring *in vitro* the geometry and pressure distribution in the human acetabulum. 1. Ultrasonic measurement of acetabular surfaces, sphericity and cartilage thickness. *J Biomech* **14**: 253–60.
4. Hodge W A, Fijan R S, Carlson K L, Burgess R G, Harris W H and Mann R W (1986) Contact pressures in the human hip joint measured *in vivo. Proc Natl Acad Sci USA* **83**: 2879–83.
5. Simon W H, Friedenberg S and Richardson S (1973) Joint congruence. A correlation of joint congruence and thickness of articular cartilage in dogs. *J Bone Joint Surg [Am]* **55**: 1614–20.
6. Roberts S, Weightman B, Urban J and Chappell D (1986) Mechanical and biochemical properties of human articular cartilage in osteoarthritic femoral heads and in autopsy specimens. *J Bone Joint Surg [Br]* **68**: 278–88.
7. Gore D M, Higginson G R and Minns R J (1983) Compliance of articular cartilage and its variation through the thickness. *Phys Med Biol* **28**: 233–47.
8. Oberländer W (1978) On biomechanics of joints. The influence of functional cartilage swelling on the congruity of regularly curved joints. *J Biomech* **11**: 151–3.
9. Sokoloff L (1966) Elasticity of aging cartilage. *Fed Proc* **25**: 1089–95.
10. Kurrat H J and Oberländer W (1978) The thickness of the cartilage in the hip joint. *J Anat* **126**: 145–55.
11. Simon W H (1971) Scale effects in animal joints. II. Thickness and elasticity in the deformability of articular cartilage. *Arthritis Rheum* **14**: 493–502.
12. Radin E L and Paul I L (1970) Does cartilage compliance reduce skeletal impact loads? The relative force-attenuating properties of articular cartilage, synovial fluid, periarticular soft tissues and bone. *Arthritis Rheum* **13**: 139–44.

13. Simkin P A, Graney D O and Fiechtner J J (1980) Roman arches, human joints and disease. *Arthritis Rheum* **23**: 1308–11.
14. Pugh J (1985) Biomechanics of osteoarthritis. *In: Biomechanics IX-A* (D Winter, R Norman, R Wells, K Hayes and K Patla, eds), pp. 135–9. Champaign IL: Human Kinetics Publ.
15. Simkin P A, Pickerell C C and Wallis W J (1985) Hydraulic resistance in bones of the canine shoulder. *J Biomech* **18**: 657–63.
16. Frost H M (1979) A chondral modelling theory. *Calcif Tissue Int* **28**: 181–200.
17. Bullough P G (1981) The geometry of diarthrodial joints, its physiologic maintenance and the possible significance of age-related changes in geometry-to-load distribution and the development of osteoarthritis. *Clin Orthop* **156**: 61–6.
18. Green W T Jr, Martin G N, Eanes E D and Sokoloff L (1970) Microradiographic study of the calcified layer of articular cartilage. *Arch Pathol* **90**: 151–8.
19. Seyedin S M, Thompson A Y, Bentz H, Rosen D M, McPherson J M, Conti A, Siegel N R, Galluppi G R and Piez K A (1986) Cartilage-inducing factor-alpha. Apparent identity to transforming growth factor-beta. *J Biol Chem* **261**: 5693–5.
20. Poole A R, Pidoux I, Reiner A, Choi H and Rosenberg L C (1984) Association of an extracellular protein (chondrocalcin) with the calcification of cartilage in endochondral bone formation. *J Cell Biol* **98**: 54–65.
21. Bullough P, Goodfellow J and O'Connor J (1973) The relationship between degenerative changes and load-bearing in the human hip. *J Bone Joint Surg [Br]* **55**: 746–58.
22. Goodfellow J W and Bullough P G (1967) The pattern of ageing of the articular cartilage of the elbow joint. *J Bone Joint Surg [Br]* **49**: 175–81.
23. Meachim G (1983) Cartilage lesions of the patella. *In: Chondromalacia of the Patella* (J C Pickett and E L Radin, eds), pp. 1–10. Baltimore: Williams and Wilkins.
24. Riede U, Muller M and Mihatsch M J (1973) Biometrische Untersuchungen zum Arthroseproblem am Beispiel des oberen Sprunggelenkes. *Arch Orthop Trauma Surg* **77**: 181–94.
25. Byers P D, Contepomi C A and Farkas T A (1970) A *post mortem* study of the hip joint including the prevalence of the features of the right side. *Ann Rheum Dis* **29**: 15–31.
26. Sokoloff L (1983) Aging and degenerative diseases affecting cartilage. *In: Cartilage, Vol 3* (B K Hall, ed) pp. 109–41. New York: Academic Press.
27. Stulberg S D, Cordell L D, Harris W H, Ramsey P L and MacEwen G D D (1975) Unrecognized childhood hip disease a major cause of osteoarthritis of the hip. *In: The Hip*, pp. 212–28. St. Louis: Mosby.
28. Macys J R, Bullough P G and Wilson P D Jr (1980) Coxarthrosis: a study of the natural history based on a correlation of clinical, radiographic, and pathologic findings. *Semin Arthritis Rheum* **10**: 66–80.
29. Marks J S, Stewart I M and Hardinge K (1979) Primary osteoarthrosis of the hip and Heberden's nodes. *Ann Rheum Dis* **38**: 107–11.
30. Maquet p (1976) *Biomechanics of the Knee*. Berlin: Springer-Verlag.
31. Radin E L, Parker H G and Paul I L (1971) Pattern of degenerative arthritis. Preferential involvement of distal finger-joints. *Lancet* **1**: 377–9.
32. Hadler N M, Gillings D B, Imbus H R, Levitin P M, Makuc D, Utsinger P D, Yount W J, Slusser D and Moskovitz N (1978) Hand structure and function in an industrial setting. Influence of three patterns of stereotyped, repetitive usage. *Arthritis Rheum* **21**: 210–20.
33. Acheson R M, Chan Y K and Clemett A R (1970) New Haven survey of joint diseases. XII. Distribution and symptoms of osteoarthrosis in the hands with reference to handedness. *Ann Rheum Dis* **29**: 275–86.
34. Frey A and Müller W (1984) Heberden-Arthrosen bei Judo-Sportlern. *Schweiz Med Wochenschr* **114**: 40–7.
35. Moran J M, Hemann J H and Greenwald A S (1985) Finger joint contact areas and pressures. *J Orthop Res* **3**: 49–55.
36. Plato C C and Norris A H (1979) Osteoarthritis of the hand: age-specific joint-digit prevalence rates. *Am J Epidemiol* **109**: 169–80.
37. Van Sickle D C and Kincaid S A (1978) Comparative arthrology. *In: The Joints and Synovial Fluid, Vol 1* (L Sokoloff, ed) pp. 1–47. New York: Academic Press.
38. Loeffler K and Bidier I (1984) Zur Frage der Umdifferenzierung der Knorpelzellen der Gelenkoberfläche am Beispiel der Synovialgrubenbildung. *Zentralbl Veterinaermed [A]* **13**: 68–85.
39. Haines R W (1976) Destruction of hyaline cartilage in the sigmoid notch of the human ulna. *J Anat* **122**: 331–4.

40. Adams M E and Billingham M E J (1982) Animal models of degenerative joint disease. *Curr Top Pathol* **71**: 265–97.
41. Svalastoga E and Reimann I (1985) Experimental osteoarthritis in the rabbit. I. Histological changes of the synovial membrane. *Acta Vet Scand* **26**: 313–25.
42. Enneking W F and Horowitz M (1972) The intra-articular effects of immobilization on the human knee. *J Bone Joint Surg [Am]* **54**: 973–85.
43. Paukkonen K, Selkäinaho K, Jurvelin J, Kiviranta I and Helminen H J (1985) Cells and nuclei of articular cartilage chondrocytes in young rabbits enlarged after non-strenuous physical exercise. *J Anat* **142**: 13–20.
44. Palmoski M, Perricone E and Brandt K D (1979) Development and reversal of a proteoglycan aggregation defect in normal canine knee cartilage after immobilization. *Arthritis Rheum* **22**: 508–17.
45. Caterson B and Lowther D A (1978) Changes in the metabolism of the proteoglycans from sheep articular cartilage in response to mechanical stress. *Biochim Biophys Acta* **540**: 412–22.
46. Candolin T and Videman T (1980) Surface changes in the articular cartilage of rabbit knee during immobilization. A scanning electron microscopic study of experimental osteoarthritis. *Acta Pathol Microbiol Scand [A]* **88**: 291–7.
47. Videman T, Eronen I and Candolin T (1981) [3H] Proline incorporation and hydroxyproline concentration in articular cartilage during the development of osteoarthritis caused by immobilization. A study *in vivo* with rabbits. *Biochem J* **200**: 435–40.
48. Palmoski M J, Colyer R A and Brandt K D (1980) Joint motion in the absence of normal loading does not maintain normal articular cartilage. *Arthritis Rheum* **23**: 325–34.
49. Salter R B, Simmonds D F, Malcolm B W, Rumble E J, MacMichael D and Clements N D (1980) The biological effect of continuous passive motion on the healing of full-thickness defects in articular cartilage. An experimental investigation in the rabbit. *J Bone Joint Surg [Am]* **62**: 1232–51.
50. Williams J M and Brandt K D (1984) Temporary immobilization facilitates repair of chemically induced articular cartilage injury. *J Anat* **138**: 435–46.
51. Williams J M and Brandt K D (1985) Benoxaprofen reduces osteophyte formation and fibrillation after articular cartilage injury. *J Rheumatol* **12**: 27–32.
52. O'Connor B L, Palmoski M J and Brandt K D (1985) Neurogenic acceleration of degenerative joint lesions. *J Bone Joint Surg [Am]* **67**: 562–72.
53. Hartz A J, Fischer M E, Bril G, Kelber S, Rupley D Jr, Oken B and Rimm A A (1986) The association of obesity with joint pain and osteoarthritis in the HANES data. *J Chronic Dis* **39**: 311–19.
54. Davis M A, Ettinger W H and Neuhaus J M (1986) Sex differences in osteoarthritis of the knee (OAK): the role of obesity. *Arthritis Rheum* (Abstract) **29**: S16.
55. Typpö T (1985) Osteoarthritis of the hip. Radiological findings and etiology. *Ann Chir Gynaecol (Suppl)* **201**: 1–38.
56. Walton M (1979) Obesity as an aetiological factor in the development of osteoarthrosis. *Gerontology* **25**: 36–41.
57. Wright V (1981) Biomechanical factors in the development of osteoarthrosis. *In: Epidemiology of Osteoarthritis* (J G Peyron, ed), pp. 140–6. Paris: Geigy.
58. Lane N E, Bloch D A, Jones H H, Marshall W H, Wood P D and Fries J F (1986) Long distance running, bone density and osteoarthritis. *JAMA* **255**: 1147–51.
59. Panush R S, Schmidt C, Caldwell J R, Edwards N L, Longley S, Yonker R, Webster E, Nauman J, Stork J and Patterson H (1986) Is running associated with degenerative joint disease? *JAMA* **255**: 1152–4.
60. Puranen J, Ala-Ketola L, Peltokallio P and Saarela J (1975) Running and primary osteoarthritis of the hip. *Br Med J* **2**: 424–5.
61. Doherty M, Watt I and Dieppe P (1983) Influence of primary generalized osteoarthritis on development of secondary osteoarthritis. *Lancet* **2**: 8–11.
62. Howell D S, Muniz O E and Carreno M R (1986) Effect of glycosaminoglycan polysulfate ester on proteoglycan-degrading enzyme activity in an animal model of osteoarthritis. *Adv Inflamm Res* **11**: 197–206.
63. Hess E V and Herman J H (1987) Cartilage metabolism in decision making for non-steroidal anti-inflammatory drug use in osteoarthritis. *Am J Med* **81**(58): 36–43.
64. Howell D S (1984) Etiopathogenesis of osteoarthritis. *In: Osteoarthritis: Diagnosis and Management* (R W Moskowitz, D S Howell, V M Goldberg and H J Mankin, eds), pp. 129–46. Philadelphia: Saunders.
65. Sokoloff L (1985) Endemic forms of osteoarthritis. *Clin Rheum Dis* **11**: 187–202.

Index